Psychiatric Treatment of the Child

Psychiatric Treatment of the Child

edited by

John F. McDermott, Jr., M.D.
and
Saul I. Harrison, M.D.

Contributing Editors:

Alfred Arensdorf, M.D.
Eric Berman, Ph.D.
Peter Blos, Jr., M.D.
Marvin Mathews, M.D.
John Werry, M.D.

JASON ARONSON, INC.
New York

Contents

Section II. Behavior Therapy

Section III. Pharmacotherapy

Section IV. Group and Milieu Therapy

Preface

Following the publication of *Childhood Psychopathology,* an anthology of classic and recent literature in child development and psychopathology, the editors intended to continue their efforts in a stepwise fashion by developing another volume in which the treatment of children was the focus. After considering a comparable collection of original classical literature, we were persuaded by the rapid changes in the field that have resulted in an increasingly wide variety of therapies to modify that approach. Instead of starting with a volume of classical treatment papers, we decided to address ourselves to the more immediate need clinicians have regarding accessibility of recent contributions from diverse sources.

With few exceptions, articles emphasizing individual psychodynamically oriented therapy, behavior therapy, family therapy, group therapy, and psychopharmacology tend to be clustered in a wide variety of professional journals, so that clinicians with specific predilections tend to subscribe to those journals consistent with their interests. It is unlikely that any of us would have been exposed to the many different journals from which the articles in this volume have been reprinted. This probably represents necessary segregation in terms of classification of knowledge that may be in the best interest of the scientific advancement of our field; but it is not in the best interest of our patients, whose clinicians need to integrate the often widely dispersed information. Thus this volume is dedicated to identifying and reprinting significant recent contributions to the field from a wide variety of journals not ordinarily read by all practicing clinicians. In an effort to accomplish this, extensive screening of treatment literature of the early 1970s was done by the two editors-in-chief as well as a board of contributing editors, all of whom are experts in special areas. Reference is made in editorial commentary preceding each section and article selected to many of the excellent papers published prior to the 1970s; this should suggest access to further reading for those interested. The present volume is the first of a series to be published on a regular basis. Subsequent ones will also attempt to extract the most significant contributions to the same broad range of literature during the previous several years.

We regret that inevitable limitations of space and, in some instances, unavailability of reprint rights, precluded the inclusion of certain papers. The same limitations of space have, in some instances, dictated that we edit and shorten articles, often by eliminating tables and graphs containing original raw data. Wherever we have abridged, however, we have generally preserved the author's original wording, and, of course, where the reader insists on consulting the original complete report, he may request a reprint from the author.

Our philosophy has been one of combining breadth and depth, comprehensiveness and attempts toward synthesis, rather than narrowness or polarity of point of view. Along with our contributing editors, we have introduced each section with historical perspective and a background review of the field to be presented there. We hope that these introductory and interstitial commentaries will help the reader gain perspective by placing the paper in context and that the references to other literature will guide the student who wishes to pursue a subject beyond the confines of this volume. In the field of treatment of the emotionally disturbed child, where so much remains unknown, the appropriate function of commentary is as much to raise as to answer questions, as much to focus on or clarify issues as to resolve them.

We are much indebted and will long remain grateful to all those who helped to make this book possible. Our special thanks to our contributing editors—Drs. Alfred Arensdorf (group and milieu therapy). Eric Berman (family therapy), Peter Blos, Jr. (individual psychodynamic therapy), Marvin Mathews (pharmaco therapy), and John Werry (behavior therapy)—who helped throughout the book generally but also had special areas of interest; to the authors and publishers of papers, who were so generous in their unconditional willingness to permit the printing of their writings; and to the colleagues and students whose reaction to and encouragement of this undertaking was so important.

JOHN F. McDERMOTT, JR., M.D.
SAUL I. HARRISON, M.D.

Introduction

Our survey has suggested that much, if not all, of the effectiveness of different forms of psychotherapy may be due to those features that all have in common rather than to those that distinguish them from each other . . . Since the leading theories of psychotherapy represent alternative rather than incompatible formulations, it is unlikely that any one of them is completely wrong. The activity stimulated by the clash of psychotherapeutic doctrines will eventually yield sufficient information either to prove that they are for all practical purposes identical or to clarify and substantiate differences between them.

—Dr. Jerome Frank, 1973.

Treatment of the child may range from the witch doctor's rituals for lifting a curse to the behavior therapist establishing hierarchies; it may vary from the short-term directive and goal-oriented therapist strengthening existing defenses and achieving symptom relief to the analyst's systematic interpretation of unconscious elements from outside in, i.e., in the sequence of affect-defense-impulse. The family therapist, utilizing a different orientation, does not focus on the child as the patient, but on the family unit, viewing the child as a barometer of family tensions addressed as the problem. The group therapist utilizes present and past interactions and transactions to influence behaviors, and the therapist employing drugs considers the symptoms, the underlying diagnostic disorder, and the developmental level of the child in formulating his prescription.

Child therapies attempt to influence the youngster in three areas— cognitively, emotionally, and behaviorally. These are the essential ingredients common to all. Some emphasize one much more than the others—some, e.g., psychodynamically oriented insight therapy, have traditionally approached the emotional and cognitive spheres expecting that behavior will change as a consequence of changes in these; the behavior therapist believes that influencing and shaping behavior itself is primary, that attitudes and feelings will change as a result.

Figure 1 may be thought of as representing a series of stages or phases flowing together to form a mainstream for all the therapies. The stages along this mainstream vary considerably as to length and importance, emphasis and time spent upon them dependent on the particular technique being considered. At times they overlap or merge, and at other times, with particular therapies, may even be eliminated or reversed in order. The elements clustering around them may be thought of as representing key variables distinguishing some forms of therapy from others. These variables represent the differences among the various treatments of children, while the core elements or commonalities are represented by the central highway, the stages of which will described below.

Identification and Assessment of the Problem, the Personality of the Child and Family

Different societies and cultures determine which behaviors and attitudes are defined as symptoms and which ones are "acceptable," i.e., to be influenced. These are selected sometimes by the child patient, but more often by those around him, especially parents and school.

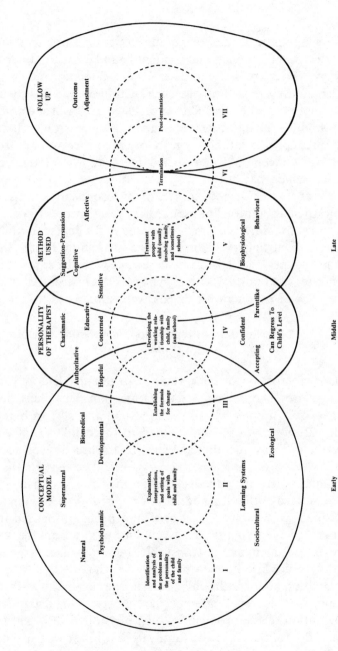

Treatment of the Child,
Universal Commonalities and Variations.

Following referral, the work of the clinicians is first to assess the child and his total life milieu and to identify and evaluate the "problem." It always relates to the youngster's life experience and involves some understanding regarding present functioning and past behavior. The examination of the child's life experience can be broad and structured (psychodynamically oriented therapy) or narrowly focused on a particular problem (behaviorally oriented therapy) according to the preferred conceptual framework of the therapist. It is the search for the "cause" which may be found by re-creating, reinterpreting events of the past with the child and family, or by proposing a cause which the clinician has diagnosed himself. Many feel that the effectiveness of the treatment to follow is ultimately related to the degree to which the child and family participate in the process of searching. That is, the degree of lasting success may correlate somewhat with the extent to which the youngster (and family) actively chooses the conceptual framework or viewpoint of the therapist or passively submits to it.

Explanation, Interpretation, and Setting of Goals
with Child and Family

The explanation or interpretation of the problem may, as with the other phases, occur over a varying time span. This phase may be more emphasized in one form of therapy than another. In many cases the explanation may also be extended to the child's family in order to prepare the way for altered behavior toward him or acceptance of change in him. In primitive systems it often entails a simple explanation that the patient is the victim of a curse or a devil because of some act that offended ancestors or spirits—a behavior that will be identified as causative. It is brief and problem-focused in behavior therapy, while lengthy in psychoanalysis, where the explanation focuses on complete intrapsychic factors which are approached gradually. If family therapy is to be the method employed, the explanation includes the child only as one element in a system; i.e., the family unit is the "patient" or "client." For drug therapy, the explanation of the problem is often physiological in nature.

In order for the child and family to be willing to learn about him and themselves and/or change, he and they must be convinced that the therapist's formulation is an acceptable one which they can adopt. This is the reason that this phase is often considered an educative or learning experience and has strong affective or emotional substance to hold it together. If the therapist and child-family's assumptions differ, they are sometimes reconciled by the one "coming around" and accepting those of the other. However, as in the previous phase, it is generally felt that therapy is most effective if the therapist's ideas are not imposed, but new ones are mutually sought and developed with the child patient and/or his family.

Establishing the Strategy for Change

The next stage establishes the formula for a solution to the problem as it has been defined, i.e, what must be done in order to "get better." It may be a prescription for the child, the family, the school, and others. It may include the number of times that something in particular must be done in order to effect improvement: i.e., the youngster and family may be told that improvement will depend upon their doing or saying certain things, within the context of a certain number and frequency of visits of behaviors inside or outside the therapeutic setting. It is during this period that behavioral components are added to the cognitive and emotional one which make up a treatment plan, so that knowledge can be put into practice.

Throughout these three stages the conceptual model of the therapist is a key variable in shaping the form and content of the phase itself (see the outer circle of variables in Fig. 1.

Developing the Working Relationship with
Family (and School)

It is obvious that this is a key phase which extends in both directions toward and into the earlier and latter stages and is only arbitrarily placed at this point in the flow of central phenomena in child treatment for diagrammatic purposes.

Different societies and cultures determine the nature of the therapist-patient relationship and, as a consequence related to this, the treatment employed. At one extreme, a society which sanctions possession by devils as the principal causative basis for emotional problems will promote exorcism as the effective treatment, and the therapist is automatically assumed to have a magical role. At the other pole, a society in which maturity and independence are valued characteristics promotes mutual investigation of the child's personality and the way he is seen by others.

Yet the young child in all societies tends to see the external world controlling him and has many magical beliefs. Therefore, he may have many more unrealistic feelings and beliefs about the therapist and the therapist's influence. Child therapists from culture to culture tend to find that suggestion "happens" more with youngsters than with adult patients. For example, the placebo effect is a potent variable in treatment programs emphasizing drug therapy with children. Furthermore, personality characteristics of the therapist become extremely important variables related to this overlapping phase, arbitrarily entitled "Developing the Working Relationship." Clusters of characteristics (Fig. 1) making up the personalities of individual therapists are dictated partly by sociocultural factors which influence both the expression of inherent and acquired personal characteristics. While these characteristics are crucial for developing a working relationship, it is also noted that they extend throughout the next phase, therapy proper, as illustrated in Fig. 1, and are also important factors in the earlier and later stages of treatment.

Hope or expectation of help, which can represent belief in a helping person, is a key to this phase. Studies have suggested that this ingredient, which is partly dependent upon the personality of the therapist and his attitude toward the youngster and family, is itself responsible for rapid and early relief of symptoms and distress independent of the type of therapy. However, significant lasting improvement in social functioning is a separate but related phenomenon which varies considerably from therapeutic modalities and is thought to be more dependent upon the length and kind of contact between the patient and the therapist.

In stage IV, we see the development of the therapeutic alliance which is dependent upon the therapist understanding and responding to the child and family and their needs, both overt and latent. It may necessitate a more prolonged phase with children than with adults because specific gratification may be needed for the youngster to develop incentive—the attitude that the therapist is a person who is important to him and who can be helpful in other ways—knows more about the "problem" than the child or his parents do, or at least knows more about how they can find out about the problem and a solution. There is a wide spectrum of the degree and intensity of "authoritativeness" either invested in or assumed by the therapist. This ranges all the way from the therapist who places distance between himself and the child and family by assuming magical or supernatural powers to one who himself regresses and operates at the youngster's own level of individual thinking and feeling. During this period the attempt is made to split off the symptoms so that the youngster can look at them separately from himself. This is true across the varieties of treatments—individual dynamic or behavioral, family, group and milieu, or even drug treatment. In achieving this the child patient may merge or identify with the "power and knowledge" of the therapist for a period of time in order to gain control over the symptoms or to encapsulate them.

It is to be emphasized that the personality of the therapist is a principal vehicle or instrument through which any technique is applied, whatever it might be. While it is not the key factor in drug treatment, it is nevertheless an important variable. Common denominators for the most effective child therapists regardless of culture are most likely to include (1) concern for the youngster, (2) sensitivity toward him, i.e., an ability to have "X-ray eyes," to get inside the youngster's head, and to think and feel developmentally with him at his own level in order to communicate effectively, and (3) an expectation of success related to the influence of his own personality. We often see young therapists of any particular school wedded to their technique, believing that the method they have learned is the most important factor in the improvement of their patient. However, as these therapists mature, they begin to become more flexible as to the use of that technique and realize the influence of their own personality as its vehicle.

The so-called "corrective emotional experience," which is so dependent upon these factors, is often a more crucial phenomenon with youngsters than with adults. It is probably a common ingredient in all forms of therapy with children—a novel experience with a new person incorporated in the youngster's life, with a reordering of behaviors in coping patterns based upon it.

Treatment Proper

Sometimes the therapeutic work is done directly and exclusively with the individual child. However, there is often a need for involvement of various family members and other elements of the child's milieu which are crucial to him, e.g., school personnel. Here the therapist participates and mediates as a helper between his young patient and the milieu he lives in, using a single method or several in combination. Sometimes the therapist indicates that the process of change is largely in the hands of those who surround the child and that they must carry the main burden of the treatment. An extreme example of this would be a purely "environmental" form of treatment in which situational change is sufficient for resolution of the youngster's problem. Other principal methods such as suggestion, persuasion, or biophysiological treatments employ a more active and directive approach on the part of the therapist and a more or less passive-receptive posture on the part of the youngster.

Those therapies in which "cognitive" factors are crucial ingredients for change employ the phenomenon of "insight" as critical, whether about intrapsychic and/or interpersonal matters. This may range from understanding complicated unconscious reasons for illness (uncommon in children), to learning that one has assumed maladaptive ways of behaving with others, or in other cultures, to understanding the nature of a curse or possession. Insight can broadly be considered to consist of an acceptance of the causative explanation of the problem. It can be experienced as self-understanding, and can be arrived at by the youngster (and family) directly, with the therapist only performing a "midwife" function of helping to "deliver" this self-understanding, or it can be achieved through utilizing the therapist's own "insight," which the patient accepts and incorporates as his own.

Other therapists employ methods which are primarily affective. In these, feeling states are released, expressed, understood, and then presumably controlled. Still other methods rely more heavily on behavioral shaping as the essential ingredient of the treatment proper, e.g., relearning and unlearning adaptive patterns. As mentioned earlier, there are undoubtedly cognitive, affective, and behavioral elements in all therapies in varying degrees of relationship and balance. However, as also mentioned earlier, some therapies presume that cognitive and emotional factors will change *after* behavior is influenced, e.g., through behavior therapy. Others rely heavily and primarily on the development of cognitive and/or emotional insight and change, assuming that behavior shifts will then follow. All these therapies include varying degrees of activity and responsibility on the part of the therapist and the patient alike in order to achieve change, translating understanding into action.

Termination

In many forms of therapy the decision for termination depends largely upon the child and family having accepted a mutually satisfactory balance of mastery over some problems, adjustment to or acceptance of others. In some forms, especially the briefer time-limited therapies, the anticipation of independence from the therapy and the therapist begins at the start and a termination date may be suggested at the beginning. This is also seen when a series of procedures or steps are outlined specifically as the treatment, and goals such as particular symptom relief are set from the beginning as the end point. The termination period depends upon the degree of self-esteem and self-confidence which the youngster and family have about their abilities to handle problems themselves, as well as the actual "changes" that have been accomplished by the treatment.

Post-termination

This last phase is a test of whether the therapeutic work has succeeded, i.e., whether improved adjustment can continue independent of the therapist's direct ongoing influence. It often constitutes a follow-up period in which the outcome is determined, but a period in which the treatment itself is still being digested, incorporated, and applied. Critical factors during this stage are the degree to which objectives have been met regarding adjustment for the child, the family, peers, and school.

Conclusions

We have attempted to produce a model which is imperfect and to some extent arbitrary. However, we hope that it can be used to provide a common framework to which the various sections in this book can be related. It must be viewed in a flexible and elastic fashion, with various clusters or cells of variables surrounding the treatment flow coming together to give a living picture of the treatment itself. Some therapists put greatest emphasis on identification and analysis of the problem, explanation in a very specific form, and formula or strategy for change. Others emphasize the working relationship as the critical and overriding phase in therapy for all children, the vehicle for the child (and/or family) "finding himself." Still others feel that the phase of treatment proper is the critical and most prolonged period, while others believe that termination, if a focus from the start in briefer treatments, is the primary representative phase of the entire treatment process. It is the editors' contention that there is no single form of treatment which is the "compleat" therapy for all youngsters, but a variety of modalities which can be used separately or blended and matched appropriately in an appropriate treatment plan for a particular youngster and his problem. In reading the papers in this volume which emphasize techniques in individual dynamic and behavioral, family, group and milieu, as well as drug treatments, we hope that the reader will consider not only their novelty and appeal, their importance in broadening his own therapeutic armamentarium with new knowledge and skills, but also the universal commonalities and variations between them which can move us further toward synthesis incorporating rather than excluding the various treatments for children—a comprehensive model which can be representative of the "compleat" child therapist.

Individual

Psychodynamic

Psychotherapy

Introduction

Many do it, some teach it, but no one has successfully defined it. Reviewing both recent and classic writings about child psychotherapy reveals that the term embraces a wide array of strategies, tactics, and techniques.

All share superficial resemblance to many of the everyday practices employed in rearing and educating children and this interferes also with tracing the history of child psychotherapy. Before the twentieth century, evidence of direct psychotherapeutic contact with children is rare. The most celebrated exception was Itard's (1801) efforts with the French boy who was assumed to have lived the bulk of his life as a savage in Aveyron. Modern child psychotherapy is generally thought to have begun with Freud's (1909) report of "Little Hans." While this case report differs from Itard's in that it is readily identifiable as psychotherapy, it is noteworthy that Hans's father was the psychotherapist, under Freud's direction. Parental closeness was assumed to be a prerequisite for such treatment with a child, so that it wasn't until 1913 that Ferenczi (1950) reported what was probably the first documented attempt by someone other than a parent to psychoanalyze a child. Ferenczi abandoned this effort because the psychoanalytic method, as then used with adults, bored the youngster, who wished to return to his toys.

It wasn't until women, who had the advantage of experience with children as well as knowledge of psychoanalysis, recognized that play should be considered a valid means of therapeutic communication that analysis developed as a direct psychotherapeutic approach to the child. Although Hug-Hellmuth (1921) published the first such report, major credit for the subsequent development of child psychoanalysis belongs to Melanie Klein (1932) and Anna Freud (1946).

In addition to the significant focus on childhood in Freud's psychoanalysis and Adolf Meyer's psychobiology, there were other simultaneous but independent developments around the turn of the century that contributed to the latter flowering of psychotherapy with children. Among these were the development of psychometry by Binet and Simon in France and the creation in Australia and in Colorado and Illinois of separate courts for juveniles. Subsequently, it was in the juvenile court in Illinois that William Healy conducted his pioneering psychiatric work with children, the forerunner of the development in the 1920s of the Child Guidance Clinic Movement from which child psychotherapy stemmed and through which it burgeoned.

Since then, the term "psychotherapy" has been used to include almost any event, method, technique, or happenstance that increases the capacity to grow, mature, develop, and expand the use of existing potential. Two decades ago Buxbaum (1954) said, "We have child analysis, child guidance, group therapy, relationship therapy, release therapy, counseling, child guidance, group therapy and a few others." Although some of the names have changed, the state of affairs is no different today; in fact, there are more varieties of psychotherapeutic intervention than ever (which constitutes the reason for this volume's existence). In addition, there is no question that fortuitous changes in connection with family circumstance, friendship, a special teacher, camp, even adolescence itself—all can have a salutary growth-enhancing effect. Psychic pain may be relieved, human relationships improved, and general functioning in the culture and society bettered. These can be accomplished also by a variety of planned interventions such as behavioral therapy, family therapy, milieu therapy, pharmacotherapy, etc., as described in other sections of this volume. But, to apply the terms psychotherapy or psychotherapeutic so ubiquitously and indiscriminately risks rendering them meaningless. To deny music therapy the title, for example, in no way should diminish the value of its psychobiological contribution. In fact, it sometimes succeeds where psychotherapy fails, underscoring the need to distinguish between effect and process.

Unfortunately, there may be a value-laden, personalized hierarchical ordering of psychotherapeutic concepts and nomenclature, stimulating intense rivalry. In many quarters, not to use the modifier *psychotherapeutic* in conjunction with a skill or technique relegates it to second place. This seems to be true in the context of theoretical battles, professional competition, or economic reward. In addition, this arbitrary pecking order has had wide-ranging effects on the design of mental health service delivery systems and clinical practice, and has inhibited vitally needed research efforts in field of psychotherapy.

Nonetheless, there is a narrower framework which can delineate more clearly and profitably the perimeters of child psychotherapy without concisely defining the term. It is these ideas which have formed the basis upon which the selections for this section have been made. With other forms of intervention, there is a sharing of common goals such as the relief of psychic pain (which children often externalize), improved human relationships, a better capacity for self-definition and functioning, increased learning and coping skills, and a reduction of impediments to ongoing development. But the psychodynamically oriented psychotherapist's approach—with etymological fidelity— focuses on creating intrapsychic change as the central pathway to psychological improvement. This requires a framework or, if you will, a basic science which includes a dynamic intrapsychic psychology, knowledge of the multidimensional interrelated sequences of child development, and an understanding of family dynamics. Among the specific requirements are conceptualizations of unconscious mental functioning, conflict, defense (A. Freud, 1946), resistance (Sandler, Holder, and Dare, 1970c), transference (Sandler, Holder, and Dare, 1970b), and countertransference. Also fundamental is the idea that putting previously unspoken affects, fears, beliefs, thoughts, or images into words contributes to coping skills and mastery (Loewenstein, 1956). Support for this assumption can be found in the fields of education (Pflaum, 1974) and psycholinguistics (Church, 1966; Blank, 1947) as well as from Helen Keller's (1954) vivid description of the development of language as contributing to the capacity for mastery of emotion and the environment. Finally, a theory of child psychotherapy should integratively encompass fantasy, reality, manifest and latent content, and a working alliance between patient and therapist (Sandler, Holder, and Dare, 1970a; Keith, 1968). From the pragmatic perspective, psychodynamically oriented child psychotherapy is a dyadic event with a procedural repertoire including play, varied forms and levels of communication (Anthony, 1964), technical maneuvers to facilitate the patients' attempts at verbal and affective expression, and a corollary capacity for the therapist to flexibly use his own personality with awareness.

Exemplifying the usefulness of such a framework is its application to classifying psychotherapy according to the manner in which the techniques are utilized in the service of specific desired effects. This should facilitate sorting out the differences and interrelationships between child psychoanalysis, psychoanalytically oriented psychotherapy, brief psychotherapy, psychotherapeutic consultation, etc. Distinctions have been based too much on time duration, despite its superficiality and inability to generate insight into the nature of the process. It would be more profitable to examine the psychotherapists' thought processes while interacting, observing, and thinking during therapeutic sessions. How the therapist selects what to focus upon from the multitude of data, the words selected to couch remarks, and what is elected to be left unsaid are all important elements of psychotherapy whatever its time duration. Elaborate insight about oneself may or may not be vital for the patient; however, it is invariably essential for the psychotherapist to understand the patient. What the therapist does with this knowledge is responsible for the difference between various modalities of psychotherapy.

Thus far, the child's real world has not been mentioned. The intent is not to ignore it but, for heuristic purposes, it is artificially segregated. Dealing with parents, schools, play groups, medication, physical illness, etc., are vital, but may be viewed as technical supporting structures which enable psychotherapy to occur. In consequence, these may constitute the greatest potential areas of confusion in the literature on child psychotherapy. Often the nature of the planned treatment for the child may be described explicitly, but at the same time something vague is said about concomitant "work" with the child's environment. The total therapeutic regimen needs description. For instance, work with parents may have the following range: (1) minimal parental involvement necessary to support the continuation of the child's individual psychotherapy, (2) interdicting contact with parents as occurs sometimes in the therapy of adolescents, (3) involvement in regular meetings to obtain detailed information about the child's background and current life outside therapy, (4) parental guidance focused on child-management techniques, (5) guidance focused on the parent-child interaction, (6) therapy for the parents' individual or conjoint needs, (7) family therapy accompanying the child's individual psychotherapy, (8) and finally, various combinations of the aforementioned possibilities.

A variety of explanatory theories pertaining to psychotherapy has evolved over the years. For many, no theory is required other than the assumption "that the individual has within himself not only the ability to solve his own problems satisfactorily, but also a growth impulse that makes mature behavior more satisfying than immature behavior" (Axline, 1969, p. 15). This assumption of nondirective client-centered play therapy leads to offering the child "the opportunity to play out his accumulated feelings of tension, frustration and insecurity, aggression, fear, bewilderment and confusion" at his own pace and his own style. The therapist's task is to facilitate this change by the consistent display of a nonjudgmental, respectful attitude which reflects only "those expressed emotionalized attitudes" (ibid., p. 18). Comparable ideas were expressed in the earliest American textbooks on child psychotherapy by Taft (1933) and Allen (1942). While admirably humanitarian, this overriding emphasis on the quality of the therapeutic relationship left much unexplored and unexplained and impressed many clinicians as being limited in applicability to rather well-integrated children.

The other extreme of complexity on the theoretical continuum involve those child psychoanalytic concepts in which detailed, elaborate theories of human development are interrelated with clinical approaches that employ verbalization and other means of communication, focusing on affect and defensive functioning preparatory to linking unconscious wishes, fears, and/or beliefs to the child's historical past and current reality. This is accomplished by the process of interpretation (Sandler, Holder, and Dare, 1970d), the sine qua non of psychoanalytically based psychotherapies. But even this point of view is not homogeneous as represented, for instance, by the major fundamental differences between Anna Freud and Melanie Klein.

Despite this plethora of theories one cannot help but note the commonality in the procedures and practices within child psychotherapy pointed out three decades ago (Witmer, 1946). Much of the theoretical position-taking occurs about the most abstract concepts, those the furthest removed from the actual data of observation and which are least significant for clinical theories and clinical practice (Waelder, 1962). What we do in the clinical hour, what we think we do, and how we then conceptualize it brings the data to a refinement which may distort the commonality of what many psychotherapists actually do with children.

The issue of the efficacy of child psychotherapy deserves attention. Much of the literature in the field is devoted to single or groups of cases that demonstrate a particular method or technique which has been successful in solving the particular problems of a child or group of children. And any practitioner can cite cases which would in his mind demonstrate the efficacy of psychotherapy. But research in child psychotherapy as a field has been minimal (Levitt, 1971). In adult psychotherapy several (Bergin, 1966; Strupp, 1973; Frank, 1973; Eysenck, 1965) have struggled extensively in research efforts but results have been admittedly meager. Nevertheless, Malan's (1973) well-reasoned and thoughtful review of psychotherapy research, noting the inability of research to demonstrate that psychotherapy is effective and also the lack of impact of research on clinical practice, does not conclude pessimistically. This is because of the growing recognition that designing "outcome criteria that do justice to the complexity of the human personality . . . correlated with meaningful variables . . . cannot be based at present on anything but clinical judgment." Anthony's praise of the basic science section of *Modern Perspectives in Child Psychiatry* (1971) echoes the same idea, although he notes that there is a failure to "accomplish the mysterious leap from basic research to clinical accomplishment." Thus, at our current level of knowledge we must fall back on clinical observation, trial and error, and intuition and, for the time being, claim only that child psychotherapy is an applied healing art as we concurrently struggle to define objectively what we do and assess its value.

The Squiggle Technique

D. W. WINNICOTT, M.D.

Like several of the recently deceased Dr. Winnicott's rich con-
tributions to knowledge about children during his long pediatric
and child psychoanalytic career in England (see 1971a), his book
on Therapeutic Consultations in Child Psychiatry (1971b) has
received considerable attention from child psychotherapists. His
method—which is illustrated in the selections from the book that
are reprinted here—simultaneously encompasses a means of
stimulating free communication between child and clinician and
affords a vehicle for unleashing the child's therapeutic interven-
tion which the reader can compare with Proskauer's approach
described on pages 71-92 in this volume.

Winnicott's therapeutic consultation is centered on the
squiggle game, the primary purpose of which is to facilitate the
expression of matters from the furthest reaches of the mind of
which the child is only vaguely aware, matters of the utmost
privacy which may not appear rational and which "others" might
not understand. The resultant interchange, which may at times
assume an aura of magical mind reading, "unhitches something at
the place where the patient's development is hitched up," in
Winnicott's words. This statement, while suggesting that artistry
outweighs science, clearly conveys the author's intent: a change in

the balance of psychic forces allowing the natural, inherent developmental impetus and the influences of the "average expectable environment" to work. This represents a philosophy of clinical work in which "cure" is not the object, as represented by Winnicott's comments about one of his case reports: "I was contented to leave him using life itself in the solution of . . . his personal problem" (1971b, p. 160). Although the selections reprinted here and the volume from which they were taken do not emphasize the roles of work with parents, school consultation, continuing support and advice by the family's general physician or case worker, these and similar factors do seem to contribute considerably to the final outcome although subsumed under the rubric of the "average expectable environment."

The mechanics of the squiggle game can be described in Winnicott's own words introducing the method to a youngster: "I shut my eyes and go like this on the paper and you turn it into something and then it is your turn and you do the same thing and I turn it into something" (1971b, p. 12). There are no other rules for either child or clinician who, despite their age differences, function with an equality that might constitute a unique experience. Skill in drawing is not necessary, respect for impressions and ideas is mutual, and clarification and understanding of subjective mental experiences are sought together. The intimate associative give-and-take atmosphere contributes a great deal to this mutuality. There are aspects remindful of projective testing, but the striking differences in the clinician's responsivity and expressiveness are crucial. He must have the ability to allow his imagination free rein accompanied by the courage to venture into an unknown fantasy land that lacks neatly demarcated boundaries between the child's and the clinician's intrapsychic processes as they take turns in producing a series of drawings with a dreamlike quality.

Readers may question how much of this work is a reflection of Winnicott's unique qualities and how much can be taught, learned, and replicated. Some clinicians have found initial efforts with this communication technique to be difficult because of a stiffness in visual imagery. Since this does not generally inhibit children to the same extent, the clinician may request the child's assistance when help is needed in perceiving something in a squiggle. The clinician may wonder also as to which issue to address and how to introduce it, but, with the increased relaxation and freedom that come from experience, it may prove to be a remarkable way to penetrate beneath the manifest problem and find out what is really troubling the child, what is on his or her mind. It need not have the magiclike feel that reading Winnicott may suggest, enabling the technique to be considered alongside other expressive modes such as doll-play, free drawing, storytelling, puppetry, drama, and other forms which encourage the communication of fantasy. Winnicott's method, of course, takes it much further in that he succeeds in expressing himself, discussing directly with the child some of the most primitive hidden facets of the mind, based on selection criteria that are not made sufficiently explicit.

Seeking exciting therapeutic outcomes like those reported by the intuitively gifted late Dr. Winnicott conceivably could entail risks. How did he avoid intervening in ways that could be more than the child could tolerate? How did he avoid risking overwhelming ego disruption in vulnerable children or pushing other children into a stonewalling retreat motivated by self-defense? Hopefully, future volumes of this series will be able to reprint reports of experience with this fascinating technique that will contribute explicit information regarding diagnostic criteria of applicability, selection of foci for interventions, and outcome of this promising technical innovation.

This concerns the application of psycho-analysis to child psychiatry. To my surprise I find that my experience over three or four decades of the analysis of children and adults has led me to a specific area in which psycho-analysis can be applied in the practice of child psychiatry, thus making sense of psycho-analysis in economic terms. It is obviously not useful or practicable to prescribe a psycho-analytic treatment of every child, and the psycho-analyst often has found himself or herself in

Introduction and "Case XV 'Mark' at 12 years" from *Therapeutic Consultations in Child Psychiatry,* by D. W. Winnicott, pp. 1-11 and 270-295, © by The Executors of the Author's Estate, Basic Books, Inc., Publishers, New York.

difficulties when attempting to put what has been learned to good use in child psychiatric practice. I have found that by full exploitation of the first interview I am able to meet the challenge of a proportion of child psychiatry cases and I wish to give examples for the guidance of those who are doing similar work and for students who wish to make a study in this field.

The technique for this work can hardly be called a technique. No two cases are alike, and there is a much more free interchange between the therapist and the patient than there is in a straight psycho-analytic treatment. This is not to decry the importance of the long analysis in which the work is done on the day-to-day emergence into the clinical material of unconscious elements in the transference, elements in process of becoming conscious because of the continuity of the work. Psycho-analysis remains for me the basis of this work, and if I were asked by a student I would always say that the training for this work (which is not psycho-analysis) is the training in psycho-analysis.

If only we knew how to select properly we should know how to choose those who are suitable for doing the work that I describe in this book even when psycho-analytic training is not available. For instance, one can say at once that there must be evident a capacity to identify with the patient without loss of personal identity; there must be a capacity in the therapist to contain the conflicts of the patient, that is to say, to contain them and to wait for their resolution in the patient instead of anxiously looking around for a cure; there must be an absence of the tendency to retaliate under provocation. Also, any system of thought which provides an easy solution is of itself a contra-indication since the patient does not want anything but the resolution of internal conflicts, along with the manipulation of external obstructions of a practical nature which may be operative in the causation or the maintenance of the patient's illness. Needless to say the therapist must have professional reliability as something that happens easily; it is possible for a serious person to maintain a professional standard even when undergoing very severe personal strains in the private life and in the personal growth process which, I hope, never stops.

An extended list of desirable qualities of this kind would leave a big proportion of people who could come forward with an urge to do professional work either in psychiatry or in social work, and for me these things are even more important than the very important training in psycho-analysis. An experience of long deep-going personal analytic treatment is as near as possible essential.

If I am right, then the type of work that I am describing has an importance that psycho-analysis does not have in meeting *social need and pressure* on clinics.

My technique in these reported cases usually takes the form of what could be called the Squiggle Game. There is nothing original of course about the squiggle game and it would not be right for somebody to learn how to use the squiggle game and then to feel equipped to do what I call a therapeutic consultation. The squiggle game is simply one way of getting into contact with a child. What happens in the game and in the whole interview depends on the use made of the child's experience, including the material that presents itself. In order to use the mutual experience one must have in one's bones a theory of the emotional development of the child and of the relationship of the child to the environmental factors. In my cases described here an artificial link is made between the squiggle game and the psychotherapeutic consultation, and this arises out of the fact that from the drawings of the child and of the child and myself one can find one way of making the case come alive. It is almost as if the child, through the drawings, is alongside me, and to some extent taking part in describing the case, so that the reports of what the child and the therapist said tend to ring true. There is also a practical significance of the squiggle or drawing material in that there can be a gain from taking the parents into one's confidence and letting them know what their child was like in the special circumstances of the therapeutic consultation. This is more real for them than if I report what the child says. They recognize the types of drawing that adorn the nursery wall or that the child brings home from school, but often they are amazed when they see the drawings in sequence, drawings which display personality qualities and perceptive abilities which may not have been evident in the home setting.

Naturally it is not always good to give parents this insight (that can be so useful). Parents might perhaps abuse the confidence that the therapist has placed in them and so undo the work that depends on a kind of intimacy between child and therapist.

My conception of the special place of the therapeutic consultation and the exploitation of the first interview for reduplicated first interviews arose gradually in the course of time in my clinic and private practice. There was a point, however, which could be said to have been of special significance, in the mid-twenties when I was a practicing paediatrician, seeing many patients in my hospital practice and given the opportunity for as many of the children as possible to communicate with me and to draw pictures and to tell me their dreams. I was struck by the frequency with which *the children had dreamed of me the night before attending.* This dream of the doctor that they were going to see obviously reflected their own imaginative equipment in regard to doctors and dentists and other people who are supposed to be helpful. They also reflected to a varying degree the attitude of the parents and the preparation for the visit that had been made. Nevertheless here I was, as I discovered to my amusement, *fitting in with a preconceived notion.* The children who had dreamed in this way were able to tell me that it was of me that they had dreamed. In language which I use now but which I had no equipment for using at that time I found myself in the role of subjective object, which rarely outlasts the first or first few interviews, the doctor has a great opportunity for being in touch with the child.

There must be a relationship between this state of affairs and that which obtains in a much less useful way in hypnosis. I have used this in the theory that I have built up in the course of time in explanation of the very great confidence which children can often show in myself (as in others doing similar work) on these special occasions, special occasions that have a quality that has made me use the word sacred. Either this sacred moment is used or it is wasted. If it is wasted the child's belief in being understood is shattered. If on the other hand it is used, then the child's belief in being helped is strengthened. There will be those cases in which deep work is done in the special circumstances of the first interview or interviews and the resulting changes in the child can be made use of by parents and those who are responsible in the immediate social setting, so that whereas a child was caught up in a knot in regard to the emotional development, the interview has resulted in a loosening of the knot and a forward movement in the developmental process.

In a proportion of cases, however, the work done in this kind of an interview is simply a prelude to a longer or more intensive psychotherapy, but it can easily happen that a child is only ready for this *after* experiencing the understanding which belongs to this kind of interview. The child may of course feel to have been more understood than in fact he or she was understood, but the effect will have been to have given to the child some hope of being understood and perhaps even helped.

One of the difficulties arising out of this kind of interview is that, when it is successful in terms of understanding, the child may easily expect to go straight on from there into an intensive therapy, with the kind of dependence on the psychiatrist or social worker which makes frequent sessions over a period of time essential. This is not what usually happens.

There is a category of case in which this kind of psychotherapeutic interview is to be avoided. I would not say that with very ill children it is not possible to do useful work. What I would say is that if the child goes away from the therapeutic consultation *and returns to an abnormal family or social situation* then there is no environmental provision of the kind that is needed and that I take for granted. I rely on an average expectable environment to meet and to make use of the changes that have taken place in the boy or girl in the interview, changes which indicate a loosening of the knot in the developmental process.

In fact, the main difficulty in assessing cases for this kind of work is a difficulty of assessing the child's immediate environment. Where there is a powerful continuing adverse external factor or an absence of consistent personal care, then one would avoid this kind of procedure and would feel inclined either to explore what would be done by "management" or else to institute a therapy which would give the child the opportunity for a personal relationship of the kind that is generally known as transference.

If the reader should *enjoy* reading the details of a series of these cases it is likely that there will emerge in the reader a feeling that I as the psychiatrist am the constant factor and that nothing else can be predicted. I myself came out in these case descriptions as a human being not exactly like any other human being, so that in no case would the same result have been attained if any other psychiatrist had been in my place. The only companion that I have in exploring the unknown territory of the new case is the theory that I carry around with me and that has become part of me and that I do not even have to think about in a deliberate way. This is the theory of the emotional development of the individual which includes for me the total history of the individual child's relationship to the child's specific environment. It cannot be avoided that changes in this theoretical basis for my work do occur in the course of time and on account of experience. One could compare my position with that of a cellist who first slogs away at *technique* and then actually becomes able to play *music*, taking the technique for granted. I am aware of doing this work more easily and with more success than I was able to do it thirty years ago and my wish is to communicate with those who are still slogging away at technique, at the same time giving them the hope that will one day come from playing music. There is but little satisfaction to be granted from giving a virtuoso performance from a written score.

The test of these case descriptions will hang on the word enjoyment. If they are a labour to read then I have been too clever; I have been engaged in displaying a technique and not in playing music. I am of course aware that this actually does take place from time to time in the case descriptions.

Undoubtedly the best cases for this kind of work are those in which there is already parental confidence in myself. It would seem to me that this is a state of affairs that can be expected; that is to say that in general people are willing to believe in the doctor they have chosen to consult, often after a great deal of discussion and after the overcoming of natural doubts. If in fact things go well, or a child does make some changes, this immediately puts the consultant in the position of someone that the parents believe in, and a benign circle is set up which operates favourably in terms of the child's symptomatology. In assessing results it is necessary, however, to make allowance for the fact that parents would naturally rather believe in the consultant than find their effort has been wasted. They are therefore, some of them, liable to report favourably if they possibly can do so. The parents' report, which is the report which has to be used in many cases, is highly suspect as an objective account and in the assessment of results, and this must be always remembered. I am not so naive as to take what the parents tell me as a final assessment. I wish to emphasize, however, that my aim in presenting these consultations is not to give a series illustrating symptomatic cure. I am rather aiming to report examples of *communication with children.*

I wish to draw attention to one other thing about these psychotherapeutic interviews. It will be noted that interpretation of the unconscious is not the main lecture. Often an important interpretation is made which alters the whole course of the interview, and there is nothing more difficult than to account for the way one finds oneself making no interpretation over a long period of time, or throughout the whole interview, and then at some point using the material for an interpretation of the unconscious. It would seem almost as if one has to tolerate the existence of two contrary trends in oneself. For me, there is some easing of the problem here in that when I make an interpretation, if the child disagrees or seems to fail to respond, I am immediately willing to withdraw what I have said. Often in these accounts I have made an interpretation and I have been wrong and the child has been able to correct me. Sometimes of course there is a resistance which implies that I have made the right interpretation and that the right interpretation has been denied. But an interpretation that does not work always means that I have made the interpretation at the wrong moment or in the wrong way, and I withdraw it unconditionally. Although the interpretation may be correct I have been wrong in verbalizing this material in this way at this particular moment. Dogmatic interpretation leaves the child with only two alternatives, an *acceptance* of what I have said as propaganda or a *rejection* of the interpretation and of me and of the whole set-up. I think and hope that children in this relationship with me feel that they have the right to reject what I say or the way I take something. Actually I do claim that it is a fact that these interviews are dominated by the child and not by me. The work is easy to do for one, two, or perhaps three sessions; but, as the reader will be only too well aware, if the interviews become oft-repeated all the problems of the transference and of resistance begin to appear and the treatment must now be dealt with along ordinary psychoanalytic lines. One thing that will be noticeable to the reader is that I never (I hope) make interpretations for my own benefit. I have no need to prove to myself some part of the theory that I use by hearing myself verbalize the material of this case. I have done all the interpreting that I want to do for my own benefit. I have nothing whatever to gain from converting someone to a point of view. Long psycho-analytic treatments have had an effect on me and I have found that interpretations that seemed right ten years ago and that the patient accepted because of awe turned out in the end to be collusive defences. A very crude example could be given. One might have a slight propagandist tendency to think of all snakes as penis symbols, and of course they can be. Nevertheless if one has to get to early material and the roots of what a penis can mean to a child one has to see that the child's drawing of a snake can be a drawing of the self, the self not yet using arms and fingers and legs and toes. One can see how many times patients have failed to convey a sense of self because a therapist has interpreted a snake as a penis symbol. Far from being a part-object, a snake in a dream or phobia can be a *first whole object*. This example gives a clue which a student can use in reading these case-histories and no doubt there will be many examples in my attempt to give honest reports in which I have made just exactly this kind of mistake. I give this as an indication of the way in which the material of these cases may be used in the student-teacher situation.

Finally, I hope it will be recognized that in presenting these cases I am not trying to prove anything. The criticism that I have failed to prove my case would not be appropriate as I have no case. I would add that it would always be better if the student could gather the material for himself or herself from personal contact with children instead of from reading my descriptions, but this is not always possible, especially for a student. At the lowest assessment this kind of attempt at honest reporting may have lessons for the student, whether social worker, teacher or psychiatrist, who tries to grow on the experiences collected by work done in the field of dynamic psychology.

* * *

Case XV 'Mark' age 12 years

In this next case there was a marked clinical change following the therapeutic consultation, and it would appear that this change was more the result of the communication between the boy and myself than of a change of attitude towards the boy in his family. It will be observed that this boy had a preoccupation with water and that eventually he established his identity by going to the sea.

I propose to give as far as posssible all I know about this case[1] in illustration of the way in which one can work in a limited area and in this way avoid the infinite amount of detail which inevitably clutters up a psychotherapeutic treatment. It is this delimitation of the area of operation that makes it possible for a child psychiatrist doing this work to carry a very heavy caseload, whereas the psychotherapist, and in particular the psycho-analyst, works with only a few cases at any one time. It is possible for the child psychiatrist doing this work to be involved in 100 or even 200 on-going cases, and this brings the work into a relationship with social pressure.

It will be understood, as I have repeatedly stated, that in my opinion the basis for the training to do this work is a thorough grounding in long-term psychotherapy of individuals, even psycho-analysis involving daily sessions over a number of years.

Family History

Girl	16 years
Mark	12 years
Boy	8 years
Boy	7 years

---

[1]Except where it is necessary to distort or omit in disguising the case.

Mark was brought to me at the age of 12 years by his parents. The father was a colleague, a member of the university staff. In this case I first saw the two parents together as they wished to get my help in orientating to the problem. Much detail emerged in the usual way of an interview that takes its natural course.

The family was intact. The following significant landmarks in Mark's emotional development were reported:

> Mark was breast-fed and *difficult to wean*. 'He resisted weaning very strongly.'

This is a matter of considerable theoretical interest. In my experience when a baby is 'difficult to wean' there is not infrequently a disturbance in the mother, either a difficulty in the area of ambivalent feelings, or else a depressive tendency. These two states are of course related, but in depression there is a more massive repression of the conflict.

The parents continued with what they wanted to say about the boy:

> Mark *had never been truthful*. (Later the parents said that this had been a fixed characteristic from 2 years.)

> Mark became at 7 (or earlier) a boy who '*if he wants must have*.'

> Mark started *to steal at 8 years*. (See below for minor correction of this detail.) This happened when he was away staying with friends. At 10 years he was taking money from his mother's bag and telling lies. There was the usual story of refusal to confess. Recently (12 years) serious stealing had taken place. This was associated with his passion for fishing. Stealing was from father's wallet and elder sister's bag and in amounts of £ 5 and £ 10. He swore he had not stolen, and by doing so he incriminated his brother to whom he was devoted. He confessed only when confronted with finger-print evidence. Then he bought a fishing rod and elaborate tackle. He spoke of 'my dealer' and claimed he would be given a special fishing rod on his birthday by this dealer. He had in fact bought two rods

and had hidden them. He had taken elaborate precautions against detection.

The family's attitude was reasonable, which was possible since the general relationships in the family were good. If Mark confessed he was never punished, but the parents were especially puzzled by the compulsive lying. Also they marvelled that all these troubles produced no unhappiness in the boy.

At last, after further incidents, the father, who was at a loss to know what to do, put Mark in disgrace; he must have his meals in the kitchen, and fishing was stopped. Mark remained without a sense of guilt, and continued to say his prayers.

The parents went on in the interview with me to build up a history of Mark's early life.

He was happy. In fact at 2 years he said: '*I'm so happy to be alive*,' conscious of a love of living.

There is probably a tie-up here with the parents' philosophy of life, which includes a 'cultivated joy of life.'

Mark chose to live at home, rather than to continue at his preparatory boarding school. School reports said: 'Mark could do better if he tried.' He was good at games and was thought to have average ability. Eventually he went to a grammar school as a day-boy and there he made an attempt to 'redeem himself by hard work.' Mark was very fond of nature study and had an incredible knowledge in this specialty, using books intelligently.

When I asked about sleep techniques, the parents reported: '*Mark adopts incredible postures* in his sleep. He is like a log. On going to bed he sleeps immediately and he has never told his dreams.' Also Mark had a twitching face recently, including blinking.

Mark had many friends, they said, but no bosom friend; also he was attractive to older people. He had been sensibly informed in regard to sex by his father. When excited Mark would sweat and work his face, and in this way he became thought of as nervous. Mark liked handwork but showed no special artistic ability. He had taste, however, and could be moved by beauty. A feature in his life was the brilliance of his older sister. He was well aware of this, and possibly associated with this feature was a fear of his father which developed over a phase in which he was doing badly in school.

Mark was courageous physically, swimming being his favourite sport. In fact, *Mark's main interests concerned water*. He was set on going into the Navy from 3 years to 8 years, but he temporarily lost this (at 9 and 10 years) when he was told he would have to work to get accepted.

The parents brought out the point that he was affected by the new baby boy, born when Mark was 5. He called him 'our baby,' and he has always been especially fond of him. They now said that it was *when he shared a room with this boy* (*at 6 or 7*) *that he first stole from his mother* (Previously the mother had dated the first theft at 8 years.)

The day after the consultation with the parents I had the first of three significant interviews followed by one (not described here) subsidiary interview with Mark. Although I knew a good deal about him it would have been valueless to have worked on the basis of this knowledge. What was needed was a history-taking of a different kind, a history revealing itself in terms of the boy's communication with me. A great deal happened during this first session, but that which can be reported here centres round the 'squiggle game' which we played together.

The First Interview

In my first personal contact with Mark, I adopted the squiggle game technique. He was pleased to play this game, a game with no rules.

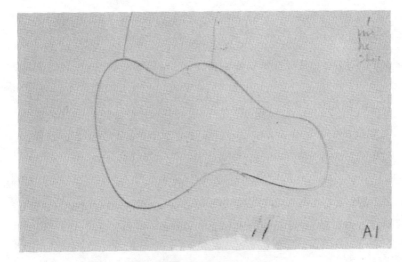

(1) My squiggle which he turned into a shoe.

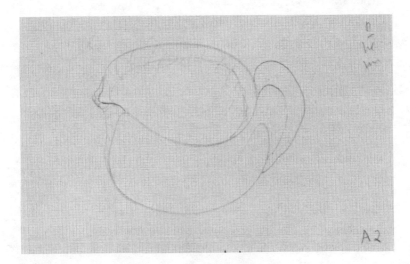

(2) His squiggle which I turned into a jug.

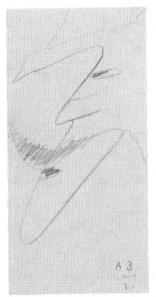

(3) My squiggle which he turned into a man with a moustache (rather fantastic).

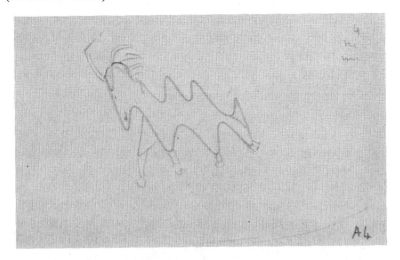

(4)   His squiggle which I turned into a kind of animal.

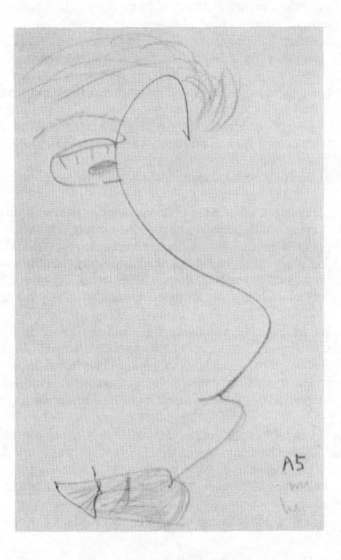

(5)   My squiggle which he turned into a face.

(6) His squiggle which I turned into two worms close to each other.
      There was a good deal of conversation about this, including a
      discussion on his part of the function of the 'saddle.' He
      indicated on the drawing the way in which worms copulate.

(7) My squiggle which he turned into a curious kind of a man's face.

Here I was already aware of the boy's tendency to undervalue
fantasy. This corresponds to the parents' statement that 'he sleeps like a
log and has no dreams.'

(8) His squiggle which I turned into a schoolmaster.

(9) A drawing of his of a man. This resulted from my talking about
      my using the imaginative part of the drawings to introduce the
      subject of dreams. He seemed surprised that I should talk about
      dreams and the drawing of the man indicated a dream figure
      which gradually lost definition from the waist down. I spoke
      about the stealing at this point, using a word that he supplied:
      impulse. I said that in stealing he was acting out ideas which
      were in his mind, like dreams. He had spoken about forgotten
      dreams, and I had said that when dreams become unavailable
      there may be a need to recapture them through acting on
      impulse so that the dream dominates what happens, and in this
      way reappears in the person's own life and conduct.

I now knew of Mark's ability to make use of my approach to the
unconscious and to dream material; this approach was somewhat new
to him, partly because of his own defense organization and partly
because of the family pattern. Nevertheless we could communicate in
this way.

After this first consultation the mother wrote:

After leaving your house with Mark last week my husband made
only casual inquiries, avoiding direct questions. The boy showed no
reaction of disturbance or pleasure. Later on in the evening he spoke
to me at some length about his visit to you, and quite spontaneously.

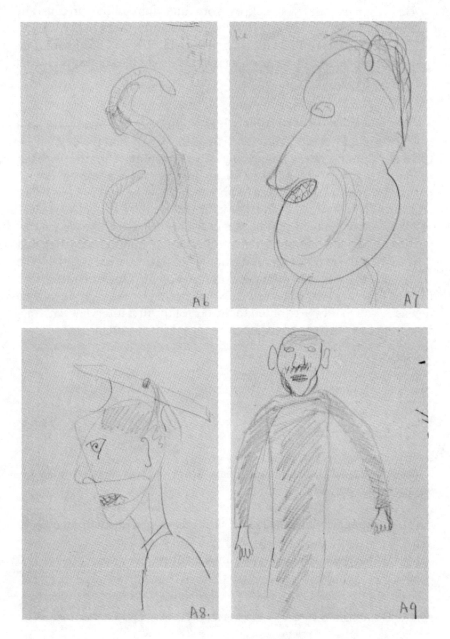

He was particularly struck by your questions about dreams and their meaning. He seemed puzzled by the importance of dreams and by your insistence on this point. I hope all this will be of some use. His comment about the toys was that it would be a 'paradise for his young brother.'[2]

(There were toys in the room which are used by younger patients.)

A fortnight after the first interview with the boy and the day before the second interview the father rang me up to report. After the first visit to me Mark was not allowed to go fishing. He wanted to take a particular boat to the pond with his brother and he said to his mother that it was a present for his birthday. Could he have £1 to get it? He was so obsessed by the boat that he had only one idea, which was to get this particular one immediately. The mother was firm in refusing. He had already told the brother about the boat. The parents were struck by the way in which eventually he gave in and so accepted the frustration and did not buy the boat. This seemed worth noting by them because of its newness, which they attributed to the fact of the first interview with me. It will be seen that water is again involved in this incident.

The Second Interview

On the second occasion that I saw Mark, he was ready to play the squiggle game again.

(1) My squiggle which he rather skillfully turned into a human head.

(2) His squiggle which I made into a tortoise.

---

[2] In this oblique way he referred to his own need to make a link with himself at a younger age.

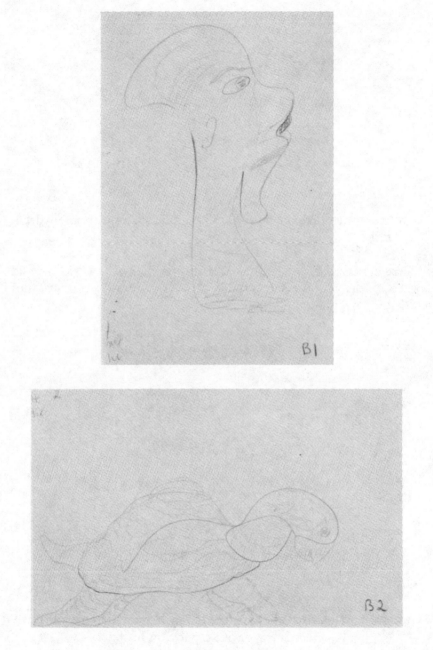

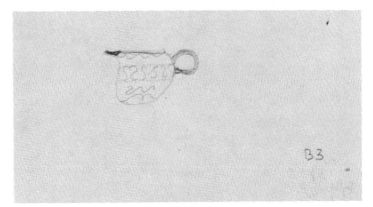

(3) He turned his own squiggle into a teacup, appropriately decorated.

Here appeared his wish to take full responsibility for a drawing and for the ideas that lie latent in it. Rather naturally, this was not markedly imaginative.

(4) My squiggle which he turned into a man very precariously climbing a rock surface with a pack on his back.

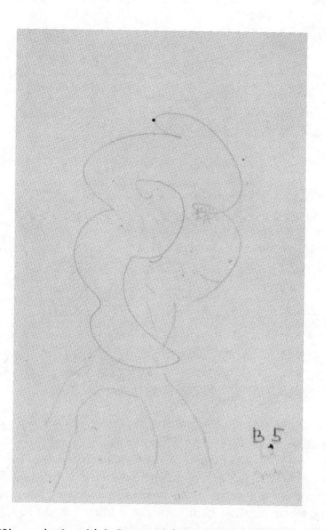

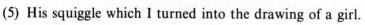

(5) His squiggle which I turned into the drawing of a girl.

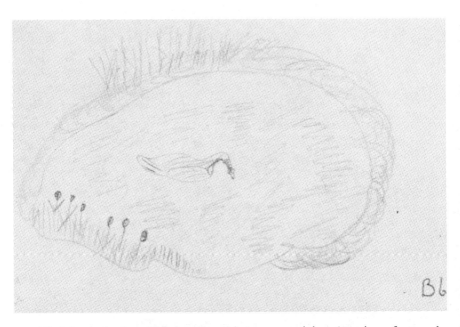

(6) My squiggle which he turned into a surprising drawing of a pond
     with bulrushes and reeds, and a water-fowl enjoying the scene
     and just about to dive its head down for food.

Here was a picture. This showed me Mark's integrative capacity and
also his capacity to love. The whole symbolized the persisting love
relationship (both instinctual and dependent) with his mother, his
fondness for water and his concern with nature generally and fertility.[3]
It also gave me a glimpse of his special knowledge. The strength of
Mark's ego organization being evident, I knew I had the right to go
ahead with interpretation of material presented.

---

[3] One could guess here that he was able through water to make positive use of his mother's
depression (sad tears).

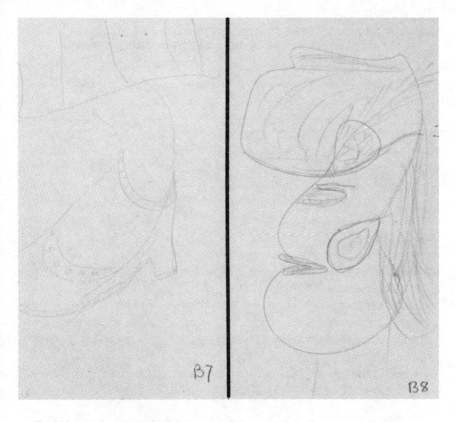

(7) His squiggle which I turned into a lady's foot and shoe.

(8) My squiggle which he turned into a most extraordinary and
    fantastic face.

Here fantasy was appearing again in the form of the fantastic which
is not free dream material. Along with all this there was a good deal of
talk, not particularly about anything. Mark could feel, however, from
what happened, that I was interested equally in fact and in fantasy,
whichever should turn up. Also he could understand my appreciation
of the picture.

The Third Interview

At the third interview we again played the squiggle game.

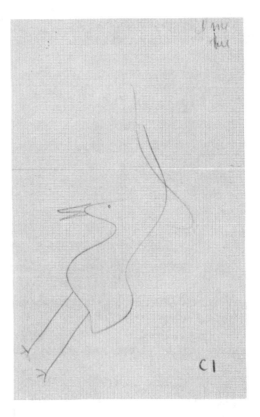

(1) My squiggle which he turned into a bird with long legs.

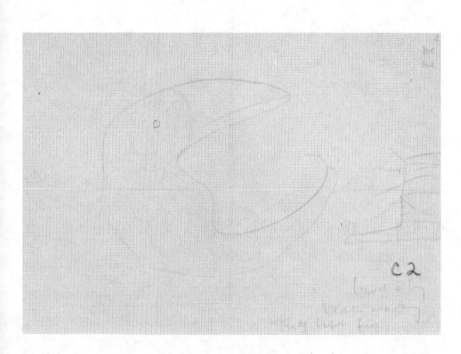

(2) His squiggle which he turned into a bird with a big beak warming
     itself before a fire.

The game had led Mark to express fantasy without feeling foolish
about it. The picture which he had in front of him was entirely his and
the whole idea came unexpectedly to him from his own unconscious.
My function here was not to interpret. The main therapeutic factor was
that the boy had found a bridge to the inner world in a way which was
quite natural. This drawing was like a dream that has value because it
has been dreamed and remembered.

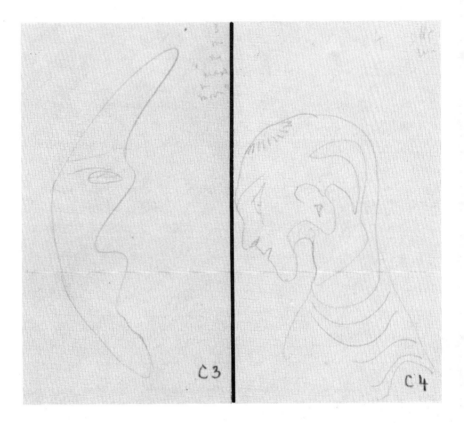

(3) My squiggle which he turned into the man in the moon. Fantasy continues.

(4) His squiggle which I turned into a head and shoulders.

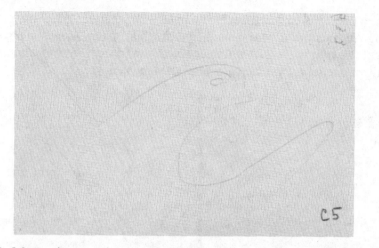

(5) My squiggle which he turned into a bird rather effectively flying upwards. He did this with a minimum of additions and got a good deal of satisfaction from the movement portrayed.

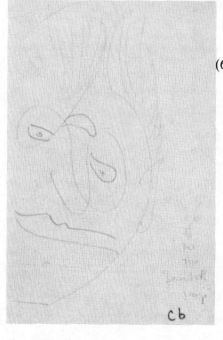

(6) His squiggle which I made into a face and he named it 'Mr. Facing-Both-Ways.' He justified this by a quick drawing of what would be eyebrows from my point of view. From his point of view it was a mouth, the mouth that I had drawn being eyebrows from his point of view. This was all done in a flash.

Here was indicated the dissociation in Mark's personality, relative to stealing. At this point Mark reached a stage at which he was nearly aware of the split in himself which enabled him to steal without shame or guilt or anxiety. I made no interpretation of this.

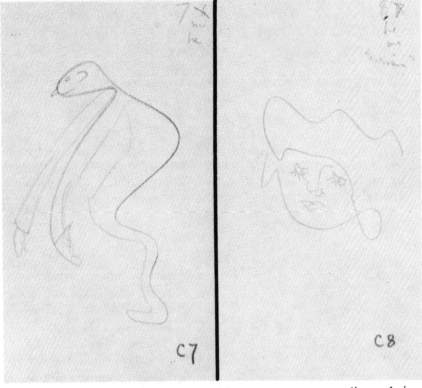

(7) My squiggle which he turned into a most extraordinary being with arms and one leg, a floppy sort of individual rather bird-like, and the drawing was certainly humorous.

Here came, along other things, a sense of humour, always a sign of freedom affording elbow room, so to speak, and in this way assisting the therapist.

(8) His squiggle which I made into a face and which he called an Eskimo.

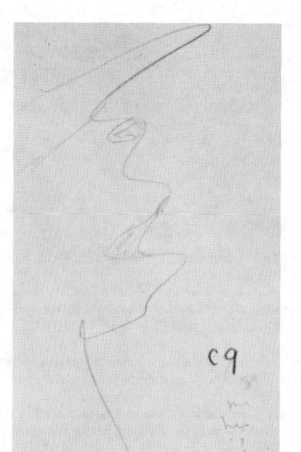

(9) My squiggle which he turned into a weird face of a man. At this point it was easy for me to ask him about dreams. He said: 'I forget them. In any case they are only ridiculous,' and he was obviously afraid of being laughed at, if he should remember them. He did, however, start to draw the next, which was not based on a squiggle.

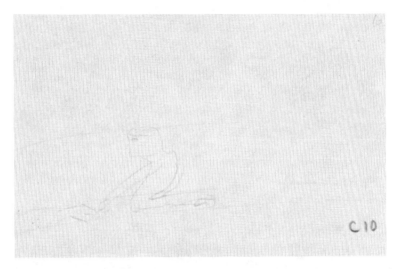

(10) Here he is kneeling in the road making squiggles in the dust. This
was a dream.

*This was a significant moment. The drawing led to the subject of
depression.* He called this 'feeling bored.'

He said: 'I only feel it for a few seconds just when I am waking up. I
often think it is a strange life; perhaps life is a dream.'

Here he was a very serious person. Instead of being in a state of
dissociation he had here become a unit, and a depressed person.

In answer to a question as to whether he had ever felt really down, he
referred to a time when he had stayed away from home because his
sister had measles. *He was perhaps 8.* He said he was homesick, sad
and lonely.

Here, as is commonly found in this work, the patient takes the
therapist to the date of the period of maximum strain. At 8 years Mark

had intolerable dreams and a nightmare that indicated a severe depressive mood. The mood indicates ego organization and maturity, and some capacity to cope with the threat of disintegration of the personality.

I referred to *the love of his mother* which was at the back of his sadness in parting from her, remembering the history of difficulty weaning. His comment on this was: *'If mother's away things are different.'*

We then talked about fishing. The love of his mother was the thing that he clearly expressed and in a deep way as it came out of his remembering feeling depressed. Hence the extent of his hopelessness at being parted from her.

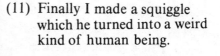

(11) Finally I made a squiggle which he turned into a weird kind of human being.

He was now ready to go.

General Comment

In this series of three psychotherapeutic consultations there came about a natural development of a bridge between Mark's conscious and unconscious, or a bridge between inner and outer realities. If asked about dreams at the beginning he would not have been able to remember any. ('He sleeps like a log and never reports dreams.') By the end of the third interview Mark was able to tell me about his period of maximum strain, which he remembered because of a dream that brought him right into the depression that was reactive to his separation from his mother. This was at the age at which he started stealing (except that he had stolen once before, from his mother, at the time when he first shared a bedroom with the baby brother).

Naturally, there are precursors to all this. In Mark's case the antisocial tendency indicating a continuing reaction to a deprivation reaches back to the actual weaning from the breast. (No doubt the mother's psychology needs to be taken into consideration here, since it is almost always true that the mother of a baby that is difficult to wean is herself somewhat depressed at the time, or somewhat depressive by nature.)

The antisocial tendency was represented by:
(a) Pseudologia fantastica (from 2 years).
(b) 'What I want I must have' (from 7 years).
(c) Stealing from the mother (8 years).

Discussion

This case illustrates three main themes:

(1) The first interview with the parents gave a clear picture of the case, which enabled the parents to re-orientate to the problem. It was not for use by me in therapy.
(2) The three interviews with Mark gave me a new view of the same problem, and gave me opportunity for doing fairly deep psychotherapy. All the essentials were in the material, and in usable form:

A mother fixation, first evident at weaning.

A significant separation at 8 years.

Stealing as a reaching across the 'weaning' gap and between the dissociated personality structures, and from external to internal psychic reality, to and fro.

An underevaluation of fantasy.

The splitting defense, pseudologia, which cleared up as a result of the consultation.

Rediscovery of the fantastic, and then of fantasy.

Unification in the personality, bringing with it a depressive dream and a sense of concern.

A sea fixation, which alternated with a water obsession and which proved to be a satisfactory sublimation of the mother-fixation.

(3) The case also illustrates the theory of the antisocial tendency as a reaction to deprivation (not privation), and appearing clinically along with hope in regard to object relationships. In this case the stealing was related to a manic defense against the depression felt as such at 8 years, and was also related to a split in Mark's personality which made him clinically two people, one who had a compulsion to steal and the other who had strong moral principles and a wish to be like his parents and to do well in the world (in Mr. Facing-Both-Ways).

According to the theory on which all this work is based, the boy in stealing was unconsciously looking for the mother from whom he had the right to steal; in fact from whom he could take because she was his own mother, *the mother that he created out of his own capacity to love.* In other words, he was looking for the breast-feeding from which he had been weaned and yet not weaned. His difficulty in weaning was turning up again in the present in the form of impatience at frustrations and the need to steal in order to circumvent frustrations by claiming rights.

Result

There was a clinical improvement following the first interview, which showed as a new acceptance of reality. After a month the father wrote:

> Mark is in very good condition in every way, so far as we can see. In particular, he is far more interested in his work at school than ever before and he is taking it much more seriously, with improved results. He has started to learn a wind instrument, which was his own idea; and he is very keen on it indeed. He formerly learned the piano, but was indifferent to it and had to be pressed to practice whereas he is eager to practice the wind instrument.

> We took him away for a couple of weeks at Easter to stay with a relative by the sea. He did not ask to fish, which he knows is still forbidden, but was nevertheless exceedingly happy by the seashore. He has transferred his interest in fishing to sailing model boats. He makes these boats quite skillfully, but he shows signs sometimes of becoming obsessed by them, and this makes us a little anxious, as the previous trouble arose (it seemed to us) from an obsession with fishing. He wants to talk incessantly about them and about his expeditions to the pond.

After a further three months the father wrote:

> We have been very pleased with Mark's progress this term. He has done very well at school, came out top of his form, and had an excellent report in all respects. He seems stronger morally and appears to derive strength from a habit I have got him to adopt of saying to me each morning that he will put honesty and truthfulness first today.

We are just about to send him off for a long summer holiday at a boys' camp under suitable supervision. He is greatly looking forward to it. After that he will go to stay for a week with an old friend of mine and I have told him that—for the first time—he can resume fishing while he is there if he feels strong enough to be sensible about it. He says he does. We shall see how it works out. He has been very happy again.

Here the father shows that he has continued his active technique for instilling moral strength, which is part of the family pattern, and which I made no attempt to alter. Also he has played a more vital role in Mark's life, and corresponding with this the boy's mother has stepped somewhat into the background since the time of the first consultation. I found that there had been a complete cessation of the stealing, and lying was no longer part of his way of life.

The father wrote again eight years after the first series of therapeutic consultations. Mark being now 20 years old.

Thank you for your letter. I am very glad to give you an account of Mark's progress during the past four or five years.

He has pursued unswervingly his chosen vocation as a sailor, and this very week he has completed his four years' apprenticeship as a midshipman in the ——— Line. He always goes to the Far East and is usually away for several months on a voyage. He has a deep satisfaction in the life at sea, although he found it involved great physical and emotional hardship, especially in the early years. He faced it with great fortitude.

He has of course developed in every way and is much more mature. He has great pride in the line in which he serves and also a sense of duty and of responsibility.

Our home means a great deal to him, and he spends the whole of his leave here. He obviously feels this to be the stable element in his life at present. He appreciates frequent letters from the family more than anything else and he writes to us and to his brother and sister from every port. This is a notable fact considering that he is not a literary type in any way. He is very affectionate in his letters; but he appears rather casual outwardly when he is at home. He has one great friend whom he knew and they are inseparable when he is at home.

Mark is much attracted by girls and enjoys going to dances with them when ashore. He talks freely to myself and my wife about his girl friends and brings them to the house. He talks openly about wishing to get married when he has qualified as an officer, though I don't think he has found a girl he wants to marry.

The timeless quality of life at sea seems to appeal to him. He often writes in his letters about the days slipping past, and of time moving past him in an effortless passage. At sea there is a fixed routine, but no pressure of time, no sense of the day of the week or of the date, all of which he finds very irksome on land.

He has become much more sensible about money. He sends me an allotment of his pay every month and I accumulate this for him. He brings home from the East very generous presents and to do this means a great deal to him.

When he is at home, he needs an unplanned life without obligations or engagements, except for dates with girls. His room is always in great disorder, in contrast with the strict neatness imposed on midshipmen in regard to their cabins. But he is very careful about his personal appearance and always wears smart clothes, whereas as a boy he was particularly neglectful of his clothes and appearance.

We are expecting Mark home next month after a very long absence of ten months and he will then be at home attending a navigation college for about three months. It will be interesting to see how he reacts to a very different kind of life from the one he has been leading.

If there is anything else you would like to know, please do not hesitate to mention it. So far as we can see, the lad is getting on satisfactorily. If you have any advice or warnings to give us, we should naturally appreciate your giving them to us.

In a final follow-up, in 1962, the father reported that Mark had continued to follow his calling, and to be successful in it. He was then 26 years old.

This is a satisfactory child-psychiatry result: the treatment did not over-tax the parents' resources, and it put but little strain on the psychiatrist. The parents did the bulk of the work and provided the continuity of management that was essential.

Essential, however, were the three significant psychotherapeutic interviews which I have described here, and which gave Mark the opportunity to get rid of the dissociation in his personality which made him lie and which led to his being antisocial without sense of guilt.

Focused Time-Limited Psychotherapy with Children

STEPHEN PROSKAUER, M.D.

There is a tendency to compare brevity of endeavor either favorably or unfavorably with length, as if either less or more were inherently better rather than equally good for different purposes. This has interfered with considering short- and long-term therapies as separate, albeit related, processes seeking to achieve different goals. Although novels and short stories are both literature, the nature and specificity of each form enables the writer to achieve with one what could not be accomplished with the other. The same should pertain in the field of psychotherapy, except the forms are not defined and delineated with a comparable degree of specificity nor are they as well developed. We are far less certain than are writers of literature when to employ which form in psychotherapy because we have a dire need for more and better delineation of specific predictive diagnostic criteria for differential therapeutic planning.

The development of brief, time-limited, focused psychotherapy has probably been handicapped by the evolution of a biased value system that has resulted in many clinicians misperceiving brief therapy as nothing more than an incomplete fragment of what would have been long-term therapy if only the circumstances had been better. From such such an unfortunate perspective, patients in brief therapy are inevitably perceived as short changed despite well-known reports by highly regarded clinicians demonstrating the value of brief therapy (Witmer, 1946). Hopefully, this bias is being put to rest by articles like the one reprinted here and representing an upsurge of positive interest in brief therapy, stimulated in part by theory that views crises as both inevitable and as a fruitful opportunity to be constructive.

Brief therapy requires accurate assessment and rapid delineation of a circumscribed therapeutic focus. Proskauer seems to determine the therapeutic focus primarily from symbolic expressions in individual sessions with the youngster while another clinician works with the parents. Rosenthal and Levine (1971) on the other hand reported that in 85 percent of their 'brief therapy cases, family members other than the identified 'patient' were seen as often or more often than the patient in the brief therapy time period." A comfortably flexible skill with a variety of therapeutic techniques is of considerable value in brief therapy. This should be accompanied by calm deliberateness on the part of the therapist so that he is not pressured into using a melange of techniques, thereby maximizing the risk of ending up in confusion. This blend of flexibility and steadfastness of purpose is easier to maintain if the therapist has a considerable capacity to tolerate crisis and ambiguity (M. Stein, 1970).

It seems logical that a systematic conceptual framework would facilitate the determination of a therapeutic focus and the vital decisions about subsequent interventions. This framework should encompass more than asserting that bried psychotherapy is based on the notion that the shift in the balance of forces enables the child's progressive developmental push for maturity to continue on its own power. A corollary of this notion is that brief intervention can be most effective if solidification and deep entrenchment has not occurred and there are sufficient energies available that are not engaged in sheer survival. Also, therapeutic intervention at the actual time of crisis facilitates changes in the balance of forces providing the youngster's capacity for basic trust is sufficient to develop a positive working relationship with the therapist and to perceive early termination, probably discussed at the outset of therapy, as a positive growth experience rather than as abandonment. Additional attention is generally required to ascertain that the new alignment of forces have continuing support, which Proskauer accomplishes with follow-up visits, while others (Rosenthal and Levine, 1971) have encouraged the family to continue at home, with the therapist's guidance, discussions of issues raised in therapy. Although Berlin (1970) relates his description of brief intervention techniques to theoretical constructs, much of what he reports seems derived from extensive experience and considerable empathic capacities. If this is a valid observation, the process may be difficult to teach other than by means of identification at our current level of knowledge. Note that in the article that follows, Proskauer is insufficiently explicit about means of determining the therapeutic focus from the symbolic material in the first session. Hopefully, future volumes in this series will be able to reprint increasingly explicit and coherent contributions to the theoretical bases for brief therapy. These should enrich further development of technique as well as facilitate clarification of the vital selective judgments that are so critical in brief therapy.

The purpose of this report is to describe a brief individual psychotherapy with disturbed children and to delineate the process, technique, supervision, and selection criteria pertinent to this treatment approach.

Comments on the Literature

Papers on brief psychotherapy with children all describe effective short-term interventions, but each one advocates a different treatment approach with varying specificity as to methods and indications.

Reprinted from *Journal of the American Academy of Child Psychiatry*, Vol. 10 (1971), pp. 619-639.

A few clinicians have discussed the use of psychodynamic theory and developmental principles in limiting therapeutic intervention to a specific problem which must be resolved in order to permit resumption of healthy emotional growth. Rank (1946) described effective treatment of a 5-year-old boy in approximately 20 interviews wherein she "picked out a single thread . . . and followed it strictly," making specific use not only of selected clarifications and interpretations but also of the child's positive regard for her by encouraging him to move in healthy directions. Several recent authors have also advocated choosing a focal issue to which therapeutic attention is directed (Lester, 1968; MacKay, 1967; Proskauer, 1969).

In various papers on short-term treatment of children, "brief" therapy has means from as few as 3 (Alpern, 1956) to as many as 50 (Schmideberg, 1949) sessions. Several authors employ a prearranged *time limit* (Proskauer, 1969; Rosental and Levine, 1970), while the majority of short-term treatment procedures aim toward an early termination without specific limits imposed from the outset (Lester, 1968; MacKay, 1967; Schmideberg, 1949).

The family's expectation that treatment will be brief has often been singled out as an important influence on the course of therapy. Stabilized motivation of the family (MacKay, 1967) reduced likelihood of premature withdrawal from treatment (Parad and Parad, 1968), effective limit-setting due to the clarity of structure and purpose in therapy (Phillips and Johnston, 1954), the family's assumption of a major share of responsibility in the treatment process (Rosenthal and Levine, 1970), and a potentially useful heightened ambivalence regarding separation and loss (Proskauer, 1969) have been mentioned.

There seem to be two schools of thought regarding indications for brief treatment. Some authors recommend short-term therapy for children with reactive disorders but not for those suffering from severe or fixed psychopathology (MacKay, 1967; Lester, 1968). Others describe good results with children assigned a variety of diagnoses (Rosenthal and Levine, 1970).

Most authors find an association between major family instability or marital disharmony a poor prognosis for brief intervention (Lester, 1968; MacKay, 1967; Rosenthal and Levine, 1970). Stein et al. (1970), however, emphasize the usefulness of brief therapeutic interventions even with disorganized multi-problem families.

Treatment Method

For the purposes of this report, focused time-limited therapy is defined by the following conditions: (1) therapy hours total from 6 to 20 and are distributed over a 2- to 6-month period; (2) a specific issue is chosen to be the focus of therapeutic attention from the beginning of treatment; and (3) the date of the final therapy hour is established at the outset and known to the treatment team, the child, and the parents from the start of therapy.

In a previous paper, I discussed similar treatment conditions and emphasized three specific issues of technique: "(1) definition of a focus of treatment by therapist and child together through symbolic play; (2) use of the therapist's insight more as a guide to developing the optimal relationship with each child than as a basis for direct interpretation to him; and (3) management of termination as the most pressing reality and potentially the most fruitful issue in the time-limited situation" (Proskauer, 1969, p. 169).

Further experience has shown that the therapist's insight is important not only to understand the child's symbolic communications and to manage the relationship therapeutically, but also to select and effectively impart needed clarifications, confrontations, and interpretations to the child throughout the treatment process. Recent cases have also demonstrated the value of follow-up contacts with children and families by means of which the therapist serves as a mental health consultant helping others to facilitate the child's emotional growth.

During the course of my training in the Boston University Division of Psychiatry, I had the opportunity to study Mann's technique of time-limited therapy with adults, in which treatment is confined to 12 hours by prearrangement with the patient and a focus is explicitly stated to that patient at the beginning of therapy (Mann, 1967, 1969, 1971). Many of Mann's principles, based upon psychoanalytic theory, have proven applicable to children and have valuably enriched my work.

Clinical Material

Eighteen latency-age children and 4 adolescents were treated at the Boston University-Boston City Hospital Guidance Center and the Douglas A. Thom Clinic for Children in Boston.[1] The majority of the children came from inner-city families with major socioeconomic problems.

The 22 cases fell into the following categories by GAP diagnosis: reactive disorder, 3; psychoneurotic disorder, 9; developmental deviation, 3; personality disorder, 7. In 9 cases, marked improvement occurred and was maintained during the follow-up period (3 to 30 months); 11 more children showed some sustained improvement without complete remission of symptoms; 2 children failed to progress at all with focused time-limited therapy.

7The average duration of treatment was 4 months (13 interviews). The time allotted for therapy was flexibly determined, both to permit tailoring of the treatment plan to the particular needs of each family and also to suit the schedules of child and therapist (e.g., termination date could be selected to correspond with school vacation or therapist's departure).

The Therapy Process

The course of therapy can be divided into three phases, each of which involves certain overriding issues for the child and specific tasks for the therapist.

Phase I: Forming a Relationship and Defining the Focus

It is striking that once time-limited psychotherapy has begun and the child is aware of its early termination, he himself will often bring up in

[1] Therapists: R. Almeida, D. Cotter, A. Greenfield, I. Stamm, R. Tyrell, E. Weeks, and the author. Supervisors: S. Kaplan, S. T. van Amerongen, B. Vaughn, and the author.

explicit or symbolic form a major issue which can be sufficiently resolved in the time allotted. The therapist must be alert to the significance of the child's early productions in order to use them wisely in guiding his own thinking about the focus of treatment.

It is unnecessary in most cases, and especially so with younger children, to confront the child with a verbal statement of the focus. The focal issue serves best as a guiding and organizing idea in the therapist's mind, enabling him to intervene selectively throughout therapy. With adolescents, however, both the time limit and the focal issue are best negotiated explicitly from the start, with the patient having some say about how many months and how often to meet. Thereby resistances related to the normal adolescent ambivalence toward external authority can be minimized.

As in all forms of therapy, it is important for the therapist in the first phase to allow the child to develop as positive a relationship as possible with him. Unnecessary frustrations of a child's wishes are thus avoided, and all opportunities are taken to demonstrate a helpful and respectful attitude toward the child.

Mark, an 11-year-old boy, was referred because of uneven school performance and angry outbursts when faced with minor frustrations or disappointments. Mark's development had been unremarkable except for temper tantrums at age 2, about the time his younger sister was born, and transient episodes of poor school performance since age 8. Also beginning at age 8, there had been several operations to correct a squint. Mark continued to be noticeably cross-eyed and was sensitive about it. His father had a history of depression, severe enough to prevent him from working for 2 years when Mark was 3 to 5 years old. At the time of Mark's treatment, his father acted impatient and intolerant of his behavior. Besides two younger sisters, Mark had a brother one year older who was regarded as much more mature and successful than Mark. The sibling rivalry was quite intense. When he was observed interacting with his mother just prior to therapy, Mark appeared very active and impulsive, reacting to his mother's indecisiveness by quickly taking charge.

At the beginning of the first session, Mark searched the playroom for food. He discovered a bag of candies and tried to buy them from the therapist. He then devoured them all at once, disregarding the suggestion that he could save some so that there would be something left for each of his remaining interviews. Later in the session, Mark drew a picture of a monster with many teeth greedily trying to steal some candy. The therapist commented that Mark didn't seem to expect he would get enough except by stealing.

At the end of the hour, Mark organized a bowling contest in which he traded off being scorekeeper and pinsetter, demonstrating a healthy capacity for participation in competitive games. Every time he fell slightly behind in the game, however, he became anxious and acted as if he were sure to lose. The therapist pointed out that his anxiety was unrealistic, since he would have plenty of opportunity to catch up later in the game.

Throughout the first phase of treatment (the first 4 of the 11 sessions), Mark made repeated demands for food whenever he began to lose at games. The therapist gratified these demands and commented that food made Mark feel better when he was disappointed in himself.

Mark presented himself in this first interview as a boy with fragile self-esteem and a propensity for regression at the slightest sign of defeat. Rather than to encourage the elaboration of the oral-aggressive fantasy material, the therapist chose to accept the needy, greedy monster as a symbolic representation of Mark's poor self-image. (Mark gave evidence for the accuracy of this interpretation in a later interview when he wrote "I'm dum" over the picture of the monster.)

The goal of therapy would be to improve Mark's self-image by making Mark aware of his potential for competence. It would also be important to build up his frustration tolerance and to increase his ability to postpone gratification so as to give stability to the improved self-image.

This strategy would also constitute an appropriate opening phase for long-term treatment in those patients for whom increased self-esteem is required before dealing more directly with anxiety-provoking repressed material. In Mark's case, improved self-esteem appeared sufficient in itself to permit resumption of healthy emotional development, since his tantrums abated within 6 weeks of starting therapy, his relations with father and playmates improved, and his schoolwork returned to honors level, where it has remained during the 2½ year follow-up period.

Phase II: Facilitating Change in a Limited Area of the Child's Functioning

Children commonly use the symbols or games chosen in the first phase throughout the remainder of therapy, establishing a limited repertoire of communication modes suited to their personalities and to the focal issue. Some children engage in symbolic play activities almost exclusively, with little direct verbalization of conflicts. The therapist can help these less verbal children adhere to the focus by having the previously selected play materials on hand at each session.

During the middle phase, the therapist limits his interventions to the chosen central issue while at the same time demonstrating to the child adaptive alternatives in thought, word, and act.

Once the relationship was well established, the therapist began to encourage Mark to delay his forays to the kitchen and to finish his games. At first, Mark felt he had to cheat when he was losing; then his skill improved and he won several times at Parcheesi. Mark's impulsivity declined, he became more relaxed, his span of concentration increased, and his snacks at the end of each hour took on the quality of shared happy experiences with a friend rather than frantic attempts to compensate for feelings or worthlessness.

On the occasion of losing a hard-fought game to Mark, the therapist commented that the game had been more enjoyable than a previous, less exciting game which the therapist had won. It was a useful experience for Mark to learn that victory need not be the only gratification from a game. Without satisfaction in the activity itself, "regression is sure to occur since phase-appropriate success is rendered impossible by the child's maladaptive defenses against possible loss of self-esteem" (Meeks, 1970, p. 163); for Mark, cheating, quitting, and regressing were the maladaptive coping modes.

In time-limited therapy it is especially valuable to handle unexpected developments in such a way that they can contribute to the resolution of the focal problem.

In the 8th interview, Mark arrived with his brother, who had just been released from the hospital after a biopsy of a benign tumor. Mark asked to have him come in for the therapy session. The therapist discussed this with Mark briefly and learned that he had been worrying about his brother and had missed him. They agreed to have his brother come for part of the time. Mark recalled his own operations, and the two boys talked about how scary hospitals and anesthesia had been for them both. Then Mark took pleasure in beating his brother and the therapist at Parcheesi.

After his brother returned to the waiting room, Mark had his usual snack. He put some of the cookies in his pocket to give to his brother. The therapist then produced Mark's drawing and said, "Look, Mark, the greedy monster needed all the candies for himself, but today you could share, and, what's more, you had fun!" Mark smiled happily as he went out to rejoin his brother.

Adhering to a more traditional technique, the therapist might not have allowed Mark to bring his older brother into the playroom and might have encouraged him to discuss his anxiety over his brother's safety, guilt about aggressive wishes toward his brother, or fears of injury related to his own operations. With Mark, however, the therapist did allow the brother to participate and restricted comments to those aspects of the situation which could contribute to resolution of the chosen treatment focus: Mark's poor self-image. Mark's wish to include his brother was welcomed for its positive value (evidence of a wish to share and of enough inner security to *permit* sharing), rather than treated negatively as a resistance. Such selectivity with emphasis upon positive aspects of the child's behavior is essential to time-limited therapy technique, especially during the middle phase.

Phase III: Termination

The goal of prime importance in the final phase is the stabilization of gains the child has made, in such a way that the child can sustain them after the loss of the therapist. Resolution of inevitable ambivalence toward the therapist is necessary to prevent a bitter feeling of abandonment from tainting the child's memories of a positive treatment experience.

When both the focus and time limit have been adhered to, feelings and fantasies about approaching termination frequently emerge with startling intensity. The actual amount and duration of emotional work prompted by termination pressure seem to be determined in each case by the degree of difficulty or deficiency in important past and present object relationships. Mark, for instance, had suffered from a relatively distant and negative relationship with his father and, therefore, had a significant reaction to leaving his therapist. Some children who have actually lost a parent have reacted more strongly than Mark, while others who have had more secure parental and peer relationships have shown relatively little concern about saying good-bye to the therapist.

Often symbolic indications of growing termination anxieties begin to appear during the middle phase, sometimes more than a month before the final interview, without conscious prompting from the therapist.

At the end of the 5th session, Mark asked to take home a magic marker. The therapist told him he could keep it when treatment was over in 6 weeks, but until then it would be left in the playroom for him to use. He agreed reluctantly and, at the start of the next hour, said, "This is our last time, isn't it?" When he was corrected and questioned about this, he explained that he'd misjudged the time because he wanted to take the magic marker home sooner.

Mark attempted to maintain this defense during further discussion of termination in the 7th interview. When he repeatedly pocketed the magic marker, the therapist finally asked him if he doubted whether he would actually be given the marker at the end of treatment. "No, but I want it *now*. Good-bye!" Mark answered emphatically. "So it would be *you* who said good-bye and *me* who would be the sad one," the therapist commented. Mark nodded in agreement. "But really we will *both* be sad to say good-bye," added the therapist. Thereupon, Mark fell silent and looked depressed. He became restless and unable to settle down in any activity, just as in the first 3 sessions. He frequently asked, How many minutes are left?"

As the end of the hour drew near, Mark pretended a beanbag was a time bomb that would explode in 2 minutes and started a vigorous game of catch with it. The therapist commented on the bigger "time bomb" that would go off in 4 weeks when time would come to say good-bye. After this interpretation, Mark calmed down and invented a game of shooting into the wastebasket with the beanbag. The session ended in playful laughter, and on the way out, the therapist commented, "We had so much fun just then with the beanbag that *we* forgot it was a time bomb." Mark smiled and put his arm on the therapist's shoulder as he handed over the magic marker, which he had stealthily concealed in his trouser pocket!

This play sequence demonstrates a typical temporary retrogression to maladaptive patterns of coping in response to termination pressure. Mark dealt more openly and comfortably with these feelings following the interpretation utilizing his own symbol of the time bomb.

Early fantasies about separation are often mobilized and can be dealt with during the termination phase, provided the therapist sticks tenaciously to the issue.

In Mark's 10th (second to last) interview, he typed out an epitaph, "Here lies a bully who wasn't very wise, he picked on a fellow who was his own size." Noticing that he looked angry and depressed, the therapist suggested that a kid might feel afraid to be angry if he thought somebody might die. Mark replied that it was not that he might die, but that somebody would kill him. The therapist agreed that it was hard to feel free about expressing anger if he was scared he'd be killed for it, even if he knew better.

Then Mark typed sadly, "Go away rain: rain, rain, go away, come again yesterday," and he acknowledged that rainy days were indeed dreary, sad times. The therapist connected these feelings with the approaching good-bye. The need to put the sadness behind him ("Come again *yesterday*") indicated how painful and strong the termination affects had become.

Toward the end of the same hour, Mark played Parcheesi. As he made a blockade, he said, "I'd like to hold you up forever." When the therapist captured two of his pieces, Mark growled, "I'd like to kill you!"

Primitive fear of retribution for the aggressive side of his ambivalence had been clarified in the light of the coming separation, leaving Mark freer now to express both the longing to hold on to his therapist forever and the wish to do away with him. Since ambivalent feelings excluded from conscious awareness can produce a fall in self-esteem and thus depression, the therapist was both concluding the essential work on the chosen focus and preparing Mark for termination by helping him articulate his ambivalence.

In the final phase of time-limited therapy, the focal issue frequently becomes intertwined with termination material, making it possible to work on both together with great therapeutic impact. This occurs most readily when the focus has to do with a real or symbolic loss.

Jeremy, an 8-year-old boy, suffered from an obsessional and depressive neurosis with a learning inhibition. His mother was a cold compulsive taskmaster who had forced his father to leave the home during Jeremy's oedipal period because of the father's alcoholism and associated marital strife. Symbolic material in the first interview suggested that much of the difficulty had to do with intolerable guilt-laden ambivalence toward his father related to the father's departure at a crucial time in Jeremy's development. It was the goal of treatment to render this ambivalence conscious and acceptable to Jeremy so that it would interfere less with his functioning.

Jeremy asked some obscure questions early in therapy about the hospital administrator, whom he imagined to be a very nasty man. He played out a fantasy of killing the administrator and his secretary. It was only during the termination phase that he revealed what his motive had been: "Since you are too nice a guy to stop seeing me, it must be that awful hospital administrator who is making you stop." When he was told that the termination date had in fact been the therapist's decision, Jeremy shook his fist in the therapist's face, smiling warmly at the same time. The therapist acknowledged Jeremy's mixed feelings and related them to similar emotions which Jeremy had experienced toward his father.

The therapist can help a child focus on termination feelings by "counting down" the last 5 or 6 sessions and by encouraging the child to plan for his final hour. Oftentimes, special activities or refreshments chosen by the child, or a carefully selected gift from the therapist, have symbolic meaning which can be utilized in dealing with feelings about loss in the last session. Some children can be told explicitly why the time limit was set and can recognize the positive aspects of their needing only a brief period of treatment.

It is especially important to stress what the child has learned and has made his own, that which belongs to him and is relatively independent of further contact with his therapist. Likewise, it helps to ask the child about other adults to whom he can turn for a trusting relationship and to give him permission to transfer his positive feelings out of the therapeutic situation into other current and future relationships. The therapist should actively avoid leaving the child with a feeling that he has just said good-bye to the only giving, trustworthy adult in the world!

In the final session, the therapist gave Mark a Parcheesi game as a gift. Mark was told that this was something fun he could take away with him, but much more important were his feelings and memories about his work in therapy: he could always recall how he learned to enjoy activities without having to feel so bad about losing that he had to get food for comfort. "Yes, I'll keep that in my heart," Mark responded. As Mark left the playroom, the therapist asked him what should be done with the monster picture on the table. Mark replied, "You keep it; I don't need it."

Thus, Mark communicated his recognition of internal change and readiness to retain corrective knowledge from the treatment experience. The picture of the greedy monster no longer represented his image of himself and could be left behind.

Follow-Up

While formal therapy terminates at the end of a few months, the therapist's responsibility to help the family does not. He can use his knowledge of and rapport with the child to provide consultation to the family and agencies involved with the child as long as such help is needed.

In essence, the therapist's work is divided into two stages. First, in the therapy proper, he helps the child make positive use of a relationship for working out a central conflict issue to a point of relative mastery. Second, he arranges for the child's environment to provide maximum opportunity for growth through other positive relationships and experiences, so that gains made in therapy will be supported rather than undermined.

Follow-up interviews can be set up at 3- or 6-month intervals. The child is thereby reassured of the therapist's continuing interest, while the therapist can assess the child's progress and recommend further interventions when needed. This follow-up approach has facilitated informal assessment of treatment effectiveness for extended periods following termination of weekly contact and has permitted continued observation of the children as they move ahead into new developmental phases.

Work with Parents

In many cases, parents have been seen regularly during the period of the child's time-limited therapy. In other instances, parents came in for periodic conferences with the child's therapist, but did not undertake treatment themselves. The parents' needs for services following the child's termination were assessed, just as they were for the child. Weekly interviews generally terminated at the same time as the child's formal therapy.

Focal issues in treatment of parents were not restricted exclusively either to the parent's pathology or to the parent's relationship with the child. An issue could often be found which was a source of difficulty for the parent, both in relation to the child and in relation to other aspects of the parent's life, so that he could feel his own needs were being met in treatment, as well as those of his child. Guilt and anger displaced onto the child from the spouse or other figures in the parent's family often made useful foci for time-limited work with parents.

Criteria for Selection

Clinical experience thus far indicates that children assigned a wide range of diagnoses can profit from focused time-limited psychotherapy. Five criteria emerged from study of early cases which seemed important in determining the clinical outcome and which were applied in selecting subsequent children for this method of treatment. The criteria do not have to do as much with diagnosis per se as with key issues which cut across diagnostic lines but appear to be important to the effectiveness of the specific treatment modality.

1. *Is the child capable of rapidly developing a positive working relationship with therapist?*

A passive, schizoid or severely depressed child may require so much time to establish a functioning therapeutic alliance that time-limited therapy seems futile. Usually this problem is evident early in diagnostic contact with the child. What is usually referred to as the child's "motivation for therapy" is included in this criterion.

2. *Can a focal dynamic issue be identified which is central to further healthy emotional development and which can be sufficiently resolved in a 2-- to 6-month period of psychotherapy?*

Short-term intervention need not be synonymous with symptom removal or behavior modification. Alteration of attitudes and maladaptive styles of coping are as much the subjects of concern in time-limited therapy as in more extended forms of treatment. Promotion of positive shifts in character development is an essential goal of the technique.

The focus in most cases fell into one of four groups: unresolved feelings about an important object loss, anxiety about body damage or illness, low self-esteem, and maladaptive modes of coping with anxiety or aggressive impulses. The focus was thus formulated in affective terms (e.g., Jeremy's ambivalence about his father) or in adaptive terms (e.g., Mark's regressive pattern of coping with threats to his self-esteem). While a child could not work through all the ramifications of his oedipal conflicts or pregenital strivings in a few months, a derivative expression of some basic conflict might be defined on an affective or an adaptive level and effectively dealt with in time-limited therapy (e.g., Jeremy's ambivalence about his father as one facet of an unresolved oedipus complex). Crippling feelings or distorted notions resulting from separation or loss have made especially effective issues for time-limited intervention because of the opportunity for reworking the loss during the termination phase.

If a child spontaneously delineates an appropriate focal issue during the diagnostic interviews, it is worth considering the possibility of time-limited therapy on that basis alone.

3. *Are the child's defenses neither too rigid nor too brittle in the area of the focal issue and does the child's character structure permit rapid resolution of the issue?*

If, for example, massive denial defends a child against recognition not only of the feelings, but even of the historical facts about the death of a parent, one might be cautious in committing oneself to a direct onslaught upon this primitively defended area. The potential dangers involve either mobilizing even more rigid defenses (making the child more resistant to change) or leaving the child vulnerable to more severe symptoms after collapse of a flimsy defensive screen against overwhelming feelings and fantasies.

The two children for whom time-limited therapy proved ineffective exhibited well-entrenched passive-aggressive character traits with underlying strongly held omnipotent fantasies. Such character pathology slows the pace of the therapeutic process and forces the therapist to take a passive role to avoid encouraging an unproductive sado-masochistic relationship with the child. The imposition of a time-limit prevents the therapist from following the child's pace in such areas.

4. *Has the child acquired sufficient basic trust so that early termination can be experienced more as a positive growth experience than as yet another abandonment?*

This criterion can be very difficult to assess. If a child has suffered multiple early losses and exhibits marked impairment of object constancy, time-limited treatment may be a difficult venture, even if one is prepared to spend all of the time working on feelings about termination. Nonetheless, time-limited treatment in modified form may prove useful, provided emphasis is placed on helping the child learn to use limited givers.

There are two specific modifications in planning which can be helpful when this criterion appears unfavorable. First, plans can be made from the start to continue follow-up appointments at relatively frequent intervals for a long period, so that the child experiences dilution of contact with the therapist rather than abrupt termination after therapeutic work is completed. Second, steps can be taken to arrange for a more permanent person to continue a positive relationship with the child as the therapist bows out. This alternative may be especially useful for fatherless or motherless children whose upsetting symptoms, ambivalence, or unrealistic expectations would prevent them from forming successful relationships with a Big Brother or Big Sister prior to a brief period of therapy aimed at partial resolution of these problems.

Martin, a 10-year-old fatherless boy with symptoms of running away and stealing on a neurotic basis, received time-limited therapy focused on his longings for a father. His symptoms disappeared within the 3-month prearranged treatment period, but termination was postponed for 6 months until a Big Brother was assigned to the boy and a good relationship had been established between them. The clinical team felt that assurance of a continuing relationship with a caring male figure was mandatory for Martin to maintain his improvement. The therapist saw him each week during the first 3 months, but only irregularly (about every 3 weeks) during the 6-month "holding period." Martin was able to shift his positive regard for the therapist to his Big Brother at the end of treatment. He continues to do well 2 years after termination of therapy.

5. *Can the child's environment be (or be made to be) sufficiently supportive so that treatment efforts will not be undermined by pathogenic forces in the child's home, school or community?*

This question must be answered before any form of outpatient psychotherapy is undertaken, but it is especially relevant to brief modes of intervention which will not involve the child directly and intensively beyond a certain point in time.

It is noteworthy that time-limited therapy can be effective with so-called disorganized or multi-problem families, provided the treatment team chooses goals realistically, assesses the family's inherent strengths accurately, and capitalizes on these strengths to the fullest.

Martin's mother was a paranoid character who reacted to emotional stress by launching into hostile diatribes against anyone available, including school personnel and the treatment team. Also in the family were a retarded older brother and a married sister who was subsequently hospitalized for suicide attempts. There were frequent household moves, a series of unlisted phone numbers, and inappropriate demands on the clinic staff. Despite these and other serious difficulties, Martin's mother was clearly interested in his welfare. She would search for him diligently whenever he ran away and saw to it that he came to his appointments, even at some trouble and expense to herself. In treatment, the team avoided dealing directly with her paranoia but focused as much as possible on her mothering functions with her son, enlisting her as a vital person in his treatment and supporting her self-esteem as a caring mother. In time, her paranoia subsided and her outbursts became much more moderate. This shift was crucial to her eventually tolerating and being tolerated by an untrained Big Brother working with her son.

Special Applications

There are at least three special situations in which principles of time-limited therapy may be usefully applied in modified form. The first might be called the "trial of therapy." Frequently, a family appears to need treatment, but there is reason to believe an open-ended commitment to therapy would be too threatening. In such cases, it is possible to suggest a trial period of perhaps 3 months, at the end of which time everyone will get together to reassess the situation. If things do not seem to be going well, the treatment can be modified or terminated. In a "trial of therapy," termination may not be managed the same way as in time-limited therapy proper, but the selection of and adherence to a focal issue present similar problems in both situations. A particularly useful goal for a time-limited trial of therapy is modification of a defensive or maladaptive position which may stand in the way of positive participation in extended therapy.

The second situation is preparation for residential treatment. Usually there are delays of months in bringing about residential placement after the recommendation has been made. Reality defines for the family a clear focus: anticipation of a forthcoming separation. The precise termination date cannot usually be specified until just a few weeks before it is to take place, but otherwise the situation is similar to time-limited therapy.

The third special situation could be termed "time-limited therapy by necessity" because the therapist or the family plans to depart in a few months. All the principles of time-limited therapy "by choice" will apply, and a decision must be made whether brief treatment or none at all is better for the child. Forced brief treatment must be a very common situation in training facilities which have a flux of trainee therapists passing through every few months in need of treatment cases, and in clinics which serve highly mobile populations.

Considerations for Training

A prearranged time limitation tends to increase the investment of energy, inventiveness, and active involvement of the clinical team. Members of the team find themselves planning and communicating together extensively. Greater clarity regarding events in the therapy process often results, to the particular benefit of inexperienced trainees. As Mann has stressed, time-limited therapy also offers an early opportunity for trainees to confront some basic problems of all psychotherapy which may not emerge as quickly or dramatically in open-ended treatment.

There are at least three technical problems which have special import in time-limited therapy. The first of these is sticking to the focus. The inexperienced time-limited therapist can easily find himself exploring far afield from the focal issue on the one hand, or, on the other, pressuring the child to give up whatever he is doing in order to talk explicitly about the focus. The work seems to progress best when the therapist follows the child's lead, selectively commenting or participating rather than intruding or coercing. The therapist watches and listens, wondering always, "What does all this have to do with the focal issue?" If he sees a useful connection between some seemingly remote material and the focus, the therapist can construct a symbolic "bridging" intervention which synthesizes the material with the focal issue in a constructive way for the child. If no connection is evident over most of an interview or beyond, either the therapist is missing something, or the focus has been poorly selected, or the child is in a state of resistance. In the latter case, the resistance should be interpreted at the earliest opportunity.

A pair of 11-year-old identical twin boys were treated by different therapists for pathological reactions to the death of their father 4 years previously. One twin (F.) had difficulty with unresolved longing for his lost father, while the other (T.) was guilty about his angry feelings toward his father. Early in treatment, T. became preoccupied with using the typewriter. In mid-therapy, F. suddenly began asking to use the typewriter and borrowing other activities from his brother T.'s therapy sessions. At this time, F. stopped responding to questions from the therapist about his father. When F.'s therapist realized that F. was using activities which he had heard about from his brother as a resistance to further work on the focus, he interpreted the resistance. F. at once returned to the issue of painful longings for his dead father.

The second distinctive problem for the therapist is overactivity, often stemming from ambivalence about the time limitation. The therapist may feel it will be possible to effect a magical cure of all the child's problems, while at the same time fear that he cannot help at all in so short a time. He may then resort to overly active interventions in an anxious effort to avoid total failure or to achieve an impossible therapeutic triumph.

The third problem for the time-limited therapist is resistance to bringing up and working on termination issues. Since separation and loss are painful, many therapists have a tendency to underestimate, avoid, postpone, or repress the fact of the approaching termination and provide little help to the child in facing the inevitable discomforts of saying good-bye.

Supervision

Like the therapist, the supervisor of time-limited treatment faces specific tasks at each phase of the process. In the first phase of therapy, the supervisor's primary responsibility is to help the therapist decipher the symbolic data and begin to formulate the focus. It requires a clear understanding of developmental psychology as well as psychopathology in childhood to choose that facet of the child's problem which lends itself best to brief treatment, taking into account both the child's personality structure and the phase of psychic development through which he is passing.

Ronny, a bright 10-year-old boy, was brought to the clinic because of poor school performance, recent episodes of minor delinquency, and refusal to obey whenever his father was away on business trips. His mother related all these problems to the father's severe alcoholism during the preceding 2 years.

In the first interview, Ronny described how he once planted some flowers in the garden; then the landlord got drunk and pulled them all up; Ronny remembered feeling mad and hurt but couldn't say anything because "children have to respect their elders."

Because of Ronny's constricted fearful quality and some explicit phobic concerns in the diagnostic interview, the therapist had planned to focus on helping him with his fears. The supervisor suggested, however, that a direct focus on fears would be too threatening for a boy who had had so much realistic concern about father (and other men) losing control and behaving destructively. The supervisor proposed an alternative focus on management of aggressive impulses, an approach which would emphasize Ronny's mastery of the impulses rather than his fear of them. Dealing with control rather than fear would not only provoke less anxiety and resistance in treatment but would coincide with the normal latency developmental strivings for mastery. The new focus was adopted and proved effective.

During the second phase of treatment, the supervisor helps the therapist stick to the focus by demonstrating ways in which the child's material is related to the focal issue. He tries to clarify any tendencies to overactivity and may suggest potentially fruitful ways to intervene.

At some point during the second phase, the emotional tone shifts, usually quite suddenly, and the therapist may express doubt that short-term treatment will be sufficient. The therapist's anxiety usually indicates that the child is beginning to communicate discomfort about the approaching termination. The therapist can be reassured that anxiety usually indicates that the child is beginning to communicate discomfort about the approaching termination. The therapist can be reassured that anxiety is expected at this point.

Once termination work begins, the supervisor can help the therapist identify the child's defenses against ambivalent feelings and see possible relationships between the focal issue and the child's reactions to termination.

It is also important for the supervisor to raise questions about suitable arrangements to promote the child's continuing development following termination. If planning starts relatively early in treatment, a risky hiatus between the final therapy session and the start of a supportive program for the child can be avoided. The therapist, however, tends to get involved in the details of the therapy process and may need prompting from a supervisor to think about long-term planning.

In several cases, individuals having no previous experience with or clinical training in psychotherapy with children have conducted effective time-limited therapy under the supervision of an experienced clinician. The application of specific technical guidelines, in supervision as well as in therapy, may enable a variety of interested persons to carry out focused time-limited treatment, provided they have a capacity to make empathic contact with children and have access to a supervisor experienced in the technique. It is yet to be determined how much previous professional background, if any, is essential for carefully supervised therapists. This question has far-reaching implications in planning community mental health services for children.

Summary

This paper defines a specific form of brief psychotherapy with children in which the duration of treatment is known to all concerned from the beginning and therapeutic interventions are deliberately directed toward resolution of a specific focal problem.

Using this method, favorable results were obtained with 20 of 22 children assigned a wide variety of diagnoses. The therapy process is described in three phases and illustrated with case vignettes. Five criteria are outlined for selecting children who are likely to benefit from focused time-limited therapy, and special applications are described. Finally, technical guidelines are suggested for therapists and supervisors using the method.

Treatment of Boyhood "Transsexualism": An Interim Report of Four Years' Experience

ROBERT GREEN, M.D.
LAWRENCE E. NEWMAN, M.D.
ROBERT J. STOLLER, M.D.

This paper was selected for inclusion for two interrelated reasons. It is a description of an apparently successful psychotherapeutic approach to effeminate boys. The authors label them "transsexual" carefully and appropriately enclosed in quotation marks to indicate that there is no prospective evidence that these boys are or will become transsexuals. In addition, the retrospective historical data derived from adult and adolescent transsexuals suggesting that these boys may be a risk for the development of transsexualism if of questionable reliability. A second reason for including this paper is that it is a vivid example of multidimensional therapy, derived from the authors' considerable study of the development of gender identity and its problems. The work with parents, for instance, combines counseling, instructual, and role-modeling modes. Firm advice is given and strong pressures are applied to parents to comply with instructions and expectations, arousing parental anxiety as a means of motivating change. The clinical contacts with the young boys also illustrate a multifaceted approach in which clear direction is given, positive identification with the male therapist is fostered and encouraged, corrective emotional experiences are sought, and a strong overtly persuasive stand is taken that feminized behavior is undesirable. Although the role of unconscious motivation and interpretation appears deemphasized, it is evident in the authors' comments about helping the youngster see the projected fear of his own aggression and encouraging the youngster to expose his fantasy life, since this can provide, in the authors' words: "rich insights into motivations for his behavior." Consistent with the multidimensionality of the therapy, the principal use of these psychodynamic formulations lies in directing behavior change.

Some will question whether the relationship and identification with masculinity could have been as effectively supplied by a paraprofessional in the form of having the boy meet with a young man, e.g., a child-care worker, educateur, or a "Big Brother" under professional supervision. This vital issue regarding the use of therapeutic personnel so as to expand the professional's impact is clearly beyond the scope of this paper, which focuses on utilization of research findings. The authors do demonstrate persuasively, however, that no matter what is done directly with the youngsters, the subtle and covert sanctioning and encouragement of feminine behavior in the home must be dealt with directly and overtly with the parents.

As in therapy that purports to be unidimensional, it is even more striking in this multidimensional approach that uncertainty remains as to what proportion of change is a consequence of which intervention—the insight derived from a psychodynamically oriented interpretation or a behavioral prescription based on psychodynamic formulation; identification with the therapist or direct suppression, suggestion, and encouragement to stop the symptomatic behavior; and the like.

We have previously described the behavior of very feminine young boys. Based on retrospective reports of childhood behavior given by adult males who want sex-change surgery, there is reason to believe these boys are pretranssexuals. These young boys, just as the adult

Reprinted from *Archives of General Psychiatry,* Vol. 26 (March 1972), pp. 213-217.

male-to-female transsexuals recall, strongly prefer dressing in girls' clothes, strongly prefer girls' games, toys, activities and the companionship of girls, take only the role of a female in games, state their wish to be a girl, and steadfastly avoid activities typical of boyhood. As long-term follow-up data are not yet available we cannot state with certainty that these boys, if untreated, would mature into adult transsexuals. However, because (1) there are no reports of adolescent or adult transsexuals who have successfully reoriented their profound crossgender identity by any psychiatric or psychologic treatment modality and (2) because males with an extremely feminine identity in our culture undergo considerable social hardship, at all ages, we have attempted psychologic intervention during boyhood. As we have reason for cautious optimism, we here report our first, tentative findings.

General principles of therapy are aimed at accomplishing four objectives: (1) Development of a relationship of trust and affection between the male therapist and the boy. (2) Heightening parental concern about the problem so that parents begin to disapprove of feminine interests and no longer covertly encourage them. (3) Promotion of the father's, or a father-substitute's, involvement in the boy's life. (4) Sensitization of the parents to the interpersonal difficulties which underlay the tendency of the mother to be overly close with the son and for the father to emotionally divorce himself from family activities.

Clinical Material

Case 1 (Treated by L. E. N.)

This boy, now 9, has been in treatment since age 5. Mother says his first feminine behavior occurred when, less than 2 years old, he began regularly putting on her high-heeled shoes. By 3 he was enticing his older sister to dress him in her dresses and to apply make-up to his face. His mother said, "From the very beginning he preferred being a girl and acting like a girl because he felt he was very pretty." He insisted that she buy him feminine dolls and she willingly complied because she did not want to "see him develop a tantrum." His maternal grandmother, a powerful woman, helped him obtain jewelry and admired his interest in "artistic things."

By 5 the boy was dressing completely in feminine clothing whenever possible, applying cosmetics to his face, and openly insisting that when he grew up he would become a woman. At this point, just prior to therapy, neither parent thwarted this femininity. His mother, an intelligent, competent, and overpowering person, had not found his behavior disturbing. She admired his ability to perform like "a female impersonator." "I really don't have anything against homosexual men. If he grows up to be a homosexual man, that's not a sin, is it?"

This mother had been extremely close to her infant son during his first year of life. She carried him around with her, pressed against her body almost constantly during the first 12 months—behavior described by Stoller as etiologic for male transsexualism.

His father was a passive man who preferred to spend his waking hours away from home, involved in professional work or hobbies. He disliked family interaction and described himself as a "loner." Although troubled by his son's femininity, he never actively disapproved of the behavior or weaned the boy away from the influence of his mother, sister, and maternal grandmother.

Treatment objectives proved difficult to attain. During the initial half-year of treatment the boy avoided eye contact with the therapist, had a great deal of difficulty in separating from his mother to enter the playroom, and insisted on playing with feminine dolls and creating feminine fantasies with toys. Despite her heightened awareness of the problem, the mother continued covertly to support the little boy's femininity at home. For example, she bought him feminine clothing— robes and capes, even dolls—without telling the therapist. When she finally admitted to these things, she attempted to rationalize them and minimize their importance. Despite intensive efforts, the father continued to avoid contact with the therapist (often forgetting his appointment) and declined to become more involved with his son. When under great pressure he finally began to come home earlier in the evening to spend the dinner hour with his family, he developed anxiety attacks and returned to his former, distant position.

During the second year of treatment the boy began to show more affection for his male therapist and began to emulate him. He loved to tell the therapist horror stories in which murder and physical aggression took place, yet was afraid of exerting himself physically in the real world. The therapist was able to point out successfully, to the boy, his fear of his own aggressiveness. Eventually, he became more aggressive and began to strike his sister and even his mother at home. The development was supported by the therapist and the mother's fears of it were allayed. (If the therapist had not intervened strongly at his point, it is likely that the mother's covert pressure against such behavior would have resulted in the boy again returning to a passive posture.)

Despite the above change the boy continued to produce pictures in which males were feminized and women appeared as strikingly beautiful, potent, and powerful figures. For example, on one occasion he drew a little boy standing with his sister. Both were dressed in identical miniskirts, high-heeled shoes, and jewelry. The patient explained that although the children looked alike, actually one was a little boy—a little boy who "wanted to grow up to become a girl." The patient insisted that such a transformation was possible. Many months later, referring to the same picture, the patient insisted that his feelings were exactly the opposite of that little boy's in the picture. "He is feminine, but I want to be masculine." With this statement he seemed to bask in the therapist's approval.

Therapy for the little boy consisted of actively approving any signs of masculinity in his fantasy life or in his actual playing and real world activities, while at the same time, actively disapproving of his feminine play behaviors. Certain behaviors such as crossdressing were actively disapproved of and suppressed. The patient was told in no uncertain terms that such behavior was "no good for him" and after a continuous battle the mother began to adopt this attitude also, despite the temper tantrums which initially took place.

By the third year of treatment, the patient, although remaining somewhat feminine in gesture and mannerisms, was displaying a clear-cut interest in masculine activities. An excellent artist, he produced many drawings in which masculine men became more and more prominent. He began to talk about growing up to become an actor. He actively renounced the wish to grow up to become a woman and when talking about the earlier years when he loved to crossdress said, "Oh, that was all baby stuff. I was just mixed up. I must have thought I was a girl or something. Now I don't."

The patient seems to have repressed the active, conscious transsexual yearnings although continuing to dislike physical sports and not enjoying even sedentary games with masculine boys his age. Efforts to alter the family dynamics, to bring the father closer into the family scene and resolve his difficulties with the mother, have proved unsuccessful and have been abandoned. Therapy at the present time concentrates itself in the work with the child directly.

Case 2 (Treated by L. E. N.)

The second case, that of a 7-year-old feminine boy, responded much more quickly to therapy. Within 18 months he renounced his feminine orientation, gave up his feminine gestures and interests and became masculine in behavior, game preference, and fantasy life. Two factors may account for this rapid improvement. The first was the atypical family dynamic picture. Frequently such families contain a mother who is somewhat mannish in manner and appearance and excessively close with the little boy while the father is distant and passive. In this family a different situation existed. The mother, although competent and energetic, was feminine in appearance, enjoyed pretty dresses, and was attractive. The father, a strong quiet man, did not distance himself from the family. Nor was there a history of exceptional closeness between the mother and son. The second factor, related to the first, was the speed and ease with which both parents involved themselves in therapy and were able to accept the guidance of the therapist in relating to the child. In this case example, the intense early feminine orientation seemed related not so much to the influence of the mother's closeness as to the envy by the little boy of his older sister.

Clinically the boy appeared similar to others in our series. The mother's initial description focused on his femininity: "When he was a lot younger he preferred playing with little girls . . . playing house, which is a normal thing for boys and girls but it just has become more and more until now he doesn't want to do anything but dress up in girls' clothing and completely take the female role when he plays with other children. If they're playing house he wants to be the mother, and if my daughter wants to be the mother then he'll say 'well, then I'll be the grandmother'; he won't ever be the father or the son. He always wants to wear girls' clothing and his best friend, next door, is a little girl and she has a 'Barbie' doll and wigs and high-heels and all this to dress up to and that's all he wants to do. Whether she wants to do it or not, he is constantly over there because I don't make it available for him at home . . . lately, now, he's kind of sneaking it. He has a robe that I found out now he has changed into a mink coat, and he will put it off his shoulders and say that this is his mink coat. Last night he said he was Cinderella . . . He's said, 'I don't want to be a boy. I want to be a girl.' "

This boy's therapy took a different course because of the ready involvement of the parents. In contrast to the first mother, she was impressed with the therapist, admired him and seemed eager to bring her son to treatment. This had an unmistakable effect on the boy. He also enjoyed coming and, although initially reluctant to engage in masculine activities with the therapist (such as ball playing), soon began to participate and after a while seemed to enjoy his visits.

In the psychotherapy sessions a warm and friendly relationship was established. The patient was told clearly that his feminine behavior was "not right" for a little boy and that the therapist would like to see him give it up. Within six months the parents reported a remarkable decrease in his feminine interests and in his seclusiveness. He now began to look for boy friends on the block and soon was engaged in typically masculine activities.

The father, who initially had been pessimistic about his son, responded well to the therapist's directions and actively engaged the boy each evening in masculine interests. He spent weekends with his son, teaching him to play ball and fight and enjoying other activities together. The change in his son's interest pattern spurred the father on to greater efforts.

One of the most important aspects of the therapeutic intervention was the direct attack on the initial parental pessimism. Before therapy began both parents admitted to their secret belief that their son was destined to become a homosexual and felt helpless to do anything about it. As a result they both avoided their son, especially the father who did not conceal his contempt and clearly preferred the other children. By contrast once the parents realized that there was a great deal that they could do about the problem the boy responded quickly. Two years after the completion of therapy, reports from the family indicate that the patient is continuing to be masculine in all respects.

Case 3 (Treated by R. G.)

This boy was first seen 4 years ago at age 6. He improvised women's clothes whenever he could, played only with girls and with girls' games, and said he wanted to be a girl. His interest in crossdressing dated to age 2 when he would improvise an apron from a dish towel and follow his grandmother about the house (she invariably wore an apron). During the first year the boy and his parents were seen together once a week in a playroom. An opportunity was thus afforded for observing the boy at play, his parents' reacting to his behavior, and the parents relating to each other.

There were two focuses in the treatment. One was directed at the relationship between the parents. In this family, the mother was the controlling influence in decision-making. Not only did she take responsibility for minor and major decisions but her husband willingly abdicated to her control in these matters. The father's authority and prestige was repeatedly undermined by his wife in a variety of ways. Descriptions would be given of events in which the family rights would be violated in some way (e.g., a neighbor boy throwing a rock through a family window) and in which father would be berated by mother for not standing up for the family rights (complaining to the neighbor boy's father). If anyone in the family would protest, it would be the mother. Thus, the son would invariably see his mother as the influence within the family which carried power and protection.

In the playroom the boy's aggressive play would be discouraged by his mother, and the father's frail efforts to allow such behavior were of no avail. Also, the mother, in the context of registering a complaint about her son's feminine behavior, would act out the boy's gestures while displaying considerable positive affect, thus transmitting a mixed message to her son. The therapist, by his actions of giving support for the boy's rough-and-tumble activity and standing up to the wife, furnished the boy with a new set of responses to his behavior and provided for the father an alternate style of family interaction.

This extended period of family observation furnished information with which to proceed in a more concerned effort, on an individual basis, during the second year. The boy was seen in the playroom alone and the parents were seen together. The therapist and boy engaged in a variety of "father-son" activities in which an effort was made to give the boy more confidence and pleasure in doing boy things. The therapist was available as a father-surrogate interacting in a manner in which the natural father had been unavailable. It was emphasized that, even if the boy did not feel comfortable in athletic or aggressive behavior, he could still relate as a boy in less competitive activities, rather than withdrawing to female companionship. Thus he could build, hike and do handicrafts, rather than dress as a girl and play with dolls.

In sessions with the parents an effort was made to reset the power balance so that father would be more involved in making decisions and providing rewards for the boy. Considerable time was spent focusing on the father's passivity in representing the family to the outside world and the effect on the boy's emerging identity of seeing his mother as family defender with father being the continuing object of mother's beratement.

Ways in which the boy's masculine-type behavior was being discouraged by maternal attitudes were scrutinized. An example of this occurred during the second year of treatment. The boy was in front of his home, dancing about with a water hose in a style reminiscent of a water sprite, all the while shrieking in a girlish manner. A neighbor boy riding past on his bicycle observed him and called him "sissy." The patient turned the hose on the boy, knocking him from his bicycle, perhaps his most "phallic" gesture to that time. The mother, witnessing the series of events through a window emerged from the house and chastised her son for knocking the boy from his bicycle (not for the feminine behavior). In spite of repeated efforts by the therapist at clarifying the implications of her penalizing the boy for rough-and-tumble boyish behavior, the mother's own needs for law and order in the boy's life have continued to hamper therapeutic progress.

Father's passivity has also remained an unrelenting obstacle to restructuring the boy's milieu. Much of the father's hostility toward his son was eventually seen as a displacement of similar feelings toward his wife. He had found himself in a marriage about which he had grave misgivings. The feminine boy, in contrast to his younger masculine brother, bore a physical resemblance to his mother. This caused the father to withdraw from him early in life and provided him with an object for directing otherwise unexpressible hostile feelings for his wife.

Behavioral change in the boy has been only modest. He no longer crossdresses, states his wish to be a girl, or plays with dolls. He associates more readily with boys. However, he remains somewhat effeminate in his mannerisms, is fearful of boys, and occasionally drapes himself in robes in a girlish manner. His relationship to his father remains very distant while that with his mother is currently hostile.

Case 4 (Treated by R. G.)

Since age 2 this boy said he wanted to be a girl, had consistently shown feminine gestures, would take only the role of a female in fantasy games (including being a pregnant woman and having a baby), and strongly preferred girls as playmates. In this family, mother was clearly boss as defined in the parental roles and attended roles and attested to by the son's statements. Mother and son spent much time together in contrast to father's time commitment to business. When father would return home from work he would be too tired and disintegrated to spend time with his boy. His weekends were used to peacefully relax, without interruption. Father's image was frequently undermined by his wife. For example, when driving a new route, if a choice he made took longer than the alternate, he would be berated by his wife in the presence of his son.

This family has been seen for three years. The boy was seen from the outset in play therapy sessions and the parents individually, in rotation, on successive weeks. With the boy, a role-modeling approach was utilized in which the male therapist and patient engaged in activities such as kick ball, basketball, running and climbing, went for long walks together, and participated in a variety of games. The advantages of being a boy were emphasized by words and deed. A warm relationship developed in which both the boy and his therapist genuinely looked forward to sessions with both enjoying them immensely.

An effort was made to convince the parents of the influence on their son's emerging gender identity and gender role preference of having role models in which father's position was second best. This family, very insightful, and exceptionally motivated to effect change in their son, did a remarkable job during two years in reworking their relationship. Decisions were, at first hesitantly, and later naturally, taken over by the father. He became increasingly comfortable in relation to his son and their enjoyable participation in joint activities increased considerably. The mother, who had during her childhood competed with a twin brother, gradually relinquished the family reins and channeled her need for competitiveness and efficiency into a professional activity. The boy shifted his perception of parental roles. Early in treatment he would say to father, "You can't tell me what to do—mommy is boss." Subsequently, these same words came to be directed at mother. The extent of his earlier identification with mother was apparent in many ways. For example, when on a family picnic he would sit by his mother and eat only the foods displayed on the picnic table which his mother would first choose. Progress was dramatically documented two years later when his father, with great pride, described a recent picnic on which the boy had selected foods from the large array of possibilities spread on the table, not only on the basis of *type*, as selected by father, but also for *quantity*. Both these observations had been made entirely without the boy's awareness.

The boy has made a considerable shift in his gender-role orientation. He no longer crossdresses, no longer improvises feminine costumes, and never takes the role of a female in games. When he draws pictures, they contain men, whereas previously they had always been of women. He plays well with boys and is accepted by them, no longer being an object for teasing. He fantasies himself, in the future, as a husband and father. Residual feminine identifications are evident in an occasional feminine gesture and an interest in long, silky men's bathrobes and other clothing which can take on a flowing gown-like quality; however, he is decidedly masculine and comfortable in his new role.

Case 5 (Treated by L. E. N.)

This is a 12-year-old boy who had been extremely feminine in his gestures, interest pattern, and sense of identity since earliest childhood. At the age of 5 he had loudly insisted he would grow up to become a woman. When his mother told him he was a boy and would grow up to become a man, he cried and screamed. Thereafter he continued to insist he would grow up to be a woman and would accept nothing to the contrary. By 9 he was taking the part of a girl in classroom plays and enjoyed dancing like a "ballerina." At school the other children called him "girl," "sissy," and "Maybelline Eyes," designations he did not seem to mind. He tended to be an isolate, had few friends and would spend much time in his room drawing pictures of beautiful women.

When first evaluated the boy's pronounced femininity was unmistakable. Though he stated that he did not want to be a girl anymore (he remembered wishing to be one when he was younger) the examiner had the impression that he did not have considerable interest in being a man. For one thing, he was preparing himself in no way for a masculine existence. Interests and clothing preferences had remained profoundly feminine and he had difficulty fantasying himself in an adult male role.

After discussing the implications of the behavior with the parents the therapist explained the urgency of the situation to the patient. He was told that if he wished to renounce his femininity he would have to do it now, before adolescence. He was told that if he continued to fantasy and behave in a feminine way he might become trapped in a situation in which, at a later date, a masculine role would be impossible. After several weeks of consideration, he announced he wanted to make every effort to "become normal like the other boys." Though expressing the feeling this might be impossible, the therapist strongly assured him that it was not. Therapeutic efforts were aided by the patient's strong religious commitment. Like the other members of his family he was deeply religious and would not "tell a lie." When he "gave his word" that he wanted to give up his femininity and become masculine, strong inner moral pressures compelled him to do so.

The boy had been going on shopping expeditions to women's clothing stores with his mother. The family was instructed to discontinue this activity and the patient agreed; instead, he began to spend more time with his father. Since both were temperamentally reticent, often hours went by in which neither said a word. They felt uncomfortable, but, under the pressure of the therapist, persisted.

During therapy sessions the boy related his earlier interest in feminine things and discussed his efforts to develop masculine interests. As in other cases, pessimism about becoming masculine and his secret belief that he was destined to live as a feminine person were continually challenged. Gradually, he began to doubt his former certainty that his femininity was inborn and unchangeable. Under the therapist's direction he learned to box and, although he did not enjoy it, his ability to handle this masculine role made a strong impression on him.

The patient's inner sense of femininity was strongly supported by his physical appearance. He was small, slim, and feminine in features. Even more importantly, he walked, talked, crossed his legs while sitting, and gestured in a feminine manner. He had assumed for as long as he could remember that his feminine mannerisms indicated he was secretly a girl, despite his male genitalia. To counteract this, he was told by the therapist that human gestures are not the result of an underlying biology but reflect early identifications—in this case particularly with his mother, since his father had been away at war during the first three years of the patient's life. He was also told that his learned feminine gestures could be unlearned with effort. Somewhat reluctantly, he agreed to try. Exercises were designed which encouraged masculine postures in sitting, standing, and walking. Instead of assuming his natural sitting position the patient was instructed to study the way his father sat at the table and to emulate him. When running he was to control the excessive roll of his hips and "run like a boy." After a year of persistent exercises, improvement in his body posture had a significant effect upon his identity as a male. This patient may represent the oldest age period in which treatment of extensive crossgender may be effected.

Comment

Our rationale for treating these boys developed gradually as one of us (R. J. S.) began seeing the most feminine of males, adult and child, and their families whenever possible in a search for etiology. The first clues of the family dynamics appeared, and it was an obvious thought that these dynamics could be found more clearly—or ruled out if the parents and their sons could be treated in extended therapy. The desire to gather information while the causative process was still active in the family (i.e., in the boy's early childhood) was paralleled by familiarity with the work of child psychiatrists on other severe pathologies of childhood. They had long since taught that one needs to work not only with the child but the parent and the sooner and more intense the treatment, the better.

With this in mind, Green took into treatment our first feminine boy and worked out a plan of therapeutic intervention that has evolved to its present form.

We feel the therapist should be male for two reasons. By the nature of his authority, prestige and capacity for providing approval and disapproval, he will be available to the boy as an appropriate object for identification. Additionally, the companionship provided by an adult male in many cases fills a void in the boy's experience left by an absent or psychologically unavailable father. The male therapist substitutes as a role model. The boy and man may involve themselves in activities which are typically boyish and within reach of the boy's ability. These may involve kicking and throwing a ball, running, climbing or just going for walks. In this context, these activities are not competitive or threatening to the boy as they might be with the feminine boy's more aggressive male peers.

Generally, parental attitudes toward the boy's feminine behavior have previously been positive, in the sense that it evoked laughter, or brought increased parental attention of a not unpleasant nature. Children have been posed and photographed in girls' clothes and shown off to friends and relatives. Many parents think such behavior is cute. Fathers, even more than mothers, tend to dismiss the behavior as "nothing to worry about," perhaps because femininity in their son is seen as a failure on their part to serve as an adequate model for male identification. Approval, implicit or explicit, must be interrupted. An attitude of disapproval must be consistent. Some parents state they are displeased with their boy's feminine behavior but, recognizing his compelling drive toward feminine activity, are hesitant to frustrate him. They need to be able to withstand signs of frustration as in any other disciplinary area for behavior which carries significant social consequences. Cessation of reinforcement for girlish behavior should be accompanied by enhancement of approval for boyish activity. The mothers of feminine boys we have seen are frequently ill at ease with rough-and-tumble, boisterous, messy behavior, and have difficulty permitting its expression. They may be able to accommodate to such behavior if stress is laid to the importance of allowing such expression for *their* son in consequence of his already emerging feminine orientation. The fathers we have seen are themselves frequently disinclined to participate in many masculine activities such as rough-housing, ball-playing, or other outdoor activities. Again, they may be better able to generate motivation for such ventures if the special nature of their son's needs are emphasized. Male peer and father-son contact may be considerably augmented by participation in a local Indian Guide Program. While some fathers are averse to such participation, others truly enjoy the time spent outdoors with a group of boys, away from the tedium of work and family. Many of the activities are of a group noncompetitive nature such as excursions, hiking, outdoor cooking (with other men, not mother), and handi-crafts.

   Parental role division may be such that the boy sees mother as the prime provider of rewards, protection and sustenance. Father's role may be undermined overtly or covertly in the boy's presence such that the male role comes to be seen as second best. Again, the special nature of the boy's behavior may be used as leverage to effect some redistribution of influence. Some fathers have considerable difficulty in overcoming their passivity and have married women whose assertiveness complements their own retiring personality. However, in our experience, there are couples who at first uncomfortably, and somewhat stiltedly, but later naturally, can modify role relationships.

Where investigation of the boy's behavior reveals the presence of companions who appear to promote feminine activities, this can also come under some control. Some parents actively discourage play with boys who are characterized as too rough or dangerous. Some report that dressing up and girlish game preference is considerably enhanced when the boy plays with neighbor girls, or in the presence of an overgratifying grandmother. Nonoverly aggressive male peers can be invited home after school or on weekends to provide a not-so-threatening peer relationship for the feminine boy, perhaps not available in the immediate neighborhood.

Some boys reveal their feminine identifications through physical gestures. By the time they are seen in consultation much of this display is unconscious or automatic. In order to bring it under volitional control, the child must be sensitized to when he is walking, sitting, or using his hands "like a girl." Parents should be instructed to consistently point out to the boy when such behavior occurs. In his contacts with the boy, the therapist does the same. The boy may also need actual instruction in modifying these gestures.

When boys feel unable to compete in rough-and-tumble, aggressive play, they may, with the logic of early childhood, choose the only alternative—being with girls and adopting their behavior. But another choice is available: they may build, draw, hike, camp-out, read, play board games, and play with boys who are themselves not wholly sport and rough-house minded. Swimming is one sport in which these boys can perform coordinated gross-motor activity without fear of body injury or undue competition.

Much of the above guidelines is consistent with principles of behavior modification as practiced by behavior therapists. Additionally, however, establishing a trusting, empathic relationship between therapist and patient can provide dividends beyond what can be accomplished by a purely behavioral modification or "shaping" approach. Providing the child with the comfort required to share his fantasy life with someone he trusts and feels he can confide in, outside the family, can provide rich insights into *motivations* for his behavior which provide an additional source of material for behavior change. Furthermore, the empathic, trusting relationship which develops between the male therapist and young boy is a considerable asset in prompting a more masculine identification. The therapist's pointing out of the advantages of being a boy, plus the pleasure he shows in his own life and work, by word and deed, underscores the advantages of manhood and perfuses the entire relationship. We see these as indispensable components of a comprehensive therapeutic approach.

We have documented and attempted to reorient signs of crossgender identity. We have much less evidence of what are harbingers of later homosexual object choice. The extent to which the latter inherently follows from the former is poorly understood. We do now know the extent to which they evolve as independent or related phenomena. The question remains as to what effect puberty with its surge of genital sexuality will have on these boys' behavior. Our study of them at early puberty may help clarify the development of both gender identity and later sexual object choices.

Lest it be misunderstood that we have ascribed an inherently higher value to masculine over feminine behavior, in closing, we will emphasize that it is rather the deleterious effect on social interaction, with the considerable resultant distress emanating from a crossgender identity, which motivates us. These boys are already, by the nature of their behavior, ostracized and teased. As adolescents and adults their social unacceptance becomes an increasing personal hardship. While privately, one might prefer to modify society's attitudes toward crossgender behavior, in the consultation room with an unhappy youngster, one feels far more optimistic about modifying the behavior of that one child than the entire society.

Our experience with treating feminine boys, though more than heretofore reported in the literature, is still in a preliminary stage. Our own thoughts have undergone revision during the preceding four years and evolution will continue. We report our observations at this time to serve as tentative guidelines to others who would join us in the venture. The treatment of boyhood "transsexualism" is at present a psychiatric frontier.

Amy: The Intensive Treatment of an Elective Mute

MORTON CHETHIK, M.S.W.

Silence, a frequent occurrence in the therapy of most children and adolescents of both sexes, is illustrated vividly in the two papers that follow, in which the youngster's problems are manifested primarily by the symptom of silence. Both papers are reprinted because they each contribute to knowledge about means of handling a thorny problem that is insufficiently discussed in the literature, where case reports that are not primarily focused on silence can describe agonizingly long silent periods in a printed sentence or two. The many meanings of silence have been discussed by Arlow (1961), Blos, P. Jr. (1972), and Zelings (1961), who illustrate that, while silence in the therapeutic session is often a resistance, it may simultaneously convey significant nonverbal communication. Although Amy in Chethik's case report, which follows, was mute throughout therapy she was able to communicate nonverbally, giving the therapist many indications about her inner thoughts and feelings. On the other hand, the two adolescents described below by Kaplan and Escoll offered relatively few hints about their inner experiences.

One of the interpretative techniques employed by Chethik entailed storytelling that the reader might compare with

Gardner's structured mutual storytelling technique described on pages 181-195 in this volume. Chethik's story about the "gobble-gobble" feelings communicated vital but difficult information Amy in a displaced, metaphorical context about a little girl other than herself. While displacing the commentary away from the patient, it is abundantly clear that the therapist is talking about Amy, but in a manner that enables her to accept the inter-pretation as having reference to herself (although she was often unable to accept direct, focused comments about herself).

Both articles underscore the effect of silence on therapists, who typically find it difficult to sit in a room with a nonverbal child, whether the latter is compulsively playing with his back to the therapist or pleadingly staring at him. It is not easy to have our presence completely denied repeatedly nor do we relish having the impotence of our presence accentuated over and over again. Defensively, our minds may wander, we may be unwisely silent in retribution, or our attempts to contact the patient may have an insensitive, intrusive aura, making us acutely aware of what happens to the word therapist if it is separated into two words by putting some space between the e and the r. (Perhaps this is the point to note: while the three patients reported in the two papers that follow are all female, silence in therapy is not limited to females, whether it is the occasional ubiquitous variety that occurs in almost every psychotherapy or whether it is the presenting problem, such as in elective mutism.)

Both of these articles illustrate youngsters who have major problems with verbal communication but the lessons from it can be applied to psychotherapy in which silence is neither the primary nor a major problem. For instance, the silence generally has multiple determinants and can represent a variety of meaning at different times. It is the therapist's task to try to understand which of the several overdetermined meanings has primary significance, while remembering that countertransference distor-tion may facilitate interpreting silence as a hostile resistance, and while neglecting that it may be a communication of silent love, longing, regressive symbiosis, etc.

Techniques to deal with the primarily silent patient or the appearance of silence in other patients are manifold. As Chethik illustrates, alternate forms of communication may be creatively utilized. Without noting the extent to which the ideas are derived from observations in the hospital milieu or from other sources, Kaplan and Escoll illustrate the employment of the therapist's ideas about the patient's concerns and preoccupations as the basis for the therapist's monologue in the presence of the patient. It should be emphasized that all of these are therapeutic guesses and should be done in a way that does not introduce an aura of magical mindreading.

Although therapists generally prefer verbal confirmation of hunches about what the patient is thinking, Chethik's experience of ending therapy with the speech inhibition improved everywhere except when with the therapist is not an unusual one. The fact that psychodynamically oriented therapists commonly end effective therapy with electively mute children with this central transference manifestation unresolved in the therapeutic situation, and that behavior therapy of mutism may entail the use of aversive reinforcers (Shaw, 1971), which behavior therapists prefer to avoid, suggest that there is a great deal about silence that we do not understand.

In order to understand the dynamics of elective mutism as a symptom in children whose basic problem is primarily neurotic, a number of authors have attempted to link very specific *individual* psychosexual phase conflicts to this pathology. For example, Browne et al. (1963) and Loomie (1961) correlate anal conflicts, stubbornness, and *silence*, while others (Parker et al., 1960) link mouth trauma and mouth injury specifically with the inhibition of speech. More recently, however, particularly in the psychoanalytic literature (Arlow, 1961; Zelings, 1961), authors have emphasized the accumulated meanings of the silence, and the ways in which the symptom often synthesizes conflicts

Reprinted from *Journal of the American Academy of Child Psychiatry,* Vol. 12 (1973), pp. 482-499.

from many different developmental levels. Amy, the patient presented in this paper, illustrates the multiple and layered meanings of silence: silence that touched every phase of development, and silence that was not only used in the service of defense, but also for intense gratification. A major purpose of this presentation is to highlight the enormous variety of "silence-uses" as it unfolded in the treatment.

Silence is clearly fertile ground for countertransference, for it creates intense emotional "wear and tear" in the therapist. What should the "therapeutic posture" be toward the symptom? What techniques are available to the therapist in the course of his work? What is the nature of the internal experience the therapist endures? These are areas I shall be describing during the course of the presentation and more fully in the later discussion of the case.

The Patient: Her History

Amy B. was 6½ years old when she began treatment, and she had had her "talking problem" throughout her life. In her kindergarten school experience, she had not spoken to her teachers or the other children for the entire year. At home she whispered occasionally to her parents and siblings, but never communicated verbally to street friends, adults, or relatives. The most general characteristic that Amy evidenced was a stubborn, passive, withdrawing quality which was evident not only in her speech difficulty, but in many areas of her life. She ignored or passively refused to comply with the normal demands in the house (dressing, washing, chores, etc.) and therefore was difficult to manage at home.

In addition, Amy had a number of prominent fears. She evidenced strong anxiety about dogs, and at times avoided going out in the street because she was terrified of being bitten. She also had many bedtime fears. Amy was very frightened of being alone, and she established many rituals and procedures before she was able to remain in bed. Enuresis was a symptom that reappeared during stress, and there were some occasional periods of soiling.

Amy's parents also expressed concern about the vividness of her fantasy life, which they felt had persisted beyond an appropriate age.

Amy would become involved without any speech with younger children, usually playing animal games; during this play, she often showed a very intense excitement and aggression.

Amy was a member of a large family, the 5th child of 6. Her father was on the faculty of a large midwestern university, and he reflected the qualities of the typical absent-minded professor. He was eternally preoccupied, highly intellectualized, lost in work and theory building. The mother was an obese, unkempt woman, overwhelmed by the reality demands of her household and children, and filled with rage that was primarily self-directed.

As the mother described Amy's history, for the first half year of her life she seemed to be a very contented baby. Mrs. B. noted that when Amy was about 6 months old, she began to "scowl," and this seemed to coincide with the beginning of the mother's next pregnancy. It seemed harder to get Amy to smile, and this "scowling" characteristic was maintained throughout Amy's childhood. The birth of Brad, the next child, came when Amy was 16 months old, and this was in general a difficult time for the family. There was much illness and mother was depressed. Amy developed many reactions during this period. She became a severe feeding problem. She fought with her mother refusing to feed herself, and her mother angrily left the food for her to take. Amy's "will" seemed strong, Mrs. B. noted, and at times she went for many days eating almost nothing.

In addition, Amy became overtly hostile toward the new baby, who had to be protected from her physical assaults. Amy also could not bear to be separated from her mother; she screamed and could not be comforted even with the father present. She refused to stay in her crib and consistently fought sleep and naptime.

Toilet training began at 2 years of age, and the pattern of fighting and stubborn refusal (as with the food) continued. Mrs. B. had a "potty time" which Amy avoided; she hid from her mother, and would place her movements only outside of the potty chair. The mother was severe with Amy; she used spankings and forced her to remain on the chair for long periods. Slowly Amy seemed to yield, though there were many "accidents" between 2 and three. The toilet-training struggle spread to other areas. Amy dawdled a great deal, refused or was slow to dress, and messed with and shredded papers for the mother to clean up.

During Amy's 3rd year her mother became concerned about the child's aggression toward herself. She scratched herself endlessly; for instance, chicken pox lesions were made into sores, and became sources of skin infections which lasted for months. In a similar way, she picked on all bites and scratches so they were unable to heal. During this period of self-injury, a dangerous and frightening accident occurred. Amy fell into a pool, was unconscious for several minutes, and was revived by resuscitation.

Amy's difficulties seemed continually to compound as she grew. When she was 3, she became acutely ill with a lung infection (a legacy of her pool accident) which did not respond to any medication. Amy was hospitalized for about a 6-week period, in which there was a time when the doctors did not think she would survive. There were extensive medical procedures which Amy endured, and she was physically immobilized for long periods of time. Amy was described as "submitting herself" to his experience: she never uttered a word or a cry. Throughout her hospitalization she never spoke, and she refused to eat to a point causing serious concern. Amy regressed in her partially completed bowel training, and upon return home from the hospital did not speak with anyone including members of the family. The mother noted that Amy had never really recovered from the hospital experience: her eating had since remained poor and her talking markedly restricted, as described above. The growing concern of parents and school finally led to the referral for treatment.

The Treatment Process

Despite the fact that Amy was totally silent throughout the 2-year period of treatment, many forms of vivid communication slowly developed—drawing, writing, intense play, body gestures, and finally sounds. Amy was a very appealing little girl with very pleasant features, blue-eyed, blonde, and tall for her age. But her face was like a mask, appearing rigid and very strained. It was apparent that she struggled with enormous effort to control all feeling from having any visible effect on her. Similarly, early in the treatment, Amy's body was characteristically stiff; she moved and walked with little freedom, particularly during her office visits. Only her hands seemed relatively active and expressive, especially through crafts, which became an important medium in the treatment.

When I met Amy for the first time, she separated easily from her mother and surprisingly took my hand as we walked down the corridor to my office. I have since felt that this gesture was a compliance, like a submission and giving in to a dreaded experience. Once inside my office, Amy kept to one corner of the room, looked furtively at the toys, and would not touch them. I commented several times that she seemed very frightened. After a few minutes she completely lost control of her urine and wet herself and the chair completely. She was so uncomfortable and soaked that I took her to the bathroom where her mother helped her clean up. I arranged subsequently for the mother to be in the room with us if this became necessary, but she never had to do so.

For the first few weeks in her sessions, Amy became very involved in compulsive play in *her* corner of the room. She rolled long, even, successive strands until she used up all the red clay. She made neat little piles of tiny pellets out of the yellow clay. This was a safe, absorbing activity which completely denied my existence. Any question or comment I made evoked absolutely no response.

At times in these early meetings, she showed evident distress about some minor messiness. She might smear herself with some of the clay or wipe her nose on her dress and become quite concerned about the spot. She accepted a tissue from me and seemed to listen when I explained where the bathroom was. This was the first accepted communication.

Slowly, Amy ventured out to use the doll family. In her silent play the children drove off in a car and left the adults, waving good-bye; or the children walked off to another house, while the parents were busy. Each separation in her games was followed by a loving reunion. The mother picked up each child in turn and hugged and comforted them. I noted how glad the children seemed to be to get back with their mother, and commented how scary it must be to come to my office. Then, since she had had several pediatric visits in this period, I wondered if she worried that I was like a doctor or a hurting person. Amy, however, would not glance in my direction.

Amy seemed to go to great length to maintain this early control. One day, another child screamed loudly near my office window. While I was startled, Amy remained absorbed in her clay work. I used this incident to point out how she needed to keep from seeing or hearing anything. It seemed safer for her not to allow anything to affect her. Perhaps she had seen or heard some very scary things before, when she was younger.

Slowly there were signs of gradual relaxation. There was a fleeting but pleasant smile when Amy entered. She assumed a certain possessiveness over her toys in the office (they were so foreign at first). She wrote her name and grade on the crayon box and arranged her toys carefully when she left. She also wanted some drawings hung on the bulletin board, and she somewhat resisted leaving when her session was finished.

Amy began to use the scissors in the office, and her scissor work absorbed most of the time. At first she cut out all sorts of drawings, mostly animals. Then she began to trace the scissor itself on sheets of paper, and she constantly cut out scissor replicas. She began a game which she at first hid from me; she put the scissor near her mouth and simultaneously opened and closed both scissor and mouth. At times, she slid from the chair and she became a fearsome four-legged animal with a mouth-scissor. (I learned that at this time she was using a scissor inappropriately at home, cutting up her sister's doll clothing and making attempts to cut her own hair.) I began to point out to Amy that she was showing me that she felt sometimes that her mouth was like a cutting or biting thing. Maybe this was one reason why she was so afraid to talk. Did she get mixed up that if she talked, it would be like biting or hurting someone? Was this why she kept her mouth closed Amy's only response was to intensify the animal game.

Shortly thereafter, she developed trouble re-entering the office; she delayed getting into the car at home; resisted leaving the waiting room at the start of sessions. She went back to her isolated games, doing schoolwork and making believe she was in class rather than in the office. In her doll play, again mother comforted and hugged the children. Amy was anxious and frightened and I began to note with her that she seemed scared of me. At this point she began to draw pumpkins. In her series of pumpkins, all of which were very large, the mouth and teeth were very prominent. I began to note sometimes children made pretend games; children pretended people were all sorts of things. I wondered if she was making believe that I was something else than a Mr. Chethik—someone maybe like a pumpkin with a big scary mouth. Maybe Amy worried sometimes that I could get angry. Would I have a big mouth and bite? Could this be why she was scared of coming? Though Amy rarely looked in my direction when I made an interpretation, her work now stopped. In response to the mouth interpretation, she drew a series of pictures of dogs, all with blood spots on them, and I commented that maybe Amy was showing me that she had so many biting worries. It seemed as though her original fear of her own oral aggression in the sessions had become projected. She became worried that I, as the therapist, might retaliate by biting, and therefore she feared the treatment for a period of time.

During these first few months, the parents remained quite ambivalent about the treatment, despite the child's immediate gains. The mother reported that Amy was talking much more elsewhere. The implication was, "Why go on?" One day, when Amy asked her mother why she had to come to see me, the mother replied, "You just have to." It seemed like a dreaded obligation. The mother seemed to fight and control any progress that Amy made. For instance, Amy began to express a desire to use the telephone for the first time, and she actually made her first calls to relatives. Rather than showing pleasure and delight, the mother immediately curtailed the number and length of calls Amy could make, not wanting to impose, she said, on the relatives' time.

Payments for the treatment were in arrears, and a pattern of lateness to hours continued. When I discussed these things with the mother, she felt I was just creating an issue, and Amy would only react because I made it so important. As I underscored the fact that she had a great deal of question and doubt about the treatment, grievances emerged. Their friends felt they were silly and were wasting so much money. With 6 children, Mrs. B.'s practical problems were enormous, and there was reality to this complaint.

Slowly, however, Mrs. B. brought out her *enormous* fury with Amy, how this little girl was so capable of getting under her skin. She described how she could not stand her daughter's deliberate dawdling whenever there was someplace to go, which happened every day. She reacted with rage to her daughter's deliberate whining and baby talk, and she also felt very guilty about her punishments and slappings. There was evident intense relief as Mrs. B. described her tremendous fury with her child. Material also emerged about her strong anxiety that Amy would follow in Mrs. B.'s sister's footsteps. Physically, Amy closely resembled Mrs. B.'s sister, who had been hospitalized several times for breakdowns. I was able to interpret to Mrs. B. how excessively upset she must become when she saw any "danger signs" or problems with Amy, with the shadow and the specter of her sister in the background.

I found in my work with the parents throughout the treatment that when they were confronted with their interference and ambivalence, we would come to understand and work out the immediate impending forces. But there remained a strong tendency for them to act out their resistance, usually through bringing their child late for sessions, and this became an index and barometer of underlying feelings.

After about 6 months of work, Amy continued to be very busy with her schoolwork during her session. She practiced the alphabet and numbers, but there was a very different quality to her affect. This seemed no longer to serve as a safe flight from the dreaded therapist, but had a very strong teasing quality. The teasing became more apparent around her use of speech: she spoke loudly to her mother in the waiting room, practically shouted at her mother upon her return, but was mute the moment she crossed the threshold into my office. I began to tell Amy the story of "little miss opposite," which she enjoyed immensely. The little girl always does the opposite: her mother tells her to dress and she takes her shoes off; the father tells her to eat and she leaves everything on the plate; Amy is supposed to spend the hour with me and she makes believe I'm not here; she is supposed to talk and she doesn't let a single peep come out of her mouth. Following this kind of discussion, I would comment how sad it was that she had to make such a fight about the talking, and I would describe the painful and difficult events of the week which had been told my by her mother (dog fears, night worries, or loneliness), the worries that she didn't let herself get help with.

After some of these early interpretations about her withholding (which was a repeated theme in the treatment), Amy became much less of an adversary for a period of time. She began to write on her pictures, to inscribe "This is a picture of Brad and Amy," in an effort to tell me more. She indicated she wanted to play Tic Tac Toe, and we also began some silent word games. She then began a series of frightening drawings, many of which she drew while shuddering. These were evidently her nighttime worries. They were robot monsters which chased frightened little girls. She acknowledged by nods or writing that there were night fears, indicated how sad she felt by adding tears onto the girl's face. All sorts of sharp, sticking projections came from the monsters, they were often drawn in haste with much anxiety. We began collecting these pictures and put them in a special "talking" folder, for use when Amy would be able to talk. Amy was quite eager to place these important drawings in the folder. I pointed out to Amy during this period how much a *part* of her wanted me to know her worries and help her get rid of them, but that another part stopped us—the part that kept her from talking.

The idea of adding drawings to the talking folder pleased Amy, and she brought a new series of drawings. These were huge animals, like dinosaurs and alligators, with open mouths. These mouths were at times so large that they extended beyond and could not fit on the page. But these were not only frightening or aggressive animals; the accompanying affect was primarily pleasure and growing excitement. Red birds began appearing in her drawings, flying in squadrons, and all had the characteristic of the open mouth. Amy controlled the mounting excitement of these drawings by abruptly stopping the activity and going to her compulsive play. But even in her defensive play, eating was the major theme. Amy carefully seated all of the doll family around the table and made huge mounds of food out of clay. She divided the portions equally and proceeded to stuff each doll with excessive amounts of food. When she went back to these bird drawings, she giggled and laughed. Over a series of sessions, she began creating a mural; this was filled with fleeing red birds with open mouths. Behind them were some hunters, who were firing bullets from their guns. When I asked why the hunters were after the birds, Amy wrote in enormous letters, large enough to cover a page, to "EAT THEM."

I began to feel that, as Amy developed more positive transference feelings, she was struggling with impulses of oral incorporation. I began to tell Amy the story of the Gobble-Gobble feelings. Sometimes girls become afraid when they begin to like places and people they come to. This was because the gobble-gobble feelings came up inside. They would worry, in their pretend games, that because of their liking feelings they would want to eat everything all up, even to swallow up the people they liked. Even though the gobble-gobble feelings were from long ago and were *only ideas*, sometimes they were such a worry that they made children keep their mouths shut very tight.

Amy seemed to show a similar mechanism to that we observed with the scissor material. At first she showed the eating, oral, devouring impulses which she feared in herself. Then the impulses were projected onto the hunter in the mural, and onto the therapist who sought to eat the birds and who began to frighten Amy in her sessions.

As the positive feelings for the treatment increased, and as her wish to show me her problem drawings grew, there was also an increase of a great deal of guilt within Amy. There were many feelings of being disloyal toward her family. She became very provocative at home, deliberately courting punishment by such open acts as standing on the living room chairs, and this was followed by frightened questions like, "Do you still like me, Mommie?" I could handle some of these problems with Amy directly. She had a big worry that, as she began to like me, her mommie wouldn't like her so much. But the parents themselves reacted strongly. The lateness returned rather consistently, and there was a critical cancellation with little reason, at a point when Amy was making a particularly strong effort to communicate. (This was immediately after Amy announced on a weekend for the first time she wanted to talk to Mr. Chethik.)

In the session after the missed appointment, Amy dramatically removed all of her pictures from her "talking folder" and took them home. There seemed to be very strong "going away feelings," I noted with Amy. She was obviously worried that the treatment might soon end, and we learned shortly thereafter that her fears were not totally unrealistic.

The mother herself was quite upset by Amy's actions. She cried and felt responsible, but seemed to indicate that she was growing more depressed herself. Several days later I received a call from the father who told me in a faltering tone that they had failed to inform me that Mrs. B. was "in circumstance," which for the B. family meant "pregnant." Not only was Mrs. B. pregnant, but she was in the latter part of her 6th month and this was not easily apparent because of her obesity. It then emerged that the parents (especially the mother) had, for the past months, a growing question about whether she could realistically carry the burden of the treatment with the added demands of a new baby, and this question was looming larger and larger. It seemed to come as a great relief when we were able to work out a new schedule by which I could see Amy late in the day, and the father, by changing his work schedule, took on the responsibility of chauffering Amy. At that point there was a positive shift in the mother-child relationship, and striking changes in their interplay, which I shall discuss later.

During the beginning of the 2nd year of work, the earlier teasing and anal withholding seemed to reappear strongly. Amy sang again in the hallway as she approached my office, but silence ensued when she entered. When she did write to explain her pictures more fully, she wrote in such small letters that it was impossible to make out the words. In addition, she had all the members of the family dolls talking to each other in tiny, whispering, inaudible voices, but no sound came out directly toward me. I began to attempt to reconstruct for Amy the earlier toilet-training situation. I felt that Amy was showing me in the office an old struggle, the old feelings she had when she was 2 and 3 years old when her mother used to chase after her to get her to go on the potty, how she used to hide under the bed and in the closet. It must have become sometimes an exciting, teasing chase with her mother and now I felt she was trying to make a very exciting, teasing chase with me: she was trying to have me chase after her words. I also discussed how she was coming to see me the *same time* every day to talk, and that *must* remind her of the special potty time that her mother had each day—when she was supposed to make her BM. Now 5:00 every day must feel like a new potty time for her. There were times, I also knew, when Amy used to put her BMs *everywhere*, except in the potty, where her mother wanted her to; and now she was showing me she could talk *everywhere* except in the right place—here in the office. It seemed as if the old 2- and 3-year-old feelings were controlling her much of the time.

Amy became preoccupied with the bathroom furniture; she stuffed the toilet full of clay, and she had each member of the family go to the potty several times a session. She then began a game in which she attached many items together with clay. The purpose of the game was to move the long attached train without losing any of the parts. I talked with Amy about the worry that little girls had when they were small, the worry about losing their BMs in the potty. When children were really young, they felt that their BMs were very important to them, and very, very precious. They had a big wish to keep them and they didn't want to see them going out of them. Could Amy now have this worry about her words? She had given up her BMs, but maybe now she just didn't want to give up her words. In this period Amy made her most active direct attempts to bring up words. There was a strong desire to tell me about some pressing worry. She opened her mouth to say something to me, and quickly covered her mouth with her hand. This was a striking struggle, and her anguish and terror were difficult to watch. When she failed and no sound came out, she went to the table to draw the worry instead—the robot monster or a witch—and wrote to tell me more about the worry. These desperate attempts to bring out words were repeated throughout the treatment; at times she turned pale, used her hands to pull something from her mouth, or writhed on the floor in her efforts. The anxiety was very severe, and Amy was most frightened.

After about a year and a half of treatment, I spoke with Amy and her family about the fact that I would be leaving the community in about 6 months. We decided to postpone a decision about further treatment until the end of our work. Amy reacted by temporarily withdrawing into severe compulsive play, but at home she spoke directly of her sadness and anger.

In the last phase of the treatment, Amy seemed to focus on her problems of excitement. Throughout the treatment Amy had struggled with many feelings about having a male therapist. Amy showed a marked sudden increase in hyperactivity related to her father. She seemed constantly to find things to fight about with him in the waiting room. She would act like a puppy dog, sitting in front of him, climbing on the furniture, and at times directly on him. Sometimes I also could hear the commotion the other children were making with the father while Amy was in her session. Amy's drawings reflected this theme— little animals climbing higher and higher, one on top of the other; or a big elephant was lifting little ducks on his back. A new consistent game with the dolls was introduced, in which a man in one car was chasing children in another car in a big race. The accompanying behavior was giggling, much bodily twisting and turning, and at times holding of genitals. I noted with Amy how much excitement there often was when her father brought the children. Sometimes I could see he didn't stop them and they could get very excited. I thought she must also worry that things might get too wild and excited in the office, and that I might let her do things like her father. Maybe it was hard for her sometimes because I was a man, like her daddy. But I reassured her I wouldn't let things get too exciting in the office because I knew this would scare her and not help her.

During another period of animal-climbing drawings, she brought in a picture of a boy. This was Alfred, her 9-year-old-brother, whom she wrote she *hated*. A series of drawings showed him attacked by the robot monsters and thrown into the sea to a nest of hungry sharks. From the mother I learned that Amy was doing acrobatics and exercises with Alfred, and at times she was provoking Alfred to wrestle and fight. The mother then felt she had to supervise and limit their play.

In this period I clearly became the direct object of Amy's excitement. She was much more coquettish in her general manner, and she began to come to the sessions much better dressed and groomed. A new femininity emerged. Sometimes her dress seemed accidentally to slip too high. She had renewed desires to play Tic Tac Toe and word games, but she was so apparently stimulated that I had to stop the games, telling her that now they just seemed to make her excited. She attempted to have me touch her or stop her physically by scribbling on the desk or beginning to take a chair out of the office, but an anticipatory interpretation that she wanted to make an exciting fight with me seemed to stop her at the moment.

Pregnancy and birth fantasies were present. Amy drew a series of pictures showing me how a cornstalk grew from seed planting through maturity. She presented me with elaborate drawings of Easter eggs, writing on the back of the page "For Mr. Chethik." I noted sadly that she showed me she had many questions and thoughts about how things grow, but it was hard to understand all her ideas from her drawings alone. She sought sexual knowledge from her mother directly, which enormously pleased the mother.

On one occasion she wet herself as she approached my office. I wondered with Amy if one of the problems that kept her from talking was her big worry that so many excited feelings would come out. She showed me, by her wetting, that she sometimes had a very hard time controlling these excited feelings. Maybe she was very afraid that a whole flood of excited words and ideas would come out if she opened her mouth.

During the second year of our work, Amy's general adjustment markedly improved. Slowly, her speech inhibitions lessened and disappeared outside of the treatment. She became increasingly able to participate in class, including volunteering and contributing her own ideas to the group. She made many friends in class among the girls, and spoke to, visited, and played with a number of them after school. She began to talk with neighbors for the first time and found much pleasure in being able to call extensively on the phone.

The most striking area of change was the difference in her relationship with her mother. Her mother felt she understood Amy much more, and extensive and sympathetic discussions occurred between them. Amy discussed her night fears and dog worries with her mother. She increasingly became able to express her affects with her mother. For a period of time she responded to her mother's sensitive remarks by sobbing in her lap for protracted lengths of time. It was, indeed, with her mother that she worked on our final separation. She was particularly worried that I was leaving because she had so consistently been unable to talk with me. Amy showed increased desires to help her mother in the kitchen, she learned to cook and shop, and she became the mother's major helper with the new baby in the family. The family decided not to transfer Amy to another therapist, but instead had Amy's oldest brother (who had learning problems and problems in sexual identity) enter treatment. Amy's gains appeared to be stabilized during her latency years, which was the period I was still able to keep in touch with the family.

Discussion

It quickly became evident, as the treatment unfolded with Amy, that her silence was a complicated symptom, and inhibition primarily with a complex developing structure. We worked on conflicts related to oral, anal, and phallic strivings at various points in the treatment. The primary vehicle for our work was through the transference. It became necessary, despite the lack of direct verbal material, to attempt to analyze the affects, defenses, conflicts, and fantasies that had been responsible for the formation of the symptom.

First, I would like to focus on some of the technical problems the silence evoked. Though Amy communicated fully at times, the lack of verbal material provided some evident limitations. I felt particularly handicapped when we attempted to work on her sexual fantasies. There seemed to be a specificity that was necessary for adequate interpretation, and her behavior and drawings could not fully articulate these conflicts. Similarly, I felt unable to reconstruct the experience of the hospital trauma. Again, I felt we lacked a vehicle that could provide for the particulars and details of those events, though there were times in the treatment when Amy clearly brought in the hospital atmosphere and problems. In fact, I was able to reconstruct and resurrect experiences that the mother more fully amplified in our parent sessions together. It is my impression that the above gaps in our work contributed to the inability to resolve fully the transference problems (reflected in Amy's inability ever to speak directly in her treatment sessions). While change was evident and dramatic outside of the treatment hour, the concern remains that silence can be re-employed during intense stress, since it continued to be maintained within the therapy.

There were many concerns about technique that I encountered during the work. The problems related to the process of interpretation were twofold. There was, on the one hand, a major concern about inaccuracy. Was I "shooting in the dark" or using insufficient data in describing a conflict? During silences, the associations of the therapist proliferate, and I had to make deliberate efforts not to develop fully and use my own constructions without adequate confirmation from Amy. But there was also the problem of adequate interpretation. I felt that, at times, Amy was awed by my ability to understand her from her nonverbal material and action fragments. It was as though I had a "touch of magic" at such times, and the ability to see through and literally read minds. This created anxiety in Amy throughout the treatment, and when it seemed appropriate, I explained rationally how I came to understand what she was feeling.

Silence easily promotes rage and feelings of frustration in the therapist. During those periods, I could quickly move from a former empathy with her desperate anxiety, and instead focus on the secondary gains she was experiencing. I would suddenly perceive her as a controlling, manipulating, provocative youngster. My tendency at times was to give her a taste of her own medicine, by countersilence and a revengeful silent treatment of my own. The silence also served a special form of gratification for Amy. At times it was an invitation to a special intimacy, which one had to dilute throughout the work. It seemed easier, without the boundary of words, for Amy to make me a silent partner in a shared clandestine meeting, or to invite me to an emotional experience that I had little control over by a magic gesture.

In reviewing this case, I feel it is also important to reconceptualize some of our diagnostic assessment. While it is clear that treatment was focused on dealing with neurotic conflicts on every level of development, the intractability of the speech problem (within the transference) suggests the possibility that there were more fundamental difficulties involving Amy's ability to neutralize instinctual energy, questions of ego arrest, and some failure in object constancy.

Despite Amy's considerable symptomatic improvement and her ability to resume normal developmental progress, I was left with the concern that her ego functioning was not totally free from conflict, from regression, and that under stress (e.g., adolescence), these ego achievements could perhaps be reversed. There is certainly ample evidence, in Amy's history material, of problems in early object development. Many authors (e.g., Kernberg, 1966) link significant speech deviations with pathology involving internalized object relationships and defects in secondary ego autonomy.

Despite many areas of trust, Amy's capacity for a close, non-dangerous, and confident relationship with her analyst was somewhat limited. There appeared to linger underlying omnipotent fantasies and belief in the magic of words and thoughts (her talking was still equated with killing in the transference). During times of stress, it appears that Amy's object development can regress to narcissistic "splitting" (in Kernberg's sense of the term) where object and/or self could become the magical destructive slayer (bad object).

Similarly, there was a fragility in Amy's ability to test reality. She was unable to discover during the treatment (again within the transference) that some of her most primitive fears of and wishes for destruction could not come about. It was clear, at the termination of treatment, that some primary process thinking remained accessible to Amy, and Amy also maintained some disturbance in the neutralization of her aggressive drives.

In our work with children with "lifelong talking problems" it is clearly important that we attempt to differentiate between disturbances in which there is primary neurotic conflict, and those in which early problems of object development and neutralization of instinctual energy are suggested.

Despite the evident limitations, Amy's healthy desire to communicate through the alternate means she effectively erected within the therapeutic alliance distinguishes her from many elective mute patients who promote total silence.

Treatment of Two Silent Adolescent Girls

STUART L. KAPLAN, M.D.

PHILIP ESCOLL, M.D.

A form of initial resistance frequently encountered in a wide variety of adolescent parents is prolonged silence. This paper reports two case histories of adolescents with an initial and prolonged psychological inability to speak with their therapist. Except for an occasional comment, neither had spoken to her family for 1 to 3 years prior to seeking treatment. These cases represent symptom formation at the extreme of a behavior spectrum, the midpoints in such a spectrum are frequently encountered in the passive-aggressive, the depressed, and the constricted adolescent (Rinsley and Inge, 1961; Martin, 1963; Noshpitz, 1957). The phenomenology and dynamics of the behavior will be described. Techniques for managing the silence, often a vexing problem for the therapist, are presented, and this behavior in adolescence is compared with childhood elective mutism in order to clarify the significance of the adolescent's use of prolonged periods of silence.

Case Presentations

Presenting Features

Although an inability to speak under a wide variety of circumstances was a conspicuous part of each adolescent's behavior prior to

Reprinted from *Journal of the American Academy of Child Psychiatry*, Vol. 12 (1973), pp. 59-72.

treatment, it was not mentioned as a problem by the patient, the family, or the referring agencies. As will be discussed, the intense feelings of shame that the silence evoked in both patients and those involved with them may have led to this oversight. The chief complaints that led to treatment included suicide attempts, stealing, and conversion reactions

A problem with talking was a symptom that had to be discovered by the therapist himself. In each of the two cases the silence began during one of the first 3 interviews in the same way: the patient responded to specific questions, but there was no spontaneous offering of information. During the session in which the patient was to become silent, replies became terser. Finally, the patient was silent. A "yes" or "no" question asked at this time was answered with only a barely perceptible nod of the head. The patient's eyes were tearful and her body rigid with tension. She behaved as if a large dose of unnecessary pain had been added to what must have been an already difficult adolescent existence. The therapist responded by feeling that he had blundered inexcusably. Except for an occasional response, the silence in individual therapy remained intractable for months.

The patients were as persistently silent with their families as they were with their therapists. They were not moved to speak by the family's entreaties, pleas, bribes, or angry accusations. This symptomatic silence antedated the therapeutic encounter by 1 to 3 years. With both patients, the onset of the speech refusal began in adolescence. One patient became progressively mute at age 14 following an appendectomy. She had restricted her speech to her mother. During her prolonged hospital course, when she felt that her mother was not visiting her frequently enough, she stopped speaking to her mother as well. The second patient had had only sparse communication with her father throughout her life. Left alone with him at age 12 following the sudden death of her mother, she found herself unable to speak with him.

In both cases, it was easier for the patients to talk with peers than with the therapist or family members. Peer relations were characterized by excessive shyness, which in stressful situations often deteriorated into mutism. Both patients had one close friend of the same sex whom they described as very quiet.

Past History

The past histories of both adolescents included several similar features. Infantile colic and poor feeding followed by vomiting were among the early milestones. More recently, wide swings in weight and occasional periods of complete food refusal were noted. No difficulties in learning to talk were recalled.

In early childhood both youngsters had sustained a traumatic loss, either through divorce of the parents, or death of a parent. During latency, conscious feelings of depression and isolation were present and peer group relations were poor. No history was elicited of refusing to talk to peers, teachers, or families until adolescence. There were difficulties in separating from mother to attend school; this led to mild school phobic behavior. Both patients made an overt or secretive suicide attempt at some point prior to treatment. From latency onward each had had a great deal of age-inappropriate responsibility thrust upon her. This included complete responsibility for housework as well as rearing younger siblings.

Although depression and passive aggression were significant features in these cases, they are most accurately diagnosed as Hysterical Personality Disorder #301.5, according to DSM-II.

Case 1

Miss Z. is a 15-year-old, white, 10th grade student who was admitted to a psychiatric inpatient unit with a 9-month history of being bed-ridden in a succession of general hospitals because of hysterical ataxia following an appendectomy. The abdominal pain that led to the appendectomy was factitious. During those 9 months she was listless, apathetic, lost 25 pounds, because of food refusal, and declined to talk to anyone except for brief exchanges with her mother.

Past history. Except for colic and vomiting, birth and developmental landmarks, including speech development, were within normal limits until the age of 5, when her parents divorced. She began school at this time and had considerable difficulty separating from her mother. This led to mother's remaining with her in class for the first 6 months of school. Each year of elementary school she had an illness that necessitated her missing large blocks of time. At age 8, her parents remarried each other. She then developed "rheumatic fever." She told her therapist that she had often told the doctor she had joint pain when, in fact, she had none. She gained 30 pounds during this period and was started on appetite-depressant pills at age 9. She remained at 135 pounds until the appendectomy.

From the time of the divorce until her appendectomy, Miss Z. assumed major responsibility for the care of her siblings 2 and 3 years her junior. In addition, she did virtually all of the housecleaning and laundry. The family referred to her with pride as the "little mother."

Observations of the family. The parents were seen once a week, usually alone, but sometimes with Miss Z. The father was a 42-year-old shipping clerk who was prone to rage reactions that had a paranoid flavor. Each visitors' day at the hospital, father and Miss Z. greeted each other as if they were reuniting lovers. Their tight embrace ended with a pat on the behind from Mr. Z., although his daughter refused to favor him with speech.

Mrs. Z. appeared as a desperate, anxious, immature woman who had been very close to her daughter until the time of the appendectomy. When Mrs. Z. was angry at her husband, she refused to speak to him for weeks at a time.

The marital relationship was characterized by mutual hostility and disappointment. Mr. Z. was angered by Mrs. Z.'s frigidity. Mrs. Z. felt she could not turn to her husband for support in time of distress.

Both parents were angered at Miss Z.'s refusal to speak in family sessions. They used her silence to scapegoat her severely. Paradoxically, however, their anger increased to full-blown rage when she did begin to talk. When Miss Z. began to socialize with ward patients, her mother became very agitated and strenuously attempted to abort any of her efforts to develop peer relationships on the ward. Both parents attempted to denigrate and interrupt the relationship between the daughter and her therapist.

Individual treatment. Since Miss Z. was unable to talk, the therapist assumed this responsibility for her. She often began a session with a few cryptic comments, only to lapse into a tense silence. The therapist used her opening remarks as the theme of a sympathetic monologue he delivered for the rest of the session. The therapist interrupted his monologue from time to time to elicit a response from the patient. Early in treatment the patient responded only with silence or some nonverbal behavior such as a nod, a tear, or an expression of disgust or despair. Toward the end of treatment, it became possible to involve the patient in a dialogue for increasing periods of time. Eventually, the patient's opening remarks became more extensive until they began to last half of the session. However, her verbal flow would usually "dry up" in any given session, and the therapist would have to take over for the rest of the session. If she did talk for an entire session, she was completely silent the next session. "I always feel worse after I talk to you, so why should I? I know that talking will help me, but I don't feel that I deserve to be helped; that is why I don't talk more." Thus, her low self-esteem and the guilt she felt because of talking with her doctor became clearly delineated. Early in individual treatment the therapist interpreted this in terms of breaking unwritten family rules against relating to anyone outside of the family. Later, some of the oedipal implications were explored.

Any interruption of treatment caused by the therapist, such as a vacation, was followed by the patient's return to silence. Regardless of the content or character of a session she always became tearful and silent at its end. Thus, separation as an important precipitant of her silence could be discussed meaningfully with her.

Six weeks after admission, Miss Z. was walking, talking, eating, and socializing. She was discharged to the care of a psychiatrist in her hometown, but had to be readmitted 2 months later with a return of her silence and depressive affect.

Her second hospitalization lasted 6 months. She improved slowly over a 3-month period until the therapist took a vacation. From the moment he left, she made a dramatic improvement and on his return she immediately became silent again. This led to her verbalization of strong positive feelings for the therapist and the wish to maintain her illness to preserve that relationship. Thus, silence as a defense against positive feelings became clearly delineated for the patient. Guilt about positive feelings and the use of illness to maintain a close relationship were explored. This was partially resolved in therapy when the parents terminated treatment.

Six-month follow-up, made by telephone, yielded the information that the patient is in school and doing well at home.

Case 2

Miss F. is a 17-year-old, white, high school student. An only child, she lived at home with her widowed father. When she made 3 suicide attempts in rapid succession, Miss F. was admitted to the hospital after 9 months of twice-weekly psychotherapy. Her silence with the therapist was intractable and her depression deepened during the course of treatment.

Past history. When Miss F. was 12 years old, her mother died suddenly from a cerebral vascular accident. With her father and grandmother, who had lived together with Miss F., the family then moved into a maternal uncle's house. The patient had never been close to her father and, following the mother's death, the estrangement increased. When Miss F. was 15, she and her father moved out of the uncle's house into an apartment, leaving the grandmother with the uncle. Miss F. resented the move, but she was not consulted and raised no objections. Miss F. was given total responsibility for running the new household. Although she performed the cooking and cleaning without complaint, she and father rarely spoke to each other. They lived in a world of silence. They both had agreed that "there was nothing to say."

During this period, Miss F. had occasional dates. Her sense of loneliness and isolation would often intensify on these outings and she found herself with as little to say to her date as to her father.

Miss. F.'s earliest memories are of being forced to eat by her mother and grandmother. After this, she would self-induce vomiting. She was confined to her backyard during childhood and could play with children only if they came to visit her. When they did visit, Miss F. was unsure how to behave with them.

She made her first suicide attempt at age 9 in the school ladies room with a bottle of shoe polish. She reportedly took a small sip. She made several more suicide gestures between the ages of 9 and 15, but kept them a secret. She usually took only a few aspirins.

Family observations. The father is a small, thin, 50-year-old man, who appears chronically depressed. He works as a helper in a small grocery store, a job of which he is ashamed. When his wife was alive, he felt completely dominated by her and her mother. He felt it necessary to represent himself to his daughter as a man with no outside contacts aside from her. However, he had a small network of friends and relatives whom he visited regularly. He concealed these visits from Miss F.

During the family sessions, he pleaded with his daughter to speak with him and repeatedly lamented that he could only be happy if Miss F. could be happy. His pleas served to drive Miss F. deeper into her silence.

Individual treatment. Miss F. was seen 4 times a week as an inpatient for 30-minute sessions. She became tense, hostile, tearful, and silent after the 3rd session. She complained during that session. "There is nothing more to say, and besides you are not listening anyway." Although she listened carefully for the next several weeks of therapy as the therapist talked, she would only nod her head imperceptibly if pressed for a reply to a direct question. At the end of each session her eyes filled with tears. She complained to ward personnel that treatment made her feel worse. After 6 months of treatment the therapist was transferred to another institution. Although Miss F. was talking freely at this time, the only acknowledgment of separation feelings was the same tearful silence that had precipitated her admission.

Comparison with Childhood Elective Mutism

The syndrome of childhood elective mutism provides a useful frame of reference for a discussion of the dynamics and behavior of the two adolescents we have presented. For purposes of easy comparison we shall refer to our two cases as Adolescent Elective Mutism. Table 1 summarizes significant contrasts.

Table 1

	Childhood Elective Mutism	Adolescent Elective Mutism
Onset	Before age 6	After age 12
Partial Mutism	With peers, strangers, therapist	With family and therapist
Chief Complaint	Does not talk	Stealing, conversion reaction, suicide attempts
Dynamics	Preoedipal	Preoedipal, oedipal genitality

Childhood elective mutism is the selective refusal of a child to converse, for an extended period of time. Except for close intimates and members of their family these children are abnormally silent in all social contacts. The onset of the disorder occurs between 2 and 5 years of age. Browne et al. (1963) regarded trauma at the time of learning to speak as significant, while Pustrom and Speers (1964) saw the separation experience at kindergarten as a precipitating event. The problem of separating from mother was reflected in school refusal, excessive clinging behavior, and difficulty in leaving mother to accompany the therapist to treatment sessions. Elson et al. (1965) and Pustrom and Speers (1964) viewed the refusal to talk as a defense against the expression of hostile impulses. Elson et al. (1965) suggest that hostility is displaced to a third person outside of the family, thereby reducing anxiety over the hostile impulses. Elson et al. (1965) and Reed (1963) comment on the secondary gain of special attention that results from the silence.

There has been some study directed toward the families in which childhood mutism is found. Browne et al.(1963) found severe marital difficulties between the parents. Mother and the silent child in an excessively close and mutually dependent relationship formed a coalition against the father. Pustrom and Speers (1964) found that these children knew family secrets. The children had the impulse to reveal these secrets as an aggressive retaliation for the separation experience represented in beginning school. Since the price for revealing the family secrets might be total abandonment, the children solve the conflict with silence.

Zuk (1967) has reported on silence in schizophrenic patients who do not speak to their families. He views the index patients as having been silenced by the family in order to serve as an object for the family projections. The parents wish to prove to the patient that he needs the family. The patient may discover that by remaining silent he can reduce the family to a state of helpless agitation, and thus he can dominate and control them.

Dynamics of Silence
in the Two Adolescent Cases

The literature on childhood elective mutism emphasizes preoedipal factors such as dependency, separation, and anality as important determinants of partial mutism. In our adolescents, these factors remained central, but in addition the understanding of sexual conflict proved to be crucial in elucidating the etiology of the silence.

Each of our cases was an attractive middle adolescent female placed in a sexually overstimulating position vis-a-vis her father. The normal adolescent pattern of turning to heterosexual objects outside the family in order to defend against increased oedipal feelings was not available to either patient.

One reason this solution was not available was that neither patient had adequately worked through the preoedipal problems of mother-child separation-individuation (Mahler, 1963). Both of our patients had had overprotective mothers, suffered significant object losses, and had displayed school phobic behavior. Blos (1967) has discussed the significance of separation-individuation in adolescence. However, there is another sense in which separation is a problem for these adolescents: it was as if the entire family had agreed that there could be no significant relationships with anyone outside of the family (Haley,

1959). Mrs. Z.'s frantic efforts to prevent her daughter from speaking with other patients on the ward and Mr. F.'s attempt to conceal from his daughter his visits with other people illustrate how the family operated as though there were a law forbidding them to associate with people outside of the family.

A normal defense that adolescent girls use to manage positive oedipal feelings is anger and derogation of the parent of the opposite sex in order to maintain psychological distance. This defense was difficult for our two youngsters to use, since there was a strong family prohibition against the expression of anger toward father.

Silence solved the problem of separation, the problem of the prohibition against the expression of anger, and the problem of excess stimulation of sexual feelings toward the parent of the opposite sex. The adolescent could remain in the family, but deny her entrapment by not talking. She could leave the family, but deny her separation from them by not talking with her peers. She could both deny to herself and to other members of the family any feelings of anger toward them. At the same time she could provoke them into angry tirades toward her because of her silence. Anger on the father's part would make the threat of sexuality easier to tolerate because it made for greater psychological distance between them.

Similarly, the patient's silence partially solved these same problems for the family. As long as the patient was silent, the family rules against separation, and against the expression of anger and sexuality, could be maintained to some degree. Furthermore, the patient provided the family with a scapegoat. When the patient began to speak, however, the threat of breaking one or more of these rules became imminent. The parents' paradoxical increase in anger and disorganization as the patient began to improve may be understood in terms of this threat.

Identification is important in the choice of silence as a symptom. In both of our cases one parent intermittently used prolonged silence as a significant part of his or her interpersonal repertoire. A dramatic illustration of the importance of identification as a determinant in the patients' use of silence occurred in the first case. Infuriated over her daughter's silence, Miss Z.'s mother frequently threatened to cease speaking to the therapist until her daughter began to speak to her.

Recommendation for Treatment

Except for diagnostic interviews early in treatment, it is best to exclude the silent adolescent from family sessions. The provocative quality of the patient's silence provides an excellent target for scapegoating. Seeing the patient and family separately tends to make concrete the psychological problem of separation for the family and the index patients. When both the patient and the family have reached a stage of readiness to relinquish the restraining relationships that have bound them so closely together, the patient can then be reintroduced.

In individual therapy the initial tactics of the therapist are predicated on the thesis that the central issue with the silent adolescent is separation, i.e., both intrapsychic separation anxiety based on the infantile fear of the loss of the mother and the family rule against having significant relationships outside the family.

Both girls attempted to structure the therapeutic situation around the issue: is the therapist clever enough or seductive enough to induce her to talk? If the therapist accepted this definition of treatment, the patient would defeat him, and remain silent. However, if the central issue for the therapist is separation, speech is no longer the central focus of treatment. Instead, the problem becomes one of establishing a relationship with the adolescent. The patient's first step in negotiating separation from the family is to establish a relationship with a therapist. For this crucial step to occur, the patient does not have to talk.

Instead, the therapist must talk for the patients when they are silent. One could assert that the therapist should remain silent and wait for an indeterminate time until the patient's mounting anxiety propels her to speak. There are several reasons against this strategy. The first is that these patients had amply demonstrated an apparently limitless capacity to tolerate silence by their lengthy periods of mutism prior to treatment. Furthermore, if the therapist remains silent, the patients are provided with an opportunity to assign whatever meaning they wish to the therapist's silence. With an adult neurotic patient who is talking, this opportunity might be considered a necessary condition of therapy. However, with our silent adolescents, whatever meaning they might assign to the silence is not amenable to reality testing or interpretation, since the meaning is not verbalized. Also, it seems to us that there is an element of countertransference acting out in a therapist's remaining silent in this situation—a wish to do to the patient what she is doing to the therapist.

The therapist's comfortable, sympathetic acceptance of the patient's silence without angry accusations is a relief for the patient. The therapist may give her explicit permission to be silent. Although our two adolescent patients did not talk, they were perceptive listeners. Much of the therapy time was occupied by long monologues delivered by the therapist. These monologues consisted of one-sided discussions of what the therapist considered to be the central dynamic issue at the time. The patients were quite content to allow the therapist to speak endlessly about issues which were of no concern to them. Hospitalization and family therapy diminish the possibility that the therapist will too often be off-target in his monologues. He knows the events that are of concern to the patient. The therapist asked frequent questions. When the patient refused to answer, the therapist, in effect, offered a list of possible answers from which the patient could choose.

Shorter (30-minute) but more frequent sessions (3 to 5 times per week) were found to be preferable to longer sessions in which the tension that developed could become unbearable for both patient and therapist.

The therapist who talks for the patient must be aware of the potential risks for extremes of dependency and infantilization that may arise in such a situation. Initially, the therapist removed the responsibility of speech from the patient. As the work went on, he periodically encouraged speech and induced discomfort in the patient because of her silence. This tended to set limits to the dependency that developed, and provided the patient with an opportunity to talk which she used when she was ready.

As the adolescent began to talk in treatment, the therapist was careful not to overvalue the patient's speech. Speech was accepted in the same sympathetic manner as the silence.

The silent adolescent may seem hostile and disappointed with treatment. Yet, the transference is usually positive, although she will be careful to conceal this from the therapist. After one in a long series of silent interviews with Miss Z., in which all she offered was apparently hostile, continuous, disappointed silence, she returned to her hospital room, flopped on her bed, and was heard to sigh, "Oh, I love him!" The remark was assumed to refer to the therapist.

As in any therapy, countertransference may be a problem. The silent patient can stimulate fantasies with the same facility as the silent therapist. The anger these youngsters evoke was reflected by a tendency on the part of some members of the hospital staff to diagnose them as schizophrenic. The therapist was not immune to anger and it may have led him to be somewhat defensively overprotective and excessively gentle in interpretation. The patients tested the therapist's sense of therapeutic competence. The therapist, the hospital staff, the parents, and the patient may collude in the belief that it is the psychiatrist's task to get people to talk. When this does not occur, all may be prone to a sense of failure. The ensuing anger and the challenge to the therapist's sense of competence can lead to the development of guilt in the therapist. This can take the form of either excessive inhibition on the one hand, or a countertransference-provoked attack on the other. The central guideline in treating these cases was a firm commitment to understanding the patient rather than simply to induce speech.

Summary and Conclusions

Two case histories of adolescent females who had not spoken to their families for 1 to 3 years prior to treatment are presented. With the initiation of psychotherapy at the time of psychiatric hospitalization, they maintained their silence with their families and with their therapists.

The major dynamics of our patients were separation, a prohibition against the expression of anger from adolescent to parent, and a sexually stimulating relationship between adolescent patient and father. The patient's separation anxiety along with an implicit family rule forbidding social relationships outside of the family made it insurmountably difficult for these adolescents to utilize the adaptive defense of turning to heterosexual objects outside of the family. This intensified the anxiety-provoking closeness between father and adolescent daughter. With silence the adolescent could both remain in the family, but deny her entrapment, and leave the family, but deny her separation. he could deny any angry feelings on her part both to herself and to other family members; but she was able to provoke angry tirades from them because of her silence. The father's anger made the threat of sexuality easier to tolerate because of the psychological distance the anger created between father and daughter.

In individual treatment, the initial task of the therapist was to shift the focus of therapy from the patient's silence to the issue of separation. This was accomplished by the therapist speaking for the patient when she was silent. Explicit permission to be silent was given. The therapist offered a wide variety of answers to his own questions, from which the patient could indicate her choice nonverbally. The hazards of this approach to treatment are discussed and some of the countertransference issues that arose are considered.

In family therapy, the embittered attacks to the patient's silence evoked from the parents necessitated working with the parents and adolescent separately for a period of time before they could meet together productively.

Children Who Cheat at Games

JOHN E. MEEKS, M.D

Cheating in games is something that occurs in the psychother-apy of many children. Meek's study of this phenomenon also underscores a basic cornerstone of child psychotherapy: What occurs in the session between the child and therapist must be viewed not only as a phenomenon of the manifest relationship but also from the perspective of what its latent motivational content reveals about that youngster.

In the illustrative paper that follows, cheating expresses an extreme intolerance to losing (anxiety), an incapacity to work in order to increase skill level (reality distortion), a poor sense of self-esteem, and an impotent feeling of inherent inability. In other words, persistent cheating reflects difficulty in the phase-specific development tasks of the latency period, specifically, a capacity to work, a lessening need for magical thinking, and the develop-ing capacity for the internalization of social values.

Youngsters are usually only vaguely, if at all, aware of such matters and often strenuously avoid confrontation with such knowledge. An adult's usual spontaneous reaction toward a child who cheats is an educative response, communicating to the child in a variety of ways that cheating is undesirable, reiterating the rules and stressing the advantages to all of adhering to them. The article that follows, focusing on psychotherapy, does not address itself to the range of responses which parents, teachers, counselors, and peers may have to cheating behavior. Even for those youngsters in psychotherapy, it is our opinion that the outside world should support the reality principle in a firm and unambivalent manner. Despite those events in the adult world that lead children to question the reliability of the adage that "cheaters never win," cheating should not be overlooked or condoned and its potential unpleasant consequences should not be ignored. This goes beyond issues of fairness and morality which are important in and of themselves; it also supports the youngster's developing abilities to do well without needing to cheat.

Meek's paper, on the other hand, focuses on cheating in exploratory psychotherapy. In consequent, he suggests that cheating be allowed to develop and unfold in the therapeutic situation preparatory to gently confronting the child with the fact of his cheating, the uncontrollable urge and need to cheat, and what this reflects about the youngster's view of himself. This stems from the principle that exploratory psychotherapy involves the unfolding of maladaptive behavior in such a way that the youngster tells us in action what he cannot yet communicate in words. Whether a child plays an age-appropriate game or reverts to one more appropriate for younger children, whether he regresses from a game which requires skill, such as checkers, in favor of a game based entirely on chance, whether he tells a story, makes up a puppet play, or draws a series of pictures—these are all the raw materials of psychotherapy. What the therapist does with this grist is the essence of the process. He may reflect an affect. He may point out the self-defeating role of the defense. He may enunciate an unexpressed wish. He may encourage latent skill development utilizing capacities unrealized by the youngster. He may reflect the realistic consequences of specific behaviors. But whatever he chooses to do with the material it should be determined by the short- and long-term goals of the treatment with that particular patient.

The role of food (Haworth and Keller, 1962), gifts (Levin and Wermer, 1966), and/or games like checkers (Loomis, 1957) are some of the common ingredients of psychotherapy which have been discussed in the literature. The manifold dynamic meaning may be explicitly stated in the therapy, may be communicated nonverbally with or without later interpretation, or simply left unspoken as the therapist uses the knowledge as a basis for other therapeutic interventions. Other common elements that have been addressed in the literature are silence (see the previous selections in this volume), configurations, language usage, and the use of body language and other nonverbal forms of communication. Therapists are interested not only in the content of the fantasy, the drama, the play, but also the form it takes and the style used. Why does this child utilize the distortion form of cheating rather than lying? What is the youngster telling us when the form of his building changes from flat, heavy, bomb shelters to complicated, elaborately decorated, upright structures in which people enjoy a constructive life? The paper that follows focuses on some of these issues by means of a detailed study of one style of playing in therapy.

Peller (1954), in her classical paper on the meaning of play, clearly ties the preference for playing organized games to the latency of development. She states, "Strict rules are the backbone of games, and the players recognize them as absolute for the duration of the game. Their meticulous observation gives independence from external superego figures." The developmental thrust behind the interest in such games is, then, the reduction of oedipal preoccupations and the learning of techniques for group cooperation and competition according to specified rules, roles and limitations. This is the first step in the development of autonomous personality functioning within the confines of prescribed social roles, a task which will reappear throughout latency and adolescence in increasingly complex re-editions which

Reprinted from *Journal of the American Academy of Child Psychiatry*, Vol. 9 (1970), pp. 157-170.

gradually approximate the requirements and possibilities of the adult society. Peller contrasts this latency play with that observed during the oedipal period, in which idiosyncratic fantasy and magical elements predominate. She states that the goal of the oedipal play is to deny that the child cannot enjoy those things which adults enjoy. Oedipal play, therefore, is more fanciful, charming, and unrealistic because of the child's imaginative efforts to pretend that he is adult. Peller also notes, "The mood pervading oedipal play is usually one of happiness, even of triumph, of a naive invincibility."

The different dynamics involved in the organized games of latency may account for the somewhat different mood which often accompanies these games. Latency children, rather than demonstrating a sense of "naive invicibility," often show a serious, doubtful, and almost strained approach to the competitive games which they enjoy and prefer. The competitive nature of the game implies, for healthy children, that they should attempt to improve their skill and attempt to win. This, too, is in contrast to oedipal play, in which victory is merely a state of mind achieved by a wish.

Since this type of play is characteristic of the latency child, it is not surprising that in child psychotherapy sessions, youngsters in this age range often wish to occupy themselves with checkers, chess, card playing, or other games typically enjoyed by this age group. The reluctance of these youngsters to enter into the more imaginative and fanciful play characteristic of younger ages leads many therapists to feel that they are not interesting in treatment, and that they are more defended than is the oedipal child. This is an unfortunate state of affairs, since in many clinics the peak ages of patient referral fall in the latency range. Therefore, we are called upon to treat large mumbers of children who are considered by some therapists as less interesting and more difficult to reach.

Loomis (1957) has pointed out the value of checker games in "disclosing the presence of resistances, aiding in analyzing them, and helping to discover their inner meaning." His paper is one of the few which discuss the value of utilizing structure games in therapy. His delightful brief communication suggests that working around a game need not be dull or unproductive.

The Cheating Syndrome

Many latency age children seen in psychotherapy, however, do not show the acceptance of game rules typically demonstrated by their age group. In fact, many of them cheat at games. Often the diagnostic information collected from the parents includes references to the child's inability to lose at a game, perhaps accompanied by observations that the youngster often cheats to avoid defeat. At times the parents state that this behavior appears only with siblings or close friends of the same age. This history seems to be more common in youngsters who are having school difficulties, especially in the area of academic learning.

Typically, cheating at games appears in psychotherapy only after the child has become moderately comfortable in the therapeutic relationship. If such behavior is not interrupted, cheating becomes more and more frequent, and the child establishes a pattern of beating the therapist at every game. This behavior is often accompanied by high-spirited, gay bragging, which may become quite arrogant and at times even belligerent. The child often behaves as though he had no inkling of the therapist's awareness of his cheating, even when the cheating has been quite gross and apparent. The child seems to regard himself as having legitimately proved his superiority to the therapist, and may become quite condescending and belittling in his attitude.

If this behavior is permitted to reach its peak, there is often a remarkable response when the child is confronted with the fact that his victories are based on cheating. The child typically becomes quite angry, often accuses the therapist of being the one mistreated.

These observations suggest that cheating at games, at least in a psychotherapeutic relationship, has strong emotional roots which may be useful in the therapeutic understanding of the child. The strong feelings which accompany these activities, the interpersonal intensity between therapist and child, and the response to confrontation suggest that cheating at games is a "transference" behavior or, to use Erikson's classification (1940), represents an example of "macrocosmic play." In other words, the child is utilizing the therapist as an important object that facilitates externalization of an intrapsychic conflict. It is this conception of the meaning of cheating that suggests that the therapist should permit full elaboration of the cheating process before actively intervening. Early prohibitions against cheating tend to force the child to manage his wish to cheat entirely by superficial conformity. The underlying fantasies and meanings are then lost to understanding.

Cheating and the Reality Sense

Cheating represents an inability to accept the formalized and ritualized structure of the game. Organized games are structured to provide open competition within a mutually acceptable framework. This permits a high level of friendliness to exist concurrently with overt competitive attitudes.

If the game depends on skill, the rules control the conditions of rivalry and the best man is to win. If necessary, a handicap may be given to equalize the competition. If the game depends purely on luck, each player must accept his fate as determined purely by chance.

Paul Morphy, the chess genius (Jones, 1931), said that the game "should be received in a friendly manner; that it should be ascribed to worthy motives; and that it should be regarded as a serious and grown-up activity." This describes well the general attitude of the latency child toward an organized game. It is very upsetting to a youngster if his opponent in the game is "not trying" of if he demonstrates unsportsmanlike behavior in response to loss, thus suggesting that the game was not friendly.

Of course, children often see their "gentlemen's agreement" to abide by the rules dissolve in a rising flood of accusations of cheating which may mount to a tide of unstructured hostility. Sublimation may fail entirely, as when checkers are angrily launched as very personal missiles rather than being utilized as proxy warriors on the traditional and regulated checkerboard battleground. The effect, of course, is to end the game. Latency children will not continue to play with a child who consistently is unable to stay within the structure and "play fair" without "losing his temper." The latency attitude toward ritualized combat can occur only with successful resolution of the oedipal conflict. The striking feature of the behavior in children who cheat is that it retains the magical and destructive competitive attitudes which characterize the oedipal child. The child who cheats is demonstrating motives which are clearly unworthy: he cannot be seen as friendly toward his opponent, and his attitude toward the game is neither serious nor grown-up.

The persistence of oedipal conflicts may account for the attitude of gleeful invincibility which the cheating youngster often demonstrates toward his unfairly defeated competitor. The resultant anxiety and guilt over magical, destructive fantasies may be one factor at work in producing another observable feature of the cheating pattern, namely, that the child often shows self-defeating behavior in games and may actually, at times, even cheat against himself. There are other reasons why "cheaters never win" (or win only erratically); these relate to the chronic erosion of ego skills, which may result from a prolonged reliance on cheating.

The acceptance of irrefutable and irresistible laws of reality is an essential precondition to successful adjustment to that reality. This is especially important in the area of learning, as George Gardner (1966) and Plank and Plank (1954) have emphasized. In other words, if one does not admit the existence of an objective reality, unaffected by one's wishes, skills in dealing with that reality are unlikely to develop. An acceptance of the general laws of chance are also necessary to good reality adjustment. If magical thinking prevails, the child continually makes decisions which oppose the odds in a given situation. For example, in a Monopoly game, such a child will continually sink all his money in a few properties, ignoring the likely possibility that he will be caught short before his investment can pay off. He may continually neglect doing homework, relying on the slim chance that the lapse will not be detected. Of course, youngsters with this view often resort to cheating in order to escape the blind finality of chance.

Superficial observation of the cheating syndrome might suggest that it represents merely a carry-over of the omnipotent attitude toward competition characteristic of the oedipal child. However, this would not account for the fact that children who cheat are well aware of the rules and of the fact that they are cheating. They do not, as the oedipal child does, simply remain unaware of reality restrictions and limitations, but admit them to awareness and then rebel against them under certain circumstances. After all, one has to know the rules in order to break them to one's advantage.

Of course, some children do not appear even to acknowledge the rules. This pattern commonly is observed in youngsters with strong symbiotic ties to a parent whom they regard as omnipotent. This implies strong preoedipal fixation points. They seem to be truly unconcerned with the rules of games, and often show no interest in even learning how to play properly. A child of this type may, for example, make random moves which are totally divorced from any game pattern, and simply announce after a series of such moves that he has won the game. This demonstrates a more primitive attitude toward reality, quite different in its dynamic implications from the more typical cheating described above. It is a pattern often observed in borderline psychotic youngsters and in those with severe impulse disorders.

We can return now to consider one other feature of the youngster who cheats, namely, his inability to accept losing without a severe drop in self-esteem. It would appear that youngsters of this kind can feel satisfied with themselves only when they can maintain a fantasy of omnipotence. This observation suggests an underlying sense of inadequacy arising from unfavorable oedipal comparisons and a regressive identification with the omnipotent parent fantasied at an earlier stage of development. They can only visualize two alternative positions, either omnipotent control over all situations or total helplessness. This conflict can often be observed in their academic efforts, where they often pretend to possess knowledge that they do not have and approach areas of new learning with anxiety and avoidance techniques. It may be that cheating for these children represents a compromise between their emotional need to be omnipotent and their growing recognition of reality limitations. Only by cheating can they venture into true competition, keeping their anxieties at a manageable level by holding the possibility of cheating in reserve. The attitude might be paraphrased as follows, "I will cautiously explore the possibility that I can deal adequately with competition within reality, but if things become too frightening I can always resort to magic. I can cheat." Perhaps it is only in this way that the child can permit himself to become aware of the constrictions of reality at all.

Unfortunately, this developmental compromise or transitional phase tends to be self-perpetuating. As mentioned above, the remnants of magical destructiveness which persist at a fantasy level tend to produce guilt with consequent self-punitive and self-defeating behaviors. In addition to these dynamic reasons for losing, there is a loss in the opportunity for development of cognitive skills. To take chess playing as an example, it is impossible to develop a wide range of strategic possibilities if one is not clearly aware of the rules and limitations regarding the possible movement of the pieces. If there is a possibility for resorting to magical solutions, solutions in reality are not actively sought and learning and skill do not progress. The end result is that the child tends gradually to become truly inept and inadequate in comparison with other children who have made this effort. Magical solutions must be sought with greater frequency and the tendency to avoid confrontation with realistic problems increases. Regression is sure to occur since phase-appropriate success is rendered impossible by the child's maladaptive defenses against possible loss of self-esteem.

Therapeutic Management of Cheating

The therapeutic aim in dealing with cheating at games is to increase the child's acceptance of his real capacities and limitations. This goal requires the therapist to deal tactfully with several aspects of the syndrome of cheating: (1) the child's fragile mechanism for maintenance of self-esteem; (2) the child's magical interpretation of successful performance, both in the therapist and himself; (3) the self-defeating characteristics of a reliance on cheating.

Because these children have a marked narcissistic vulnerability, it is impossible to approach the cheating behavior until the therapist is viewed by the child as a reliable source of narcissistic supplies. This implies an understanding of the permissive atmosphere of psychotherapy, so that the child sees the therapist as noncritical and nonjudgmental in his approach. The child will often signal his readiness to explore his cheating behavior by expressing some feelings of guilt, a sense of his unfairness, or by questioning why the therapist permits him to cheat without correcting the behavior. In some youngsters it may be necessary, paradoxically, to encourage them to go ahead and express their impulses to cheat. These situations arise when the child is obviously feeling a strong wish to cheat, but is strongly bound to acceptable social behavior while in the presence of an adult. This is analogous to encouraging a younger child to "go ahead and pretend' or encouraging free association in the adult.

Full development of the cheating syndrome permits direct observation of the child's magically oriented fantasy life, a view which the latency youngster may otherwise attempt to conceal from his therapist. These children may not discuss the omnipotent daydreams which occupy them in the classroom and usually deny their humiliation because of their failure to learn, but the same issues are clearly demonstrated within the therapy relationship by their cheating. They may be unwilling to discuss their deceitfulness at home and school, their petty stealing and other techniques to avoid awareness of reality demands, but they cannot avoid awareness of what they reveal in their play.

In order to expand this dim awareness, extreme tact and careful management are necessary. This management must include realistic praise and acceptance of the child's adpative skills and capabilities at playing games. Children with problems of this kind need to have their good moves recognized and their increments in skill played up to a maximum only barely short of flattery. Since their performance falls so far short of their omnipotent expectations, the youngsters are often unable even to recognize, much less accept, the approved, gradual improvements in their performance.

The therapist can also be helpful by clearly conveying his own stable self-esteem, even in the face of repeated defeats. Children often test this area by making derogatory comments regarding the therapist's failures to win, with aspersions on his intelligence and his general worth as a human being. If the therapist responds only by inquiring if it makes the child feel stupid and worthless when he loses at games, therapeutic gains may be encouraged. It goes without saying that these youngsters should be permitted to win some games when they play fair, even if they play rather poorly.

The management of the child's projection of omnipotence onto the therapist is also clearly related to this issue. Many of these youngsters have no real conception of why the therapist is more skillful at most games than they are. The concept that the therapist's expertise is related to learning and experience is alien to their world view, or at least poorly grasped within it. They tend to believe, at least at an unconscious level, that the therapist's skills represent magic endowments and are without limitations. In addition to clarifying these matters at a factual level, it is sometimes useful for the therapist to recall his early ineptitude at the game in an attempt to convey the learned nature of his ability. At times it is also useful to place the therapist's relative skill in perspective, especially in regard to games such as checkers and chess, where a combination of intelligence and serious application can lead to a level of skill much greater than the therapist's. In addition to these approaches, it is, of course, important to recognize evidences of magical thinking when they occur in overt form. As Buxbaum (1954) said of her goals with a cheating girl patient, "She had to learn self-control, to work instead of cheating, to go to school instead of truanting, to dress and work instead of running around like a ragamuffin." In short, these patients need to accept the idea that achievement is based on patient effort which gradually leads to improved performance, and not on a wishfulfilling, magical attitude toward the environment. Naturally, in order to adopt this point of view, the child's belief in his capacity to perform adequately must be strengthened.

The final technique in dealing with cheating, as it represents a commitment to unreality, is to make it ego alien by clarifying its futility. Obviously the approaches described above lay the groundwork for this final step, since the child must be given extensive help before he can be expected to consider relinquishing a major defensive position. Once this groundwork has been laid, the therapist can begin to point out that the child is following a "no-win" policy, since victory achieved by cheating can never be a source of legitimate pride. The child can be reminded that even when his cheating is not detected by others, there is an inner awareness that the victory was not real, so that he will always doubt his own capacities. Children can often come to see how they are thus cheating themselves, especially if the therapist is generous with his encouragement and support of their capacity to win by fair means.

Of course, the presence of guilt and anxiety leading to self-defeating behavior of a more direct type must also be recognized and interpreted in the course of treatment.

Unfortunately, any attempt to formulate therapeutic strategies cannot adequately deal with the problems of timing, appropriate wording, and emotional tone which are at the heart of any successful therapeutic approach. The intent in offering these suggestions for therapeutic management is not to provide a stereotyped approach to an isolated problem, but attempts to conceptualize dynamic forces involved in a common form of clinical interaction. This conceptual skeleton must be filled out with the living flesh of personal skill and therapeutic sensitivity. It is also beyond the scope of the paper to discuss the parental attitudes and behavior which may have produced or aggravated the leaning toward unreality (Meeks, 1968; Millar, 1968). Often progress can be made only with collaborative, family-oriented therapy.

Case Report

Charles, the oldest of three brothers, was referred at age 9 because of poor school performance and general immaturity. His professional parents stated that he was preoccupied with fantasy, mostly involving war and other forms of violence. His IQ was bright average (Full Scale 116) without significant scatter, and there was no evidence of neurological dysfunction. Despite his intellectual potential, he was a full grade behind the national averages on an achievement test. The psychologist said of Charles, "He seemed anxious in the testing situation, but he handled this by attempts at humor. He was not task-oriented, and his motivation was not always optimal. He seemed more concerned with the reaction of the examiner than goal-directed behavior. He had a tendency to try to redefine the situation so as to make himself more comfortable rather than to follow directions."

There were no significant behavioral problems in school or at home. A high level of sexual curiosity had been noted since his mother's pregnancy with his younger brother. He continued to ask many sexual questions, especially of his mother, at the time of referral.

The father was in the early stages of professional training at the time of Charles' unplanned and unwanted conception. The presence of a child produced major economic difficulties for the parents. The mother returned to work when Charles was 6 weeks of age. She continued to work until he was 6 years old. He was cared for at the home of a kindly lady who kept several youngsters. The parents noted that she was good to Charles, but could offer him very little individual attention.

Charles was reportedly weaned from the bottle at 6 months and was toilet trained prior to 2 years of age. However, the parents moved to another city when Charles was 2 and left him with his grandmother during the move. When they came for him after a week with the maternal grandmother, he was back on the bottle and in diapers. The parents felt that the grandmother "didn't like to cross him" and said that it took Charles several weeks to "come around."

Charles's relationship with his two younger brothers was pleasant except for the normal amount of arguing. He was said to get along well with other children except that he tended to "give in" to them. Though he enjoyed sports, he refused to join any organized team. He once told the parents, "They wouldn't even let me on *my* team." The parents felt this was an unrealistic appraisal, since Charles was actually moderately adept in athletics. His father felt Charles avoided overt competition in any form.

Therapy

Weekly psychotherapy sessions were scheduled. Initially, Charles regaled the therapist with the adventures of his "gang." These clearly fanciful forays were always directed against the gang's mortal enemies, little girls. He swore me to secrecy, since he said his mother would kill him if she knew about the gang's attacks on lemonade stands, tea parties, and other sinister female gatherings. He assured me that he hated girls. After a few sessions I agreed that boys his age did dislike girls in many ways, but suggested that most boys were also very interested in girls and women. Charles vehemently denied this. His father reported that following this interview, Charles' sexual curiosity became insatiable. At this point, however, his questions were directed to the father rather than to the mother. At school his teacher was surprised to find Charles circulating a crude picture he had drawn of all his classmates in the nude. The boys and girls alike wore prominent and substantial penises!

In therapy Charles dropped the tales of raids on the girls. He became very passive, talked little, and insisted that I decide what he should do during his sessions. When I suggested that Charles could do what he wished, he said, "Okay, let's go blow up the school." He became reluctant to come to the sessions and sometimes "lost his way" coming to the playroom and was late. He told his father that he did not like coming to therapy any longer. The father encouraged him to discuss this with me.

Finally Charles was able to discuss some of his negative feelings about me. When I recognized and accepted his anger and anxiety, he entered the "game playing" phase of his therapy.

He was openly competitive. He would "murder" me. I would wish I "had never seen a checker!" In a poker game he would "win the shirt off your back." "You'll go out of here in a barrel," he warned.

When he was near losing, Charles would cheat. A mischievous grin would appear and he would jump off the checker board, back on again and then backward, accomplishing a triple jump that turned the tide of the game in his favor. After winning he would taunt me and chant, "Ya, ya, ya, ya, ya."

After this went on for some weeks, I commented that winning seemed very important to Charles. In a tone of mock solemnity, Charles said, "If I lose, my father will kill me." Later he stated that his father had told him, "It's not how you play the game that counts, it's whether you win or lose."

This was certainly Charles' credo. In card games he switched the cards he did not want. In darts he hand-carried the missiles to the bull's eye whenever he needed points. Needless to say, he won all the games. He also continued to be a very bad winner, gloating and reviling me. His parents reported that he was now eager to come to his sessions and was beginning to show an interest in doing his homework. However, his previous attitude toward his brothers disappeared. He was very aggressive toward them and was especially critical of their "baby" behavior.

Abruptly he dropped his interest in games and wanted to exchange ghost stories during his sessions. He insisted that I take turns spinning the scary yarns. I chose "ghost" stories which turned out to have reality explanations. Charles told stories of people brutalized and killed by malevolent supernatural forces which could not be resisted. The victims in his stories were always brave, daring boys! I commented that Charles seemed to think that brave boys who tried to show how well they could do things would be hurt or killed. He replied, "How did you ever guess?" His tone suggested that it was about time I caught on.

He began the next session by drawing an aviator falling from his plane, which had been shot down by an enemy. Without commenting, I added a parachute and had the aviator shout, "Help," in a cartoon balloon. Charles drew another falling flyer, again *without* a parachute. He had this one point to the other flyer and comment, "And *he's* shouting *help?*" I commented that Charles felt like the guy without a parachute. A further suggestion was offered that Charles cheated at games because he felt he did not have the equipment to win fairly. I said firmly that Charles had it, but was afraid to use it, just as he was afraid to take a chance at school. Charles listened quietly, then asked, "You really believe that?" Cheating appeared periodically, usually accompanied by "clowning," in later sessions, but became increasingly rare.

His favorite game for several weeks involved an argument about what "me" spelled. He would show me the word and ask what it spelled. I would say, "Me." No," Charles would argue, looking at the paper, "it doesn't say 'you,' it says 'me.'" The game would at times be elaborated by forcing me to agree at gunpoint that Charles was right.

Later Charles would manage to get the gun into my hand and then hasten to capitulate, pleading for mercy and promising never to argue again. This would go on and on, with first one, then the other in control.

I commented that Charles really could not be satisfied either way. He did not like to be wrong, but he did not like for me to be wrong either. I suggested to Charles that we were both right and simply had our own points of view. Charles accepted this eagerly. I also suggested that this situation might also prevail with his teachers. Maybe they were really on the same side, but had somewhat different viewpoints in regard to homework. Charles was not so eager to accept this, but he did admit reluctantly that he had decided school was not as bad as he had thought. Actually his school performance was gradually improving during this period. At this time Charles returned to checkers, which he insisted on playing at least once each session until termination. He became interested in learning to play more skillfully. He did not cheat, but would often pretend that he was going to do so, recalling, "Remember how I cheated before?" He was very pleased that he was able to beat his father at times. Defeat remained hard to bear, but was tolerable to Charles. I was actively supportive, saying that when two good players tangled, you could never be sure who would win.

Discussion

Charles' developmental history and later playroom behavior suggest several reasons why he tended to rely excessively on omnipotent fantasy in dealing with reality. The early separation from his mother accompanied by a strong push for precocious independence did not permit the gradual emergence of a sense of mastery based on realistic ego skills. To avoid massive anxiety, he had to "fake it," pretending he could master any situation and avoiding those which might reveal his vulnerability.

His belief in the omnipotence of thought, however, was a two-edged sword. It made it impossible to resolve his oedipal feelings. His death wishes and sexual fantasies were all too real. He had to convince himself that he hated females or that women did not actually differ from males. His projected hostility made his father a frightening figure despite his actually gentle and kindly characteristics.

Therapy gave Charles the opportunity to re-experience some of his competitive anger within the framework of games. Through the management of his cheating, he came to recognize the safety and feasibility of depending on himself rather than on magic.

Summary

A pattern of behavior frequently observed in latency-age chidren, especially those with learning problems, involving a tendency to cheat at organized games, appears to be related to a compromise between efforts to compete realistically and unrealistic wishes for omnipotent control. The dynamics of the cheating behavior are related to a wish for a more mature behavioral pattern which can be attempted only if the child can reassure himself that he can return to a reliance on magical devices when he is faced with personal inadequacy. The end result of such a transitional state is to perpetuate a weakened sense and to interfere with the development of coping abilities. Therapeutic intervention should aim at bolstering realistic self-esteem, clarifying the futility of magical thinking, and encouraging a reliance on personal growth and the gradual emergence of ego skills.

Books in the Playroom: A Dimension of Child Psychiatric Technique

CARMEN R. GOLDINGS, M.D.

HERBERT J. GOLDINGS, M.D.

Since psychotherapy often occurs in rooms designed specifically for therapy with children, it is noteworthy how little has been written on the layout and content of such space. Lowenfeld's (1935) and Axline's (1947, 1969) descriptions relate primarily to school-type situations, and Beiser's (1955) and Scott's (1961) descriptions of rooms and materials for psychotherapy impress many as describing more elaborate layouts than most seen, used, or discussed. Many practitioners and teachers seem to be of the opinion that the equipment necessary need not be ornate or voluminous. In general the less structured the toys and materials, the greater the opportunity for the child to creatively express fantasy.

In the paper that follows, Goldings and Goldings discuss a particular type of equipment in the playroom which is usually not there because it is typically not considered suitable to psychotherapy, namely, the book. Often books may be seen as providers of fantasy and utilized in a defensive manner to restrict the coming to consciousness of one's own fantasy. Or, they may be used to convey information and avoid discussions as in the classical example of the parent giving a child a book about sex rather than offering to answer questions or having a discussion about it face to face. However, as we will be seeing in the following paper, books can be used creatively in the playroom to test the ability to read, to reveal the defenses and reactions to a disclosure of one's inability to read, to provide structure, as a source of information, and as a tool for mastery. That a child or adolescent may bring a book to read during the hour as a demonstration of resistance is a common experience, but as we all know any material can be used either for expression or containment. The authors illustrate the truism that a variety of materials can be utilized by the patient and therapist as a way to begin and sustain communication. They stress the importance for the therapist of having ideas about what it is that he hopes to achieve by the use of a book as opposed to some other play materials, which of course entails a need for familiarity with all items in the playroom.

There is a psychotherapeutic approach called bibliotherapy which stems primarily from the librarians of children's collections and attempts to match the child in need with a helpful book. The premise that certain emotional or practical or life experience problems which are worked through in the story, whether fiction or biography, opens a wider arena of options to the youngster to cope with a situation. There is no doubt that books have successfully contributed to the development in the lives of many youngsters, but we as therapists rarely hear about such cases. It is probably the normal problems and strains of growing up which respond to a variety of solutions provided by the "good enough" (Winnicott) parents and school.

Many examples could be cited from outside the usual range of experience, such as the toddler who utilized read-out-loud books as a controlled way to deal with extended debilitating illness threatening the life of her mother. The mere familiarity this little girl had with the book and its story allowed anticipation of what was coming next. Turning the pages controlled the rate of input, and of course she could always stop the reading and continue later. All of this contributed to some sense of mastery in an overwhelming traumatic situation in which no other recourse was available to her.

One of the authors of the selection that follows recently stated in a review of "Mental Health Books for the Modern Child" (1974) that the constructive stories which focus on particular feelings states in specific difficult situations are insufficient by themselves. Such books must be utilized as an auxiliary to an interpersonal communication whether as an introduction, an intermediary source of content, or as a conclusion, but they cannot be considered sufficient to do the job alone. Hospitalization, fear of death, a visit to the physician or the dentist, the birth of a sibling, or recognition of sexual differences require personalized and direct communication. Although books can serve only to lend technical assistance, they merit far more consideration than they have typically been given as an addition to psychotherapeutic playroom equipment.

". . . and what is the use of a book," thought Alice, "without pictures or conversations?"

—Lewis Carroll, *Alice in Wonderland*

In this paper we shall examine the use of books as part of the equipment in the child psychiatrist's playroom and as an aid in diagnostic and therapeutic work. A number of classical and modern studies have dealt witht the subject of children's literature, stories, and reading in the psychological development and mental life of the child (Freud, 1913; Friedlaender, 1941; Peller, 1954, 1959). Studies on the role of the fairy tale (Heuscher, 1963), sex differences in children's reading preferences (Peller, 1958), and the impact of modern social trends on the literature produced for children (Goldings, 1968;, Pickard, 1961) have all helped to draw the child psychiatrist's attention to the fact that, for many children, books and reading play a vital part in

Reprinted from *Journal of the American Academy of Child Psychiatry*, Vol. II (1972), pp. 52-65.

development (Pitcher and Prelinger, 1963). Shopper (1969) has recently drawn our attention to the use of classical children's stories in the teaching of child development concepts. None of these studies, however, nor studies of play therapy technique, has dealt specifically with books as vehicles for play and for fantasy development in the child psychiatrist's office; it is to this subject that our present attention is directed.

The use of books as part of the equipment for the diagnostic and therapeutic work with children is governed by the same general considerations which apply to the use of other play materials (Woltmann, 1955). Play materials are used to facilitate the child's expression and delineation of himself, his conflicts, and his inner life, and as a vehicle for the communication of ideas and affects between doctor and patient. Books should not be used as clever "gimmicks" or as mere entertaining diversions in child therapy. They should not be pressed upon the child to the exclusion of other freely available play materials; they have no "intrinsic" diagnostic and therapeutic value per se, and in no sense are the authors advocating some sort of "biblio-therapy." The value of particular books in any instance will be determined by the familiarity and practiced skill of the psychiatrist in their use, his sense of the timely and apt in the therapeutic strategy, and the suitability and receptivity of the specific patient to this medium. Like other items in the playroom, books used there must be "expend-able." This is no place for rare, precious, or irreplaceable editions, only for inexpensive copies or solid volumes which can tolerate hard use. The doctor's own adult reverence for "Books" and any efforts to protect them against childish handling must similarly be put aside.

We shall demonstrate, by means of descriptions and case vignettes, some of the range of situations in which we have found books useful in clinical work. We shall cite specific titles as illustrative of the *type* of books that meet the needs of particular clinical situations. We find that child psychiatrists tend to be insufficiently familiar with children's books. Annotated annual catalogues of children's books are available (4, 18),[1] but a regular visit to the children's book department of a

Numbers in parentheses refer to the List of Children's Books appended to this paper.

library or bookseller is even more valuable. We hope the examples in this paper will encourage the psychiatrist to examine specific children's books more closely and to consider adding some of them to his diagnostic and therapeutic armamentarium.

The Assessment of Language Abilities

The most obvious use for books in the playroom is to help in the assessment of the child's language skills: *Can* the patient read? *How* does he read (phonetically, by look-say, linguistically)? and *How well* does he read for his intelligence and his academic background? How effectively can the child use what he has read? If he cannot read, what skills does he have in the translation of graphic and pictorial material into sequential prose having grammatical and affective syntax? If there is a defect or abnormality in language usage, e.g., a dyslexia, reading efforts in the playroom may serve to define and illustrate this more fully.

A detailed and rigorous assessment of reading skills is usually undertaken by the clinical psychologist who has at his disposal a variety of standardized test materials. It is, however, clinically useful for the psychiatrist to have at hand two or three simple books at fairly early grade levels (3, 5, 6, 29), including a storybook with no words at all (12). He may invite the child directly to make use of these books, or he may make a more indirect assessment of reading and language functions by means of observing the child's ability to read and follow written instructions on a variety of games and puzzles. The Uncle Wiggily cards, for example, and some of the Dr. Seuss stories (25, 26) are demanding tests of particular reading skills; similarly, puzzles and "Make and Do" books offer a partial assessment of the reading skills and capacity for comprehension.

Sam, an 8½-year-old boy, was referred for psychiatric evaluation because of very poor schoolwork, failure to learn to read, distractibility, tearfulness, and irritability. Mental retardation was strongly suspected by his teachers and parents. In his first two interviews he showed a marked immaturity in visual and motor coordination in drawing, and a tearful, panicky rejection of any invitation to read formal books. He was familiar with the Uncle Wiggily game and his participation in this activity was especially revealing. "White cards" (cards bearing a numeral and a few lines of printing) were handled with great confidence; Sam could read the numerals flawlessly and count out the prescribed number of steps, ignoring the written material. The "red cards" (which lack numerals) were a great trial to him; he would not attempt to read them except for two-letter words which he frequently read incorrectly. Yet he looked at each card closely hoping it would be a "good" one. From closer observation we could see that the "good ones" were cards containing an instruction to proceed to a certain point on the game board. From the jumble of letters Sam was able to pick phrases such as "doghouse," "cluck-cluck henhouse," "five-and-ten-cent store," etc. and match them with the appropriate places printed on the Uncle Wiggily board without any other interpretation of the literally symbol. Thus the child showed a serious dyslexia, a facile number sense, and a prodigious memory, clearly indicating that his reading deficit was surely not on the basis of mental retardation. Serious and disabling emotional reverberations, related to his awareness of his reading shortcomings, complicated his performance.

Reading as "Sedative" Play

Keith, age 4 years 2 months, was an extremely anxious, aggressive and hyperactive child who for several months was unable to separate from his mother to come into the psychiatrist's office alone. His 2-year-old sister has a recently fractured leg in a cast and often came to the clinic with him. In his first hours, themes of violent, sadistic, and punitive aggression and related fears of retaliation poured forth with little control by the child and little mediation by the psychiatrist. By the 4th hour, Keith became increasingly reluctant and fearful about coming to the clinic and entering the doctor's office. The psychiatrist elected to introduce reading *with* and *to* Keith as a collaborative and quieting activity, choosing for this purpose *A Hole Is to Dig* (7). This is a very simple illustrated storybook of early definitions and includes the familiar, the humorous, the childishly concrete, and the surprising and the absurd. It is a small book (5 by 7 inches) with each page containing a few words, an attractive illustration, and a "complete" idea. This activity was something in which the child could participate with pleasure and a sense of excitement, safe and free from the aggressive-retaliatory excitement of the earlier play which was too threatening to be dealt with at this beginning point in therapy.[2]

For Charlie, a 6½-year-old hyperactive boy in psychoanalytic treatment, reading served as a frequent and deliberate regressive retreat from the anxiety about specific aspects of the therapeutic situation. At times, during the 4th to 7th months of analysis, when Charlie's most fundamental personality defenses were undergoing a dissolution, this highly intelligent and linguistically competent child took a series of nursery rhymes of the "This is the house that Jack built" type to read by himself. At times he would shout these rhymes at the doctor from a point of retreat beneath the analytic couch or from within the closed toy closet. Lines containing rhythm, cadence, repetition, and regularity were chanted as a ritual by the patient to counteract his own fears and experiences of internal disorder. Confirmation of the specific dynamics of Charlie's anxiety came later when, from "The house that Jack built" (1) he changed to "For want of a nail," and "I had a cat," and finally to "This is the key of the kingdom." (In that kingdom is a city, In that city is a town, etc.) This latter rhyme was converted by Charlie to a chant of his own:

> In the world there is a building,
> In the building there is an office,
> In the office there is a couch,
> Under the couch there is a boy,
> In the boy there is a [sic] ass-hole.
> ... Ass-hole in the boy,
> Boy under the couch,
> Couch in the office,
> Office in the building,
> Building in Boston,

[2] The authors are indebted to Dr. Gregory Rochlin for this example demonstrated during a continuous treatment seminar.

Boston in the world,
World in the universe.

From this and subsequent material it was possible to develop
Charlie's hypomanic and grandiose wish that his "ass-hole" (key-hole)
would be the center of the universe and his equally strong fear of a
sadomasochistic attack and seduction by the analyst.

As a therapeutic technique, the book of rhymes provided a channel
for defensive regression, "private" for the patient, to which he could
safely go without pursuit when his own defense or impulses were in
such disrepair. Much later in the analytic treatment, Charlie wrote
some "books" of his own as vehicles for more active mastery of specific
anxieties and as a means of communication with the doctor.

Books in the Active Mastery of Anxiety

With a less disturbed child and in a more superficial therapy some
exercise in the more active mastery of an anxiety may be attempted
through reading together. An effective book, for this use, should focus
specific issues or affects succinctly. The book, while clearly fantasy,
should contain enough of the child's primary process in plot and
illustrations to strike a note at once fearsome and yet familiar. It
should include a hero (or heroine) with whom the child can identify.

Myra, age 5 years and 2 months, had been through a number of
frightening hospitalizations for study of an abnormality of the
genitourinary tract. An additional psychological trauma was the
illness and aftercare of a 2-year-younger brother who had an un-
heralded and life-threatening attack of idiopathic thrombocytopenic
purpura. Myra was a restless, fearful child who cried easily and had
severe difficulties in going to sleep. Ogden Nash's *Adventures of Isabel*
(15) had an instantaneous appeal for her, and she chose it for reading
and rereading many times during the middle period of her psychotherapy. In this book, following each of the series of fearsome
situations, fetchingly illustrated, the reader is told over and over in
rhyme: "Isabel, Isabel didn't worry, Isabel didn't scream or scurry,"
and Isabel's own aggressive and humorous solution in action to a

potentially overwhelming threat is described. As is so frequently the case, Myra discarded the book when she no longer needed it and remained completely indifferent to it when her therapy moved on to other areas. (Maurice Sendak's *Where the Wild Things Are* (24) can be used similarly for a somewhat older child. In this book the hero is a boy and the entire story is a single adventure rather than a series of 2-page, 8-line episodes.)

The Withdrawn and Inhibited Child

At quite a different pole from the child who throws himself anxiously, chaotically, and unreservedly into the playroom situation, there stands the withdrawn, inhibited child, sometimes guarded and suspicious, who parries every invitation with passivity or resistance.

Lauren, age 8 years and 3 months, was a severely obsessional child whose emotional expressiveness at home was limited to quiet, solitary weeping and rare furious outbursts at her younger sister. In the playroom she was often mute and wooden, watching closely, saying little or nothing, sitting tightly hunched with her face averted from the doctor. For parts of many hours she listened attentively as the doctor read from *Charlotte's Web* (31), offering nothing of her own: neither comments nor elaborations but clearly listening and often enjoying the activity. It was finally agreed that when *Charlotte's Web* was finished, in a few sessions, it would be up to Lauren to choose the next book. After much tentative searching in the office Lauren selected Udry's *Let's Be Enemies* (28) and an important turning point was reached in her therapy. Not only did she choose it, but she read and reread it with the doctor many times, reaching eventually into her own feelings of hating and being hated as the major emotional interchange between herself and others—the one which she had best perfected and was most disturbed by.

In this example the doctor took the initiative in the responsibility for selecting a "neutral activity" which won first the attention, next the interest, and finally the active participation and elaboration by this inhibited patient. Reading was the activity chosen in this instance; the subject matter, an animated spider portraying, with other animals, a variety of human emotions and experiences, was also of the doctor's choice. The same end might have been served by the use of a number of other play techniques. Later in her psychotherapy, Lauren sometimes used reading and books as resistance. Bringing a book from home, she would hide behind it during the therapeutic hour. Under pressure she would read aloud but more to put off the doctor than to include him. The resolution of this defensive activity was often aided by reminding her of our earliest reading sessions when the doctor saw her fear and anger and touched it through reading. "It looks like Mary Poppins (or whatever other book the child was using as a defense at that moment), but it sounds to me like *Let's Be Enemies* all over again," the doctor often said.

Books for Information

At times children need books for "information." Such use of books in scholarly activity is more properly pursued within the school setting or at home. There are, however, a few special information books which are often useful to a child psychiatrist.

"Sex books," books dealing pictorially and verbally with the reproductive process, can be valuable, provided the physician bears in mind that they should *not* be used in any manner which will shut off, obscure, or impede the use and elucidation of the child's own feelings and ideas on these important matters. Rarely in child psychiatry or child analysis is mere factual knowledge about the phenomena of sexuality the key to a cure; still more rarely is the child actually innocent of most of the true "facts." Uneasy and "sophisticated" parents frequently ask the doctor to "recommend a book" which they can give the child in lieu of a direct interaction with the child in this area. Such books are numerous and of highly variable quality. Despite the child psychiatrist's reservations and cautions about giving out books to parents for children, he would do well to be both forewarned and forearmed with firsthand knowledge of some of the presently available books in this area, and have some choices about which ones he might wish to use himself. A good "sex book" is written for specific developmental level; hence separate books written in a series (such as that published by the American Medical Association for the preschool,

school-age, and adolescent child (10)) incorporate this important principle. Another useful feature is the inclusion of a "parent's section," which attempts, in part, to assist the parent to return to this important scene with the child rather than to encourage him to escape it (8, 9, 19).

Before we go to the direct use of sex books, however, and for more general use, there are some simple and well-illustrated books about the human body and how it works (23, 32). For the child to have access to such physical information in concrete form within the playroom is both appropriate and helpful in furthering the course of many therapies.

"Hospital" books represent a second kind of special information book useful to the child psychiatrist. Two of the best known of these, *Johnny Goes to the Hospital* (27) and *Curious George Goes to the Hospital* (20), were specifically designed to help prepare the young child for some of the reality situations which he will encounter in an elective hospitalization. In *Curious George*, a monkey, who is a well-known friend to most present-day children, is a patient, and the child reader accompanies him on a delightful hospital adventure in which a swallowed jigsaw puzzle piece is successfully retrieved and all is well at the end. How successful such "preparations" are for the average child is difficult to know. What is more striking to the child psychiatrist is the usefulness of hospital books *post hoc*, that is, in the review and recovery of hospitalization experiences in psychiatrically ill children. For this purpose the authors prefer a simpler book, *The Hospital* (17). Here a variety of hospital procedures, paraphernalia, and personnel are portrayed without the charm or distraction of a formal or familiar hero and a clever plot. *The Hospital* is a book most frequently rejected when first offered a child with a significant hospital history, but one to which he very likely returns as his therapy progresses.

Reference Books

Two standard reference works are sufficiently useful to warrant a permanent place in a child psychiatrist's office. A dictionary at the high school or collegiate level is a piece of external reality and authority to which both the child and the doctor may sometimes appeal when those vital tools of their work together—words and their meanings—become obscure and in dispute. The use of the dictionary can give the late-latency and preadolescent child a new dimension in which to exercise his growing mastery over words and his burgeoning curiosity.

Kenneth, 9 years and 2 months old, an aggressive and destructive child, being treated in a residential setting, was regressively ensnared in a preoccupation with 4-letter words, the meaning of which he usually knew quite accurately. His mother was a philologist and linguist, his father a scientific writer. Much time was spent in Kenneth's repeatedly looking up "shit," "crap," "cock," etc., copying down their pronunciation, definition, sometimes derivation, and illustrating them, and in speaking or shouting these productions at the doctor. Kenneth became increasingly irritated as he tried to find obscenities which were not in the office dictionary. As an aspect of his work in therapy he became involved in compiling his own more complete "Dictionary of Dirty Words." He was pleased and excited that the doctor not only allowed him to do this but even helped out with spellings and definitions. Kenneth was able to accept and eventually to understand the doctor's single restriction about his new book; namely, that it must remain in the office until both Kenneth and the doctor were sure that Kenneth really knew these new words and how to use them. The doctor's reason for this rule lay in the general principle that powerful instinctual images and affects represented by the words should be subject to the exercise and judgment of the ego. Without this, the entire activity would flood the child with both burdensome anxiety and "social" reproof.

A second useful standard reference work is a book of rules for games (e.g., *Hoyle's Rules of Games* (13)) to serve not only as a source of information but also as an objective arbiter of how things such as these should be done: an authoritative set of rules which will bind both parties equally and from which both doctor and patient will sometimes mutually agree to depart.

Books of Skills and Secrets

For children in the mid- and late-latency age, a few books providing "secret" knowledge and special skills, which can be shown off to others, are useful adjuncts to therapy. We have found that a book of simple magic tricks (21), a book on codes and secret writing (16), a book on general paperfolding (14) (not Origami, which is too complex and demanding for most young children), and a book of paper airplane techniques (2) fill the requirements well. A simple book of puzzles, jokes and brain teasers (22, 30) is widely useful in addition. Especially useful is a book of visual illusions (11), providing for the obsessive child an often much needed graphic illustration that "things are not always what they seem," a general moral which is a goal in much therapeutic work.

The Child as Author

Even more valuable for the individual child than any of these published books cited above are the "books" which some children may be encouraged to produce and review during the course of therapy. Kenneth's "Dictionary of Dirty Words" has already been cited as one example. Charlie, the 6½-year-old hyperactive child cited above, confined his fearsome monsters to the analytic situation by means of his own "Child's Own Book of Monsters" dictated to the doctor, illustrated by the patient, returned to repeatedly, and revised in several editions. It was finally replaced by the "Child's Own Book of Superheroes" as the neurotic obstructions to Charlie's phallic development underwent resolution. Myra described her real and ideal relationships with her despised younger brother in a diary type of notebook produced during the therapeutic hours.

The presence of "real" books in the playroom and the doctor's readiness to make use of them may act as in incentive to the child to use his own book as a type of play in which to express the form and fabric of his fantasy as well as his daily life experience in the real world. Such use of the child's own books clearly illustrates the function of book authorship as a "projective" technique. However, even in his use of standard, published books, the child, by his selection of material, by his emphases, and by his associative elaborations beyond the printed text, provides data which are of projective quality and which partake of the same richness and validity as other associative and fantasy materials. Not all children are able to use books in this way. Certainly not all children should be required to try. Nor is it always essential that the doctor come to an ultimate, objective understanding of what the child produced.

George was an 11-year-old borderline psychotic child of superior intelligence. In one of his earliest hours he sat totally absorbed with a flattened tablet of plasticene on which he made line upon line of meticulous marks with a wedged-shaped stylus. At the end of the hour and only with considerable urging on the part of the doctor, George said that this was "cuneiform writing in secret code of the whole terrible story." He gave it to the doctor to hold onto, saying, "Maybe someday I will translate this." George did not ask for the tablet again, and during the next 2½ years of visits for psychotherapy the doctor brought it forth several times hoping for further elaboration or explication. On each occasion, George would reject the tablet instantly and say, "No, it's not time yet." The patient improved considerably during his treatment; in his final therapy hour, the doctor again reminded George, now 13½, of the cuneiform tablet that he had written during the earliest part of his treatment. George's eyes shone and he eagerly asked to see it. He held it in his hands, scrutinizing it closely, turning it on its side, and then turning it upside down. "You know, Doc, I can't make anything out of this crazy thing. Maybe it's not important at all . . . but you know it is important that you kept it for me all this time."

Summary

In this paper we have presented a description of some of the ways in which books may be a useful part of the child psychiatrist's playroom equipment. Specific descriptions and case vignettes have been offered to illustrate the use of books for the clinical assessment of language, sedative play, active mastery of anxiety, and as an initial activity with the withdrawn and inhibited child. We have also discussed the use of information and reference books, books as sources of special skills, and the child as the author of books used in his own therapy.

We wish to emphasize our opinion that books should not dominate either the tone of the treatment or the physical layout of the playroom.

Indeed, all of the books cited in this paper together occupy less than one linear foot of shelf space. The doctor must be especially watchful not to succumb to the use of books as a diversionary device or as a "pleasant" way of avoiding or glossing over difficult issues and resistant periods during child psychotherapy. The use of books is governed by the same canons that apply to the use of other play media and are subject to the same limitations. These limitations are determined by the doctor's familiarity and skill in the medium, the timeliness and suitability for a particular patient, and the child's own ability and inclination to use such materials.

List of Children's Books

1. Anderson, R. L. & Bradford, J. (1964), *The House That Jack Built and Other Favorite Jingles.* New York: Dell Publishing (Harlan Quist).

2. Barnaby, R. S. (1970), *How to Make and Fly Paper Airplanes.* New York: Bantam.

3. Bemelmans, L. (1968), *Madeline's Rescue.* New York: Scholastic Book Services (Originally: Viking Press, 1953).

4. *Best Books for Children* (Annual). New York: R. R. Bowker.

5. Cook, B. (1964), *The Little Fish That Got Away.* New York: Scholastic Book Services (Originally: Crocket Johnson, 1956).

6. Friskey, M. (1964). *Indian Two Feet and His Horse.* New York: Scholastic Book Services (Originally: Children's Press, 1959).

7. Krauss, R. (1952). *A Hole Is to Dig.* Pictures by Maurice Sendak. New York: Harper and Row.

8. Lerrigo, M. O. (in consultation with Michael A. Cassidy) (1964), *A Doctor Talks to 9-to-12 Year Olds.* Chicago: Budlong Press.

9. Lerrigo, M. O. (in consultation with G. Lombard Kelly) (1962), *What Teenagers Want to Know.* Chicago: Budlong Press.

10. Lerrigo, M. O. & Southard, H. (in consultation with M. J. E. Senn) (1961/62), *Sex Education Series: Parents' Responsibility, A Story About You, Finding Yourself, Approaching Adulthood, Facts Aren't Enough.* Chicago: American Medical Association.

11. Luckiesh, M. (1965), *Visual Illusions: Their Causes, Characteristics, and Applications.* New York: Dover.

12. Mayer, M. (1967), *A Boy, A Dog and a Frog.* New York: Dial Press.

13. Morehead, A. H. & Mott-Smith, G. (1963), *Hoyle's Rules of Games*, 25th Ed. New York: New American Library (Signet paperback).

14. Murray, W. D. & Rigney, F. J. (1960), *Paper Folding for Beginners.* New York: Dover.

15. Nash, O. (1963), *The Adventures of Isabel.* Illustrated by Walter Lorraine. Boston: Little, Brown.

16. Peterson, J. (1966), *How to Write Codes and Send Secret Messages.* New York: Scholastic Book Services.

17. Pyne, M. (1962), *The Hospital.* Boston: Houghton Mifflin.

18. *Reader's Choice* (Annual). Catalog of Paperback Books published by Scholastic Book Services, 904 Sylvan Avenue, Englewood Cliffs, N.J. 07632.

19. Rey, H. A. (n. d.), *Where's My Baby?* Boston: Houghton Mifflin.

20. Rey, M. E. & Rey, H. A. (1965), *Curious George Goes to the Hospital.* Boston: Houghton Mifflin.

21. Ripley, S. (1955), *An Introduction to Magic: 141 Professional Tricks You Can Do.* New York: Sentinel Books.

22. *Ripley's Puzzles and Games* (1966), New York: Simon and Schuster.

23. Sanders, L. P. (n. d.), *Your Body and How It Works.* Chicago: American Medical Association.

24. Sendak, M. (1963), *Where the Wild Things Are.* New York: Harper and Row.

25. Seuss, Dr. (1965), *I Had Trouble in Getting to Solla Sollew.* New York: Random House.

26. Seuss, Dr. (1965), *Fox in Socks.* New York: Random House.

27. Sever, J. (1953), *Johnny Goes to the Hospital.* Boston: Houghton Mifflin for Children's Medical Center.

28. Udry, J. M. (1961), *Let's Be Enemies.* Illustrated by Maurice Sendak. New York: Harper and Row.

29. Vinton, I. (1961), *Look Out for Pirates.* New York: Random House.

30. Wiegle, O. (1959), *Jokes, Riddles, Funny Stories.* New York: Grosset and Dunlap.

31. White, E. B. (1952), *Charlotte's Web.* New York: Harper and Row.

32. *The Wonderful Human Machine* (1967), Chicago: American Medical Association.

Mutual Storytelling Technique

RICHARD A. GARDNER, M.D.

The mutual storytelling technique, a contribution to the technique of psychotherapy with children is, as Gardner asserts, neither therapy in itself nor a method to be used in isolation. Rather, it is part of the therapist's vast technical armamentarium. Readers will note also that it embodies elements which are present in many technical maneuvers within child psychotherapy. Fortunately, Gardner's structured "Make-Up-A-Story Television Program" method calls for the use of a tape recorder, so that verbatim transcripts of what the child and the therapist said are readily available. The almost one thousand page book from which the following excerpts have been reprinted contains many detailed examples of recorded mutual storytelling (accompanied by an ingenious, helpful "patient index," enabling readers who wish to do so to follow patients sequentially through different sections of the book). Information regarding what transpired before the storytelling in a particular session or what followed afterward when the child and therapist took up other modalities of interaction is not presented in comparable detail.

Like many maneuvers in child psychotherapy, this technique is easily categorized into two central elements. It is a way to elicit the child's inner thoughts and feelings comparable to techniques developed by Lowenfeld (1935), Levy (1939), and Erikson (1940). Through the child's metaphorical communication of fantasy, for instance, the therapist develops an appreciation of the particular child's problems and concerns. This insight leads to the second element: the therapist's intervention, which in the examples that follow entails interpretive communication to the child of what the therapist has learned in a way that is constructive and useful for the child, and which Gardner accomplishes through the therapist's corrective story embodying alternative adaptations and solutions.

While Gardner is explicit and direct in communicating through metaphor, it should be noted that any play interaction in which the therapist voices a participant's concern, feeling, or perception, entails addressing the child metaphorically. Readers who wish to read more about metaphoric communication in psychotherapy, particularly with psychotic children, can consult Ekstein (1965) and Cain and Maupin (1961). In the present volume, Chethik's paper illustrates the therapist communicating therapeutic interventions to the child in the form of a story without using Gardner's structured technique.

Among the issues of intercommunication in psychotherapy are the content of what we wish to communicate and at what level of the child's psychic organization and conflict we wish to address these communications. Many therapists agree, for instance, that it is generally unwise to immediately interpret to a child in gross terms oedipal drives and their related conflicts, such as wanting to kill one parent and marry the other, even if the child's play and other communications make this abundantly clear to the therapist at the outset. In the exploratory psychotherapies interpretations are generally aimed at a level which is just below the child's awareness, endeavoring to avoid depth that the child can dismiss as a "nutty idea from the shrink." Another issue in level of communication might be referred to as determination of dosage. Although Gardner does not refer to this explicitly, it is clear that he has it in mind when he uses the child's moral as a clue to what it is in this particular story at this particular time with which the child is most concerned. Dosage has to do also with the level of emotionality which the youngster can tolerate, e.g., telling a youngster that he is "terrified" or "scared" may too easily provoke denial, whereas initiating the same intervention with less charged words such as uneasy makes it easier for the youngster to acknowledge the affect.

 Gardner makes an assertion in his introduction which deserves further study: "Few children are interested in gaining conscious awareness of their unconscious processes let alone utilizing such insights therapeutically." While agreeing that such children are in the minority among those who need our help, investigation is needed to enable clinicians to more reliably assess which children do not need to talk explicitly about the specifics of their problem in order to gain marked and lasting changes because the same can be accomplished more readily by communication within a metaphor. How can these children be distinguished from those in whom it is vital to explicitly show them the conflicts which are unwittingly expressed in their everyday lives, directly connecting their unconscious processes with their reality in order to effect changes or to render the changes lasting. Hopefully, a future volume of this series will report the results of research regarding this question that will enable clinicians to make this decision on bases other than those that seem to be currently prevalent, i.e., the therapist's predilections and unrelated external circumstances such as willingness and ability to continue therapy instead of basing the decision on the youngster's specific individual needs.

Eliciting stories is a time-honored practice in child psychotherapy. From the stories children tell, the therapist is able to gain invaluable insights into the child's inner conflicts, frustrations, and defenses.

 A child's stories are generally less difficult to analyze than dreams, free associations, and other productions of the adult. His fundamental difficulties are exhibited clearly to the therapist, without the obscurity,

Reprinted from *Therapeutic Communication with Children: The Mutual Storytelling Technique*, Jason Aronson, Inc., 1971, pp. 17-18, 25-31, 36-39, 939-940.

distortion, and misrepresentation that are characteristic of the adult's presentation. The essential problem for the child's therapist has been how to use his insights therapeutically.

The techniques described in the literature on child psychotherapy and psychoanalysis are, for the most part, attempts to solve this problem. Some are based on the assumption, borrowed from the adult psychoanalytic model, that making the unconscious conscious can itself be therapeutic. My own experience has been that few children are interested in gaining conscious awareness of their unconscious processes, let alone utilizing such insights therapeutically. Children do, however, enjoy both telling stories and listening to them. Since storytelling is one of the child's favorite modes of communication, I wondered whether communicating to him in the same mode might not be useful in child therapy. The efficacy of the storytelling approach for the imparting and transmission of values and insights is proved by the ancient and universal appeal of fable, myth, and legend.

It was from these observations and considerations that I developed the Mutual Storytelling Technique, a proposed solution to the questions of how to utilize the child's stories therapeutically. In this method the child first tells a story; the therapist surmises its psychodynamic meaning and then tells one of his own. The therapist's story contains the same characters in a similar setting, but he introduces healthier adaptations and resolutions of the conflicts that have been exhibited in the child's story. Since the therapist speaks in the child's own language, he has a good chance of "being heard." One could almost say that here the therapist's interpretations bypass the conscious and are received directly by the unconscious. The child is not burdened with psychoanalytic interpretations which are alien to him. Direct, anxiety-provoking confrontations, so reminiscent of the child's experience with parents and teachers, are avoided. Lastly the introduction of humor and drama enhances the child's interest and pleasure and therefore his receptivity. As a therapeutic tool, the method is useful in combination with traditional techniques. It is most useful for children who tell stories but who have little interest in analyzing them. It is not a therapy per se, but rather one technique in the therapist's armamentarium.

* * *

Although drawings, dolls, puppets, and other toys are the modalities around which stories are traditionally told in child therapy, these often have the effect of restricting the child's storytelling or of channeling it in highly specific directions. The tape recorder does not have these disadvantages; with it, the visual field remains free from contaminating and distracting stimuli. Eliciting a story with it is like obtaining a dream on demand.

In order to show in detail how the technique works, the tape recorder will be utilized. The same method, however, can be employed—with some modifications—with dolls, blocks, drawings, and other play material.

I introduce the child to the game by first pointing to a stack of tapes, each of which has a child's name clearly written on the end of the box. I tell the patient that each child who comes to my office has his own tape for a tape recording game which we play. I ask him if he would like to have a tape of his own. The child generally wants to follow usual practice, and having his own tape enhances his feeling of belonging. If he assents, I take out a new tape and let him write his name on the box.

I then ask the child if he would like to be guest of honor on a make-believe television program on which stories are told. If he agrees—and few decline the honor—the recorder is turned on and I begin:

Good morning, boys and girls. I'd like to welcome you once again to Dr. Gardner's "Make-Up-A-Story Television Program." As you all know, we invite children to our program to see how good they are at making up stories. Naturally, the more adventure or excitement a story has, the more interesting it is to the people who are watching at their television sets. Now, it's against the rules to tell stories about things you've read or have seen in the movies or on television, or about things that really happened to you or anyone you know.

Like all stories, your story should have a beginning, a middle, and an end. After you've made up a story, you'll tell us the moral of the story. We all know that every good story has a moral.

Then after you've told your story, Dr. Gardner will make up a story too. He'll try to tell one that's interesting and unusual, and then he'll tell the moral of his story.

And now, without further delay, let me introduce to you a boy (girl) who is with us today for the first time. Can you tell us your name, young man?

I then ask the child a series of brief questions that can be answered by single words or brief phrases such as his age, address, school grade, and teacher. These simple questions diminish the child's anxiety and tend to make him less tense about the more unstructured themes involved in "making up a story." Further diminution of anxiety is accomplished by letting him hear his own voice at this point by playback, something which most children enjoy. He is then told:

Now that we've heard a few things about you, we're all interested in hearing the story *you* have for us today.

At this point most children plunge right into their story, although some may feel the need for "time to think." I may offer this pause; if it is asked for by the child, it is readily granted. There are some children for whom the pause is not enough, but who nevertheless still want to try. In such instances, the child is told:

Some children, especially when it's their first time on this program, have a little trouble thinking of a story, but with some help from me they're able to do so. Most children don't realize that there are *millions* of stories in their heads they don't know about. And I know a way to help get out some of them. Would you like me to help you get out one of them?

Most children assent to this. I then continue:

Fine, here's how it works. I'll start the story and when I point my finger at you, you say exactly what comes into your mind at that time. You'll then see how easy it is to make up a story. Okay. Let's start. Once upon a time————a long, long time ago————in a distant land————far, far away————there lived a————.

I then point my finger, and it is a rare child who does not offer some fill-in word at this point. If the word is "dog," for example, I then say, "And *that dog*————" and once again point to the patient. I follow the statement provided by the child with "And then————" or "The next thing that happened was————." Every statement the child makes is followed by some introductory connective and by pointing to the child to supply the next statement. That and no more—the introduction of specific phrases or words would defeat the therapist's purpose of catalyzing the youngster's production of his *own* created material and of sustaining, as needed, its continuity.

For most children, this approach is sufficient to get them over whatever hurdles there are for them in telling a story. If this is not enough, however, it is best to drop this activity in a completely casual and non-reproachful manner, such as: "Well, today doesn't seem to be your good day for storytelling. Perhaps we'll try again some other time."

While the child is engaged in telling his story, I jot down notes, which are not only of help in analyzing the child's story, but serve also as a basis for my own. At the end of the child's story and his statement of its moral, I may ask questions about specific items in the story. The purpose here is to obtain additional details, which are often of help in understanding the story. Typical questions might be: "Was the fish in your story a man or a lady?" "Why was the fox so mad at the goat?" "Why did the bear do that?" If the child hesitates to tell the moral of his story or indicates that there is none, I usually reply: "What, a story without a moral? Every good story has *some* lesson or moral!" The moral that this comment usually does succeed in eliciting from the child is often significantly revealing of the fundamental psychodynamics of the story.

For the younger children, the word "lesson" or "title" may be substituted for "moral." Or the child might be asked: "What can we learn from your story?"

Then I usually say: "That was a very good (unusual, exciting, etc.) story." Or to the child who was hesitant: "And you thought you weren't very good at telling stories!"

I then turn off the tape recorder and prepare my story. Although the child's story is generally simpler to understand than the adult's dream, the analysis of both follows similar principles. At this point, I will present only a few fundamentals of story analysis. My hope is that the reader who is inexperienced in dream and/or story analysis will, by careful reading of the numerous examples of story analysis to be presented in this book, become adept at story interpretation.

I first attempt to determine which figure or figures in the child's story represent the child himself, and which stand for significant people in his environment. It is important to appreciate that two or more figures may represent various facets of the *same* person's personality. There may, for example, be a "good dog" and a "bad cat" in the same story, which are best understood as conflicting forces within the same child. A horde of figures, all similar, may symbolize powerful elements in a single person. A hostile father, for example, may be represented by a stampede of bulls. Swarms of small creatures such as insects, worms, or mice, often symbolize unacceptable repressed complexes. Malevolent figures can represent the child's own repressed hostility projected outward, or they may be a symbolic statement about the hostility of a significant figure. Sometimes both of these mechanisms operate simultaneously. A threatening lion in one child's story stood for his hostile father, and he was made more frightening by the child's own hostility, repressed and projected onto the lion. This example illustrates one of the reasons why many children see their parents as being more malevolent than they are.

Besides clarifying the symbolic significance of each figure, it is also important to get a general overall "feel" for the atmosphere and setting of the story. Is the ambience pleasant, neutral, or horrifying? Stories that take place in the frozen tundra or on isolated space stations suggest something very different from those which occur in the child's own home. The child's emotional reactions when telling the story are also of significance in understanding its meaning. An eleven-year-old child who tells me, in an emotionless tone, about the death fall of a mountain climber reveals not only his hostility but also his repression of his feelings. The atypical must be separated from the stereotyped,

age-appropriate elements in the story. The former may be very revealing, whereas the latter rarely are. Battles between cowboys and Indians
rarely give meaningful data, but when the chief sacrifices his son to
Indian gods in a prayer for victory over the white man, something has
been learned about the child's relationship with his father.

Lastly, the story may lend itself to a number of different psychodynamic interpretations. In selecting the theme that will be most
pertinent for the child at *that particular time*, I am greatly assisted by
the child's own "moral" or "title."

After asking myself, "What would be a healthier resolution or a
more mature adaptation than the one used by the child?" I create a
story of my own. My story involves the same characters, setting and
initial situation as the child's story, but it has a more appropriate or
salutary resolution of the most important conflicts. In creating my
story, I attempt to provide the child with more *alternatives*. The
communication that the child need not be enslaved by his neurotic
behavior patterns is vital. Therapy must open new avenues not considered in the child's scheme of things. It must help the child become
aware of the multiplicity of options which are available to replace the
narrow self-defeating ones he has chosen. My moral or morals are an
attempt to emphasize further the healthier adaptations I have included
in my story. If, while I am telling my story, the child exhibits deep
interest, or if he reveals marked anxiety, which may manifest itself by
jitteriness or hyperactivity, then I know that my story is "hitting
home." Such clear-cut indications of how relevant one's story is are
not, of course, always forthcoming.

After the moral to my story, I stop the recorder and ask the child
whether he would like to hear the recorded program. In my experience,
the child is interested in doing so about one-third of the time. Playing
the program makes possible a second exposure to the messages that the
therapist wishes to impart. If the child is not interested in listening to
the tape, then we engage in other therapeutic activities.

The therapist's attitude has a subtle, but nevertheless significant,
influence on the child's ability to tell a story. Ideally this attitude
should be one of pleasurable anticipation that a story will be

forthcoming and surprised disappointment when the child will not or cannot tell one. The child wants to be accepted by those who are meaningful to him, and if a productive therapeutic relationship has been established, he will try to comply with what is expected of him.

Peer group influence is also important. When the child gets the general feeling that storytelling is what everybody does when he visits the therapist, he is more likely to play the game. Seeing a stack of tapes—with each child's first name prominently displayed—tends to foster his desire to tell stories "just like the other kids do." In my typical session, the mother and child are seen together for a few minutes. The mother then leaves, and the child and I start our time together with the storytelling game. The rest of the session is devoted to other therapeutic activities—most often initiated by the child. In this way, there is a pattern set down which both of us routinely follow. It is a *matter of course* that we proceed to the tape recorder (which is conspicuously placed in my play area) as soon as the child's mother leaves. If the child is disinclined to play the game he must break an expected pattern. Since this is hard for most children to do, he generally goes along with the game and finds it not only less anxiety-provoking than he anticipated, but pleasurable as well.

* * *

Steve, and eight-year-old boy who was a disciplinary problem in school, told this story in his first session:

> I have this friend named Andy. We get into a fight. Then we decided not to have a fight. Then Andy and I met with a big boy and we both didn't want to fight the big boy. We ignored him.
>
> We met with this monster. It tried to burn us. Then he (the monster) got himself all smoked and burned. The fire from his nostrils went the wrong way.
>
> Moral: never try to get into a fight unless you know what the victim is, how tough or weak.

The first part of the story reveals Steve's ambivalence over expressing his anger. The two boys get into a fight and then decide not to.

When the boys meet a big boy—probably the patient's father—they decide not to fight him. Again, the notion of fighting is considered and then rejected.

In my opinion the monster symbol serves a double purpose. It represents the patient's father as well as Steve's own projected hostility. He sees his father as basically malevolent. As is so often the case, he perceives his father's rejection as hostility, and, in addition, he probably anticipates his father's retaliation for his own unconscious resentment of him. He protects himself from his father's fury by preventing its outward expression. The fire from the monster's nostrils goes the "wrong way," becomes directed internally, and he burns himself. A more poignant representation of the internalization of anger is hard to conceive of. By the father's self-traumatization, the patient's hostile impulses toward him are also gratified. It is as if Steve could say: "He did it to himself; I had nothing to do with it." In addition, the monster, as the projection of the patient's own rage, reveals his fear of such external expression. His wrath must be disowned via projection and even then repressed and internalized. The moral epitomizes Steve's fear that overt expression of anger can be dangerous.

This story, like most, contains many themes which could reasonably be selected for elaboration in my version. I usually try to develop in my story that issue which is most dramatically emphasized—the theme, that is, which appears to be at the forefront of the child's imagination. Concentration on this element increases the probability that my story will be meaningful to the child. I attempt to reach the child at the level that is most significant. This level is not necessarily "deep," for significance and depth need not be identical. For example, in this child's story, the hostility toward the father suggests that oedipal problems are being dealt with. The most impressive element exhibited, however, was the dramatic representation of the repression of rage— the monster internally directing his own fire—and so this aspect was selected for amplification in my story:

Once upon a time there was a dragon. This dragon never noticed that he was different from other dragons in that he did not breathe out smoke and fire like the others. When the other dragons were bothered by someone, they would say to them, "Get out of here." And if those who were bothering the dragon did not go away, then the dragon would breathe out smoke and fire and that usually worked and he wouldn't be bothered again. When this dragon was bothered, however, he said nothing; did not breathe out smoke and fire and kept it all inside himself.

One day this dragon began to complain of aches and pains in his chest and stomach. He went to his doctor. His doctor examined him and then asked him what he did when he was bothered by others. He told the doctor that he said nothing and held his feelings inside himself. The doctor then said to him: "I know what's wrong with you. When other dragons get angry at someone, they tell them to stop bothering them and if that doesn't work, they breathe out smoke and fire, and that usually stops people from harming them. But you keep the smoke and fire inside you and that's hurting your lungs and stomach. I suggest that when somebody does something that bothers you, you tell them about it. If that doesn't work, then let out your anger, let out your smoke and fire, and that will usually help."

The dragon went home and thought a lot about what the doctor had said. He realized that the advice was good and he then tried to follow it. It was hard at first because he had never done such a thing before in his life. In fact, he was quite afraid to do such a thing. But the more he did it the less afraid he became. He had to return to the doctor once in a while for further instruction and advice, but he gradually learned how to do it and the pains in his stomach and chest went away.

The moral of this story is: if somebody is doing something which bothers you, tell them about it. Let out your anger. Don't keep it inside. If you do that, most often things will be better for you.

As can be seen, in my story I did not touch upon the sources of the child's anger because I could only guess them at this early point in treatment. I did know, however, that he was significantly inhibited in the expression of hostility, and I tried to help him in this regard.

Anxiety-provoking communications such as these can best be digested piecemeal; too much at once only overwhelms the child and increases his anxiety and resistance.

* * *

On being introduced to the Mutual Storytelling Technique many therapists have said, "It sounds like a good idea. Are you sure no one else has done it?" I had similar thoughts when I first came upon the idea. It seemed so obvious a thing to do. Children enjoy telling stories; they love hearing them; and communicating with them through stories is an ancient tradition. And yet, I was unable to find any articles in the literature describing a therapeutic procedure in which the *therapist* systematically tells stories, each of which is *specifically based on what has been elicited from the child*, and each of which is designed to introduce therapeutic messages *pertinent to the particular issue (s)* raised in the child's story. I cannot imagine, however, that others— somewhere, sometime—have not used it. What is possibly original is my systematization of it, and my detailed recording of the process.

I wish to emphasize my point that mutual storytelling is not a therapy per se, but rather one technique in the therapist's armamentarium. It is a valuable treatment modality but should be used along with other approaches if the child is to derive maximum benefit from his treatment. The method is primarily useful for verbal children with neurotic and characterological problems. It may be of value in borderline children, but would be contraindicated in most psychotic children—such patients need reality confrontation more than fantasy stimulation. It can be useful in drawing out the subdued and repressed child or the child with borderline intelligence. It has little place in the therapy of children below the age of four or four-and-half because such children generally do not consistently produce material which lends itself well to story formation by the therapist. The five-year-old, who represents a borderline age for the utilization of this technique, usually provides enough meaningful fragments for the therapist's story formation. He is also old enough to listen with interest to the therapist's tales. The pubertal period is the upper age limit for effective use of this method; the adolescent is usually too self-conscious to verbalize his fantasies freely and considers the game childish.

The efficacy of the Mutual Storytelling Technique is not due only to the more efficient and effective communications that it provides. Other benefits are derived by the child in a more subtle way. The telling of the stories is genuinely creative and therefore ego-enhancing. The therapist himself usually finds the procedure both enjoyable and challenging, and this affords the child the salubrious feeling that he is a person who can provide meaningful satisfactions for the therapist's needs. All too often therapists involve themselves in activities with children which they themselves find onerous or boring. When this happens, the child unerringly picks up the therapist's resentment and the activity thereby becomes psychologically deleterious, even to the point of compromising the treatment.

The Mutual Storytelling Technique, which is imaginative, constructive, and pleasure-giving, is the kind of fulfilling and rewarding experience that is salutary and meaningful in both therapeutic and non-therapeutic relationships.

It has been my purpose in this book to acquaint the child therapist with a technique which has proved valuable to me as a treatment method. My hope is that it will prove equally valuable to the readers of this book. Those of us who do utilize the method to the benefit of our child patients can enjoy a unique sense of accomplishment. When such children leave it is as if they said to us, in the words of William Cullen Bryant:

> Deeply hath sunk the lesson thou has given,
> And shall not soon depart.

A Psychoanalytic Viewpoint of Behavior Modification in Clinical and Educational Settings

GASTON E. BLOM, M.D.

Much of the interaction between psychodynamically oriented therapists and behaviorally oriented therapists has been characterized by dogmatic polemics emphasizing distinctions and contrasts between the two points of view. The growing gulf has resulted in an extreme segregation that would enable the same patient to be discussed in two different case conferences as if the same person were two different people. In one conference attention might be focused exclusively on intrapsychic factors, while external behavioral considerations were dismissed as an irrelevant distraction for the clinicians. In the other case conference the same person's behavior could be discussed as if it were of exclusive significance and regulated only by external factors, while internal factors were viewed as either insignificant or inevitably so complex that they should be dismissed as an incomprehensible distraction. Since this volume is dedicated to the minimization of such artificial barriers, it is appropriate to conclude this section devoted primarily to individual psychodynamically oriented psychotherapy, with Blom's paper which follows, as an integrating transition to this volume's behavior therapy section. Blom's paper endeavors to construct such a bridge and in so doing he has performed a valuable service by examining the merits, interactions, and congruity between the psychodynamic and behavioral points of view.

Blom's paper is significant also because of its focus on children and the extent to which his thinking is derived from the educational tradition (see Blom et al., 1972). Others have made similar attempts but from perspectives that were less child-focused (Alexander, 1963; Dollard and Miller, 1950; Feather and Rhoads, 1972; Marmor, 1971; Mowrer, 1950; and Sloane, 1969). Simultaneously, nonprofessionals know without debate or equivocation that most children are reared and educated with behavior modification techniques applied spontaneously, informally, and without structure by caring parents and/or teachers who may be sensitive to conflicts between the child's inner needs and the external world and to conflicts within the child and between various parts of the child's inner self. Ekstein's (1965) characterization of "the love of learning" being preceded developmentally by "learning for love" says it eloquently.

It is not as easy for the clinician to integrate both points of view because that requires assessment of the balance of forces at any particular time and the determination of which therapeutic influence or how much of each could most parsimoniously and reliably be effective. Blom takes a step in the direction of outlining criteria for specific therapeutic prescription. Much more investigation is needed to enhance our ability to differentially employ various therapeutic modalities, either exclusively or in combination, but with appropriate forethought, deliberation, and discrimination.

Changes in therapeutic approach probably stem too often from clinicians' discouragement with lack of therapeutic progress. While this may entail an appropriate correction of an inaccurate assessment resulting in the application of an inappropriate therapy, there are many other instances in which this state of affairs should be a cause for concern. Obviously, clinicians wisely prefer to avoid making decisions for negative reasons. More significantly, our discouragement may reflect countertransfer-

ence more frequently than it may be correlated with inappropriate therapy. Many clinicians have experienced that stick-to-itiveness in the face of apparent futility can prove amazingly effective in certain instances.

Although our current level of knowledge leaves us less skilled in making positive determinations as to which therapeutic modality or combinations thereof are the most appropriate in specific instances, there are some long-established therapeutic approaches in which there is considerable experience in making such differential assessments and basing the therapeutic strategy on a combination of modalities. In the treatment of preschool children via their parents (Furman, 1957), regardless of the mode of intervention (counseling focused on the parent-child interaction, conjoint marital therapy focused on parental interactions, exploratory psychotherapy for one of the parents seeking to effect intrapsychic change in that parent, etc.), the favorable effects on the child inevitably are a consequence of altered behavioral interactions between the child and the parent.

In residential treatment, as Noshpitz (1957) has pointed out, there is a "Ping-Pong effect" in that behavior change is initiated within the residential setting while its repercussions are discussed concurrently in the individual psychotherapeutic sessions, so that the action in one arena and the information derived from it augments and illuminates what goes on in the other. McDermott, Fraiberg, and Harrison (1968) vividly described a case illustrating that what occurs in the residence enhances the understanding of the individual psychotherapist and what transpires in the individual therapeutic session contributes to the formulation of management techniques for the milieu treatment that comprises the child's real-life world while he is in residential treatment.

As Blom says in what follows: "Behavioral change is viewed as capable of being accomplished both from the inside out and the outside in."

The Day Care Center of the University of Colorado Medical Center is a psychoeducational facility in the Department of Psychiatry which has been in operation since 1962. It serves a population of 16 to 18 elementary-school-age children whose social and academic problems are particularly manifest in the school setting. These children attend the Center from 9:00 a.m. to 3:00 p.m. daily for a period of 1 to 2 years with the goal of their returning to public school programs. The staff consists of teachers, psychologists, psychiatrists, social workers, pediatricians and auxiliary personnel, and trainees in the indicated professional disciplines. A special education program is provided together with psychoanalytically oriented therapy for the children and their parents. In addition to this intramural activity, the Center conducts consultation and inservice training programs in a number of public elementary schools. The Center also functions as a research facility in special education and treatment methods for children and families.

The Center, an environmental resource, has made it possible to program corrective and remedial efforts for troubled children. Such children have had to struggle not only with personality disturbances but also with difficulties arising from a deficit in developmental skills and competencies. In this setting it was assumed that the environment could foster maladaptive behavior patterns when it responded in a haphazard, random, and inconsistent fashion.

Children with emotional and learning problems have been approached through an interaction of intrapsychic and environmental methods. Behavioral change is viewed as capable of being accomplished both from the inside out and the outside in. Indeed, it has been the Center's experience that an approach to an understanding of intrapsychic dynamics does not necessarily produce alternative behaviors and skills. Not infrequently behavior achieves an autonomous and syntonic status that makes it markedly resistant to change (Freud, 1926). There are also behaviors that are not the consequences of inner conflict but which arise from the lack of inner structures within the personality.

Reprinted from *Journal of the American Academy of Child Psychiatry*, Vol. 11 (1972), pp. 675-693.

Behavior modification has provided one of the means by which one could deal with environmental influences in a more systematic and thoughtful manner. These methods have the potential for establishing cycles of positive behavior: they deal with consequences of behavior which have a powerful influence on its continuation, even though this behavior originally arose from antecedent conditions and current intrapsychic causes.

From our experience at the Day Care Center with the usefulness of behavior modification, we have developed a point of view which encourages us to make use of its methods. This presentation will consider some of the principles, orientations, issues, assets and limitations of behavior modification methods (Lundin, 1963). A number of clinical examples will be given to illustrate both its usefulness and its limitations.

"Behavior modification" is a term used to describe methods of altering characteristics of the environment so as to modify existing human behaviors and to facilitate development of new alternative behaviors. Those associated with this field are for the most part from the professions of psychology and education, with some notable medical exceptions (Clement et al., 1970; Wolpe, 1969). Within this field, there is an extensive and expanding professional literature in psychology, special education, and educational psychology with particular emphasis on schools and learning situations (Snow and Brooks, 1970). In some special education programs behavior modification has become the central methodology (Haring and Phillips, 1962; Hewitt, 1968).

In view of its popularity, of the reports of success, and of its application to a variety of social and academic behaviors of children at various ages (Bandura, 1969; Bradfield, 1970; Ullman and Krasner, 1965; Yates, 1970), it is important for psychoanalysts and psychiatrists to have a viewpoint about his discipline. It may in fact provide an impetus for progress in psychoanalytic ego psychology and in methods of practice (Porter, 1968). However, it is difficult to examine this question dispassionately and rationally: controversy (Arthur, 1967; Barrett-Lennard, 1965; Murray, 1963), extreme positions, partisanship, dogma, polemics, claims, and derogations are not unusual with voices speaking both for (Eysenck, 1964; Rachman and Eysenck, 1966) and against (Glover, 1959; Porter, 1968) behavior modification. Some professionals have been disillusioned with psychodynamic therapies and critical of the use of the medical model in diagnosis, etiology, and treatment, and such people may regard behavior modification as a solution to clinical problems they find inadequately solved (Yates, 1970).

The controversy is not unlike another which arose a number of years ago labeled "clinical practice versus social competence" and which developed as a consequence of many Great Society programs emphasizing the acquisition of skill and competence by training and educational methods. In conjunction with this emphasis, criticism was leveled at clinical practice methods and at the concepts on which they were based. A constructive response to this controversy has been to explore how educational and training methods could be integrated more effectively with clinical and therapeutic methods (Blom, 1967a). At the Day Care Center this integration has been called a psychoeducational approach, a term more commonly used in special education than in clinical settings (Blom, 1967b).

A psychoanalytic orientation to childhood emotional disturbances views manifest behaviors as symptoms of underlying conflicts at manifest levels, the psychoanalytic therapist expects them to change to the degree that underlying conflicts and states are resolved. As this solution occurs, adaptive patterns of behavior are expected to develop in relation to environmental opportunities. There is considerable evidence that these expectations are often not fulfilled, often enough, in fact, that many individuals have challenged both their efficacy and their basic propositions. This leads to a consideration of other views of and approaches to behavior such us: the consequences of behavior, its autonomous and syntonic nature, the lack of inner conflict, the absence of inner structures, and the lack of natural environmental opportunities for change. In considering the latter one can question another tendency in therapeutic work with children, i.e., the reluctance to provide advice and guidance to parents about changing the child's environment. The widely held impression that such measures will fail unless feelings and relationships are fully understood and modified may often reflect an unjustified bias; again, an unrealistic expectation exists that adequate parental responses will emerge as underlying problems are resolved. While we recognize that parental feelings are important, many of us have learned that intrapsychic change can become too exclusive an emphasis so that parent education is neglected in the course of therapeutic efforts. One aspect of this complex problem is that rigid and somewhat unskillful application of technical concepts and measures may be adopted which do not do justice either to the technical ideas or theoretical constructs proposed, and which then are criticized when they do not appear sufficiently useful.

In this discussion of behavior modification, we may not be able to satisfy either psychoanalysts or proponents of behavior modification. In talking with school personnel about behavior modification approaches to problem children, one finds that educators often view these methods as practical and precise, but not humanistic. Under these circumstances, they frequently want to explore latent meanings of behavior, family relationships, and the like. In contrast, when teachers are presented a psychodynamic explorative method of understanding and approach, they ask for specific suggestions and practical advice. The dilemma is a common one, and in a sense, represents a value conflict. It may also reflect the difficulties of the early stages of a process of coming to understand and to use new concepts and techniques.

One should recognize that behavior modification is an outgrowth of academic and experimental psychology and that it does not originate from clinical and naturalistic observations and studies. It is rooted in the behaviorism of Watson and of Skinner, which was and is concerned with those aspects of behavior that are directly observable and measurable. Traditionally, inner mental behavior has not been its concern, although recently more and more attempts have been made to deal with these elements (Stoyva, 1970). Laboratory experiments with animals under restricted stimulus and response conditions have led to generalizations which were then applied to animal and human behavior in natural environments. The theoretical framework of behavior modification is stimulus-response learning theory, which is extended to all aspects of behavior. The definition of stimulus is anything that has an effect on the organism, and the definition of response is any action of the organism. The theory tends to exclude what goes on inside the organism not only between stimulus and response but also within the organism itself apart from the environment. One may view the theory as dealing with behavior in simplistic, parsimonious formulations, but such a stance does not mean that it has no value or utility: it may have explanatory value for some aspects of behavior without dealing with other aspects.

In the development of learning theory two main classes of learned behavior have received attention (Bijou and Baer, 1967):

1. Classical conditioning: this approach is associated with Pavlov, who paired neutral stimuli with unconditioned stimuli to produce conditioned responses, i.e., responses become conditioned to the previous neutral stimuli.
2. Operant conditioning: any behavior which can be conditioned has an operant level of occurrence. One can produce the behavior at will by reinforcing; and reinforcing events can weaken or strengthen the probability of a response occurring.

It is not always clear whether a given learned behavior is classically conditioned or operantly conditioned. In most situations it is probably a combination of classic and operant conditionings. In this presentation the primary focus will be on behaviors developed through operant methods, since this is the area on which we have focused and in which we have had clinical experiences.

In applying behavior modification techniques one must be familiar with certain principles. The focus is on overt behavior, with less concern for latent and less measurable behaviors. One looks at the frequency aspect of a behavior rather than its qualitative characteristics. Syndromes or nosological categories are ignored. The focus is on individual behaviors that are maladaptive. The goal of treatment is symptom removal or modification. Alternative behaviors are considered and methods are used to generate them.

In describing the ingredients of a behavior modification program one can be caught up in the nature, schedule, and timing of reinforcement, which, although important, may miss a crucial aspect, i.e., problem analysis[1]—the careful observation and description of behaviors in the here and now, their frequency, the response to the behaviors, and the settings in which they occur. From this analysis a behavior is selected for modification. Steps in this modification and in the generation of alternative behavior are considered. Progress, or lack of it, is carefully followed and modifications of the program are made as one proceeds. In itself, problem analysis offers opportunities for clearer understanding of behavior. It also illuminates forms of intervention other than behavior modification, such as medication, focal inquiry and others. Moreover, altering contexts of and responses from the environment may in itself be sufficient to change behavior.

Having decided on behaviors to modify and/or generate, one considers the kind of reinforcement and the specific person to provide this reinforcement. The person needs to be cooperative, reliable, and consistent. It is possible to use inexperienced people, including parents, after explanation is given and follow-up is provided. This makes it possible to use behavior modification in a variety of settings for children: in the classroom, residential settings, and also in the home. The nature of the program is fully explained to both the reinforcing person and the child recipient, preferably together.

What about reinforcement? One aspect is its valence; i.e., positive, negative, neutral, or some combination of these. Positive reinforcement accelerates the frequency of a behavior occurring. It encourages alternative behavior and provides information to the child about the desired behavior. It may be used alone or in combination with negative or neutral reinforcement toward undesired behavior. Negative reinforcement decelerates the frequency of a behavior occurring. It takes the form of a type of "punishment" or escape from aversive stimuli and is used to modify an undesired behavior. However, negative reinforcement may have limitations such as merely suppressing a behavior but not encouraging alternative behavior. Punishment as a reinforcer often generates complex affects such as anxiety, anger, and

[1] Some approaches also make use of careful history taking regarding the origin and history of particular behaviors and apply such findings in a therapeutic program (Bandura, 1969; Ullman and Krasner, 1965; Yates, 1970).

inhibition. It may support an undesired behavior and becomes then a positive reinforcer; for example, negative attention behavior. Yet, punishment may be needed to interfere with rigid stereotyped behavior or dangerous behavior which is seriously interfering with an individual's adaptation. Even punishment is used, positive reward can follow for an alternative behavior. A neutral reinforcement means not responding, or ignoring, or being objective, and has the possibility of extinguishing a behavior. Behavior modifiers would consider any reinforcement that leads to deceleration as a negative one.

Another aspect of reinforcement is its nature, i.e., what is rewarding to children or to a particular child. A distinction is drawn between a reward that is: (1) extrinsic—that is, the giving of candy, tokens, stars, money, time, etc. (or their withdrawal); (2) social, in the form of praise, attention, liking, scorn, threat, punishment from other people; or (3) intrinsic, in the form of positive inner feelings such as safety, gratification, and competence (White, 1963). These three types of rewards (extrinsic, social, and intrinsic) are sometimes viewed in a developmental hierarchy, both by age and by value system. They can also be used in combination. The task is to find out which is the most effective reinforcer by using inquiry, observation, or trial and error. Social rewards may not reinforce effectively and may have negative effects even when they are presented with positive valence. They may become effective later after one has started with extrinsic or intrinsic rewards. One often sees change or progression in terms of which rewards become reinforcing. Satiation may occur with specific rewards, in which case one can vary their nature and scheduling. The goal of reinforcement is to obtain natural reinforcement of adaptive behavior(s) under the usual contingent conditions of the environment (Homme, 1966).

Another aspect of reinforcement is its delivery in terms of a schedule of frequency and timing. It is usual to begin a program with immediate, prompt, continuous reward in close association with the behavior to be generated or modified. The progression usually goes from immediate reward to delay and from continuous to intermittent. Immediate and delayed rewards can be built into the program so that something now gets paid off later (tokens are later cashed in; time earned may be turned in for a later desired activity). The goal is a gradual phasing out of the rigid, planned reinforcement schedule so that natural contingencies of the environment take over and maintain the behavior (Homme, 1966).

To review, the ingredients of behavior modification include: (1) problem analysis; (2) selection of behavior to be modified and/or generated; (3) obtaining a baseline of behavior on which change can be measured—particularly in carefully designed programs; (4) selection of reward by valence and nature; (5) scheduling of timing and frequency of reinforcement; (6) selection of person to reinforce; (7) explanation of reinforcing person and recipient; and (8) goal of maintaining behavior under natural contingencies.

What are some of the issues behavior modification raises? Many of these problems and issues can be raised and have been raised with other therapeutic approaches as well. In any field in which a given method experiences a wave of popularity, one encounters extreme claims of success without adequate consideration of failures and limitations. Behavior modification advocates prefer to explain failure by inadequate program design rather than question basic issues such as the effects of rewards direct, automatic, and inevitable (Breland and Breland, 1961; Greenwald, 1966), or consider that conflict about success may play a role with particular individuals. One can also wonder whether success in a method cannot better be explained by reasons different from those proposed. Thus, suggestion, novelty, relationship influence, and other intervening factors may play a role. Success may also be more apparent than real with the patient's hiding or suppressing behavior. One can question the selection of patients on which reports are made and from which generalizations are drawn. The selection process may bias the population about the adequacy of controls, or comparison groups. Unfortunately, comparison groups may not be similar in the nature of the problem or in the outcome specified (Gelfand and Hartmann, 1968).

Another provocative issue concerns the goal of symptom removal as a main criterion for success. Here there is considerable disagreement; there are many who question the sufficiency of this criterion. Even if we consider symptom removal alone, questions are raised about the return of symptoms, the replacement of symptoms, and other psychic consequences of symptom removal. These questions have not been answered adequately by behavior modification adherents; on the other hand, neither is the expectation of undesirable consequences from symptom removal always fulfilled. In reality, one observes both types of results. Symptom removal may lead to an increase in the mastery of reality relations and to inner psychic shifts, as well as to a return of symptoms, replacement, or to psychic states that are unbound by defense operations. One should carefully consider the question of symptomatic treatment that does not deal with the dynamic sources of the symptom. However, it is hard to predict what changes will occur in a psychic system as a result of modifying a symptom. It should be recognized that behavior modification is also concerned with generating alternative behaviors and therefore provides a potential redistribution of forces within the personality. As mentioned before, symptoms represent complex considerations; for instance, some are compromise formations, others the result of a lack of stable functions, some being perpetuated by consequences, others achieving an autonomous and syntonic status. White (1964) presents one attitude toward this dilemma: "We must accept the long accumulating evidence that symptomatic treatment can be successful, but we must not overlook the equally long accumulating evidence that symptoms are in many cases the surface phenomena of more complex emotional difficulties" (p. 333). A single paradigm approach to symptoms or behavior is not sufficient but neither can we say that it is not effective on specific occasions.

Another problem which concerns psychotherapists is the way in which latent and inner behaviors and the qualitative characteristics of outer behavior are handled. To emphasize the frequency or quantitative aspect of carefully described behavior ignores its meanings, which one is being communicated, and the like. That behavior may be influenced by inner states is not taken into account. There is considerable evidence that these aspects of behavior are salient and important. Conflict situations, particularly inner conflicts, are not sufficiently considered even though the approach-avoidance paradigm from experimental behavior research is used as the theoretical explanation and basis for intervention.

One can give many examples of naturalistic reinforcement schedules and conditions in human behavior, such as whether one is paid for work by the hour, on commission, or according to piecework, or the use of extrinsic-social-intrinsic rewards in the socialization and development of children. However, these are not intellectually satisfying or sufficiently explanatory. Many other complex motivations are involved in such activities and may be far more important in determining certain behaviors. Rapaport's concept (1957) of the relative autonomy of the ego may be useful in obtaining a perspective. He points to two extreme views of man: (1) one that is totally dependent on forces and images residing within himself whereby the external world view is determined by these inner forces; and (2) another view whereby the inner images and forces arise from the impingements of the outside world. Observation confirms neither of these extreme views. Inner forces, in particular instinctual life, become safeguards against stimulus-response slavely or complete dependence on the environment. External reality as well as the constitutional ego apparatuses of reality relatedness ensure that the ego is not the slave of inner forces. Rapaport discusses special extreme situations in which there is imbalance between inner and outer forces and the relative autonomy of the ego is not maintained. The ego surrenders its autonomy and becomes extraordinarily influenced by environmental measures under situations of extreme need and dangerous attacks on a person's identity. Also, under conditions in which instinctual forces are unusually heightened and in which ego and superego structures do not receive environmental nutriment for their continued stability, the ego is overwhelmed by inner forces and is unresponsive to environmental and reality considerations. Between these two extremes lies the possibility for the environment to influence behavior without totally determining it.

Behavior modification also raises questions about values (Breger, 1969). It often focuses on extrinsic rewards, which some would consider bribery. It also makes use of a system that explicitly and deliberately selects and/or removes behaviors in terms of desirability and undesirability. This raises the issue of self-determination of behavior as compared to determination by others. Extrinsic rewards and the selection of behavior by others are not necessarily used in all programs, but insofar as they are, these questions can be raised. Such value questions pose problems in the use of behavior modification, even though value questions are also present in other therapeutic methods.

In the experience of the Day Care Center there are some situations in which we have found behavior modification useful, and others in which it is not appropriate. Here we consider the questions of treatability and by what means. The issue of criteria for treatment method needs far more emphasis than it receives. It is possible to consider behavior modification along with other methods, as is our practice at the Day Care Center. However, in other settings it is not always possible to offer such approaches in combination. One may have to select an approach for practical reasons rather than in response to specific indications. As one deals with population groups which either have not been served by child treatment and consultation or have not been helped sufficiently or effectively, one should consider methods other than those which have been traditionally practiced (Blom, 1967a).

The following are some of the situations in which behavior modification can be considered:

1. when there is a solitary symptom with little indication of general personality or developmental disturbance (e.g., a specific phobia);
2. when symptom removal or modification is indicated because of the urgency of the symptom (e.g., not eating), because of the autonomous status of the symptom (e.g., enuresis), and when the patient and/or family are symptom-oriented;
3. as a corollary to other treatment going on concurrently;
4. when alternative behaviors and skills needs development;
5. when there is a lack of internal conflict, i.e., there is a need to develop recognition of clear consequences of a behavior, or to present external conflict to the child;
6. as a first step before more extensive procedures are used, i.e., dealing with here-and-now behavior rather than past experiences which influence present behavior;
7. when relationship problems interfere in the development of skills

and one may wish at that time to bypass relationship problems;
8. when there are incomplete and unstable ego functions, i.e., there is a need for structure, predictability, clarity and stability from the environment;
9. in learning situations when there is a need for novel and different instructional approaches rather than for continuing procedures which have failed;
10. practically, when professional help is not available, when resistance to professional assistance exists, and when follow-through is not anticipated.

Some of the situations in which behavior modification does not appear applicable are as follows:

1. when symptoms reflect inner states and emotions that need uncovering, expression, insight, and working through (e.g., grief);
2. when past experiences clearly influence present behavior so that reconstructive efforts in treatment are indicated;
3. when relationship issues need to be approached directly;
4. when inner conflict exists and persists;
5. when the patient displays psychological awareness and eagerness to understand issues associated with the behavior;
6. when goals other than symptom removal or abatement are desirable, achievable, and desired by the patient;
7. when insight is available to the patient;
8. when feeling issues interfere with the actual application of the procedure.

These criteria of applicability and nonapplicability are not sufficiently inclusive, nor should they be considered too specifically. They are presented as guidelines. Some examples of the use of behavior modification from the experiences of the Day Care Center staff may help clarify indications and use.

One illustration concerns Terrance, a borderline psychotic boy of 7, who was diagnosed as autistic. While he possessed language, he rarely used it to communicate meaningfully with others. He was hyperactive, distractible and constantly in motion. In observing his various behaviors, we noted one that particularly impressed us as significant to learning situations and communication, namely, his attention span. It was actually timed at 45 seconds! The problem was posed: could he be programmed for this attention span and would success follow and become reinforcing? At the start of this program, Terrance stayed only 1½ hours at the Day Care Center. When he was given an instruction or a required task, it was always structured within his attention span—45 second bits. Therefore, he received and did 45-second bits. In between times he would crawl on the floor, make noises or go under his desk; but each time when there was an instruction and learning period it was 45 seconds long. We had the managerial problem of containing behavior between instructional bits. Now what happened? Of course there were many other inputs going on at the same time: 3 times a week individual therapy of a relationship type, weekly interviews with his parents, the continuous influence of peer relationships, and others. Slowly, with success at 45 seconds, it was possible to extend his attention span from seconds to minutes, and thereby to increase the duration of the school day. Other behavior became more organized as well. Toward the middle of the second year Terrance spent a full 6-hour day at school, and at the end of 2 years was placed in a public school developmental class. We were concerned about this placement since on psychological tests he functioned in the 90s, which would have made him ineligible for a special class. Fortunately, a public school psychologist, a stranger, tested him on the low 80s so that he became eligible for this program. One might characterize the behavior modification aspect of his program as structured on attention span behavior, with experienced success as an intrinsic reward, and with social reinforcement as a later reward as well.

Another example, Stuart, age 11, was heavy and large for his age. He engaged in explosive outbursts of rage in which he not only was verbally aggressive, but also would physically attack the teacher. We noted that one of the consistent occasions for this response was when his seatwork was checked. Regardless of whether he had more errors or correct responses, the situation had considerable emotional significance. It seemed to mean that he was bad ("I'm stupid") or that the teacher was bad ("I hate you." "You don't like me, you hate me.") Since a neutral machine was not available for information feedback, the teacher returned his work papers with as much neutrality as possible— no encouragement, no praise, no negatives. Stuart was at first puzzled by these teacher responses and would try to engage in negative, positive or mixed interactions. The response of the teacher remained at neutral valence both to the returned papers and his attempts at engagement. This procedure was maintained until Stuart had been able to clarify in therapy the meanings of his being bad and/or the teacher being bad. Stuart had been deserted by his mother when he was 18 months old and had an alcoholic father. The mother's brother (uncle) and his wife (aunt) reluctantly agreed to take on Stuart's care even though they had older children of their own. Unwanted by his own parents and reluctantly cared for by his relatives, Stuart had a deep sense of rejection, experienced as being no good himself and not wanted by others. His anger expressed rage and defended against depressed feelings. As Stuart worked these feelings through more satisfactorily in treatment, he talked about how the experiences in learning evoked his feelings of being bad, dumb, stupid, rejected, and his feeling toward teachers as being rejecting and disliking him. He had many previous experiences in school which had had these meanings for him. He had been referred to the Day Care Center because he was viewed as an extremely dangerous boy. It was later possible to alter the teacher's response to a more natural one and to discuss his errors and correct solutions more objectively. One could describe the behavior modification part of this program as involving neutral responses toward threat/aggressive/engagement, leading to a diminution of these behaviors.

Another illustrative example was from a school consultation about a boy, age 7, who was reluctantly to attend school. In contrast to the 2 previous cases, the approach and understanding were more superficial. Not very much was known about this child except those circumstances which surrounded school attendance; this was the focus of inquiry for the consultant. The school nurse had made a home visit while the boy was at home and found that he and his mother were not particularly concerned if he stayed home on certain days. The mother was more concerned that the school was angry at her and been insisting on written excuses. In the classroom the nurse discovered that each time the boy came to school the teacher immediately asked for the written excuse, which he never had; she would then become angry, and ask him to bring the excuse: it was the school rule. On other occasions she would write notes home to his mother, to no avail. The teacher was concerned about what the principal thought. The teacher and principal had in fact asked the school nurse to investigate what was going on because the boy's mother would not come to school, despite their repeated requests. This had occasioned the home visit.

The approach of the consultant to the nurse was to focus on the contingencies surrounding school attendance. Every time the boy came to school he was met by an upset, angry teacher who wanted his excuse; at home the boy and his mother were not particularly upset when he stayed home; the mother was also angry at the school. The following interventions were discussed: (1) that the principal give the teacher permission not to ask for an excuse; (2) that the teacher become aware of the consequences of her angry responses; (3) that the teacher provide a positive reinforcing social response to the boy when he attended, such as: "Eddie, I am glad you came to school today"; and (4) that another discussion with the mother help her become less angry about school, including the provision that an excuse was not necessary. These in fact were the procedures used: first, the contingencies which fostered poor school attendance were understood, and then the nurse explained these to teacher, principal, and mother. The response to this program was immediate and dramatic. Eddie began attending school regularly. The teacher added another dimension to her response a short time later by saying, "Eddie, I am glad you came to school rather than stay home." It was clear that more was involved in the behavior than was dealt with, but the focus on a specific behavior and on the contingencies at school and at home surrounding it made it possible to alter that behavior. This is an example of altering existing contingencies of a behavior and presenting positive social reinforcement for the desired behavior.

An example of the limitations of a behavior modification approach arose from an observation of a 13-year-old boy, Dean. He was attending a special education school which used a behavior modification approach. This consisted of an individually designed academic program so that a child could achieve 60 to 80 percent correct responses and build up credits which could be exchanged for time in a highly desired activity. School records of Dean's academic progress were impressive in that he had skills that had not existed at the time of admission a year previously. An interview was conducted with Dean that focused on his view of himself and the school. Dean was at first anxious and shy, but when the purpose of the interview was discussed, he talked easily—in fact, it was difficult to stop the discussion. He expressed his feelings about being a "retard," teased by his neighborhood peers for going to a special school. He wished that the school had recess like other schools and that he was in regular school; he spoke of liking and disliking certain teachers; he described his younger sister who could do better in school and ski better as well; and told of his reaction to a schoolmate who yelled, shouted, and hit people. He enjoyed talking about experiences in skiing when he took dramatic flops.

Dean indicated that he had come to this school because he was slow, and although acknowledging that his schoolwork had improved, he denied the necessity of attending. He ignored comments by the interviewer about his progress, and emphasized instead his complaints and feelings. He did not like the time credits: he saved them up so that he could go home. He did like science, but had not thought of using credits for science. Dean had a strong desire to talk about feelings; in spite of outward progress there was still a poor self-image; he tended to deny his problems, using his time credits to escape from school. While recognizing that he had skills available that previously were not there, Dean still had feelings which had not been altered by these competencies. One wondered about the maintenance of his skills following discharge without the continued school structure. In such a case attention could have been given to inner feelings, without having to conflict with the carefully and thoughtfully designed academic program.

There are many other examples: a withdrawn, mentally retarded girl refused to eat until gentle stroking was used as a reinforcer whenever she mouthed objects or touched her mouth; a neutral valence response in a principal's office attenuated the anxiety of a case of school phobia. Tokens without cash value can facilitate a group perceptual-cognitive training activity. A child who is afraid or has experienced failure in social and academic situations may be exposed to stress in gradual doses. At the Day Care Center a contingency at the end of the day exists: make-up time or project period—depending on sufficient performance in the day's program, which has been designed to be within the child's capability of achievement.

Based on her preliminary work with 3 children at the Day Care Center, Camp (1971) has used the Staats procedure (Staats and Butterfield, 1965) with token reinforcement for children with poor reading achievement in the inner urban community setting. The Staats procedure makes use of graded reading lesson plans (SRA) which build on one another and contain several parts: new words, old words, reading stories, and comprehension questions. Optimally, it is used in daily ½-hour sessions. Camp has been able to structure the method carefully, using tokens for correct responses. She has also been able to train, supervise, and pay community workers who work in schools and in neighborhood centers. She has both successes and failures with this approach, but a fairly large number of selected children (about 80 percent of 60 children) have been responsive to it, including some children whose relationship to adults had been seriously disturbed. With the development of some reading skill, a number of children have organized other behaviors as well and set in motion extensions of adaptive performance. These experiences and others have made us realize that while human relationships can be organizing in their influence on children, this may not always be so at the onset. Moreover, it may not easily follow even with a great deal of effort. Many times an approach that originally bypasses relationship and deals with an important skill may have an organizing effect.

Summary

In this presentation a point of view has been presented about the use of behavior modification with children in clinical and educational settings. The existence of polar positions of advocacy and opposition is discussed, and a thoughtful application of behavior modification principles to social and academic behaviors of children is suggested. It seems unnecessary that only a single paradigm approach to behavior be used: in point of fact, multiple paradigms are not only useful but commonly utilized (Marks and Gelder, 1966; Weitzman, 1967). Interest in behavior modification at the Day Care Center stems from the use of careful programming of environmental experiences for children to facilitate adaptation and change. We refer to our orientation as the psychoeducational approach—which takes into account feelings, relationships, and other inner forces of children and their families—of special interest is the development of skills, competencies, and alternative behaviors. While one can question the adequacy of stimulus-response learning theory as the base of behavior modification (Blom, 1967b; Breger and McGaugh, 1965), the contribution of its methods and the central issue of learning in behavioral acquisition and change are important additions to theory and practice.

Behavior Therapy

Introduction

While there is no commonly accepted definition of behavior therapy (or *behavior modification* as it is often called in the United States particularly with children), even among behavior therapists themselves (Eysenck, 1959; Franks, 1969; Yates, 1970; Ullmann and Krasner, 1965), there are some distinguishing features to this significant addition to the methods of child treatment:

1. It sees psychopathological symptoms as learned though this does not distinguish it from, for example, psychoanalysis. What is distinctive are the particular theories of learning employed (principally those of Pavlov and Thorndike) which are all derived from experimental psychology. While Freud's pleasure principle is analogous to Thorndike's law of effect, the intervening half-century has taken Freudian "learning theory" and those theories of experimental psychology in entirely different directions. Freudian theory is mentalistic and has been developed largely in the clinical context, whereas the learning theories employed by behavior therapists were developed in academic experimental psychological laboratories and animal derived.

2. These origins lead to a second but regrettably unnecessary distinction, namely that behavior therapy develops its technology of therapy by the experimental testing of its validity and efficacy.

3. A third though increasingly less valid distinction lies in the *focus of therapy, namely, on externally observable behavior*. While Skinner's (1957) radical definition of behavior as necessarily observable still dominates behavior therapy practice, important new directions are clearly apparent as behavior therapists attempt to deal with internal behavior or make assumptions about it as necessary for execution of therapeutic programs. The inordinate emphasis on externally observable behavior is understandable both in terms of the history of American psychology as it attempted to break away from philosophy, or *mental* science, and in terms of the prerequisite that experimental methods must be applicable to any application of learning theory in the clinical situation. It is clear, however, that there is an increasing concern by behavior theorists and therapists (Day, 1969) with the important but much more complex and difficult to measure internal behavior. This may erode some of the differences between it and psychotherapy, particularly as the latter, in turn, continues to develop its own application of experimental methods to evaluation (Bergin, 1971; Malan, 1973).

Other somewhat but not absolutely distinctive features to behavior therapy lie in:

4. The extensive use of parents, teachers, child-care workers, and other relatively untrained but widely available personnel as primary therapists, reminiscent of the origins of the child guidance movement.

5. The focus of therapy is usually naturalistic (home, classroom, camp, etc.) rather than clinical.

6. The dry, often impersonal, concentration on technique with the underplaying of the role of the patient/therapist relationship (though there are by now few prominent behavior therapists who do not believe in its fundamental importance as a prerequisite to therapy).

7. Concern with, in addition to the more common clientele of child psychiatry, neglected or difficult to treat populations and problems such as the severely psychotic, mentally retarded, the physically handicapped, the culturally and economically disadvantaged, as well as normal children with minor problems of behavior.

8. Limited but highly relevant goals, relevance being defined largely in terms of consumer (parent, teacher) definition of the problem.

Some of these differences, such as with clientele, have been forced on behavior therapy, which originated largely with psychologists in academic settings who felt denied free access to many clinics. While resistance and hostility to behavior therapy were initially quite strong (Franks, 1969) due in part to child psychiatry's early conservatism and partly to the messianiac fervor and frank intolerance of some of the early behavior therapists, there are now few child psychiatric settings which do not have a place for behavior therapy and those who practice it. Some problems remain, however, due largely to the fact that few child psychiatrists, who by and large direct clinical settings, have contributed to the development of behavior therapy, which is largely the domain of psychologists.

The muted but still real power struggle between some aspects of both psychology and psychiatry is likely to continue to be expressed in therapeutic approaches during the seventies, lending an unnatural politically derived sharpness to some of the differences in behavior therapy. Therefore, some similarities should be noted.

In reading the selections which follow, it should be clear that good behavior therapists are first good clinicians, whose practice is as ethical, humane, understanding, and relevant to patient needs as that of any good clinician independent of ideology. Second, many of the techniques of behavior therapy are refinements of long-established clinical practice. For example, there is hardly a residential treatment center which could survive if it did not have some way of isolating and often restraining a shouting, kicking, destructive child. The parlance in behavior therapy is different—"time out"—but the communality with clinical practice in general is clear. However, a note of caution is necessary. While there are necessarily similarities with long-established clinical practice (new knowledge is frequently little more than an elegant, parsimonious or useful transmutation of the old), it is quite naive to dismiss these as invariably nothing more than (simply) old wine in new casks. Some of the differences are real and substantial.

It is clear from the foregoing discussion, that the place of behavior therapy in child treatment is still fluid. It is neither the panacea proclaimed by some of its determined missionaries, any more than it is the apotheosis of evil as declared by some of its opponents (Franks, 1969).

Its coverage of patients' problems and environments for whom traditional techniques are unavailing or uneconomic gives it a legitimate place alongside older techniques recognized by child psychiatric centers. Its devotion to evaluation of outcome add an exemplary quality long lacking in child treatment. However, behavior therapists, like all child therapists, still have a large number of untreatable patients. Just as behavior therapy has helped to reduce the numbers of the unreachable, we must certainly be ready to look perhaps to biological, humanistic, or community and social approaches to reduce their numbers even further. This need for eclecticism and combinations and synthesis of approaches may be exemplified in the sadly neglected area of the combined use of pharmacotherapy and behavior therapy. Behavior therapists need to overcome their intransigence and see this as a promising new approach which will tax the skill and ingenuity of both psychiatrists and psychologists and which needs a joint endeavor for its development.

The origins of behavior therapy necessarily give it both a terminology and a technology which other clinicians find alien, and often, alienating as well. In choosing papers for this section, a number of decisions had to be made. Simple clinical papers devoid of technical terms and experimental strategies could have predominated but to do so would be to do an injustice to the therapy and its present state of development. With several hundred publications a year, behavior therapy as an addition to the treatment methods considered useful with children seems established. The literature is now vast, much, perhaps most of it, concerning children and adolescents, so that clinicians who work with children need to take the trouble to learn its language and understand its concepts and techniques. Thus certain selections are quite technical but with a little patience and persistence reading them can be informative. To assist in this, certain terms will be defined for ready reference.

Conditioning: Learning.

Contingency: The immediate environmental or other consequences of a behavior.

Discriminative stimulus: One which the organism learns to associate with a particular contingency (q. v.) such as reward or punishment or being ignored.

Extinction: Unlearning.

Generalization: Transfer of eliciting properties to other stimuli (stimulus generalization) or behaviors to other environments.

Operant: Operating on. Also the baseline or random level of a behavior.

Operant conditioning: Learning which depends on the organisms' making a choice of behavior based on an expectation of the particular consequences or contingencies (q. v.) of that behavior.

Punishment: Contingencies (q. v.) which suppress behavior. Usually unpleasant or aversive.

Reinforcement: Contingencies (q. v.) which cause learning to occur. Positive if their application causes learning (a reward) or negative if their removal causes learning (not the same as punishment).

Respondent: Behavior or learning in which the organism responds passively to an eliciting stimulus. The response is usually reflexive, involving the autonomic nervous system (including emotions).

Respondent conditioning: Synonymous with Pavlovian conditioning in which an unnatural or conditioned stimulus comes to elicit a reflex (or respondent behavior) by being repeatedly paired with the naturally occurring or unconditioned stimulus for that reflex.

Subject: Patient or client or subject of the study or program.

Time out: (1) A period of time during which the subject is prevented from exhibiting a particular behavior such as by restraint or removal from a situation, or (2) a period during which reinforcement (q. v.) cannot occur such as by removing a child from a rewarding situation. In practice it is often used loosely but too narrowly to mean putting a child in a special isolation room.

An Interview Guide for Behavior Counseling with Parents

CORNELIUS J. HOLLAND. Ph.D.

This paper is a useful introduction to behavior therapy of the operant type most commonly used. It is simple and nontechnical and serves not only to provide a method of intervening and mapping out a therapeutic program but also offers for those unfamiliar with behavioral concepts most of the basic principles in nontechnical language. Missing from this paper are details of recording progress well described in other papers elsewhere (Fixsen, Phillips, and Wolf, 1972; Hall et al., 1972; Patterson (in press); Thomas and Walter, 1973) and many of the other selections in this section. It may be noted incidentally that this protocol and the behavioral approach in general has much in common with the currently popular problem oriented approach to case records in medicine (Weed, 1969) and shows that child psychiatry is just as amenable to such an approach as other branches of medicine.

This paper outlines a procedure found helpful by the author as interview guide when counseling parents for behavior problems of their children. A modified form of the present procedure based on "The Analysis of Human Operant Behaviour" by Reese (1966) and *Child*

Reprinted from *Behavior Therapy,* 1970, Vol. 1, pp. 70-79.

Development I by Bijou and Baer (1961) was found to be readily understood by parents with secondary school educations who attended a clinical group led by the author to teach parents to apply behavioural principles, generally operant in nature, to a wide range of problems the parents were experiencing with their children.

The guide serves not only as method for the interviewer to assemble the necessary data but simultaneously as a training aid for parents, especially when used in conjunction with such a book as *Living with Children* by Patterson and Gullion (1968). When the interview guide has been completed, most of the information necessary for behavioural analysis will have been gathered as well as a selection of the procedures required by the parents to bring about change.

The points for analysis should be carried out as exhaustively as possible before the actual reinforcement program is introduced by the parents. It is better to have too much information than too little, and only with patient and repeated observation of the behaviours and the environmental conditions within which the behaviours occur will the necessary clarity of the determinants emerge. For example, behaviour such as tantrums may be a function of either positive reinforcement or avoidance. Although the topography of the behaviour is similar, it is important to locate and specify the major controlling stimuli, i.e., whether they occur antecedent or consequent to the behaviour in question, and whether they have positive reinforcing or aversive properties.

Not every point covered will be equally appropriate for every behaviour problem. With some cases such as tantrums, simple extinction procedures may be sufficient; with others, such as attempting to shift behaviour from competition to cooperation, extinction, punishment, and positive reinforcement may be indicated and subsequently used in the total program. Nevertheless, it is well to cover every point. Often a complete coverage introduces the possibility of using simultaneously two or three techniques for behaviour modification, and as such, enhances the possibility of success.

Readers will recognize the outline to be focused on the single child. However, other children in the environment present no need for additional principles. If parents experience some difficulty in modifying a child's behaviour because of the intrusions or interferences of a second child, they merely must see these intrusions as behaviours on the part of the second child and apply the same principles to them accordingly. An example of this would occur when one sibling teases another and the teasing behaviour is maintained by the reactions of the second child. In addition to reinforcing either positively or negatively nonteasing behaviour of the first child, the parents may reinforce positively the second child whenever he does not react to the teasing in his usual manner, thus indirectly instituting an extinction procedure for the unwanted behaviour.

A final point should be kept in mind. Although the author believes the outline follows the principles of reinforcement theory closely, the points covered are in a sequence which the author finds helpful to himself. Counselors who wish to use the outline may find other sequences more appropriate. It is also to be understood that the guide does not suggest the use of a mechanical gathering of information devoid of the rhythm and pace found in the counseling experience. The points covered in the guide are logical in nature and are not intended to place artificial constraints on the counselor or the parents. Neither are they intended as substitutes for the more traditional skills of a sensitive ear or a judicious tongue.

1. Have the parents establish general goals and complaints. This step usually presents no problem for the parents or the psychologist since most of what the parents say concerning their child implicitly contains the present complaints (symptomatology) and goals (what the parents want the child to do or become). Usually much of this is revealed in the first interview. Subsequent interviews may serve to clarify, but it is the author's experience that general complaints and goals are readily isolated even though not explicitly stated by the parents.

The above does not imply that the interviewer is merely a passive recipient of information. It is surprising how often parents voice complaints about their children without being able to state clearly what they want the child to do, even in the general way discussed here.

It is the job of the interviewer to make this vagueness on the part of the parents known to them so that they become more definite about it themselves. Some problems with children probably find their inception just in this area, where demands are made by parents without any clear notion of what they want their child to do. Consider the frequent exhortation from parents for their child to be "good" without clarifying the terminal behaviour which defines "goodness" for the parents. An interesting result of this clarification is that behaviour often changes to some extent spontaneously in the desired direction before the parents put into operation any of the specific procedures for behaviour change.

2. Have the parents reduce the general goals and complaints to a list of discrete behaviours which require an increase or decrease in frequency. A procedure commonly used and found by the author to be helpful is to have the parents make a list of five or ten behaviours they wish to increase and five or ten they wish to decrease, and then have the parents rank order them in terms of severity or nuisance value. It has been the experience of the author that a generalized change in the child's behaviour usually takes place after three or four behaviours have been systematically altered so that going through the entire list is unnecessary.

3. Have the parents select from the ranked list a single problem behaviour on which to concentrate their efforts. The behaviour that is selected is often the one causing the most difficulty or the one most dangerous to the child's welfare. This suggestion of focusing on a single problem while ignoring the others is one of the most important ways of bringing about some kind of manageable order into the entire attempt at behaviour modification. Often parents who make contact with a child guidance center feel overwhelmed and confused by the difficulties their children are having or causing. By suggesting a focus on one problem behaviour, the parents can be relieved of dealing with the many other problems for the present. Also by reducing the immediate requirements of the parents to more manageable proportions, it is more likely that any efforts at behaviour change will meet with success. This in turn helps develop confidence in the methods used, and more

importantly gives the parents some sense of control over what they formerly considered an almost hopeless situation.

4. Have the parents specify in behavioural terms the precise behaviour that is presently occurring and which they desire to change. This will require on the part of the parents a detailed observation of the behaviour in concrete terms. By doing so the parents get closer to the actual behaviour they want changed so that it becomes salient for them. Also, when they focus on the actual behaviour, and not on inferences from the behaviour, they are able to get a better idea of the frequency with which the behaviour occurs. It is the change in frequency, consistent with operant psychology, which is the criterion of success or failure of the program.

5. Have the parents specify in behavioural terms the precise behaviour which they desire. This rule is very similar to the requirements of Number 4, but here the parents must articulate in behavioural terms the terminal behaviour, or goal, for any problem which they wish to modify. The task for the interviewer is to help make the goals as clear and precise as possible. Not only is this rule important in terms of measuring the success of the program, but it often reveals the first step toward the goal.

6. Have the parents discuss how they may proceed to the terminal behaviour in a step-by-step manner. It is important for the parents to realize that it is often self-defeating to insist upon the terminal behaviour immediately. For various reasons the child may not be capable of it either because the final behaviour necessarily requires the foundation of prior learning, or the final behaviour desired is of an aversive nature to the child.

Also important is the implication that in proceeding in such a step-by-step fashion the parents are required to make clear to themselves what is the first step toward the final goal. Often the first step or steps are already present in the child's repertoire but are ignored by the parents and thus remain at an operant level.

It is well, therefore, as an exercise for the parents to have them rehearse the steps required by the child in moving from his present behaviour to the terminal behaviour. By doing so, the parents are less likely to insist upon too much too soon, and will also better appreciate approximations already being made by the child toward the terminal behaviour.

7. Have the parents list positive and negative reinforcers which they think will be effective in bringing about behaviour changes. Although the assumption is maintained by environmental consequences of the behaviour, it is not always easy for parents to isolate the reinforcers effective in controlling their children's behaviours. Some of course are quite common, such as candy, but others and probably the more important ones are or may be quite specific to the child, such as being given the opportunity to make an independent choice. But it must be emphasized that discovering a reinforcer as being either positive or negative is an empirical matter for the most part which usually must be tested in a trial and error fashion. One complaint by parents heard by counselors in a guidance clinic is that what they consider rewarding for their children often has the opposite effect. As an extreme example, certain forms of praise or attention if applied following behaviour may act as an aversive stimulus and thus be functionally punishing if the reinforcement history of the child were appropriate. More commonly, what are considered rewards by the parents are neutral for the children. There are, however, good guesses that can be made based on the fact that the child shares a common culture in which certain stimuli take on positive values for most of the children in it.

The task of the interviewer is to determine as completely as possible the total resources which are accessible to the parents or anyone else dispensing the reinforcers. It is helpful to explore systematically the social resources available to the parents, such as praise, attention, affection, or recognition; the physical resources available in the home such as radio, TV, games; and the activity resources available to the child, such as riding a bicycle or making a phone call. A list of these made by the parents is helpful in fitting the reinforcer to the desired behaviour in as natural a manner as possible as well as helping the parents realize the many reinforcers available to them which may be used when any unexpected situation occurs which makes immediate reinforcement desirable.

8. Have the parents discuss what deprivations are possible. The value of a reinforcer fluctuates with the child's being either deprived or satiated with it. Withholding toys, for example, will enhance the value of a toy when it is given following a behaviour which is desired. If toys are given haphazardly, they should not be expected to be effective in behavioural control. The same can be said for affection or praise or any other stimulus serving as a reinforcer.

Many parents are reluctant to deprive their children of praise or affection for obvious reasons even though an indiscriminate use of these reinforcers may actually be doing harm to the child. It has been the experience of the author, however, that children whose behaviour is being modified by these procedures do not suffer a loss of positive reinforcers in the long run; in fact, there is usually a gain when the problem behaviour begins to diminish and the parents are more comfortable with the child. It has also been the experience of the author that deprivation of such activities as watching TV or using the phone are often the only deprivation necessary to bring about desired change. More importantly, the child is usually in some deprived state already. Some piece of sports equipment that the child greatly desired but cannot have at present is a deprived state for these purposes; also such things as a pet, a watch, a toy which the child values but does not have can be considered instances of deprived states. Therefore it is helpful to discuss with the parents the usually many things the child greatly desires but does not have, or is not obtaining as often as he desires.

9. Have the parents clearly establish what they want to do, either to increase or decrease a behaviour or to do both. This information has already been determined from the ranked list of behaviours which the parents wish to change. It is introduced again because in many instances parents do not merely wish to decrease a behaviour but also increase an incompatible behaviour. It is helpful if they have clear what is required for the total modification desired. Much of the success of this method depends on the readiness on the part of the parents to act immediately, either by reinforcing or withholding a reinforcer, and a clear notion of what they desire helps them to do so.

10. Have the parents discuss the situation in which the desired behaviour should occur. The requirements for this step are to determine the discriminative stimuli for the desired behaviour. If, for example, the parents desire to change their child's behaviour from a withdrawn, isolated social style to one of more social participation with peers, the presence of the child's peers would be the discriminative stimuli at which time any increase in social participation would be reinforced. If the parents desire an increase in obedience on the part of their child, the situation or discriminative stimulus would be the verbal statement of the request or demand made by the parents. The behaviour that is desired need not occur all the time but only under certain specifiable stimulus conditions, and isolating these *stimulus* conditions allows the parents to become aware of the precise circumstances in which reinforcement is to take place.

11. Have the parents discuss the situation in which the undesired behaviour should not occur. The behaviour that is unwanted and should be decreased occurs under specifiable stimulus conditions. These also have to be made known for they constitute discriminative conditions for some positive reinforcer which they must become aware of and withhold if possible. A not uncommon occurrence is found when children throw tantrums in stores but do not do so at home. The child has learned that tantrum behaviour does not yield to positive reinforcers except under the discriminative conditions in which the mother will give in to the child in order to terminate the aversive tantrum which for the mother occasions social embarrassment.

12. Have the parents determine a situation which increases the likelihood that some form or portion of the desired behaviour occurs. If, for example, the parents desire to increase their child's obedience, it is likely that sometimes the child is obedient. It is also likely that the obedience often goes unrewarded. It is precisely at these times that the program should focus its initial efforts, for strengthening the behaviour under a structured situation will usually increase the likelihood of its occurrence under those conditions in which it is not now occurring.

Another example would be the attempt to increase cooperative behaviour between sibs who show too much hostile competition. It is unlikely that competition occurs every time the children are together. Those times in which the children are together and are either cooperative or at least noncompetitive can be used by the parents as a situation in which they introduce some structure for the desired behaviour. If the parents know, for example, that a certain toy or activity usually results in some cooperative behaviour on the part of the sibs at least for a while, this could be used by the parents as the structured situation to begin the reinforcing of the desired behaviour. If it were decided that the first step toward the final terminal behaviour of prolonged cooperation was to have one minute of cooperative or noncompetitive play, the parents would reinforce after that period.

13. Have the parents discuss how they may increase desired behaviour by immediately giving a positive reinforcer following the behaviour. This of course is a basic principle of reinforcement theory. The crucial requirement is the immediate application of the reinforcer. The efficiency of this program depends on the availability to the parents of effective primary or secondary reinforcers which can be given immediately. Parents with whom the author has worked are usually quite able to develop star systems or other token economies, a certain number of which could be exchanged for backup reinforcers.

A most effective reinforcer of course is the verbal stimuli of the parents which constitutes praise or recognition. It has sometimes been found, however, that the parents' verbal behaviour must first be paired with backup reinforcers for it to become effective as a viable acquired reinforcer in a program such as this.

It has also been found necessary at times to work out a system whereby any token reinforcer is at first able to translate almost immediately into a backup reinforcer which the child can enjoy. It is often too much to expect a child to accumulate 15 or 20 tokens in order to obtain a backup reinforcer when one of the problems the child is having is an intolerance for delay of gratification.

In any event, the parents should be instructed to give some form of praise whenever they give another reinforcer. Social reinforcers are ultimately more relevant because they are less arbitrary and less artificial reinforcers in the child's broader social world.

14. Have the parents discuss how they may increase desired behaviour by immediately terminating a negative reinforcer following the behaviour. Both positive and negative reinforcement strengthen preceding behaviour, and both can be employed effectively in the

program, although usually the positive reinforcement method is the chief instrument for change. However, if parents insist on certain activities on the part of their children, such as doing the dishes, and the child finds this to be aversive, a relief from this chore can be an important source of negative reinforcement and could be effectively used.

15. Have the parents discuss how they may decrease undesired behaviour by withholding the reinforcers which follow it. The requirements here on the part of the parents are to discover what stimuli are at present maintaining the undesired behaviour, and to institute an extinction procedure. This often runs into several difficulties. The parents themselves may be providing the maintaining reinforcer. For example, a child of nine who was a chronic complainer apparently was being reinforced by his mother's concern and her getting upset. Since she had developed a habit of responding to him in this way, it was especially difficult to have her withhold this reinforcer. Again, children are often systematically taught by their parents that positive reinforcers will occur only under forms of tantrum behaviour which are so shrill and upsetting to the parents that they cannot tolerate them for any length of time. It is important for the interviewer to show the parents that "giving in" after prolonged or especially shrill tantrums is a learning experience for the child leading to a prolonging or intensification of the undesired behaviour.

Another difficulty is that extinction procedures often increase the undesired behaviour initially. In the example cited above with the nine-year-old boy, when the mother began to ignore him, his first reaction was to increase the complaining both in frequency and intensity.

A third difficulty is that extinction is a vastly different procedure from intermittent reinforcement. Unless the parents are made to see the differential effects of each, withholding of the maintaining reinforcer may not be complete and may lead to a resistance to extinction. It is for the above reasons that the author has found extinction to be most effective when there exists the possibility of combining it with positive or negative reinforcement of incompatible behaviour.

The fourth difficulty, and perhaps the most serious, is the fact that often the parents do not have control over the maintaining reinforcer. Another way of saying that parents have lost control over their child's behaviour is to say that the undesired behaviour is being effectively controlled by other people, agencies, or circumstances. Although this situation introduces real difficulties, some of which may never be overcome, a solution can often be achieved by the reinforcement of incompatible behaviour if the reinforcer used for the incompatible behaviour is of greater value to the child than the reinforcer presently controlling the undesired behaviour.

16. Have the parents discuss how they may decrease undesired behaviour by removing a positive reinforcer. This is a punishment-by-loss technique which may prove effective in suppressing behaviour long enough for the desired behaviour to occur. Although many children who come to guidance clinics have been punished often enough already, the author believes such a procedure may at times be the only technique effective in suppressing a behaviour whose necessity to change is obvious. Behaviours such as running out into the street between parked cars, fire setting, and physically abusive behaviour toward another child readily come to mind as behaviours in which the parents cannot wait for the reinforcement of incompatible behaviour to occur, or for extinction to take place.

The threat of punishment-by-loss can also be used, the threat being seen as a conditioned aversive stimulus. It must be discovered, however, whether or not threats from the parents have actually acquired aversive properties, as often threats have not been followed up by the parents in the past and are therefore looked on by the child not as a discriminative stimulus for punishment but as neutral stimuli.

17. Have the parents discuss how they may decrease undesired behaviour by time-out. Time-out is any procedure in which the child is removed from the source of positive reinforcers. Putting the child in his room for a certain period of time or in the familiar corner is a common time-out procedure. It must be carried out in such a way, however, that the child does experience a loss of reinforcers; putting a child in his room where many of his toys are available to him could not be considered a time-out procedure.

Often when a child has been given a time-out period, at least if this has not been a common punishing procedure in the family, the child will react very strongly in a negative manner. It is well to establish at the beginning the time-out procedure as a punishment by making the relief from the room or corner contingent upon a set period of time in which none of the negative behaviour has occurred. If it does occur, relief from the time-out period should be made contingent upon the absence, for a specified period of time, of the undesired negative behaviour.

18. Discuss with the parents how they may pattern the reinforcers they give to the child. The parents should give reinforcers every time the desired behaviour occurs until it becomes strongly established, then they should give them randomly. This is the familiar shift from a continuous reinforcement schedule to a variable interval or variable ratio. There are no ready rules with which the author is familiar to move from a continuous to an intermittent schedule. It seems desirable, however, to tell the child that he shouldn't expect a reward every time the desired behaviour occurs, even when the child is still being reinforced continuously. It also seems desirable to move from a continuous through a fixed schedule before establishing a random one.

19. Have the parents discuss how they may vary the reinforcers they give to the child. The parents will have available to them a list of reinforcers which they are reasonably sure are positive for the child. The parents have options of giving different amounts of the same reinforcers or different reinforcers. Varying the reinforcers enhances the probability that desired behaviour, when it occurs, will be maintained for long periods of time.

20. Have the parents discuss how they may apply two or more procedures simultaneously. Success is enhanced by the parents having at their disposal as many procedures as can be applied to the behaviour in question. The most obvious situation is an extinction procedure coupled with positive reinforcement of incompatible behaviour, but other combinations are also possible and should be explored depending on the nature of the behaviour the parents wish to change.

21. Have the parents rehearse verbally the entire program. This will require that they are able to specify clearly each step covered by the program. Such rehearsal enhances the success of the program by making salient to them such crucial issues as the terminal behaviour stated in behavioural terms, any incipient behaviour present, the initial steps toward the goal, the discriminative stimuli involved, and the reinforcers which must be withheld or supplied.

Parent and Therapist
Evaluation of Behavior Therapy
in a Child Psychological Clinic

K. DANIEL O'LEARY, Ph.D.

HILARY TURKEWITZ

SUZANNE J. TAFFEL

In this paper, the authors look at the outcome of behavior therapy in a wide spectrum of clinical problems and age groups. It thus affords an insight as to the operation and clientele of a child guidance clinic which is wholly behavioral in orientation, and clarifies the many similarities with traditional clinics. Unfortunately, no information is given as to the demographic characteristics of the patient population; thus one should not accept this article as proof that behavior therapy is better than psychotherapy, but rather that it seems helpful in a large number of cases of a particular kind. One of the problems, of course, in child treatment is to try to fit the treatment to the patient and to get away from the idea of a panacea. For example, a great deal of the work of a typical child clinic consists in trying to match the child or family with the right helping agency, so cumbersome and intricate have these become in the average sized urban area. Other parents or children can be given little else than emotional support in intolerable but unchangeable life situations, while for still other children pharmacotherapy is the most effective and efficient treatment. Only a minority of children (about one-third) are ever given psychotherapy in most clinics (Levitt, 1971).

Other noteworthy points are the failure to find a significant incidence of symptom substitution, a phenomenon long used to oppose behavior therapy, and which now seems quite variable in its tendency to occur, certainly not inevitably; and the clear evidence of a warm patient-therapist relationship in most of the therapeutic transactions, an essential component of any treatment program generally ignored or underplayed in descriptions of behavior therapy programs or techniques. This may help to serve as rebuttal to the frequent charge that behavior therapists are irreversibly inhumane or impersonal. Finally, this paper provides a crude but simple evaluative technique which could be used in any clinic and for any treatment. While criticisms can be leveled at what improvement actually means, there seems little doubt that, for many parents, there are clearly definable things that a child does or does not do which cause them concern and which they wish to see changed. This paper illustrates a way for generating an improvement score based on change in these behaviors. While this paper still has what Franks (1969) has called the "we are better than you" stage, many more treatment techniques have left themselves vulnerable to this until they have begun to follow Levitt's (1971) advice to reexamine many of the basic assumptions involved both in patient selection and process and, even more important, address themselves to long-range outcome studies.

Several recent reviews citing a host of studies have demonstrated the usefulness of behavior modification procedures with children in home (Patterson, 1969) and classroom settings (O'Leary and O'Leary, 1972). However, the efficacy of behavior modification procedures in child outpatient training clinics has not been documented. In fact, the authors know of no published outcome data evaluating behavior modification procedures in any outpatient child clinic. Many, if not most, behavior modification projects have been conducted primarily

Reprinted from *Journal of Consulting and Clinical Psychology*, Vol. 41 (1973), No. 2, pp. 279-283. Copyright © 1972 by the American Psychological Association. Reprinted by permission.

on a research basis where the likelihood of achieving success may be greater than would be the case in strictly clinical or service work. For example, many studies with children in classrooms have involved teachers who were receiving college credit or payment from the principal investigator for their participation in the study. Such factors probably make it more likely that a teacher will implement the desired procedures. On the other hand, the behavior therapist working in an outpatient clinic does not have such incentives at his disposal to help ensure that his requests of teachers and parents are implemented. Consequently, it seemed important to the present authors to assess the efficacy of behavior modification treatment procedures in the more natural environment of a child outpatient clinic setting. Since the interns and supervisors of the Child Psychological Clinic at Stony Brook all utilize a behavior modification framework, it was decided to assess the effectiveness of this clinic; as such, this evaluation is an assessment of behavior modification procedures as implemented by graduate students in clinical psychology.

Studies evaluating the efficacy of child clinic services have used a variety of methods for determining clinic success. Levitt (1957, 1963) reviewed a substantial number of studies dealing with traditional psychotherapy with children and used as his unit of measurement "evaluations of the degree of improvement of the patient by concerned clinicians." Twenty-two studies of outcome provided an overall treatment improvement rate of 65%; this improvement rate was almost identical to the improvement rate of untreated control subjects who were defectors from treatment. Gluck, Tanner, Sullivan, and Erickson (1964), on the other hand, focused on problem description by 55 parents in their evaluations of analytically oriented child psychotherapy. Instead of having a clinician rate a child as improved or unimproved, they had the parent describe his child's presenting symptoms six months after the family's last clinic contact. The parents' narrative symptom descriptions were then rated by the authors as either improved, unimproved, or unratable. Analysis of the parent reports of specific symptoms resulted in 54% improvement rate. The present study also focused on description of problems by the parent. However, both therapists' ratings of problem improvement at the close of therapy and parental ratings of problem status at follow-up were collected. Unlike the Gluck et al. study, parents did not give a narrative description of the problem at follow-up but, rather, rated specific problem improvement or unimprovement on a 7-point scale. It was hoped that this study would not only throw some light on the efficacy of psychological services rendered by graduate students but would also assess possible differences in the therapists' and the parents' ratings of the same problem behaviors.

Method

Setting and Subjects

The study involved 70 cases who completed therapy between May 1971 and May 1972 at the Child Psychological Clinic of the State University of New York at Stony Brook. The shortest length of treatment was three sessions; no defectors or possible premature terminators were excluded from the sample. The sample consisted of 49 boys and 21 girls, aged 4-16 years. The Child Psychological Clinic provides free treatment on an outpatient basis. All children except those referred exclusively for intelligence testing are accepted for treatment. As in the case of most outpatient clinics, the presenting complaints varied greatly. The kinds of problems treated included social withdrawal, temper tantrums, delinquent acts, immaturity and lack of independence, academic retardation, self-abuse, phobias, conflicts in family relationships, and exhibitionism. Though traditional diagnostic labels are not used in the clinic, the majority of cases would be labeled unsocialized aggressive reaction of childhood, overanxious reaction of childhood, and withdrawing reaction of childhood according to the *1968 APA Diagnostic and Statistical Manual.*

As mentioned previously, the clinic has behavior modification orientation. In some cases both the child and his parents were seen by the therapist. However, particularly when young children were involved, the therapist worked primarily with the parents, and in the case of school problems, additionally with the child's teacher. With young children, the focus of treatment was on the way in which the behavior of the parents, or teacher, influenced the children's problems. The therapists helped the parents change their own behavior and attitudes so that they could deal more effectively with their children. In some cases, the parent's unrealistic expectations of his child were the targets of treatment as opposed to the child's behavior per se. In most instances, however, change in the child's behavior was of primary therapeutic concern, and treatment included consultation with the parent regarding (a) systematic use of shaping appropriate behavior and ignoring disruptive behavior; (b) time-out procedures; (c) timing of punishment; (d) modeling of appropriate behavior; and (e) the establishment of an incentive system in the home or at school. Other procedures used when the therapist worked directly with the child included (a) direct shaping of the child's behavior in the home or clinic; (b) in vivo desensitization; (c) relaxation training; and (d) direct suggestion. The total duration of treatment ranged from 3 weeks to 11 months, with a median duration of 3 months 17 days. Since most patients were seen on a weekly basis, this study is an evaluation of relatively brief treatment involving approximately 14 sessions per case.

The Child Psychological Clinic is staffed primarily by second- and third-year graduate students enrolled in Stony Brook's Ph.D. program in clinical psychology. Sixteen faculty clinicians served as supervisors for these students. Second-year students received one hour of supervision a week for each case; third-year graduate students received one hour of supervision per week for two cases. Twenty-six second-year students and 18 third-year students were the therapists whose cases were being evaluated here. Fifty-one percent of the cases were seen by the third-year students.

Therapist Rating Procedure

It is part of clinic policy to have each therapist in training rate the status of each of his client's initial presenting problem behaviors at the close of treatment. The ratings are based primarily on a verbal report by the child, parent, or teacher, although in a number of cases additional data were obtained from the parents' records, classroom observation, and home observation. All of these ratings employ a 7-point scale that ranges from "much worse" to "much improved." These ratings were collected by the authors as a measure of the clinic's success according to the therapist.

Follow-Up Procedure

A clinic evaluation form was sent to the parents of 71 children who were no longer being seen at the clinic. The form was sent in July 1972 and was accompanied by a cover letter, signed by the authors, explaining the purpose of the form and assuring the parents that their ratings would not be shown to the therapist involved. The evaluation form itself consisted of a listing of the child's presenting problems at the time of therapy. If the parent wished, it was noted that he should add items not listed by the therapist. The parent was to rate the status of each of these symptoms at follow-up on the same 7-point scale that was used by the therapists. The parent was also asked to rate how much any change in each of the problem behaviors was due to the experience with the clinic (i.e., direct contact with the therapist or consultation by the therapist with the child's teacher). A 5-point scale was used, ranging from "the clinic made the problem very much worse" to "the clinic very much improved the problem." The parent was further requested to use a 5-point scale to rate how much he liked the therapist, from "very much disliked" to "very much liked," and to describe the effect his contact with the clinic had on his understanding of his child's problem, from "I have become much more confused" to "My comprehension has greatly improved." Additional information obtained included whether or not the child was receiving professional help at the time of follow-up, and whether or not the parent would recommend the services of the clinic to a friend. The parent was also asked to describe his reactions to the clinic in terms of the personal characteristics of the therapist he liked or disliked and the aspects of therapy he objected to or found particularly helpful.

If no response was received within one month, a telephone call was made urging the parent to fill out and return the form as soon as possible. A duplicate of the original evaluation form and a second cover letter were sent to those parents who could not be contacted by telephone. These procedures resulted in replies from 65 of the 71 parents. In five of the six cases where there was still no reply, a second telephone call was made, and the evaluation forms of these five were filled out by the authors during a telephone interview. The only parent unable to be contacted had moved to another state without leaving a forwarding address. Thus, data were analyzed for 70 out of 71 cases, or 98.7% of the sample.

Results

The ratings of problem behaviors by both parents and therapists were condensed into two categories—either improved or unimproved. An improvement was defined as a score at or above 5; an unimprovement was defined as a score at or below 4. The therapists rated 140 out of 174 problems (80.5%) as improved at the close of therapy. The parents reported that 134 out of 174 of the same problems (77.0%) were improved at follow-up, and 124 problems (71.3%) improved as a result of the contact with the clinic. This difference between the reported number of problems improved and the rating of clinic-related improvement was not significant.

Since most reported clinic outcome studies have examined overall client improvement rather than problem improvement, for comparison with such studies, an estimate of client improvement was made by taking separate averages of the therapist and parent ratings of each child's problems. Clients were then designated as either improved or unimproved on the basis of their average rating. An improvement was defined as an average score at or above 4.5; an unimprovement was defined as an average score at or below 4.4. Using this improvement measure, therapist ratings indicated that 61 out of 70 clients (87.1%) were improved; the means of the parent reports resulted in overall improvement in 63 cases (90%). In addition, an average rating of clinic-related improvement was obtained for each client. Parents reported this information on a 1-5 scale, and an improvement was determined as an average score of 3.5 and above. Clinic-related improvement was reported by 55 parents, or 78% of the sample.

There was considerable agreement between the therapist and parent ratings: 77.1% of the ratings of the 1-7 improvement scale were within 1 point, and 53 of these ratings (30% of the total sample) were in perfect agreement. The correlation between the problem ratings of parents and therapists was .51 (p — .001).

The data were further analyzed in terms of the age of the child during treatment, sex of the child, duration of treatment, number of child's presenting problems, and training level of the therapist. None of these variables was significantly related to rated problem improvement by either therapist or parent. It is interesting to note, however, that of the children who were in treatment for seven months or more (n = 11), the overall client improvement rate was 100%, according to both therapists and parents. The length of time between end of treatment and follow-up, which ranged from two months to one year six months, with a median duration of six months five days, was not predictive of parent ratings of problem improvement. There was also no overall difference in ratings between the parents who returned the evaluation form soon after receiving it and those who responded only after a telephone call or second letter. However, the parents who returned the questionnaire quickly did report a greater percentage of the highest improvement ratings (six and seven) than did the group who required further prompting by telephone or letter before filling out the ratings (x^2 = 4.1, p — .05). The problem ratings of the five clients interviewed over the telephone were analyzed separately to examine whether this procedure might have increased the number of improvement ratings given. On the contrary, these parents reported significantly less improvement than the rest of the sample (x^2 = 7.6, p — .01).

Almost all of the parents reported that they liked their therapists (95.6%). The personal characteristics of the therapists most often noted by the parents were understanding, warmth, and sincere interest. The specific procedures that the therapists used that the parents perceived as most helpful were setting up behavior modification programs, giving specific suggestions and guidelines to follow, working with the child's teacher, and making home visits.

Discussion

The average improvement rate per case as reported by therapists (87%) and parents (90%) was clearly higher than that reported by Levitt (1963) in his survey of child-clinic outcome (65%). Furthermore, the specific problem improvement rate reported by parents (77%) was markedly higher than the improvement rate (54%) noted by Gluck et al. (1964). While one cannot specify the improvement rate of control subjects with problems similar to those in this sample, the improvements noted are strikingly high, and it is noteworthy that the parents in this sample specifically attributed these improvements to their contact with the clinic, as opposed to simple maturation, in 71% of the problems.

An analysis of the seven cases in which parents reported no improvement revealed that two cases involved attempts to toilet train spina bifida children.[1] Another child is now hospitalized with a diagnosis of childhood schizophrenia. Two additional cases involved reports of insufficient focus on family problems other than the target symptoms of the child, and two cases involved acts of delinquency. In only one of these seven cases, the parents reported that the problem became worse; they noted that the deterioration in the child's behavior was not a function of therapeutic intervention.

While there were no overall differences between improvement ratings by parents who returned the questionnaire promptly and those who required further prompting by telephone or letter before responding, the latter group did report a significantly lower percentage of the highest improvement ratings, and the parents who had to be contacted three times reported significantly less improvement than the rest of the sample. It is obvious that studies that obtain follow-up data only on a portion of the totally treated sample may be overestimating the efficacy of their treatment.

In 10% of the cases, new problems developed after termination at the clinic. This relatively low figure argues against the notion that behavior

---

[1] While it was recognized that many spina bifida children cannot be toilet trained, these children had received a neurological examination, and it was felt that they had some neurological potential for bladder control.

therapy results in symptom substitution. In fact, Levitt (1971) reported that 22% of children with traditional psychotherapy developed new problems ("symptoms") following treatment. It seems best to regard the onset of these new problems following treatment of any kind as simple reflecting that certain problems are likely to occur at particular ages. While it is true that 10% of the clients were receiving professional help at the time of follow-up, this does not discount the high improvement rates; it may simply reflect that further therapy was in order. Improvement rates reflect changes, not levels of adjustment. It should be noted that in several cases professional help was sought elsewhere regarding organic problems such as spina bifida and brain injury, and in one case of childhood schizophrenia (see Table 1).

Given the rather directive focus of the therapy, the emphasis on

Table 1. Additional Data Obtained from the Evaluation Forms

Item	No. clients	% of clients
Added additional problems to the therapist's list	7	10
Child now receiving professional help	7	10
New problems developed after termination	7	10
Recommended clinic to a friend?		
Yes	62	89
No	2	3
Maybe	3	4
No answer	3	4
Was there an insufficient focus on other family problems?		
Yes	6	8.6
No	52	74.3
No answer	12	17.1
Effect of clinic on parent's understanding of child's problem		
Much better understanding	34	48.5
Slightly better understanding	16	22.9
No change	16	22.9
Slightly more focused	1	1.4
No answer	3	4.3

record keeping by parents, and the specific treatment procedures usually suggested, the parent reactions to personal characteristics of the therapists were particularly interesting. The parents clearly liked their therapists, commenting most frequently that their therapists were warm and demonstrated a sincere interest in their child's problems. In addition, some insight was gained concerning the child's problems as reflected by the report of "better understanding" of the child's problems in 71% of the cases (see Table 1).

The results of this study bear on the issue of involvement of the parent in treatment. Love, Kaswan, and Bugental (1972) found that interventions that focus on parent counseling with regard to children are more effective in improving school performance than is psychotherapy for the child. In fact, they, like others (Brookover et al., 1968), found that child psychotherapy failed to result in any improvement in school grades. In almost all cases in the present study therapeutic changes in the child were effected via the parent by having the therapist consult with the parent concerning how the parent himself could change the behavior of the child. The strikingly high improvement rates found in this study, plus the Love et al. results, argue for the involvement of parents in child treatment. It has been assumed too long that child-therapist relationship factors and discussion of the child's problems with the child himself can bring about intended changes in achievement and adjustment. There are a large number of well-documented behavior modification procedures that can be effectively utilized for child problems if one is willing to focus on the parent (Patterson, 1969) and/or teacher (O'Leary and O'Leary, 1972), and the results here strongly imply that such a focus is advantageous in a child outpatient clinic.

The Efficacy of
Time-Out Procedures in
a Variety of Behavior Problems

DAVID A. SACHS, Ph.D.

The previous article discussed reward systems, but like most child treatment programs few behavior therapy programs can operate without some system for terminating seriously disruptive or aggressive behavior. The most commonly used strategy is isolating the child from the situation either by directing him to leave it or forcibly removing him. This is often referred to as time out but this definition is not necessarily accurate and if used incorrectly simply becomes a more palatable word than punishment. While there are two definitions of time out (MacDonough and Forehand, 1973)—(1) response suppression such as forcibly restraining an aggressive child, and (2) removing the opportunity to earn rewards for a specified period of time—the second use is by far the more common. Thus for the definition to apply there must be some reward system which becomes inoperative during the time out period. As the present paper shows, this can be achieved by either removing the reward (e.g., by ignoring the child) or by removing him from the rewarding situation (isolation). It also shows clearly that time out is susceptible to experimental analysis. In a review of time out in children, MacDonough and Forehand define eight parameters (such as verbalizing the reason for applying it, giving a warning, duration, etc.) needing further study. As an example, duration has been studied systematically in institutionalized classroom-based systems. Both these reviews stress that while the usefulness and efficacy of token programs is well-established, they are complex procedures which require much skill and careful supervision to avoid the many possible pitfalls. Both also point out that there has been almost no study of the continuation of the good effects after the termination of the program or the generalization to other environments where tokens are not operative. One of the most extensive documentations of the how of a token system is that by Monkman (1972) which describes in detail one implemented in a children's residential treatment center.

The selection following has been chosen because of its simple and clear description, its location in a psychiatric clinic, and its rather typical patients, all of which should make it acceptable to and easily readable by any child therapist. It also provides an interesting illustration of the necessity, stressed in the introduction to this section, of looking at possible synergism rather than the assumed antagonism between behavior therapy and pharmacotherapy. (One of the patients was amenable to the token program only when he took medication.)

In the past decade, several studies have indicated that time-out procedures—i.e., presenting discriminative stimuli for removing reinforcement of undesired behavior—will produce a reduction in the undesired behavior. Sloane, Johnston and Bijou (1967), May et al. (1966), and Wolf, Risley and Mees (1964) placed their subjects in isolation rooms after the experimentally defined undesired behavior, to remove them from the reinforcing, or at least potentially reinforcing, environment. Wetzel (1966) used a procedure which amounted to having the child stand in a corner contingent upon the undesired behavior.

The present paper presents three separate studies utilizing different time-out procedures. Study I is a multiple baseline study in which time-

Reprinted from *Journal of Behavior Therapy and Experimental Psychiatry*, Vol. 4 (1973), pp. 237-242.

out in the form of physical isolation was provided for inappropriate behaviors and no experimental contingencies were provided for attentive behaviors. Study II utilized removal of adult attention as the time-out procedure contingent upon self-stimulative behaviors. Study III used physical isolation as the time-out procedure contingent upon uncooperative behaviors.

The children in studies II and III were participants in a Child Treatment Center (CTC) for emotionally disturbed children. Generally, pairs of undergraduate students served as experimenters (E). Because the CTC was located in another city, E's were only able to work with the children on a one day per week basis. The child in study I was participant in a behavior modification class on campus at N.M.S.U. One student worked with the classroom teacher on this project, and data was collected three days per week.

Study I: Control of Inappropriate Behaviors
with a Multiple Baseline Design

Subject

Mark A. was a 10-year-old boy, medically diagnosed as hyperactive. He was one of 12 students in a class which operated on the basis of a token economy, having been referred to this class because his behaviors were intolerable in a regular classroom. His classroom behaviors defined as inappropriate were: (1) pounding on tables and walls, (2) throwing objects, (3) yelling at and threatening classmates or the teacher, (4) hitting classmates or the teacher, (5) looking up the teacher's dress, (6) exhibiting himself sexually to the teacher, (7) masturbating. In addition to the above behaviors, Mark showed a variety of distracting behaviors such as (1) squirming in his chair, (2) tapping his pencil on the table, (3) usually attending to task-irrelevant stimuli within the room and (4) walking or running around the room.

Apparatus

The apparatus consisted of a 4 ft x 6 ft sound insulated room, void of auditory, tactile and visual stimuli with the exception of a microphone, which was suspended from the ceiling and connected to a voice operated relay. Any noise emitted within the time-out room actuated the relay producing a reset pulse to a timer. The inside door handle was removed so that the child could not open the door. The room was located directly across the hallway from the classroom.

Procedures

(a) *Baseline.* Prior to initiating the time-out procedure, 25 min observations were made in the classroom for five consecutive days. Each observation period was divided into 5-min segments. The seven behaviors listed as inappropriate were recorded, as were behaviors defined as attending behaviors which consisted of (1) the absence of distracting and/or inappropriate behaviors and (2) orientating towards assigned work, including (a) eye contact with the teacher, (b) responding to questions, and (c) following directions.

(b) *Time-out.* After the last day of baseline observations, all of the children in the class were escorted to the time-out room and informed that anyone who (1) disrupted the class, (2) damaged classroom equipment or (3) injured or attempted to injure anyone else would be placed in the room and have to remain there "for 5 min straight without making a sound." Each time Mark was removed from the classroom he was informed of the specific behavior for which he was being placed out of the room and reminded that he must be quiet for five consecutive minutes. The removal of time-out was contingent on five continuous minutes of quiet behavior. When the timer operated for 5 min without being reset by the voice operated relay, a buzzer would sound in the classroom signaling the teacher to bring the child back to the classroom.

(c) *Reversal.* On day 15, the class was informed that the time-out room was "broken." This was intended as a reversal procedure.

(d) *Reinstatement of time-out.* On day 18, the class was informed that the time-out room was fixed. This was done by the teacher and student independent of supervision.

(e) *Second reversal.* Because of the premature return to the time-out procedure, it was necessary to reintroduce the reversal procedure on the 19th day and by indicating that the room was again "broken."

(f) *Final reinstatement of time-out.* On the 25th day, the teacher announced that the room was "fixed."

(g) *Added controlling stimulus.* On the 33rd day, a sign was placed on the door of the time-out room asking passers-by not to talk with the child inside the room. This study was discontinued after 40 days due to Mark being transferred to another school for administrative reasons.

Reliability data for "attending" and "inappropriate" behaviors were obtained on 8 days during the course of the study and ranged between 90 and 100 per cent.

Results

Inappropriate behaviors. During baseline (a), Mark averaged 23 inappropriate behaviors per 5-min observation. Following the introduction of the time-out contingency (b), inappropriate behaviors decreased to less than one per 5-min observation. On the first day of reversal (c), average rate of inappropriate behavior increased to 7 and decreased on the following day, when the room was "fixed" (d), to an average of one per 5-min observation. Because the reversal was prematurely aborted, it was necessary to reintroduce the reversal procedures (e). This resulted in an increase in the rate of inappropriate behavior to approximately 20 per 5-min period. Reinstatement of the time-out procedure at this time (f) did not reduce inappropriate behaviors.

On the 32nd day, it was noted that university students were stopping in the hallway outside the time-out room door and spending considerable time talking to Mark through the closed door. On the following day, a sign was attached to the door asking passers-by not to talk to the child in the room (g). The addition of the sign was followed by a decrease in rate of inappropriate behaviors to less than three per 5-min period. The data for inappropriate behavior is presented in Fig. 1.

Attentive behaviors. Figure 2 presents the data on attending behavior. Although it never exceeded 40 per cent, it directly reflects the change in inappropriate behaviors which, when reduced via time-out procedures, increased attending behavior. Increases in inappropriate behavior were associated with decreases in attending behavior.

Study II: Control of
Self-Stimulative Behaviors

Subject

Ricky was a 13-year-old boy who continually emitted a wide variety of self-stimulative behaviors such as spinning, handwaving and repetitive guttural sounds. In a free operant situation, he would spend most of his time sitting in front of a Mattel Talking-Learning Machine and jump up and down, wave his hands, and repeat the guttural sounds of the words that the machine presented. When walking across the room, he would frequently spin in circles while gazing towards the ceiling and emit loud guttural sounds. Although the staff spoke of Ricky's behaviors as autistic the experimenters defined them as self-stimulative to avoid any extraneous psychiatric implications.

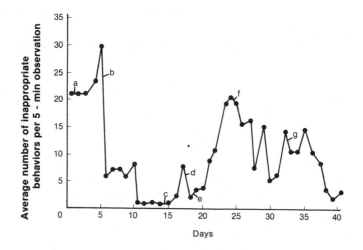

Fig. 1. Average number of inappropriate behaviors per 5-min observation. "a" indicates baseline observations, "b" denotes the introduction of the time-out contingency. "c" and "e" are reversals and "d" and "f" denote time-out procedures. "g" indicates the posting of a sign on the time-out room door requesting passers-by not to talk with the child.

Procedures

Two undergraduate students worked with Ricky 1 day a week for 8 weeks for approximately 2 hr/session. In total, six different procedural steps were used. All of the procedures were superimposed while teaching Ricky to identify numbers, shapes and words using a Mattel Talking-Learning Machine with candy and social praise used as reinforcers. Self-stimulative behaviors were recorded in 5-min intervals.

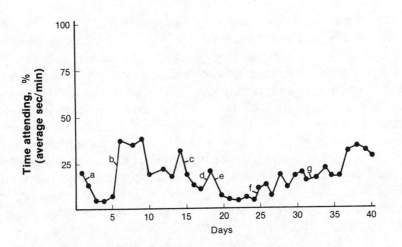

Fig. 2. Percent time attending as related to the presence of a time-out contingency for inappropriate behaviors. The letters in Fig. 2 refer to the procedures used in the time-out study. "a" = baseline; "b," "d" and "f" indicate time-out procedures. "c" and "e" are reversals and "g" indicates the posting of a sign on the time-out room door. No added contingencies were present for attending behaviors.

The six procedures consisted of: *(a)* Baseline observation during which time the experimenters did not react to the self-stimulative behaviors; *(b)* the experimenter saying "No" contingent upon self-stimulative behavior; *(c)* removing Ricky from the teaching machine and having him stand behind a piano; *(d)* having Ricky remain quietly in his seat for 30 sec while the experiementer turned his back toward him. If Ricky emitted any self-stimulative behaviors during the 30-sec time-out interval, the experimenter recycled the time period. Thus the time-out situation was removed contingent upon 30 sec of quiet behavior. The last two procedures were: *(e)* reversal of contingencies during which self-stimulative behaviors were reinforced with social praise and candy; and *(f)* replication of procedure *(d)*.

Results

The effects of these various procedures on Ricky's rate of self-stimulative behavior are presented in Fig. 3. During the baseline condition, Ricky emitted an average of six self-stimulative behaviors per 5-min period. The initial rate of self-stimulative behaviors during the baseline condition *(a)* may have been due to the novelty of the experimenter working with Ricky in a one-to-one situation, which afforded Ricky a greater opportunity for uncontrolled social reinforcement. When "No" was presented contingent upon self-stimulative behaviors *(b)*, the resultant effect was an initial marked increase in rate with an overall increase to approximately eight self-stimulative behaviors per 5-min period. Whereas the exclamation "No" may be subjectively considered to be aversive, the result indicated that, for Ricky, this exclamation was positively reinforcing.

The next procedural step *(c)* was to isolate Ricky from the potential reinforcing components of his environment by placing him behind a piano in a corner of the room and requiring 30 sec of quiet behavior before removing him from this situation. When this procedure was instituted, Ricky began screaming and pounding the piano for long periods of time and gave no indication of subduing this behavior. Because of the limited available time for working with Ricky, the procedure was changed.

Procedure *(d)*, having Ricky sit quietly for 30 sec while the experimenter turned his back on him produced an initial reduction and then an elimination of self-stimulative behaviors. When the experimenter began this procedure, Ricky would start to get out of his chair. This problem was solved by the experimenter who, while saying nothing, pushed Ricky's leg down and then withdrew his hand. Whenever this became necessary, the time-out interval was recycled.

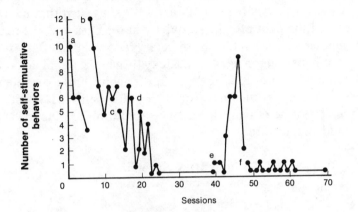

Fig. 3. Number of self-stimulative behaviors per 5-min session. "a" indicates the period of baseline observation; "b" indicates saying "no" contingent upon self-stimulative behaviors; "c" indicates the restriction of Ricky's behavior contingent upon self-stimulative behavior; "d" indicates a 30-sec time-out from reinforcement requiring only removal of adult attention; "e" indicates a reversal of procedure with self-stimulative behaviors being reinforced, and "f" is a replication of procedure "d."

Procedure *(e)* was a reversal of contingencies in which candies and social praise were delivered contingent upon self-stimulative behaviors. Although self-stimulation rate did indeed increase, it was initially necessary for the experimenters to shape self-stimulative behaviors since Ricky had ceased emitting these behaviors in their presence.

The last procedure *(f)* was a reinstatement of procedure *(d)*. The effects were similar to those obtained with procedure *(d)*. During this phase *(f)*, the experimenters also introduced new children and adults to the experimental environment and had Ricky working at a blackboard under the direction of adult volunteers. The addition of a more complex environment did not produce any change in Ricky's rate of self-stimulative behaviors, which remained at a zero level.

An anecdote to this procedure occurred when the center's secretary asked whether there was any means of stopping Ricky from turning off the light in her office whenever he walked by the door. She said that this occurred at least once, often two to three times daily, and her reaction was to shout "No" or "Don't." We suggested that next time Ricky turned the light off, she sit quietly in the dark and not react to him. When seen 1 week later, the secretary reported that after less than a minute of her sitting in darkness, Ricky turned the light back on and at last report, had not turned the light off again. This anecdote indicates how an experimental procedure which proved effective in modifying one type of behavior may be applicable to other behaviors in the child's repertoire.

Study III: Control of
Uncooperative Behavior

Subject

Mark B. was a 5-year-old boy whose behavior was characterized by a complete refusal to obey any requests and/or commands made by the staff. He spent all of his time in isolated play, typically building enclosures with blocks, and would not interact with other children. Any attempt to approach Mark met with refusal, as did non-contingent candy.

Procedures

Mark was seen 1 day a week for 4 weeks for approximately 2 hr per contact. Following several days of baseline observation, the experimenter established a contingency of placing Mark in a 5 ft x 5 ft darkened time-out room upon his failure to obey three commands. Mark was commanded to perform discrete tasks chosen by the experimenter. Attempts were made to select tasks which would increase Mark's interaction with other children by inducing play activities involving at least one of the other children. A command was repeated twice if not initially obeyed. If the command was not obeyed by the third presentation, Mark was placed in the time-out room and was required to remain quietly in the room for five consecutive minutes. Any noise Mark made resulted in the experimenter recycling the time-out period. The experimenter responded to obeyed commands with attention and verbal praise. Verbal aggression and other negative verbal response were ignored, if the command itself was obeyed.

Results

Mark's base rate of uncooperative behavior was 100 per cent, as shown by "a" in Fig. 4. The introduction of the time-out procedure *(b)* resulted in a decrease in his rate of uncooperative behavior. The first time-out lasted for approximately 10 min. Following this, Mark failed

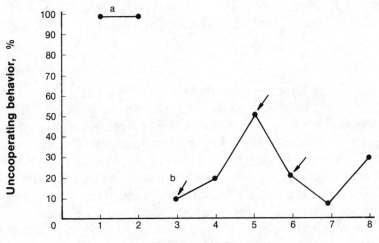

Fig. 4. Percent of uncooperative behaviors per block of 30 commands. "a" indicates baseline observation and "b" indicates the 5-min time-out procedure during which Mark was placed in an isolation room contingent on three successive uncooperative behaviors. The arrows indicate that a time-out procedure was enforced during a block of trials.

to obey only one of the following 24 commands. In succeeding sessions, few time-outs were necessary, and those that occurred lasted from 5 to 6 min, indicating that he rapidly learned both the criteria of three successive uncooperative behaviors and behaviors which would terminate the time-out interval. Although Mark continued to emit uncooperative behaviors, his rate was markedly lower (15 per cent) and the result was his emitting the commanded behaviors approximately 85 per cent of the time. It is possible that the contingency of three failures allowed sufficient latitude for maintaining some uncooperative behaviors since it was the chain of uncooperative behaviors and not merely the simple occurrence of one which produced a time-out. It was noted that following the time-out training, staff reports commented favorably on Mark's increased cooperativeness and interaction with other children. Whereas it would have been desirable to change the criterion to one uncooperative behavior, time limitations resulting from the termination of the Spring semester at the Child Treatment Center made this variation impossible.

Discussion

The three studies reported illustrate that time-out procedures provide an efficient, effective method for diminishing the rate of undesired behavior. Although time-out is often conceived as a physical isolation procedure, total isolation is not necessary. The essential feature of time-out is that the occurrence of the undesired behavior produces a signaled period during which reinforcement is unavailable, and this period is ended contingent upon a desired response. The method of implementing a time-out procedure must depend upon the behavioral repertoire of the individual, the availability of reinforcers in the environment, and the physical characteristics of the environment. If an individual can be reinforced by social attention, then simply removal of the opportunity to receive this attention may suffice, as was the case with Ricky. If social attention of peers proves to be a reinforcer, and if this cannot be controlled by the experimenter (or teacher) then it may be necessary to isolate the child from the environment, as was done by May et al. (1966).

The multiple baseline procedure used with Mark A. illustrates the effect that decreasing "inappropriate" behaviors had on "attentive" behaviors. Although no added reinforcers were provided for attentive behaviors other than those already programmed within the classroom token economy, the presence of a time-out contingency produced an increase in behavior which was amenable to reinforcement. Thus time-out may serve to potentiate the reinforcers that are present in the environment. It was only when the undesired behaviors resulted in loss of availability of reinforcement that the rate of the desired behaviors increased.

Mark A's behavior during phase (f) indicates the need continually to monitor behavior. By conversing with students in the hall, Mark A. changed the time-out environment into a reinforcing environment. The researcher or teacher must be prepared to change his program in keeping with the child's observed behavior.

The possibility does exist that the use of differential positive reinforcement alone would eventually yield the same results that were obtained using time-out procedures. However, an advantage of time-out procedures is that they establish contingencies applied to both desired and undesired behaviors. When only differential positive reinforcement is used, undesired behaviors do not systematically alter the potentially reinforcing environment. Time-out procedures provide feedback to the subject for undesired as well as desired behavior and allow for negative reinforcement of desired behavior upon termination of the time-out.

Application of a Token System in a Pre-Adolescent Boys' Group

JAMES M. STEDMAN, Ph.D.
TRAVIS L. PETERSON, Ph.D.
JAMES CARDARELLE, Ph.D.

One of the problems in behavior therapy programs based on operant systems has been to develop a reinforcement (reward) system with the following desirable features: ability of therapists to give immediate reward in any environment, flexibility for the child to choose what reward and to vary this as the whim takes him, self-auditing, not tied to such unnatural and perhaps unhealthy rewards as candy, easily adjustable so that increasingly more exacting levels of adaptive behavior can be shaped. One answer to this has been the development of token systems which are essentially monetary systems in which the therapist (rather than the Federal Reserve Bank) is the economic czar. A well-known exposition of the token economy is that by Ayllon and Azrin (1968) which was applied to adult patients in a back ward of a state mental hospital. Token systems have also been used extensively with children and adolescents such as predelinquents in a group foster home (Phillips et al., 1971), with disruptive and underachieving children in classrooms (O'Leary and Drabman, 1971), with children with various psychiatric disorders in a residential treatment center (Monkman, 1972), and in various other conditions and situations (Kadzin and Bootzin, 1972). In the case of two important critical reviews, that by Kadzin and Bootzin covers token systems, in general much of it concerned with children, and that by O'Leary and Drabman (1971) covers retarded children (White, Neilson, and Johnson, 1972) where it was found that fifteen minutes' isolation was superior to one minute but that thirty minutes offered only a little advantage over fifteen. Another interesting finding was that the power of one minute could be increased greatly if it were used after priming by thirty-minute periods. In another study (Monkman, 1972) isolation (a time-out procedure) was compared with a system of fines or response cost in a residential treatment center. While both forms of punishment were effective, isolation proved to be significantly more so. These studies may strike some readers as smacking of academic preciousness and obsessiveness, but if one accepts that time out is one form of punishment (White et al., 1972), that punishment is not necessarily antitherapeutic but one form of disciplining, that the use of punishment in attempting to control children's behavior is widespread, and that ignorance of its effects and qualities is vast, there will be less argument about the necessity for the most rigorous study of it.

Pre-adolescents would seem highly amenable to operant techniques in groups. However, the fact that there is only one report (by Gittelman, 1965) suggests that this application has received little attention. We attempted to utilize the principles and guidelines reported by Ayllon and Azrin (1969) to establish an operant motivational system (a token economy) in a pre-adolescent boys' group. This paper will report the procedures we used in establishing the system, our attempts to extend it to academic and social behaviors in the school, and its effectiveness in eliminating deviant behavior in two group members.

Reprinted from *Journal of Behavior Therapy and Experimental Psychiatry*, Vol. 2 (1971), pp. 23-29.

Method

General Characteristics of the Group

The group comprised 8 boys, ranging in age from 10 through 12.5 years, and met on a weekly basis for approximately 1 hour. The group was composed of a mixture of overtly aggressive and withdrawn types. In fact, however, the prevailing mood was one of hostile interpersonal relationships and generally aggressive behavior. Even the withdrawn and anxious children were continually drawn into hostile interactions because of the exceptionally aggressive behavior of two of the group members. Behavior, as ascribed to the boys in the "real world," followed the patterns familiar to child guidance workers. At home they acted out prevailing patterns seen in the group, manifesting aggression, manipulation or seclusion, depending on the modal behavioral deviation of the particular individual. In school, group members showed inconsistent to poor academic performance, with frequent D's or F's in conduct.

Both before and during our experiment with the token economy, the group was conducted according to an activity group orientation. Sessions began with a brief discussion of the plan for the day, with activities sometimes structured by the therapists and sometimes decided upon by group members. It was at these weekly activities that therapeutic interventions occurred.

Characteristics of the Experimental Subjects

In order to evaluate accurately behavioral changes as a function of the token economy system, two boys in the group were chosen as test subjects. Subject #1, age 11, had been diagnosed as "Unsocialized Aggressive Reaction of Childhood." Behavioral problems at home and in school included fighting with peers, temper tantrums and the use of "bad" language. At the time of his group participation he was in a special education class placement for children with minimal brain injury, receiving academic grades of B's and C's. As part of his unpredictable, for the least provocation often led to physical or verbal aggression or both. All other group members were obviously afraid of him, verbalized their feelings of relief on days he missed the group and generally regarded him as a powerful and uncontrollable boy. Before instituting the token economy, the therapists had seriously considered removing him from the group because of his disruptive influence.

Subject #2, age 12.5, carried the diagnosis of "Anxiety Reaction." His behavior both at home and in school was seen as erratic, swinging from extreme politeness and conformity to aggressive outbursts directed toward others. Moreover, teachers complained that he often made loud, disruptive noises and manifested other attention-getting behaviors. Academic grades varied unpredictably from A's to F's. This child was also receiving medication but observable effects were negligible. His group behavior was characterized by attention-getting "stunts," childish clowning and provoking aggressive reactions from others.

Prosocial Target Behaviors for the Group

Table 1 presents behavioral clusters and the "token" values for specific prosocial target behaviors. These clusters were established after informal but detailed observations of the behaviors which seemed to be most disruptive for the group as a whole and least adaptive for the particular members. After negative target behaviors were specified, we tried to restate each item positively; however, it became apparent that many behaviors needed dual specification in terms of the positive behavior expected and the negative counterpart to be avoided. Perhaps this process helps group members to differentiate positive, rewardable responses from negative, non-rewardable ones. After a process of elimination from several previous lists, the items presented in Table 1 emerged.

It should be noted that the group members themselves contributed to this item evolution process and were especially active in modifying the token schedule for behaviors outside the group. Our experience suggests that changes in target behavior lists be made in cooperation with group members for both therapeutic and practice reasons.

As inspection of Table 1 will indicate, the behaviors chosen were specific, in keeping with the basic principles of behavior modification which call for precise determination of target behaviors (Ayllon and Azrin, 1969). However, no attempt was made to specify individualized behavioral programs for each member. Instead, the therapists established an informal consensus regarding rewardable individual conformity to the items of Table 1, thereby establishing a certain degree of individualization.

Table 1. Schedule for Earning Tokens as Positive Reinforcement for Children in Group Therapy

I. Beginning Group
   1. Come to group (1 token)
   2. Stay in waiting room until group starts (1 token)
   3. Good behavior in the waiting room prior to the group (1 token)
   4. Come to place where the adult group leaders are and stay there (1 token)
   5. Take part in group decision about today's activity (1 token)

II. Cooperation In Group
   1. Participate and try in group activities—sports, discussions, hikes (1 token at beginning, middle and end of group session)
   2. Act like a friend—do not hit, pinch, call names or hurt others (1 token at beginning, middle and end)
   3. Try to help people be friends and get along—do not stir up one against another (1 token at beginning, middle and end)
   4. Stay with the group (1 token at end)

III. Cooperation In Group Discussion
   1. Listen to others—don't hog the time (1 token at beginning, middle and end)
   2. Talk about the problem—don't act silly, shout, hit others (1 token at beginning, middle and end)
   3. Make helpful comments to the other boy about his problem (1 token at beginning, middle and end)
   4. Raise hand (1 token at beginning, middle and end)

IV. Behavior Outside Group (as indicated on school report card)
   1. Same conduct grades as on previous report card period
      A, 5 tokens
      B, 4 tokens
      C, 3 tokens
   2. Any improvement in conduct grades (20 tokens)
   3. Academic grades—same and show you are trying (10 tokens)
   4. Academic grades—improved
      A, 5 tokens per grade
      B, 4 tokens per grade
      C, 3 tokens per grade

Section IV, Table 1, represents an attempt to bridge the gap between the activity group and the school room. As is obvious from inspection, reception of tokens is contingent upon academic and conduct behaviors. Though some of the items are rather arbitrary (such as Item 3—"Academic grades—same and show you are trying."), the therapist felt that a reasonably accurate subjective judgment could be made regarding a child's attempts to cope with academic work. The emphasis on conduct grades reflects the therapists' special interest in modifying social behavior.

Negative Target Behaviors for the Two Test Subjects

After informal but detailed observation, two habitual behavior patterns were chosen for each of the test subjects. For Subject 1 these were: (1) acts of physical aggression or threatening gestures and (2) acts of verbal aggression (e.g., "I'll get you," or "I am going to murder you," or "I hate you"). For Subject 2, behaviors included: (1) verbally interrupting conversations between a therapist and another child or another therapist and (2) interrupting such conversations by physical action, such as swinging hands, dropping a chair, or otherwise producing a loud noise or distracting behavior. Before we began the token system, Subjects 1 and 2 were observed for four sessions in order to establish a base line of occurrence for each of the behaviors mentioned above (see Fig. 1). One observer recorded the frequency of occurrence of these behaviors during the session. The same observational procedure was followed at the four base line sessions and at the experimental sessions after the token economy was begun.

Procedure

Initiation of the Program

Before starting the token economy, we explained the system to parents; and in view of the closeness to the supper hour, we obtained permission from the parents for a session-ending "party" with refreshments. Parents were also requested not to send money for the purchase of food from the clinic's vending machines, so that neither appetite nor the desire for a snack would be dampened.

Implementation and Operation of the Token System

At the start of the experiment, printed schedule sheets, similar to Table 1, were given to each group member and discussed in detail. This ensured that members understood the nature of the program and provided an opportunity to clarify questions regarding items on Table 1. The program was fully implemented the following week.

Inspection of Table 1 will reveal that the tokens, consisting of 1¼ in. steel washers, were dispensed according to two basic schedules. Some responses (such as I, Item 3) were reinforced on occurrence. Most of the other responses were reinforced after a fixed time interval, with receipt of tokens occurring at definite periods during the session (after 10, 30, and 45 min of the activity portion of the session). Responses reinforced after the fixed time interval required the therapists to pay particularly close attention to specific behaviors occurring during the intervals. Token dispensation was decided by therapists' consensus during each reinforcement period, and, if any deviant behavior had been noted during the interval, the group member was informed of his infraction and token reinforcement omitted. Though it is obvious that reinforcement after fixed time intervals probably led to many errors of observation, our experience suggests that the system, with the built-in correction offered by therapist caucus, produced satisfactory results.

Most tokens were dispensed according to the schedules shown in Table 1. Occasionally, however, bonus tokens were given for outstanding adaptive behaviors. For example, when one boy returned a token which a therapist had accidentally dropped, this "honest" response was promptly rewarded. Dispensing of such bonus tokens occurred after the therapists publicly consulted and agreed that a particular response constituted an obvious example of desirable behavior.

Token "earnings" were tallied at the end of each activity portion of the session (after 45 min) and recorded on a tally sheet. Tokens were then "spent" for the following reinforcing events; (1) the right to return for the next group session; (2) the right to attend the "party" during the last ten minutes of each session; and (3) the privilege of going on occasional field trips away from the clinic. The reinforcement value of Items 2 and 3 seems obvious, but Item 1 may strike some readers as inappropriate and even risky as a child might easily forego returning to the group. However, as Ayllon and Azrin (1969) point out, research indicates that any behavior with a high probability of occurrence is capable of functioning as a reinforcing event. Since all our boys had been group members for some time, we reasoned that group attendance was a highly probable event for them and, therefore, reinforcing. The problem involved in applying this reasoning to any new group member was recognized and will be discussed briefly in the results section.

At the end of the session each child was required to "pay" ten tokens for the right to return to the next group meeting, and five tokens for the right to attend the "party" during the current session. During a normal meeting, each child could earn 14 to 16 tokens. Though this amount did not allow much leeway, our experience suggests that there is some value in making the child "stretch his budget" in order to acquire Reinforcers 1 and 2. Accumulation of a "bank account" was possible through the child's participation in the group; however, most "bank accounts" were swelled considerably by tokens received for improved behavior in the school situation. Improvement was determined on the basis of report cards, and, invariably, each member earned a substantial number of additional tokens. These were "spent" for Reinforcer 3 (special field trips), for which the number of tokens required was established by the therapists before each occurrence.

Reinforcer 3 was made more attractive by the fact that group members determined the nature of each field trip.

Results and Discussion

For the Test Subjects

Figure 1 presents observed occurrence of unacceptable behavior for the two experimental subjects, under baseline and token economy conditions.

Analyses of average weekly occurrence of deviant behaviors for baseline vs. token economy conditions were highly significant (all t's, $p — 0.001$), except for Verbal Aggression exhibited by Subject 1 ($t = 1.09$, $p — 0.15$). Inspection of Fig. 1 will show that unusually high occurrences of Verbal Aggression during sessions #11 and #15 account for this finding.

Though this grouped data is of interest, perhaps the weekly behavior trends charted in Fig. 1 are more important. Inspection reveals a dramatic and marked decrease in all forms of deviant behavior, particularly on the part of Subject 2. Though our quantitative analysis was restricted to decreasing the deviant behaviors, we can report that competing, socially positive responses (the behaviors described in Table 1) were increasing for both test subjects, while their socially deviant behaviors were decreasing.

Results for Subject 1 indicate that he too reacted rather well to the structure provided by the token economy. The relapses, occurring during sessions #11 and #15, happened on days when the subject had failed to use his stabilizing medication; and on those days, he came to the meeting in a hyperactive condition and grew progressively worse. During session #11 he refused to accept tokens (the only occasion on which he or any of the other children showed disregard for the token system) and proceeded to emit physically and verbally aggressive responses at an increased rate. His behavior during session #15 was similar. The fact that verbal aggression occurred more frequently than physical aggression during both sessions might be significant, for this might indicate a tendency to use words rather than fists, a situation generally regarded as indicative of therapeutic movement in conventional treatment of aggressive children.

Lack of medication certainly seemed to contribute to decreased effectiveness of the token system during both these sessions, and reasons for this are not clear. However, it may be possible that Subject 1 arrived in such a "stirred up" state that the reinforcement system was simply not powerful enough to counteract fully expression of aggressive responses, although inspection of Fig. 1 indicates a decreased rate of responding, at least for Physical Aggression. Previously medication alone had never proved powerful enough to counteract either form of aggression in this patient.

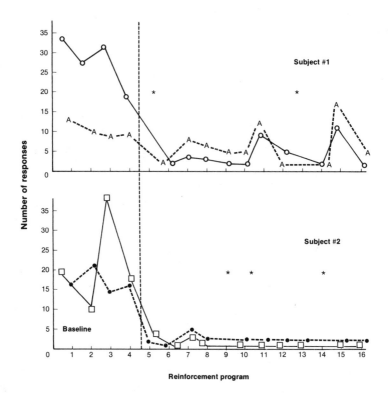

Fig. 1. Occurrence of deviant behavior for two test subjects (O Physical aggression or threatening gestures; A Verbal aggression; □ Verbal interruption; ● Physical interruption; * *Child absent for session).

The group's reaction to his behavior was interesting. In the past they had become immediately embroiled in any aggressive action by Subject 1. On these occasions, however, they made supportive statements and generally attempted to draw him back in the group. Despite their efforts, Subject 1 continued to act out and was removed from the group for a "time-out" period during both sessions. It should be noted, however, that he was able successfully to rejoin the group activity on both occasions.

There are no quantitative data for other group members. Our observations suggest, however, that the token economy system served as a positive facilitator of group therapeutic process. The children accepted the rationale behind the reward system without question or protest, and there was little or no loss of interest in group attendance or group participation. Whereas initially the "game" aspect itself offered some appeal, the children quickly accepted the system as routine and sought token with much fervor. On only one occasion did a boy fail to earn sufficient tokens to participate in the "party" at the end of the session and at no time did any member fail to earn sufficient points to return to the group the following week. Though the design of the study obviously does not take account of previous base rates for all group members (with the exception of Subjects 1 and 2, it is certainly our impression that, following initiation of the token system, the rate of socially acceptable behavior increased greatly, while socially deviant behavior declined.

Qualitative inspection of the trends in report card grades from the beginning of the token economy to the end of the spring semester suggested that five group members had either maintained adequate academic and conduct grades, or had actually improved in both areas. Two others showed mixed patterns, with some scattered improvements. One member manifested little observable change, although his group behavior improved markedly.

Though these data are uncontrolled, they at least suggest some impact on the school behaviors of some group members. We can also report that members presented their cards during each grading period and were eager to point out areas of improvement. Furthermore, at least one teacher spontaneously indicated that two of the group members (both of whom were her students) seemed very aware of the relationship between their school room behavior and receipt of tokens. Her impressions were supported by the fact that one of her students chose to fulfill an English assignment by writing a paragraph regarding the token economy aspects of his therapy sessions.

Nevertheless, Wahler (1969) has recently reported that contingency programs do not automatically generalize from one setting to another (from home to school in his case). This finding suggests that maximal behavioral improvement will occur only when all settings operate with similar contingency systems, and it implies that to be most effective, operant programs should be installed simultaneously in several settings. No doubt any attempt to modify behavior in two or more settings can best be achieved by simultaneous and systematic introduction of similar operant programs in all settings.

Finally we should comment on the difficulty involved in introducing a new member to the group. Theoretically this seems to pose a problem, as the new member presumably would not be "hooked" on the group and therefore might not experience group participation as a reinforcing event. One new member entered the group during our experiment. He and his family were thoroughly briefed regarding the structure and operation of the group; and upon entering the following week, he began to seek tokens as actively as any other member. Though this limited and uncontrolled experience with one case does not settle the issue, at least it suggests that participation in the group might be established as a reinforcing event merely by defining it as such during an intensive family session before group entry. Further research, systematically controlling all other sources of reinforcement is needed to settle this issue.

Behavioral Contracting
Within the Families
of Delinquents

RICHARD B. STUART, Ph.D.

This paper is an illustration of a particular behavior therapy technique usually called "contingency contracting," described in more detail in an easily read little book by Homme and associates (1969). Contingency contracting is one of the more significant recent developments in behavior therapy since it adopts a much more rounded and less mechanistic view of man.

Some may find it strange to read of terms such as privileges, responsibilities, and freedom in a behavior therapy paper, but this paper represents a blend of concepts from social psychology, sociology, and social work plus good clinical sense and judgment. Stuart's prior experience in these fields before coming to behavior therapy give this paper a depth and breadth which is often lacking in the technical exercises of much of behavior therapy. It illustrates clearly the maxim cited in the introduction to this section: to do good behavior therapy one must first be a good clinician. As with other selections in this section, readers will recognize in this technique many of the things that clinicians have always done with children and parents. What differentiates contingency contracting beyond the new terminology is, first, the relating of it to a theory of learning, and second, a greater degree of precision about the specification of the program and the recording of results. However, this paper lacks one of the important features in behavior therapy, an attempt to manipulate therapeutic variables in a systematic way to establish their efficacy. This would be necessary before contingency contracting can be adjudged useful and effective in delinquency.

Any intervention program intended for use with delinquents must first define a specific subpopulation as a target group. Delinquents may be subdivided according to whether their predominant offenses are or are not classifiable as adult crimes, whether they are initial or chronic offenders, and whether or not they reside in environments replete with constructive resources which can be mobilized to their advantage. For many delinquents (e.g., for 24 percent of the adolescent male wards of one Michigan county juvenile court (Huetteman et al., 1970), violations of parental authority and other uniquely juvenile offenses (e.g., possession of alcoholic beverages and failure to attend school) constitute the only "crimes" ever recorded. Many engage in chronically dysfunctional interactions with their families and schools, both of which settings contain the rudiments of effective behavior controls.

A continuum of short- to intermediate-term dispositional goals is available for working with this group (see Fig. 1). Ranging from maintaining the youth in his natural environment, through a series of semi-institutional settings, to institutionalization in correctional or psychiatric settings, the points along the continuum vary according to the extent to which they provide social structure and make use of natural forces of behavioral control in the community. Recent studies have shown that the more potent the influence of the natural environment throughout treatment, the greater the likelihood that behavioral changes will be maintained following treatment. For example, it has been shown that two groups of delinquents, who spent an average of 131.6 days in psychiatric settings or 91.8 days in correctional settings of every year that they were wards of the juvenile court, actually committed more offenses than another very similar group who were

Reprinted from *Journal of Behavior Therapy and Experimental Psychiatry*, Vol 2 (1971), pp. 1-11.

not institutionalized (Huetteman et al., 1970). Even stronger support of the need for community treatment is found in a large-scale review of many rehabilitation programs, which concluded with the finding that:

> since severe penalities do not deter more effectively, and since prisons do not rehabilitate, and since the criminal justice system is inconsistent and has little quantitative impact on crime, the best rehabilitative possibilities would appear to be in the community. [Harlow, 1970, pp. 33-34]

Community treatment for large numbers of delinquents will be possible only when techniques have been developed which (a) are effective, (b) require comparatively little time for administration, (c) can extend family influence to control behavior in a number of different situations, and (d) can be administered by paraprofessionals. It is suggested that behavioral contracting, to be described and illustrated in this paper, is one technique which meets each of these requirements and can be employed as a tactic in every instance in which efforts are made to strengthen the place of an adolescent in a natural, foster, or group home environment.

Rationale

At the core of the effort to use behavioral contracting to combat delinquency are two assumptions. First, it is assumed that the family plays a critical role in the etiology of delinquency when certain dysfunctional family interaction patterns coexist with a paucity of opportunities for acceptable performance in the community (Rodman and Grams, 1967) and when peer pressures are conducive to deviant behavior (Burgess and Akers, 1969). The family may function as a pathogen in two ways. First, the family may model and differentially reinforce patterns of antisocial behavior (Bandura and Walters, 1963). Second, the family may inadequately reinforce prosocial behavior in comparison with the reinforcement of antisocial behavior available in the community. Stuart (1970a) showed that the family of delinquents could be differentiated from the families of nondelinquents on the basis of their low rate of positive exchanges, while Patterson and Reid (1971) demonstrated that interactional patterns of coercion are more common within delinquent families than patterns of reciprocity.

The second assumption is that the family in many instances is a potentially powerful if not the only force available to aid the delinquent in acquiring prosocial responses. Over 15 years ago, Katz and Lazarsfeld (1955) clearly showed that in studies of attitude formation and change the family accounts for over two-thirds of the observed variance. Modern sociologists such as Schafer and Polk (1967) have shown that most social agencies, including schools in particular, are more oriented toward removing than rehabilitating the delinquent. Therefore it is essential to both eliminate the pathogenic elements of the family and to harness its vast power to order to mount constructive programs to aid delinquents.

Behavioral Contracts

A behavioral contract is a means of scheduling the exchange of positive reinforcements between two or more persons. Contracts have been used when reciprocal patterns of exchange have broken down within families (Carson, 1969; Tharp and Wetzel, 1969) or in efforts to establish reciprocal exchanges from the outset in formal relationships in therapeutic (Sulzer, 1962) and scholastic (Homme, Csanyi, Gonzales and Rechs, 1969) settings. Contracts structure reciprocal exchanges by specifying: who is to do what, for whom, under what circumstances. They therefore make explicit the expectations of every party to an interaction and permit each to determine the relative benefits and costs to him of remaining within that relationship (Thibaut and Kelley, 1959). Furthermore, by making roles explicit for family members, contracts enhance the likelihood that responsibilities will be met, and by postulating reciprocal exchanges within families, contracts contribute to interactional stability. Finally, because privileges and responsibilities are fairly well-standardized across families the execution of behavioral contracts in time-limited, high-pressure settings is quite feasible.

- (1) Own home, strong controls
- (2) Own home, weak controls
- (3) Foster home, strong controls
- (4) Foster home, weak controls
- (5) Structured living situation, adults present
- (6) Unstructured living situation, adult monitoring
- (7) Group home (semi-institution)
- (8) Institution

**Fig. 1. Continuum of Dispositional Goals
for the Treatment of Juvenile Delinquents.**

Behavioral contracting with families rests upon four assumptions. First, it is assumed that:

Receipt of positive reinforcements in interpersonal exchanges is a privilege rather than a right.

A privilege in this sense is a special prerogative which one may enjoy at the will of another person upon having performed some qualifying task. For example, states bestow driving privileges upon citizens who qualify for this privilege by passing certain performance tests and by driving with standard prudence. In contrast, a right implies undeniable and inalienable access to a prerogative. Furthermore, a right cannot be denied, no matter what an individual might do. In modern society there are virtually no rights beyond the right of the individual to think as he may choose. For example, people in a democratic society have the privilege to say what they think, but not to shout "fire" in a crowded theater no matter how hard it is to find a seat.

Within families it is the responsibility of one person to grant the privileges requested by another on a reciprocal basis. For example, an adolescent might wish free time—this is his privilige—and it is his parents' responsibility to provide this free time. However, the parents may wish that the adolescent attend school each day prior to going out in the evening—the adolescent's school attendance is their privilege and it is his responsibility to do as they ask. Privileges may, of course, be abused. Thus a parent might wish to know where his adolescent goes when he leaves home, but if the parents attack the adolescent when they learn of his plans, they have failed to meet their responsibility, i.e., use the information constructively. Thus it is appropriate to consider as a part of the definition of a privilege the conditions for its appropriate use.

A second assumption underlying the use of behavioral contracts is:

Effective interpersonal agreements are governed by the norm of reciprocity.

A norm is a "behavioral rule that is accepted, at least to some degree, by both members of the dyad" (Thibaut and Kelley, 1959, p. 129). Norms serve to increase the predictability of events in an interaction, permit the resolution of conflicts without recourse to power and have secondary reinforcing value in and of themselves (Gergen, 1969, pp. 73-74). Reciprocity is the norm which underlies behavioral contracts. Reciprocity implies that "each party has rights and-duties" (Gouldner, 1960, p. 169), and further, that items of value in an interchange must be exchanged on an equity or *quid pro quo* ("something for something" (Jackson, 1965, p. 591)) basis. Therefore, inherent in the use of behavioral contracts is acceptance of the notion that one must compensate his partner fairly for everything which is received, that is, there are no gifts to be expected within contractual relations.

A third principle basic to the use of behavioral contracts states that:

The value of an interpersonal exchange is a direct function of the range, rate, and magnitude of the positive reinforcements mediated by that exchange.

Byrne and Rhamey (1965) have expressed this assumption as a law of interpersonal behavior postulating that one's attraction to another will depend upon the proportion and value of positive reinforcements garnered within that relationship. In a similar vein, Mehrabian and Ksionsky (1970) have reviewed many years of social psychological research supporting the conclusion that: "Situations where affiliative behavior increases positive reinforcement . . . induce greater affiliative behavior" (p. 115).

In the negotiation of behavioral contracts, through a process of accommodation (Gergen, 1969, p. 73), each party seeks to offer to the other the maximum possible rate of positive reinforcement because the more positive reinforcements which are emitted, the more will be received. In this sense, each positive reinforcement offered represents an individual's "investment" in a contract, and each privilege received represents "return on an investment." Therefore a good intrafamilial contract encourages the highest possible rate of mutual reinforcement as represented by the following diagram (Fig. 2) in which CO_{FMA} implies the optimal choice for father, mother and adolescent, $CO_{F/MA}$ the optimal choice for father which the mother and adolescent will accept, etc., and k a value-determining constant.

The fourth and final assumption basic to the concept of behavioral contracting is:

Rules create freedom in interpersonal exchanges.

When contracts specify the nature and condition for the exchange of things of value, they thereby stipulate the rules of the interaction. For example, when an adolescent agrees that she will visit friends after school (privilege) but that she will return home by 6:00 p.m. (responsibility), she has agreed to a rule governing the exchange of reinforcers. While the rule delimits the scope of her privilege, it also creates the freedom with which she may take advantage of her privilige. Without this rule, any action taken by the girl might have an equal probability of meeting with reinforcement, extinction or punishment. If the girl did not have a clear-cut responsibility to return home at 6:00 p.m. she might return one day at 7:00 and be greeted warmly, return at 6:00 the next day and be ignored, and return at 5:30 the following day and be reprimanded. Only by prior agreement as to what hour would be acceptable can the girl insure her freedom, as freedom depends upon the opportunity to make behavioral choices with knowledge of the probable outcome of each alternative.

$$CO_{FMA} = F [CO_{F/MA} + CO_{M/FA} + CO_{A/FM}] + k$$

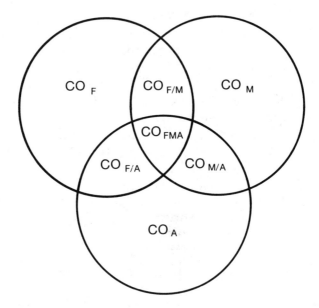

Just as contracts produce freedom through detailing reciprocal rule-governed exchanges, so must contracts be born of freedom, since coerced agreements are likely to be violated as soon as the coercive force is removed. Therefore effective behavioral contracts must be negotiated with respect to the following paradigm:

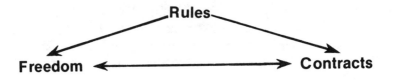

Elements of Behavioral Contracts

Good behavioral contracts contain five elements. First, the contracts must detail the privileges which each expects to gain *after* fulfilling his responsibilities. Typical privileges used in behavioral contracts in the families of delinquents include free time with friends, spending money, choice of hair and dress styles and use of the family car for the adolescent. Second, good contracts must detail the responsibilities essential to securing each privilege. Again, in the families of delinquents, responsibilities typically include maintenance of minimally adequate school attendance and performance, maintenance of agreed-upon curfew hours, completion of household chores and keeping parents informed about the adolescent's whereabouts. Every effort is made to restrict privileges to prosocial behaviors and to keep responsibilities to a minimum. The former is necessary if the family is to effectively serve as an agent of social control. The latter is necessary because the parents of teenage children control comparatively few salient reinforcements and must use those which are controlled with sufficient care to maintain desired behavior. If the number of responsibilities is increased without comparable increase in the value of privileges offered, little or no reinforcement will be provided for the new responsibilities and they are unlikely to be met, weakening the general credibility of the contract.

As an added requirement, the responsibilities specified in a family contract must be monitorable by the parents, for if the parents cannot determine when a responsibility has been fulfilled, they cannot know when to properly grant a privilege. Therefore there are some things which are beyond the scope of behavioral contracts, such as where an adolescent goes when he is not at home or whom he sees as friends. The single exception to this rule is the possibility of using school attendance and performance as responsibilities. While it can be argued that classroom behavioral management is the primary responsibility of teachers (Stuart, 1970b), it is often not possible for a behavior modifier to gain access to *any* or all of an adolescent's teachers (Bailey, Phillips, and Wolf, 1970), so he may be required to attempt to control behavior in school with reinforcements mediated in the home. When this is done, it is essential to arrange for systematic feedback to be provided by the teacher to the parent describing the teenager's attendance and performance in class. A simple card brought for a teacher's signature every day or every week by the teenager is sufficient and very practical means of securing this feedback.

The third element of a good behavioral contract is a system of sanctions for failure to meet responsibilities. While in one sense the possibility of time out from privileges should be adequate to insure the completion of responsibilities, there are obviously periods in the course of family life when this is not the case. At all times, behavior is under multiple contingency control (Stuart, 1970c), and in certain instances it is more reinforcing to violate the contract and to forfeit a subsequent privilege than to garner the rewards of adhering to the terms of the contract. At these times the existence of sanctions may tip the balance of a behavioral choice toward compliance with contractual obligations. Furthermore, sanctions have an added advantage: they provide the aggrieved party with a temperate means of expressing his displeasure. In families without explicit or understood behavioral contracts, the failure of a child to meet curfew is often met with threats of long-term "grounding." Faced with the threat of not being permitted to go out for weeks on end, the teenager is often persuaded to violate his contract even further and remain out later because the magnitude of the penalty is fixed and not commensurate with the magnitude of his violation.

When sanctions are built into the contract, they may be of two types. One is a simple, linear penalty such as the requirement that the adolescent return home as many minutes early the following day as he has come in late on the preceding day. The second type of sanction is a geometric penalty which doubles or triples the amount of make-up time due following contract violations. It is probably best to combine both types of sanctions, making certain that lateness does not reach a point of diminishing return when it would actually be impractical for the adolescent to return home at all because he would incur no greater penalty for continued absence.

The fourth element in a good behavioral contract is a bonus clause which assures positive reinforcement for compliance with the terms of the contract. Much behavior control within families consists of "negative scanning" (Stuart, 1969) or the extinction of positive responding (by ignoring it) coupled with the severe punishment of negative responding. The effect of this punishment is, of course, to strengthen negative behavior as a consequence of the facts that attention follows negative behavior and does not follow positive responses (Madsen, Becker, Thomas, Kosar and Plager, 1968). To counteract this, bonuses calling for permission to remain out longer than usual, extra money or extraordinary privileges such as the opportunity to have a party or to take a trip with friends are built into contracts as contingencies for extended periods of near-flawless compliance with contractual responsibilities.

When behavioral contracts are well executed, each member of the family is assured of receiving the minimum level of positive reinforcement (privileges) necessary to sustain his participation in the interaction. Furthermore, each party to the agreement is provided with a means of responding to contract violations and each is reinforced for long chains of desirable responses. The contract is not complete, however, unless a means is also built in for keeping track of the rates of positive reinforcements given and received. This is accomplished through feedback systems which serve two functions. First, they cue each individual as to how to respond in order to earn an additional inducement. Second, they signal each person when to reinforce the other. Furthermore, the provision of feedback in this context also sets the occasion for positive comments which themselves strengthen prosocial behavior. The exchange of feedback is facilitated by the use of a behavioral monitoring form calling for each person to check off the fulfillment of his own responsibilities (which includes provision of the privileges of the others).

Illustration

A behavioral contract constituted the primary treatment procedure in the management of a 16-year-old girl who was referred to the Family and School Consultation Project by the local juvenile court. At the time of referral, Candy Bremer[1] had been hospitalized as an inpatient at a local psychiatric hospital following alleged promiscuity, exhibitionism, drug abuse and home truancy. Associated with these complaints was an allegation by her parents that Candy engaged in chronically antagonistic exchanges within the family and had for a year done near-failing work at school. Owing to the cost of private psychiatric care, the parents sought hospitalization at state expense by requesting that the juvenile court assume wardship. After initiating this action, the parents were informed by a court-appointed attorney representing their daughter that the allegations would probably not stand up in court. The parents accordingly modified their request to a petition that the court place Candy on the consent docket affording quasi-ward status without termination of parental rights.

At the time of referral, Mr. and Mrs. Bremer were 64 and 61 years old respectively, and both were physically ill—Mr. Bremer suffering from emphysema and Mrs. Bremer from a degenerative bone disease in her hip. Both holding college degrees, Mr. Bremer performed scholarly work at home on a part-time basis while Mrs. Bremer worked as a medical secretary. Candy, the third of their three children, was 20 years younger than her oldest sister. The Bremers resided in a very small ranch-type home which lacked a basement, so privacy could only be found in the bedrooms.

Initially, Mr. and Mrs. Bremer wished to maintain virtually total control over Candy's behavior. They were reluctantly willing to accept her at home but established as conditions that she adhere to a punishing curfew which allowed her out of the home for periods averaging 2 to 3 hours per summer day. Great effort was expended to convince the parents of the need to modify their expectations and to modify a continuous chain of negative interactions. However, when both of these efforts failed, it was decided to execute a behavioral contract anyway, because the problems expected at home seemed less negative than the probable consequences of continued institutionalization and because it was hoped that a more realistic contract could be effectuated

[1] Pseudonym.

Privileges	Responsibilities
General	
In exchange for the privilege of remaining together and preserving some semblance of family integrity, Mr. and Mrs. Bremer and Candy all agree to	concentrate on positively reinforcing each other's behavior while diminishing the present overemphasis upon the faults of the others.
Specific	
In exchange for the privilege of riding the bus directly from school into town after school on school days	Candy agrees to phone her father by 4:00 p.m. to tell him that she is all right and to return home by 5.15 p.m.
In exchange for the privilege of going out at 7.00 p.m. on one weekend evening without having to account for her whereabouts	Candy must maintain a weekly average of "B" in the academic ratings of all of her classes and must return home by 11.30 p.m.
In exchange for the privilege of going out a second weekend night	Candy must tell her parents *by 6.00 p.m.* of her destination and her companion, and must return home by 11.30 p.m.
In exchange for the privilege of going out between 11.00 a.m. and 5.15 p.m. Saturdays, Sundays and holidays	Candy agrees to have completed all household chores *before* leaving and to telephone her parents once during the time she is out to tell them that she is all right.
In exchange for the privilege of having Candy complete household chores and maintain her curfew	Mr. and Mrs. Bremer agree to pay Candy $1.50 on the the morning following days on which the money is earned.
Bonuses and Sanctions	
If Candy is 1-10 minutes late	she must come in the same amount of time earlier the following day, but she does not forfeit her money for the day.
If Candy is 11-30 minutes late	she must come in 22-60 minutes earlier the following day and does forfeit her money for the day.
If Candy is 31-60 minutes late	she loses the privilege of going out the following day and does forfeit her money for the day.
For each half hour of tardiness over one hour, Candy	loses her privilege of going out and her money for one additional day.
Candy may go out on Sunday evenings from 7.00 to 9.30 p.m. and either Monday or Thursday evening	if she abides by all the terms of this contract from Sunday through Saturday with a total tardiness not exceeding 30 minutes which must have been made up as above.
Candy may add a total of two hours divided among one to three curfews	if she abides by all the terms of this contract for two weeks with a total tardiness not exceeding 30 minutes which must have been made up as above and if she requests permission to use this additional time by 9.00 p.m.

Monitoring

Mr. and Mrs. Bremer agree to keep written records of the hours of Candy's leaving and coming home and of the completion of her chores.

Candy agrees to furnish her parents with a school monitoring card each Friday at dinner.

_____
_____
_____

Fig. 3. Behavioral Contract

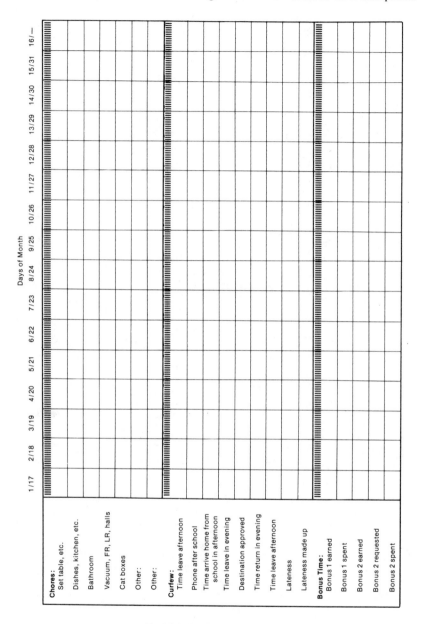

Fig. 4. Behavioral Contract Monitoring Form

as time progressed. Within 3 weeks of the start of the contract, Candy was reported to be sneaking out of her bedroom window at night, visiting a local commune and returning home before dawn. It was found that over a 24-day period there were eight major contract violations, and the probability of an extended series of days of contract compliance was quite small. While it was deemed vital to introduce more privileges for Candy, it seemed imprudent to do this as a contingency for her having violated her contract in the past. Finally it was decided to do two things. A new contract, which was far more permissive, was introduced (see Fig. 3), accompanied by a new monitoring sheet (see Fig. 4), but a new court order was requested and granted which proscribed Candy from entering the communes. Candy was made to understand that, should she be found in either commune, not she but the commune members would be liable to prosecution for contributing to the delinquency of a minor as they had been officially informed of the limitation placed upon Candy's activities.

This modified contract was quite effective, increasing the rate of compliance to the contract terms to a very respectable high rate. When court wardship was terminated and the contract was the sole behavioral prosthesis, Candy's behavior actually continued to improve.

Discussion

Behavioral contracting served as a very useful means of structuring a constructive interaction between Candy and her parents. By removing from the realm of contention the issues of privileges and responsibilites, the elicitors of many intrafamilial arguments were eliminated. When fights did occur, they tended to be tempered by the options available through the contract. The contract itself cannot account for a change in Candy's behavior; but the contract apparently served to assure the use of privileges such as free time and money as contingencies in the truest sense of the term.

The process of negotiating a contract through accommodation of each other's wishes (Gergen, 1969) might have been characterized as an "experience in form" by John Dewey. It appears to have laid the groundwork for a more effective interaction and in this case was adequate in and of itself. In other instances, it is likely that behavioral contracting could profitably be supplemented with interaction training for the parents, tutoring or vocational guidance for the adolescent or financial assistance for the family. The decision about which additional techniques should be employed is discretionary, but it is suggested that behavioral contraction be made a part of every plan to improve the interaction between an adolescent and his parents.

Some Generalizations
and Follow-Up Measures
on Autistic Children
in Behavior Therapy

O. IVAR LOVAAS, Ph.D.,
ROBERT KOEGEL, Ph.D.
JAMES Q. SIMMONS, M.D.
JUDITH S. LONG, M.D.

Lovaas needs no introduction. His work with severely autistic children has attracted more attention than any other in behavior therapy with children and was significantly responsible for making child psychiatry aware of this new type of therapy. Some of his techniques, such as the use of physical punishment and electric shocks described in this paper, evoked a considerable amount of criticism and helped to promote an image of behavior therapy as punishment and inhumane. Lovaas is identified with the most controversial aspect of behavior therapy in children, the use of physical punishment, in this case, an electric shock. As stated previously (in the introduction to the article by Sachs (p. 255), the use of punishment in the management of children is widespread in our society and there is little doubt that "psychological" punishment is used frequently in times of crisis in most residential treatment facilities for children, though it may masquerade under innocuous sounding names such as time out, isolation, etc. There are several articles which attempt to demonstrate that electric shock can be simple and effective, though finding of failure of generalization to other situations as opposed to positive reinforcement is not only well known but is actually predictable from animal studies (Azrin and Holz, 1966).

However, the simplicity, economy, and efficacy of the technique begs the issue. Recent activities by civil rights and consumer groups makes it clear that the present ethos in our society makes this treatment unacceptable except perhaps where (1) it was clear that there was no alternative treatment and (2) it could be predicted with considerable certainty that, if no treatment were given, either severe injury would result (as in the cases of Lovaas and Simmons, 1969) or the patient would suffer severely in the long run.

The danger with a simple and effective treatment process like electric shock is, that like hasty surgery, it can become an easy substitute for diagnostic and therapeutic acumen. Also, it is particularly likely to appeal to governments which wish to cut the costs of mental health and mental retardation services.

This paper has been selected (its original, technical nature and length required considerable editing of the entire Results Section) because of the historical importance of Lovaas' work and continuing interest in the long-term effects of his treatment program for this most difficult and disabling of the psychiatric disorders of childhood. It also gives an overview of the evolution of his treatment methods over a period of several years. It freely admits shortcomings in efficiency and failures of the treatment procedures, acknowledges the roots of some of the techniques in the work of others, and has useful bibliography on behavior therapy in autism.

The first succinct attempt to understand the behavior of autistic children within a behavioristic framework was carried out by Ferster (1961). Ferster presented a very convincing argument of how it was that, based on a general deficiency in acquired reinforcers, one might expect the very impoverished behavioral development one sees in autistic children. The primary contribution of Ferster's theoretical argument lies in the explicitness and concreteness in which he relates

Reprinted from *Journal of Applied Behavior Analysis*, Vol. 6 (1973), pp. 131-136, 156-166.

learning principles to behavioral development. Shortly after he presented his theoretical notions about autism, Ferster and DeMyer (1961) reported a set of studies in which they exposed autistic children to very simplified but controlled environments where they could engage in simple behaviors, such as pulling levers or matching to sample for reinforcers that were significant or functional to them. The Ferster and DeMyer studies were the first studies to show that the behavior of autistic children could be related in a lawful manner to certain explicit environmental changes. What the children learned in these studies was not of much practical significance, but the studies did show that by carefully arranging certain environmental consequences, these children could in fact be taught to comply with certain aspects of reality.

The first systematic attempt to use behavior modification procedures on more general, socially practical behaviors of an autistic child was reported by Wolf, Risley, and Mees (1964). The worked with a 3.5-year-old boy who did not eat normally, lacked normal social and verbal repertoires, and evidenced extreme tantrums and self-destructive behaviors, often leaving himself bruised and bleeding. By systematically controlling the child's environment, these investigators were eventually able to bring the child's responding toward a more normal level of functioning. Tantrum behavior was treated by a combination of mild punishment and extinction. They also reported on certain training procedures that helped the child to communicate more effectively verbally. At about this time, several other studies appeared where psychologists reported success in helping autistic children acquire certain basic and important repertoires, particularly in the area of imitation and language (Hewett, 1965; Metz, 1965; Lovaas et al., 1966a).

These behavioristic attempts to treat autistic children carried with them a promise of help and a certain optimism for the autistic child. This contrasted with the general hopelessness that had grown out of the failure that the psychodynamic therapies had encountered in trying to help these children. Kanner, who was the first person to describe and label these children as "autistic," also reported on the failure of psychodynamic therapies to effect change (Kanner and Eisenberg,

1955). Brown's 1960 study supported Kanner's data that the children were unaffected by psychotherapy. Later, Rutter (1966) provided a comprehensive review of investigations dealing with sizable groups of autistic chidren. The results of the studies that Rutter reviewed are quite consistent with one another and are quite pessimistic regarding prognosis. They may be summarized as follows: (1) Of those children who originally had IQ scores below 50, almost none acquired speech nor received any schooling, and three-fourths were in long-term hospitals at follow-up. If the child was mute and had no appropriate play before the age of five, the prognosis was particularly bad. (2) When marked improvement has taken place, it has generally become evident before the age of six or seven. From middle childhood on, the course has been fairly regular with a continuation of improvement of deterioration evident by then. (3) In almost all cases, there were declines in IQ. (4) Improvement was unrelated to whether or not a child had received therapy. When improvement has taken place, it has been described as "spontaneous," that is, independent of a professional prescribed treatment. Havelkova (1968) reviewed several other recent studies. The results have been consistent with those reviewed above.

In contrast to these very pessimistic observations, the early studies that used behavior therapy were quite optimistic. But since this form of intervention is quite new, it remains to be shown how effective it really is with autistic children. The design of the early studies left many questions unanswered. Most of the studies reported work on single subjects, which begs the question of generality across children. Little if any systematic data were presented on the extent to which the treatment effects generalized across environments, neither were data reported on response generalization. Except for the follow-up data on one child (Wolf, Risley, Johnston Harris, and Allen, 1967), there are no data that allow one to assess how well the behavioral intervention held up over time.

The primary purpose of the present paper is to present some measures of generalization and follow-up data on 20 children that we have treated with behavior therapy during the last 7 years. We hope to provide the reader with an approximation of changes one might expect to see in autistic children undergoing behavior therapy. However, it is also our belief that the results presented here probably underestimate the benefits of such therapy for autistic children because the results were influenced by our extensive efforts at measurement and replication as well as therapy.

We will try to evaluate the treatment effects along three dimensions: (1) stimulus generalization, the extent to which behavior changes that occurred in the treatment environment transferred to situations outside that situation; (2) response generalization, the extent to which changes in a limited set of behaviors effected changes in a larger range of behaviors; and (3) durability or follow-up, how well the therapeutic effects maintained themselves over time (Baer, et al., 1968).

Method

Subjects

We have treated a total of 20 children, all of whom have been diagnosed as autistic by at least one other agency not associated with this project. The majority of the children had been given more than one label, usually also being referred to as retarded and brain damaged. Our experience and that of others (see Rutter, 1966) suggests that there is considerable behavioral heterogeneity among autistic children. Therefore, it may be appropriate to describe the children we have treated in more detail. First, we have treated the very undeveloped children, that is, children who would fall within the lower half of the psychotic continuum, and whose chances of improvement were considered to be essentially zero. Most of the children had at least one prior treatment experience up to 4 yr of intensive, psychodynamically-based treatment) which had not effected any noticeable improvement. Most of the children have been rejected from one or more schools for the emotionally ill or retarded because their teachers could not control them, in addition to which their behavior was often so bizarre that it was disruptive for the other children in the class. Clinically speaking, with three or four exceptions, they seemed void of anxiety, and none had any awareness that he was considered abnormal.

Generally, the children we have treated can be described along the following dimensions: (1) *Apparent sensory deficit*, indicating that when asked to complete the Rimland Checklist (Rimland Diagnostic Checklist for Behavior-Disturbed Children, Rimland, 1964), most of the parents report that their children (a) at one time appeared to be deaf; and (b) seemed to look through or walk through things as if they were not there. Furthermore, many of the parents indicated that at one time they sought professional opinion about their children's hearing and/or vision, only to be told that the child had "normal" hearing and vision. (2) *Severe affect isolation* was a predominant feature. This means that parents indicated on the Rimland Checklist that their children (a) fail to reach out to be picked up when approached by people; (b) look at or "walk through" people as if they were not there; (c) appear so distant that no one can reach them; (d) are indifferent to being liked; and (e) are not affectionate. (3) Our sample showed a high incidence of *self-stimulatory behavior*, that is, behavior that appears solely to provide the children with proprioceptive feedback (e.g., rocking, spinning, twirling, flapping, gazing, etc.). (4) *Mutism* occurred in about half of the children in our sample. These children produced no recognizable words (their sounds consisted primarily of vowels). (5) *Echolalic speech* was present in the remaining children. These children echoed the speech of others, either immediately or after a delay, often giving the impression of non-related inappropriate speech. (6) In all children *receptive speech* was minimal or missing entirely. Some of the children would obey simple commands (such as "sit down," or "close the door"), but *all* failed to respond appropriately to more complex demands involving abstract terms such as prepositions, pronouns, and time. Most often they responded to speech in a very generalized manner. For example, they would close the door when they heard the command, "Close the door," as well as when they heard commands like "Point to the door," or statements such as "There is a window and a door," etc. (7) There was also an absence of, or only minimal presence of, *social and self-help behaviors*. For instance, most of the children could not dress themselves; most were unaware of common dangers (e.g., crossing the street in front of oncoming cars); most could not wash themselves or comb their hair; some were not toilet trained, etc. (8) A small number of these children were *self-destructive* or self-mutilatory. All displayed severe aggressive, tantrumous outbursts, scratching and biting attending adults when forced to comply with even minimal rules for social conduct. Some smeared their feces.

Treatment

When one decides to treat a child within a reinforcement theory paradigm, then one can facilitate the behavioral development of autistic children in two ways. One way would be to concentrate efforts on facilitating the autistic child's acquisition of social reinforcers, rather than on building behaviors. If his developmental failure was based on a deficiency in social and other secondary reinforcers, as Ferster claimed it was, then an intervention at this level would seem to strike at the base of the problem. A treatment program centered on the establishment of a normal hierarchy of social reinforcers would give the child's everyday social environment (his parents, teachers, peers, etc.) the tools with which to build and modify the myriad behaviors necessary for the child to function effectively within the environment. In a sense, the person's behavioral changes would "take care of themselves," provided that he returned from treatment to a normal environment with a normal reinforcement hierarchy.

When we first began to treat autistic children, we explored this alternative of enriching and normalizing reinforcing stimuli for these children. We did succeed at establishing certain social stimuli as reinforcing, using either pain reduction (Lovaas et al., 1965b) or food presentations (Lovaas et al., 1966b). Although we produced some durable reinforcers, they were too discriminated (situational) and the procedures too cumbersome to be of much practical significance.

We turned, therefore, to the second alternative: building behaviors directly relying on already effective, largely primary reinforcers such as food, essentially circumventing social stimuli. The use of primary reinforcement has several disadvantages, as compared to social, secondary ones. For example, in using primary reinforcers, special environments need to be established to develop and maintain the new behaviors. Since we have inadequate information about how to construct such environments, the gains that the child may make would probably fall short of the ideal. Despite these restrictions, however, it is worthwhile to assess how much one can accomplish using a limited range of reinforcers. Therefore, we describe the program we did develop.

Because the children were replete with interfering self-stimulatory, self-destructive and/or tantrum behavior when they entered treatment, we immediately attempted to reduce the frequency of such behavior. The procedures employed to extinguish and suppress pathological behavior (including biting and scratching of self and others, feces smearing, etc.) rely heavily on several operations: (1) contingent reinforcement withdrawal, that is, the adult simply looked away from the child when he was engaged in undesirable behavior, left the child in his room, or placed the child in an isolation room (separate from the treatment room); (2) contingent aversive stimulation, for example a slap or painful electric shock; or (3) reinforcement of incompatible behavior, such as sitting quietly on a chair. The rationale for the suppression of self-stimulatory behavior lies in the observations we have made indicating an apparent attenuation of the child's responsivity while he is engaged in self-stimulation (Lovaas, Litrownik, and Mann, 1971). Simply stated, when the child is engaged in self-stimulation, it is difficult to teach him something else. The reasons for suppressing self-destruction, feces smearing, etc., are perhaps obvious, and our intervention model does not prescribe the therapeutic benefits of their expression. A detailed presentation of data and method for suppression of self-destruction may be found in Lovaas and Simmons (1969).

Simultaneously with the suppression of undesirable behavior, the therapist attempted to establish a kind of primitive stimulus control. Usually, the therapist demanded some simple behavior from the child, such as looking at the therapist, or sitting down when the therapist asked. These behaviors could be easily prompted if the child did not already know how to respond. Usually, the therapist's first attempts to establish stimulus control elicited tantrumous and self-destructive behavior; therefore, we combined the suppression of undesirable behavior with the attempt to establish stimulus control.

Once these introductory steps had been taken, we introduced our central training program in which language training alone consumed about 80% of the child's total training. The heavy emphasis on language training was undertaken partly for academic reasons. We wanted to know how much could be accomplished using operant procedures. This was not necessarily the most beneficial therapeutic approach for all the children. Many of them have benefited more from a program emphasizing non-verbal communication.

If the child was echolalic (or once a mute child had about 10 imitative words), we introduced a program designed to make speech meaningful and functional. For example, as soon as a child was taught the label for a particular food, he could eat only if he asked for the food by name. The child was gradually moved through a series of steps designed to establish increasingly proficient use of language, including training in semantics, such as use of abstract terms (pronouns, time, etc.), and syntax, such as the correct use of tense, etc. Some of the latter levels were never reached by the mute children, but were usually obtained with the echolalics. A more detailed description of the language program exists on film (Lovaas, 1969) and in written outline (Lovaas, in preparation).

At the same time we were involved in building speech, we also initiated programs designed to facilitate the acquisition of other social and self-help skills. These programs focused on those behaviors that made the child easier to live with, such as friendly greetings and other indications of affection, as well as dressing, good table manners, brushing the teeth, etc. We have outlined a procedure based on non-verbal imitation (Lovaas et al., 1967) that has been particularly useful for these purposes.

Throughout, there was an emphasis in making the child look as normal as possible, rewarding him for normal behavior and punishing his psychotic behavior, teaching him to please his parents and us, to be grateful for what we would do for him, to be afraid of us when we were angry, and pleased when we were happy. Adults were in control. In short, we attempted to teach these children what parents of the middle-class Western world attempt to teach theirs. There are, of course, many questions that one may have about these values, but faced with primitive psychotic children, these seem rather secure and comforting as initial goals.

We selected reinforcers on the basis of their value for a particular child. Many children would work only for food and required an occasional slap on the buttocks if the therapist was to control undesirable interfering behavior. For other children, symbolic approval and disapproval were effective in maintaining the child's behavior throughout the working sessions. As we became familiar with the idiosyncracies of the various children, the reinforcers seemed easily accessible and their selection was fairly simple, despite their limited range. However, scheduling these reinforcers was a much more difficult task. A relatively untrained person can build simple behaviors, like eye-to-face contact or raise the frequency of vocal behavior. But it is unlikely that a person will be able to build complex speech unless he is familiar with discrimination learning procedures. Most people who work with autistic children are not. Therefore, it seems likely that there will be few studies in the near future to replicate the present one.

Measurement

We have employed two measures of generalization of change during treatment. First, we have attempted to assess changes in the children's behavior using a *multiple-response recording*. Secondly, we have assessed changes in the children's Stanford Binet and Vineland Social Maturity scores. The multiple-response recordings constitute the main focus of our measures and were designed to provide information both on stimulus and response generalization. The Stanford Binet and Vineland do provide similar measures, but they give less specific information. We shall first present a description of the multiple-response recordings.

Multiple-response recordings. We have previously published (Lovaas et al., 1965a) information on apparatus that allows for simultaneous recordings of several commonly occurring and everyday behaviors in free-play/observation settings. Essentially, certain behaviors (both normal and pathological) are defined for an observer who records their frequency and duration on a button-panel, which in turn is coupled to a computer tape, allowing swift calculation of the frequency, duration, and interaction of the various behaviors.

The kind of child one is studying helps decide what kinds of behaviors to record. In the case of severely psychotic children, this is somewhat simplified because of their limited behavioral repertoires. We eventually selected five behavioral categories. The presence or absence of behaviors in these categories are used to describe autistic children, and we have found they can reliably be recorded. (1) *Self-stimulation*, which denotes the stereotyped repetitive behavior that appeared only to provide the child with proprioceptive feedback (e.g., rocking, spinning, twirling, flapping, gazing, etc.). (2) *Echolalic speech*, which was defined as the child's echoing the speech of others, either immediately or after a delay, giving the impression of non-related inappropriate speech, with pronoun reversal, incorrect use of tense, etc. We also included bizarre words and word combinations in this category. (3) *Appropriate speech*, which was defined as speech related to an appropriate context, understandable, and grammatically correct. (4) *Social non-verbal behavior*, which denoted appropriate non-verbal behavior that is dependent upon cues given by another person for its initiation or completion (e.g., responding to requests, imitating, etc.). (5) *Appropriate play*, which denoted the use of toys and objects in an appropriate age-related manner.

Two of these behaviors (self-stimulation and echolalia) are pathological. Their presence, and the relative absence of the remaining three "normal" behaviors, forms part of the behavioral complex diagnostic of autism.

The multiple-response measures do to some extent assess response generalization. That is, many of the behaviors we did score (particularly social non-verbal and play) were not specifically taught during treatment. But we had no way of knowing exactly how much of these behaviors were new and novel by the child, so that the recordings are not pure measures of response generalization. The measures do, however, lend themselves well to studies on stimulus generalization.

To assess stimulus generalization, the children were observed in a room separate from, and not associated with, the training situation and in the company of an unfamiliar adult. The room was equipped, like most playrooms, with the following toys: a wagon, paper and crayons, a bobo doll, a 9-in. rubber ball, three plastic bowling pins, a plastic telephone, a magnetic board with numbers and letters that attach to it, 12 assorted wooden blocks, a 6-in. tom-tom drum, a hand puppet, and three simple wooden jigsaw puzzles. The child was observed in this room during sessions lasting 35 min each. In the first condition (the Alone condition), the child was observed by himself in the playroom. In the second condition (the Attending condition), an unfamiliar adult was present and attended visually to the child, but made no comment, interfered in no way, and did not initiate any interaction with the child. If on the other hand, the child initiated some activity that required the involvement of the adult, the adult performed those responses and made whatever comments necessary to complete the interaction. In the final condition (the Inviting condition), the adult encouraged the child to participate in several different kinds of activities. The adult invited the child to play with each of the 11 toys in the playroom in succession (1 min per toy), giving demonstrations of how to use the toy if the child appeared not to know how. The adult also attempted to initiate a simple game of "patticake" for 1 min. He also gave the child a 1-min series of simple commands that could be performed non-verbally, such as "Stand on one foot," "Touch the floor," and "Sit down." Next, the adult asked a 1-min series of questions which could be answered either verbally or non-verbally. This series consisted of questions such as "Where is your nose?" or "Which block is bigger?" A final 1-min series of questions, which could only be answered verbally, was also asked. This series consisted of questions such as "How are you?" or "Where do you live?"

We have multiple-response measures on only 13 of the 20 children we have treated. This is so because we initially had considered these measures to be inappropriate for outpatients, since we had less control over their treatment. Since 1968, however, we have obtained multiple-response measures on the outpatients as well.

The first four children (Ricky, Pam, Billy, and Chuck) for whom we have multiple-response recordings received a "before" measure (in June, 1964) and recordings were then made on a monthly basis for the 14-month duration of their treatment. Pam and Ricky were discharged immediately to a local state hospital, while Billy and Chuck spent a short time (less than 6 months) with their families before being hospitalized in the same hospital. Pam and Rick were returned to us for follow-up measures 2 yr later (1968). They were then briefly treated once more (24 hr for Ricky and one month for Pam), discharged to the state hospital again, and finally returned for a second follow-up 2 yr after that (1970). Pam and Rick received our treatment twice, interspersed by a period of no behavior therapy treatment; Billy and Chuck were treated once, but measured again 4 yr after discharge from our project (1970); they received an ABA design.

We replicated essentials of the treatment on a second group of children (Jose, Michael, and Taylor) who were hospitalized in 1965 and received 12 months of treatment, with multiple response measures before treatment and at 3-month intervals during treatment. They were returned for follow-up measures 3 yr after treatment (in 1970).

The third group (Leslie, Tito, and Seth) to receive the multiple-response recordings were seen as outpatients. They were measured before treatment (1968) and after 1 yr of treatment, and received follow-up measurements 1 yr later (1970).

A fourth group (Kevin, Ann, and James) to receive multiple-response recordings was also seen as outpatients. Measures were taken before treatment (1969), after 1 yr of treatment (1970), and with follow-up measures in 1972.

The first and second groups of children were inpatients. They received 8 hr of treatment per day, 6 to 7 seven days a week. The parents of the first group were not involved in the treatment. With the second group, however, we began to train the parents in our treatment procedures. The third and fourth groups were outpatients, and while we initiated training programs in the clinic, we otherwise served essentially as consultants (2 to 3 hr a week) to the parents, training them in shaping procedures.

Discharge procedures for these children differ for each individual case, depending on the rate of progress by the child, the skill of the mother as a therapist, and the prospects for enrolling the child in a special school. In general, our approach was gradually to phase the children out of the program. We decreased the number of sessions from three per week to once a month. After the child was officially discharged, a therapist visited the home several times during the first few months. Generally, by this time the parents had found a school placement for the child and our involvement became minimal. Parents were encouraged to call us when they encountered difficulties, and we spoke to them from time to time informally discussing the child's progress. Often, the therapist visited the school and discussed the child's case with the teacher, suggesting ways he might find effective in dealing with the child and encouraging the teacher to call on us if he encountered any difficulties.

The basic rationale for changing the treatment procedure from treating inpatients, with the parents as observers, to treating outpatients with the parents as therapists, became apparent from examination of the follow-up data.

Intelligence and social maturity. The Stanford Binet Intelligence Scale was administered before and after treatment either by an agency not associated with UCLA, or when this was not feasible, by a graduate student trainee in the UCLA Psychology Clinic. Nineteen of the 20 children received IQ testing. One child, Taylor, received the Merrill-Palmer Intelligence Test instead of the Stanford Binet. We will also present some data from the Vineland Social Maturity Scale, which was administered to the parents of the last 14 of the 20 children. The irregularities in the number of children who received the various tests does not reflect a systematic bias. Rather, in the early phases of the program we did not consider generalization and follow-up data to be significant data for our study.

Discussion

In summary, the major results of this study are that: (1) inappropriate behaviors (self-stimulation and echolalia) decreased during treatment, and appropriate behaviors (appropriate speech, appropriate play, and social non-verbal behaviors) increased; (2) spontaneous social interactions and the spontaneous use of language occurred about 8 months into treatment for some of the children; (3) IQs and social quotients reflected improvement during treatment; (4) there were no exceptions to the improvement, however, some of the children improved more than others; (5) follow-up measures recorded 1 to 4 yr after treatment indicated that large differences between groups of children were related to the post-treatment environment (those groups whose parents were trained to carry out behavior therapy continued to improve, while children who were institutionalized regressed); (6) a brief reinstatement of behavior therapy could temporarily reestablish some of the original therapeutic gains made by the children who were subsequently institutionalized; and (7) the technique utilized for recording therapeutic change was reliable. Observers were trained to be able to recognize and record specific behaviors, the presence or absence of which may be considered diagnostic of autism.

Individual Differences

While the major findings listed above characterize each of the children in the group, there has been considerable heterogeneity with respect to the degree of improvement shown by each child. The delineation of "autism" is one area that will demand considerably more work. It has not been a particularly useful diagnosis. Few people agree on when to apply it. It is not a functional term in the sense that it is neither related to a particular etiology nor to a particular treatment outcome. Our children responded in vastly different ways to the treatment; Rick learned, in 1 hr, what Jose learned in 1 yr. Since there was such heterogeneity among the patients, three fairly representative case descriptions will be presented in order to give a picture of the clinical implications of our findings: first, we present Scottie, who showed considerable gains in treatment; second, Tito, who showed moderate gains; and finally, Jose, whose progress was minimal.

Scottie, who was 4.5 yr of age at the start of treatment, spent much of his time staring into space and did not attempt to initiate interactions with people. If he was directly addressed, he would show a passive and friendly interest. When left to himself, he would self-stimulate; he was particularly attracted by spinning wheels. Scottie was echolalic, and he could label common objects, but he had very little communicative, and no spontaneous, speech. He had to be washed and dressed by others, helped when he ate his meals, and he was not fully toilet trained. He was, however, relatively free from tantrums, and he could understand simple directions. Because of his social responsiveness when approached, and occasional appropriate play, he was considered less psychotic than most of the children we have seen. His social quotient was 68.

Initial treatment sessions took place in his home, lasting 2 to 4 hr each, several days a week. His treatment plan included programs designed to teach him communicative skills, as well as the behaviors necessary for him to take care of his own practical needs, and to take a more active part in his everyday life. He was taught common abstract terms, such as prepositions, words denoting temporal relationships, as well as counting singular *versus* plural, etc. The frequency of echolalia was decreased. Meals and almost all daily activities were made strictly contingent on verbal requests for them. At first he missed several meals. He was also taught to offer materials as well as to request them. Much emphasis was placed on conversational speech. He was asked a general question about something he had done, and then was asked progressively more specific questions. Any spontaneous responses he made were reinforced socially, since he was responsive to social reinforcers. Again, the language program (Lovaas, *in preparation*) gives a rather complete discussion of these procedures. We focused our efforts on consultations with his grandmother, who was brought in to take special care of him, and who held him to a highly demanding schedule. She was different from most of the parents we had seen, since she did not tolerate withdrawal or other expressions of pathology.

Scottie is presently attending third grade in a normal elementary school. His social quotient is 100. He shows no trace of autism, and in all respects must be considered a normal child.

Tito, at admission, was a hyperactive 5-yr-old boy who evidenced an extremely short attention span. Eye contact was absent. He had many compulsive rituals. For example, he would spend considerable time arranging objects in a straight line and would become very upset if the arrangement was disturbed. He "refused" to let his parents read the

Sunday paper by becoming very upset when they removed the string that tied it in a bundle. He was untestable on intelligence tests, and he obtained a social quotient of 52. He was echolalic, but occasionally would use speech for communication. Tito's understanding of speech, however, was minimal. He resisted any involvement with people, and was unresponsive to displays of affection. He was extremely negative and clever at getting himself out of situations he did not like, often responding to the most elementary demands (e.g., "sit in the chair") with extreme tantrums.

Tito was treated as an outpatient. He was seen for three sessions per week for 1 yr. We served primarily as consultants to his mother, who was very conscientious and warm. His treatment program included two main objectives. First, we tried to teach him to deal with frustrating situations more maturely rather than engaging in tantrums. This was an extremely demanding job, and he received many spankings. Secondly, he was taught those basic skills upon which he could build more complex behaviors, particularly in language. Included in this category were pronoun usage, preposition usage, number concepts, relational concepts such as big and little, and social greetings. He was taught to comment upon his environment. He was also taught to draw, and to play more appropriately.

At discharge, Tito was observant and alert, but still appeared definitely educationally handicapped. He had made some progress in most areas, but his biggest gains were in language. His speech was quite spontaneous, and he could comment correctly on most social interactions. He obtained and IQ of 47 on the Stanford Binet and a social quotient of 63 on the Vineland. He now attends a school for retarded children 3 hr per day. His mother reports that he has continued to show improvements in most areas. He remains emotionally aloof with strangers, but is close to his mother. His future is uncertain. He may escape institutionalization if his progress continues.

Jose was 4 yr old at the start of treatment. His extreme negativism was reflected in tantrums, biting, and extreme stubbornness. He did not play with peers. He did not respond to his name or any commands. He had no speech, could not dress himself, was not toilet trained, nor did he have any other self-help behaviors. Appropriate play was essentially absent. He was found to be untestable on intelligence tests. He had a social quotient of 59. In short, he was extremely behaviorally retarded.

He was treated as an inpatient at the UCLA Neuropsychiatric Institute for 1 yr. His mother was given some limited training in how to continue therapy with him as described above. His treatment was primarily designed to overcome his negativism and to build some basic language skills. The latter included simple labeling, color discrimination, response to simple commands, and forms discriminations. Some work was also done on the reinforcement of spontaneous babbling.

We probably made slower progress with Jose than with any of the other children. At discharge, his gains in language were minimal. He would obey some commands; his vocabulary included a number of common nouns, some names, and a few verbs. He would use these words to label objects or express a desire for something, but never for commenting. He would attempt to imitate new words spontaneously on occasion. His greatest improvements were social. His social quotient of 74 reflected increases in smiling, laughing, and self-help skills. He was partially toilet trained. He was testable on the Stanford Binet Intelligence Scale (IQ = 47).

At present, Jose uses only a few words spontaneously (e.g., "car," "go to school," etc.), and what he has retained of his speech training is negligible. He can take care of himself at dinner and is fully toilet trained. His greatest gains at home have been in his play, which has become elaborate and creative, enabling him to entertain himself. He appears indifferent to people. While at intake he appeared unaware of ("blind" and "deaf" to) social contact, it now looks more as if he does not care whether anyone is there or not. He has to be watched constantly. Otherwise, he runs away from home, going nowhere in particular. His parents fear he will be killed because he is unaware of many common dangers. His parents plan to place him in a nearby state hospital. He will be able to come home on weekends and short vacations. We concur in these plans.

It is important to note that given the considerable heterogeneity among patients diagnosed as autistic, it is not enough merely to say that one has treated autistic children. Considering that some children improve without treatment, and that these children are differentiated from those who do not by certain behaviors, a good diagnostician can select his patients so that the majority of the children would eventually improve independent of the treatment offered. No doubt such pre-selection of patients, which would yield a much more favorable base rate change than is true of a nonselected group, keeps many non-functional treatments alive.

We utilized several procedures that allow us to argue with some confidence that autistic children improve with behavior therapy. First, we have performed two within-subject replications (on Rick and Pam), and in both instances demonstrated that we could establish behavioral control at will over the course of time for these patients. Therefore, we can argue that their behavior change must have been due to our intervention. Secondly, we performed several between-group replications. All replications yielded similar results. Also, each group of children was treated independently of the others, demonstrating that we could replicate out treatment effects independent of any conditions that may have been specific to one group of patients. We attempted specifically to avoid pre-selecting patients who might provide a favorable base rate of change regardless of treatment. The majority of patients were selected specifically because they displayed behaviors (IQ less than 50, mutism or no appropriate play) that were considered to be poor prognostic indicators. In addition, we did not drop any patient from treatment once we began. Finally, we consider our measures to be socially meaningful, and independent of any given theory of autism.

Further evidence that directly supports our results has been provided by other behavior therapy programs, which also demonstrated improvement with autistic children (Hewett, 1965; Risley and Wolf, 1967; Wolf, Risley, and Mees, 1964). Furthermore, Wolf et al. (1967) provided some additional data that lend support to our follow-up results. Such data suggest that replication of the data presented here is practically feasible.

Reservations About the Follow-Up Data

We have some confidence in the inferences we have drawn about the effectiveness of behavior therapy from the Before and After measures. The study was designed primarily to assess for change during treatment. But the reader should view the follow-up data with certain reservations; we did not initially design the project with follow-up assessment in mind and a number of variables were left uncontrolled. In retrospect: (1) The children should have been randomly assigned to the hospitalized versus parent-trained groups so as to minimize child characteristics associated with differential prognoses. Age of the child, testability on standard psychological tests, amount and kind of play at intake are some of the more obvious variables that should have been equated across groups. (2) We should have exercised more control over the post-treatment environments. For example, we were unable to assign children to special educational institutions, yet presence or absence of school is probably an important determinant of subsequent improvement or relapse. Similarly, future studies would do well in developing more objective assessment of the extent to which the parents are in fact continuing to implement the treatment procedures. Not all parents are equally good as behavior modifiers. The more successful parents seem to have the following features:

(a) A willingness to use strong consequences, such as food and spankings, to be emotionally responsive, showing their anger as well as their love. Not all parents can do this, some people are more "gentle" or more permissive than others, preferring to let their children "grow" or "develop" while they, as parents, assume a spectator role. Such parents do not do well with their autistic children.

(b) The willingness to deny that their children are "ill." This means that they deny the child the "need" to be sick, and, instead, give him some responsibility.

(c) The willingness to commit a major part of their lives to their children and to exercise some degree of contingent management throughout the day. This virtually rules out any professional or extensive social interests on the mother's part, requires a stable family structure, etc. Parental assistants, such as special tutors, can help out at times, but ultimately the parents must bear the major responsibility.

Despite these limitations, we have included the follow-up data because their validity seems strengthened when one considers the study as a whole. Basically, it is not surprising that the children who were "discharged" to their parents tended to improve, because these children remained in a treatment environment.

Major strengths. Behavior therapy programs for autistic children help. That is their major asset. So far as we know, despite its limitations, it is the only intervention that is effective. Our program did not give everything to each child. Sometimes it gave very little to a particular child, but it did give something to each child we saw. The improvement was analogous to making from 10 to 20 steps on a 100-step ladder. Scottie probably started at 80 and gained 20; his treatment brought dramatic changes, he became normal and his change is irreversible. Jose, on the other hand, may have started at 10 and gained 10; the change was not all that dramatic.

We have been especially successful at suppressing self-destructive behavior. In minutes, we have been able to stop the self-destruction of children who have mutilated themselves for years. The suppression was highly discriminated (situation specific), but his merely meant that we had to apply the treatment in more than one environment.

We have also been successful at rearranging behavior. For example, if the child was not mute (if he already had psychotic speech), then we could help him make large strides in his language and intellectual behavior.

The gains the children made in treatment generalized. Our multiple-response measures clearly demonstrate that we obtained stimulus generalization. We realize that sometimes the generalization was not as broad as we might have suspected. The shift in our program to teach the parents to treat their own children is a direct attempt to build greater stimulus generalization.

We were interested in response generalization as well as stimulus generalization. We do have some data on the subject, but they are limited. Response generalization, like stimulus generalization, deals with efficiency. How much behavior can one get for free? We obtained changes on the IQ tests for free; that is, we did not train the children on the test items, yet they improved. The data on response generalization are limited because psychology has little to say about it. We had no information about what changes to expect, which made it difficult to assess changes this first time around. From casual observation, during the treatment, the children looked much more "alert" and "aware" and became more effectively prosocial. It was particularly dramatic when, during the continuous demands of the therapy hour, a child would suddenly start sobbing and put his head in the therapist's lap; or when, after much hard work, a child appeared delighted over his new mastery. One does not often observe appropriate affect in autistic children.

Certain changes were difficult to assess because they seemed outside our behavioral framework. The children who were chronic toe-walkers (one of the soft neurological signs) began to walk normally after four or five months of treatment. Children who had never slept normally through the night began sleeping for 10 hr without interruption. Children who were chronically diarrhetic began having firm stools, etc. It is the search for this kind of generalized behavioral change that we feel will be particularly useful in future research.

Major weaknesses. There are many disappointments, and only a full appreciation of these will enable more realistic hopes now, and solutions in the future. We will discuss the major problems.

The most significant disappointment was the failure to isolate a "pivotal" response, or, as some might describe it, the failure to effect changes in certain key intervening variables. This means that in the beginning, we searched for one behavior which, when altered, would produce a profound "personality" change. We could not find it. We had once hoped, for example, that when a child was taught his name ("My name is Ricky") that his awareness of himself (or some such thing) would emerge. It did not. Similarly, the child who learned to fixate visually on his therapist's face did not suddenly discover people. Our treatment was not a cure for autism. But we had to start somewhere. At least the child who learned his name was then in position to learn someone else's name. When he learned to fixate visually on the therapist's face, he could pay more attention to teaching cues.

The failure to isolate a pivotal response or change a crucial intervening variable (or cure autism) can be discussed in two different veins. First, behavior therapy may not be the correct approach to treating autistic children. One could suggest in this regard that the "underlying pathology" (the intervening variable) is biochemical, and that the early detection and correction of this imbalance will enable the child to learn from his everyday environment, with little or no special educational remediation. If this should prove to be the case, our research has limited ultimate clinical value for autistic children. Behavior therapy alleviates some problems now, but the ultimate solution may involve correction of a biochemical imbalance. This is a viable alternative and intelligent people will pursue it.

Speaking of physiological variables, it is possible of course, that the pathology is structural. It could be that something is non-functional, as is the case with the blind or deaf child. The repair of this structural deficit, an attempt to "connect up" the millions of neurons in order to correct or bypass the deficit is beyond the limits of present medical technology. In this case, we must approach the problem as we approach blindness or deafness. In other words, it is sometimes the case that even where the underlying pathology is neurophysiological, the only feasible treatment may be essentially psychological. It is the early detection of blindness and deafness, and subsequent special remedial environments that allow blind and deaf children to develop normally. Without special consideration, they closely resemble the autistic children. The perceptual deficit that may underlie autism is more difficult to assess, hence it is more difficult to remediate. We will speculate on some possible basis for such a perceptual deficiency later in this paper.

The second possibility is that behavior therapy is the correct approach, and that it is the problem that is erroneously conceptualized. A full discussion of this point involves evaluations of terms like "mental illness," "treatment," etc., and that is beyond the scope of this paper. But it is important to bear in mind that "autism" is a hypothetical construct and a very shaky one at that. We have been expected, in a sense, to cure the children of someone else's inferences about them. There are no studies on "autism" that point to either a common etiology or a common response to treatment (or even a common response to experimental situations of much more limited scope). "Autism" was coined before a functional analysis of pathology.

The public and emotional appeal associated with the term, not our scientific understanding of the "syndrome," helps the term survive.

There are other conceptual problems. Consider, for example, a behavior as easy to build as "looking at the therapist's face." In data language this behavior has a very limited meaning. However, the associated theoretical structure is very extensive, implying that the child is recognizing and evaluating another person. For autistic children, the behavior of looking or not looking at another person has acquired special significance on a purely conceptual level (see Hutt and Ounsted, 1966). According to some conceptions of the problem, one would expect major changes in the autistic child who started to look at others. In our research, we have found these changes to be of minor significance.

Research Problems

We had anticipated that the children in the state institutions would regress. From the beginning, we have published studies (Lovaas, 1967; Wolf, et al., 1964) that show that when the experimental reinforcers were withdrawn, behaviors weakened. Such extinction occurred whether we employed food or fear as reinforcers, and whether the behavior was physical contact, imitation, or abstract speech. The shift from response to time-contingent delivery, the very procedure that we employ to demonstrate the effectiveness of our main treatment variable, also demonstrates our major weakness, the tenuousness with which the behavioral gains were maintained. Reversible baselines help one's research design, not one's patients.

The reversibility of the treatment effects was most dramatically observed with the first four children we treated: Rick, Pam, Chuck, and Billy. Although each one was making progress at the time of discharge, when we assessed them after 4 yr in the state hospital they appeared to have made no gains in appropriate behavior during that time, and showed large increases in self-stimulation. It is probably worth elaborating on this point, that they had learned nothing in the intervening 4 yr, but seemed to have stayed still. They gave the same smiles, the same facial expressions, the same words. This again emphasizes the point that without therapeutic, prescribed, contingent, functional reinforcers, children like these do not improve or retain their improvement; and, since we are not yet in a position to help them acquire normal, social reinforcers, their post-treatment environment has to be controlled. In our philosophy, functional contingencies are reality; if removed, any child would fail to develop.

The reversibility of the treatment effects are not peculiar to autistic children. It has been observed in a large variety of behavior therapy programs, and has led Bandura (1969) to speak of the distinction between physical and psychological treatments. The work of others illustrates these problems. For example, Tharp and Wetzel (1969) attempted to avoid discrimination and reversal problems by placing the treatment in the hands of those persons who have control over most of the patient's reinforcers. Our failure to maintain the gains made by the first four patients underscores the need for that kind of intervention. Wahler's (1969) study provided a good illustration of the need for interventions across settings. When the children he saw were treated in school, they did not necessarily change at home. When the contingencies were instated both in the home and at school, the behavior changed in both settings. Many therapists (see Patterson and Bechtel, 1970) now argue that the child's parents are essential as mediators of treatment.

The extent to the reversibility of treatment effects will probably be some function of various patient characteristics. It seems that when the primary problem centers on the child's motivation, and when treatment relies on "artificial" or experimental reinforcers (stimuli that do not characteristically maintain the patient's behavior on the outside), then one invites certain problems. Food, slaps, and accentuated social reinforcement are not the reinforcers that maintain the daily behaviors of normal school-aged children. Our use of such reinforcers set up the exact conditions for the kind of discriminations and the kind of extinctions we did not want. The necessity for using primary reinforcers, rather than everyday, more natural ones, is a probable reason why the children regressed in the state hospital environment. The state hospital, since it did not prescribe contingent functional reinforcers, constituted an extinction run.

It is implied in the above discussion that we view the problem of maintaining the treatment gains (generalization over time) as a special case of stimulus generalization. When the child stayed home with his parents who had learned our techniques he did not regress (i.e., extinguish) because the environments before and after discharge were similar (i.e., we maintained stimulus generalization). However, the child who was discharged to a state hospital entered a new environment to the extent that it did not possess (or did not program) effective reinforcers. Remember that the children had not "lost" the behaviors we had given them (some "progressive disease" had not rotted their brains), they simply did not perform, they were unmotivated, unless we re-exposed them to the treatment contingencies. The point is that it is important for research in behavior therapy to be directed towards ways of normalizing reinforcing functions so as to smooth the transition (prevent a discrimination) between the treatment and post-treatment environments.

The second major research problem centers on how to develop procedures for accelerating the acquisition of new behaviors. No doubt, the slow rate with which some behaviors were acquired was based on the children's inadequate motivation, as discussed above. However, it also seems to be the case that autistic children show deviations in attentional behaviors and that these deviations slow down their acquisition, particularly of that kind of learning that requires shifts in stimulus control. Autistic children appear to respond in an overselective manner to multiple cues. We referred to this problem as stimulus overselectivity (Lovaas et al., 1971). This finding has led us to consider redesigning many of our teaching procedures. For instance, we may well have to minimize our use of supporting prompts and prompt fading techniques, as these may provide interfering rather than helping stimuli in the learning process of these children.

Perhaps it is stimulus overselectivity that prevents or slows down the autistic child's acquisition of secondary reinforcers as well. If primary reinforcers had been used as consistently with normal children as we used them with our autistic patients, the associated environment would probably have acquired a larger range of reinforcing function. If secondary reinforcers are acquired classically (through the simultaneous presentation of neutral with already functional stimuli) then the autistic child, being overselective, may fail to respond to one of these inputs, and conditioning should then fail. Behavior therapy with the normal child, then, may not require detailed consideration of programs designed to build reinforcing function. To ensure long-lasting effects in the autistic child, the process of building secondary reinforcers would seem to require much more effort.

Finally, a major focus of future research should attempt more functional descriptions of autistic children. As we have shown, the children responded in vastly different ways to the treatment we gave them. We paid scant attention to individual differences when we treated the first 20 children. In future, we will assess such individual differences, for example, by contrasting the effectiveness of behavior therapy for very young versus older autistic children. Presumably, the very young (before 2 yr of age) child should discriminate less well than the older child, hence generalize and maintain the therapeutic gains to a more optimal degree.

It is important to remember that behavior therapy is a treatment based on research rather than deduced from theory. It is a technology for producing behavioral change through environmental manipulations. Sensitivity to new findings produces constant change in treatment techniques. Only a short time ago, imitation training procedures were developed (see Baer and Sherman, 1964). Our treatment changed and its effectiveness was greatly increased. Similar gains occurred when we developed procedures for building abstract speech. Just a short time ago, many argued that autistic children were unable to imitate, and that they were unable to form abstractions.

In closing, we should note that many of the procedures we have described are not new, but bear striking similarities to those described by Itard ("The Wild Boy of Aveyron") and by Sullivan (in Gibson's "The Miracle Worker") and recently in Clark ("The Siege"). We are especially struck by the similarity in their willingness to use functional consequences for the child's behaviors, the meticulous building of new behaviors in a piece-by-piece fashion, the intrustion of the education into all aspects of the child's life, the comprehensive, hour-by-hour, day-by-day commitment to the child by an adult, etc.

So the principles we employ are not new. Reinforcement, like gravity, is everywhere, and has been for a long time. The principles can be used to the child's advantage, or they can be used against him. What is new in behavior therapy is the *systematic evaluation* of how these principles affect the child. It is not the content of behavior therapy that is new, but its research methodology. In that sense, we have an immense and often unappreciated advantage over those who preceded us; the methodology enables us to contribute in a *cumulative* manner to psychological treatment.

Pharmacotherapy

Introduction

Many consider that psychotropic drugs are used disproportionately with children. Pediatricians are faulted for over-prescribing these medications in seeking simplistic solutions to complex behavioral and psychological problems; child psychiatrists who, as a group, infrequently use psychotropic agents are criticized for continuing an unjustified reliance on predominantly psychological treatment, precluding a method which can potentially aid in reducing symptoms and increasing acceptable behavior (Eisenberg and Conners, 1971). Nevertheless, there seems to be a rapidly growing interest and acceptance by child psychiatrists of pharmacotherapy with children, as with family therapy and behavior therapy.

It is said that in earlier centuries opium was used for a variety of pediatric diseases and was apparently also used by unscrupulous or well-meaning but ignorant nurses to quiet infants and children under their charge (Kenward, 1974). While castor oil, molasses, and other nostrums have also been long used to influence the behavior of children, the modern era of child pharmacotherapy is generally recognized as beginning in 1937, with Bradley's report on the positive behavioral effects noted in institutionalized disturbed children treated with amphetamines. Subsequently, Bender and Cottington (1942) also reported favorable results. In the 1940s and early 1950s several investigators turned their attention to the effect of anticonvulsants on children with behavior disorders and abnormal EEGs with varying results (Lindsley and Henry, 1942; Walker and Kirkpatrick, 1947; Pasamanick, 1951). In the early 1950s a few reports appeared describing therapeutic results with antihistamines, chiefly diphenlydramine (Bender and Nichtern, 1956; Effron and Freedman, 1953). Reserpine and the phenothiazines were introduced in the early 1950s and by the middle of the decade there was a rapid increase in reports describing the use of these drugs in disturbed children of widely varying clinical designation. For the most part these early studies were uncontrolled, the investigators were not blind, results were anecdotal, placebos were not used, and inadequate attention was often given to underlying psychological factors in drug administration (Grant, 1962).

In 1958, the first federal grant in child pharmacotherapy was awarded to Eisenberg and his group to evaluate the use of two phenothiazines and an antianxiety agent in children with hyperkinetic behavior disorders. They found that the medications were not superior to placebo (Eisenberg et al., 1961; Molling et al., 1962; Eisenberg et al., 1963). Then, in the early 1960s attention was turned again to study of the stimulants which had been receiving less attention, perhaps because of the faulty methodology of the early studies. Fish received the second of the child pharmacotherapy grants to study stimulant drug treatment of hyperactive children in 1961. She became a leader in classifying and developing a systematic and comprehensive set of indications for drug treatment with children (1968). Subsequently, positive results in placebo controlled treatment of hyperactive, institutionalized children with dextroamphetamine (Eisenberg et al., 1963) and methylphenidate (Conners and Eisenberg, 1963) were reported. Since that time the literature has burgeoned with studies by investigators demonstrating to various degrees the effectiveness of these agents, as well as other stimulants. Studies on neuroleptics (antipsychotics, major tranquilizers) and antianxiety drugs have also continued to appear in abundance, although the latter group, as well as the anticonvulsants, are receiving progressively less attention.

Certainly there is a rapidly growing literature, although as of 1970 there were fewer than 1,000 articles in child psychopharmacology compared to tens of thousands of adult drug studies. In reviewing the literature one is struck by the controversy, contradiction, and confusion, which seems to be in dramatic contrast to adult psychopharmacology. Fish has eloquently described the past and present difficulties in research in pediatric psychopharmacology and asked for both accurate diagnostic and developmental descriptions of the populations of children studied (1971). She decries the myth of "one child, one drug," and points out that careful diagnostic workup and classification is crucial if the appropriate drug is to be used for the individual child. She points out that stimulants are not, by definition, the drugs of choice for hyperactivity, as hyperactive children cannot be lumped together in one category. Conners has also noted the difficulties created for researchers by the "primitive state of classification in child psychiatry." When the preoccupation with treating target symptoms is added to the ethical limitations of experimentation in children, the result is a lack of knowledge as to what underlying variables are being affected by various medications (1972). (Included in the articles selected for this section is one by Conners in which he presents a step toward clarification of this problem.) Others have written on the difficulties in drug research in children, but space precludes discussion here (Minde and Weiss, 1970; Eisenberg and Conners, 1971; Werry and Sprague, 1972; Werry, 1973).

Although most articles to be found in the literature are basic pharmacological research, clinical drug studies, reviews, overviews, and commentaries, there are some sources which offer practical suggestions on prescribing psychoactive agents for children in clinical practice. These sources deal to varying degrees with the mechanics, general principles and psychological factors in drug treatment (Fish, 1968; Conners, 1970; Eisenberg, 1971; Eisenberg and Conners, 1971; Shapiro, 1975).

The purpose of this section is to present selected articles from the literature which will be of interest and relevance to the clinician actively involved in treating and/or supervising and consulting in the treatment of children. The choice includes articles on the philosophy of drug treatment, those which review the treatment of specific disorders or groups of disorders, clinical drug studies, and those which provide a critical view of the use of stimulant medication.

Principles of Drug Therapy in Child Psychiatry with Special Reference to Stimulant Drugs

LEON EISENBERG, M.D.

Eisenberg, one of the child psychiatrists best known as an advocate for better understanding of the biological origins of emotional problems in children, has written an important paper dealing with the philosophy and principles involved in drug therapy. While it does not specifically focus on technique or specified drug therapy, it sets the stage and puts into perspective the articles to follow in this section. Eisenberg squarely addresses the ethical issues involved in the use of medication with children—the "control" of behavior, the question of "normality" and its relation to chemical influence, as well as the problems of poorly understood but increasingly recognized long-term side effects on childhood growth and development. His plea is for careful assessment of all the variables in the administration of drugs, and a balanced view of their usefulness as part of a total treatment plan, not viewed as a miraculous cure for underlying disorders of all kinds nor, on the other hand, denied to those youngsters whose difficulties are at least partially responsive to them in a relatively brief period of time.

Let me state at the outset what pride of authorship constrains me to call Eisenberg's First Law of Psychopharmacology: the less the evidence on which an opinion is based, the firmer the conviction with which it will be maintained. Once this fundamental concept has been mastered, one will be better prepared for the polemics, the obfuscations, and the personal vendettas that beset the field. But I would prefer to emphasize issues rather than persons. It seems to me appropriate to begin by considering four dilemmas: the therapeutic "orphaning" of children; the problem of long-term effects; the issue of who is being treated; and the problem of social cost. Let us consider them seriatim, before turning to an outline of principles of treatment.

I. Therapeutic Orphans

The pediatrician, Harry Shirkey (1968), coined the term "therapeutic orphans" to refer to the anomalous situation in which the reluctance to test drugs in children results in insufficient data on efficacy and safety so that the drugs are labelled in a fashion that precludes their use in many children who might be expected to benefit from them; hence, children become the orphans of pharmacology. Since about 1962, the drug package insert approved by the Food and Drug Administration has contained the clause "not to be used in children, since clinical studies have been insufficient to establish recommendations for its use." This statement, it should be noted, is to be distinguished sharply from labelling that contains the phrase: "contraindicated in infants or children on the basis of studies showing it to be unsafe or ineffective." The latter is based upon data that make prescription unwise; the former reflects the lack of data as of the time the package insert was prepared. Most pediatricians would agree with the position of Modell (1967) that the insert is a useful guide, but nothing more; its recommendations should be evaluated together with other information available to the physician. What remains unclear, however, is the legal status of prescribing a drug not yet approved for use with children. While official "approval" of a drug does not protect the physician from liability for consequences subsequent to its use, there is considerable

Reprinted from *American Journal of Orthopsychiatry*, 41 (3) (April 1971), pp. 371-379.
Copyright © the American Orthopsychiatric Association, Inc. Reproduced by permission.

uncertainty, in the absence of recorded test cases, as to whether a physician who prescribed a drug in good faith (based upon available clinical evidence) might be placed in jeopardy, should an undesired effect occur, precisely because of the influence of the language of the package insert on judge and jury. It is likely that many physicians, as well as clinical investigators, are reluctant to innovate with drugs in children because of the putative danger arising from this warning. Such physician behavior can only result in denying useful medications to children.

At the heart of the problem lies the dubious ethic of experimenting with drugs in normal children. Whereas it would appear legitimate to secure adult volunteers who are willing to undergo a potential hazard after being informed of the risk because of their conviction that they are contributing to medical knowledge, few of us are convinced that parents should be asked to "volunteer" their children under similar circumstances. My department, for one, has never seen its way clear to such an undertaking despite our very great interest in the information that might be so obtained. The fact that stimulant drugs reliably produce enhanced attention and diminished purposeless motor activity in hyperkinetic children permits no informed conclusion as to what such drugs would do in normal children. Such knowledge would give us a better basis for interpreting the findings in the disturbed child. Nonetheless, we have not undertaken such studies; nor has anyone else, to our knowledge. Investigation has been limited to the use of a drug in children with a behavior disorder thought to be responsive to its administration.

Thus, the usual sequence has been thorough testing in a variety of animal species followed by investigative use in the sick child. That situation has as its corollary the necessity to gather as much information as possible in studies with pediatric patients. The problems of interspecific comparison and the remarkably different effects related to developmental age point to the necessity for far more extensive programs in pediatric clinical pharmacology than are now in existence. The child, it should not need pointing out here, is not a miniature adult. Differences, both quantitative and qualitative, in drug response distinguish the developing organism from the adult; these differences are greatest in the youngest epochs—fetal, premature, neonate (first month) and infant (up to two years) but also characterize children and adolescents.

The relevant variables are multiple and complex. Rate of absorption is influenced by the efficiency of transport across the intestinal villi, the time of transit is affected by the length of the GI tract, the recumbent posture and differences in diet and GI contents. Body distribution is influenced by differences in the percentage of lean body mass as opposed to fat and water, by the relatively greater body surface area in the infant, by the immaturity of the bloodbrain barrier and by kinetics of protein binding. As one example of the latter, the injudicious use of sulfonamides displaces bilirubin from protein thus rendering it far more toxic at the same total blood level (Odell, 1959). Further, detoxification mechanisms, in particular conjugation with glucuronic acid, are far less effective in the newborn, thus altering the effective half-life of ingested drugs. Excretion of drugs is affected by the fact that the immature kidney is relatively low in glomerular filtration rate and tubular clearance so that a substance such as penicillin G persists in the circulation for a period considerably longer than in the adult (Barnett, 1949). Finally, one anticipates differences in end-organ responsiveness. These topics have been reviewed in detail elsewhere (Conference, 1967); it will suffice to call them to attention as a backdrop for further deliberations.

II. Long-Term Effects

The immediate problem for the toxicologist in both adult and in child therapeutics is the here and now toxicity of a new drug, that is, what are its immediate consequences for morbidity and mortality? In the adult, if the period of administration is brief, there is usually little reason for concern about subsequent effects. However, in the child, what is given even briefly at a particular developmental period may have unforeseen long-term consequences. As one example, consider the effect of tetracycline on children even to the age of eight in producing dental staining in deciduous and permanent teeth. The chronic use of drugs raises many problems in adults as well, but in children we have particular concern with drug effects on growth and development, as evidenced by the growth retardation produced by the long-term use of steroids.

What we do not know, but all of us fear, is the possibility of behavioral long-term consequences. Animal data suggest that the administration of sedatives to pregnant animals or to the newborns themselves alter the behavior of the offspring when they are mature at a time when the drug is no longer detectable. We are all aware of the potent effects of miniscule doses of sex hormones given at birth on the sexual behavior of the mature animal. It is now likely that human development is so readily influenceable, given the much longer periods available for learning and the lack of phenomena strictly comparable to "imprinting." Nonetheless, we are becoming ever more aware of how widespread are drug actions on the biology of the organism at points far removed from the target of their administration. The effect of phenobarbital on liver enzyme systems or of many drugs on the adenyl cyclase system (the so-called second messenger) are cases in point. For most of the issues with which this paper is concerned, few relevant data are available on long-term effects, but by analogy to what is known, the available data urge caution upon us.

III. Who Is Being Treated?

The third of our dilemmas refers to the issue of patienthood. The adult generally volunteers himself as the psychiatric patient. He may at times have been an unwilling "volunteer" coerced by family, community or court but most often it is he who suffers the discomfort that leads him to consult the physician. Although exceptions do exist, the child rarely volunteers; ordinarily, he is brought by his parents, sometimes at the behest of his teacher or the courts. Is the child designated as "patient" because his mother is anxious about behavior that on a normative scale would be considered average? Is he brought for treatment because his teacher is angered by normally assertive behavior that threatens her authority? Does the court designate his problem "psychiatric" simply because alternative ways of dealing with it are unavailable even though the pathology is social (as is all too often the case in children found to be neglected or delinquent)?

While mothers may be unduly anxious, teachers insecure and courts at a loss, there is evidence that children designated as patients are indeed deviant. Shula Wolff (1967) has shown this in a comparison of patients with the general child population. Lee Robins's (1966) followup of child guidance cases into adulthood indicates clearly that former patients are at significant risk for adult psychopathology when compared with classroom controls. Rutter (1970) and his co-workers have carried out an epidemiologic study on the Isle of Wight that indicates that clinicians can reliably identify children in need of help.

This is not to deny the possibility of abuse. It does serve to emphasize the importance of a careful clinical evaluation before starting any treatment program. Psychiatrists should not allow themselves to become the agents of disturbed mothers, inadequate teachers or uninformed judges. If they adhere to the basic tenets of their professional training, they will not be. The risks of abuse can be contained only if drug administration is recognized to be a medical responsibility and if the physicians empowered to use drugs are appropriately trained and ethically responsible.

IV. Social Cost

Pharmacology is accustomed to weighing risk against benefit. Benefit is assessed in terms of the condition being treated, the outcome in the absence of treatment and the differences produced by the treatment. Risk is measured in terms of morbidity and mortality from drug action. In the case of children, one has to consider both the risk and the benefit in terms of long-term consequences as well as immediate ones. The behavior disorder may appear to be time-limited (as in the overactivity of the hyperkinetic child) but the risk of other and more serious subsequent disturbance has also to be weighed. If the apparent overactivity and distractibility do fade with time (even in the absence of treatment), must we not also take into account the cost to the child of not having learned during that time span because of the interference with learning produced by the symptoms? And what of the secondary consequences, both of being labelled as "bad" and of being blamed for failing to learn: the poor self-concept and the antisocial behavior that may well result?

A hidden component of cost is the problem presented by any effective treatment; namely, the possibility that its very success will diminish the social zeal for prevention. For example, the availability of methods for treating lead poisoning may have been a factor in the failure of the medical profession to take the leadership it should have exerted in public campaigns to remove lead-containing interior paints. It is not so much that physicians would not wish to see this hazard removed as that they have not been as aggressive in social action as they might have been. I am not arguing that any are completely satisfied with available treatments (which fall far short of reversing the patient's illness) but rather that preoccupation with treatment and its refinement has absorbed energy that might more effectively be aimed at removing causes. There are major research problems still to be solved in treating lead poisoning but there is no lack of data about the source of that poisoning; yet physicians put more energy into the refinement of treatment than into preventing the disorder by condemning slum housing (Anderson, 1971).

In like fashion, it is at least arguable that the relative ease with which symptoms of overactive and impulsive behavior can be treated with stimulant drugs might lead to a diminution of efforts to prevent those conditions which, in part, bring it about: complications of pregnancy and parturition; post-natal infection, malnutrition and trauma; crowded homes and crowded schools; poorly trained and poorly motivated teachers; in addition to the unknown factors that require to be searched out.

It has been suggested (Lennard, 1970) that ours is a drug oriented society that relies on substance use to alter the sensorium in place of attempts to make life more rewarding for those troubled by it. Whether or not this indictment is correct in all respects, any reader of medical journals can point to pharmaceutical advertisements that imply that unhappy housewives or harassed executives should receive this or that tranquilizer—without even so much as a suggestion that the fundamental problem is the life style that produced the unhappiness or the harassment. To the extent that physicians subscribe uncritically to this philosophy, then, indeed, the cost in toxicity from tranquilizing drugs is likely to be far greater than can be measured by counting what are customarily listed as side effects. The most costly (and uncounted) "side effect" will have been the diversion of effort from a direct attack on the sources of the symptoms, much as the prescription of aspirin for a headache caused by a meningioma allows the tumor to grow unchecked by diminishing the signal warning of its presence. More specific to our topic, restlessness in an inner city classroom can be diminished by feeding the children, since many come to school without breakfast and exhibit restlessness resulting from hypoglycemia. Let there be no misunderstanding of my view: it would be a criminal abdication of medical responsibility to treat such children with stimulant drugs. If drugs are used indiscriminately in response to symptoms rather than to the underlying medical disorder, just such abuses will occur. Moreover, every clinician (and every school teacher, for that matter) knows that behavior in the classroom is a function of the teacher's effectiveness, which, though not the only relevant variable, is an important determinant of children's behavior. Were a child to be referred for impulsive and distractable behavior from a class led by an incompetent teacher, drug administration would be counter productive as contrasted with steps to restrain or replace the teacher. The fact that abuse can occur accents medical responsibility for diagnosis; it is a poor argument for abandoning drug use, thus denying treatment to those who might profit from it in order to spare those whom drugs might injure.

The basic clinical problem stems from the fact that behavior symptoms are a final common pathway for the expression of multiple causes. A tremor may result from simple anxiety, from hyperthyroidism or from disorders of the basal ganglia. The appropriate treatment of the same manifest behavior is different in each case. With such symptoms as overactivity and distractibility, diagnostic differentiation is more difficult since we lack pathognomonic signs and symptoms. We can, however, rule out identifiable causes and reserve symptomatic medication for the cases for which no alternative remedy is available.

But what of the accusation that the hyperkinetic syndrome is nothing more than "the normal exuberance of childhood"? This statement was attributed to a distinguished physician in a newspaper account of Senate hearings. Are drugs, as alleged by Congressman

Gallagher (1970), "being employed to induce conformity, rather than creativity, in the classroom?" Or, in the words of the Brown-Pembroke SDS (1970), are they used for "stifling rebelliousness and maintaining the status quo" in the classrooms for black children?

As I have been at pain to point out, the possibility of abuse does exist. Teachers all too often do prefer conformity; physicians at times do abandon their responsibility for diagnosis and prescribe in response to parental pressure; black children are victimized by American society. But none of these admissions constitutes evidence for a nationwide conspiracy to drug children into insensibility nor contravenes the reality of a behavioral syndrome for which proper medication can produce dramatic benefit.

In 1967, the World Health Organization assembled psychiatrists and epidemiologists from France, Japan, Norway, Peru, the United Kingdom, the U.S.S.R., Austria, Italy, Belgium, Switzerland, the Netherlands, Portugal, Spain, Formosa, Australia and the United States to discuss the diagnosis and classification of psychiatric disorders in children. That expert group agreed unanimously on the need for a category termed "hyperkinetic syndrome" whose chief characteristics were described as "extreme overactivity which was poorly organized and poorly regulated by the usual social controls, distractability, short attention span, impulsiveness, and often also, marked mood fluctuations and aggression. Such disorders were much commoner in boys than in girls; there was often a characteristic response to drugs such as amphetamine, and frequently, too, there were associated perceptual difficulties and problems at school. While these conditions were sometimes associated with organic brain pathology, it was generally accepted that this was often not the case and that certainly this could not constitute any part of the diagnostic criteria" (Rutter, 1969).

Agreed, the reality of a clinical disorder is not established by vote, it does seem noteworthy that a world panel of psychiatrists, trained in different schools of thought, functioning in different cultures, and speaking different languages, all agreed on the existence in their home countries of children who exhibit the hyperkinetic syndrome and who benefit from stimulant drugs. Surely, this is a far cry from the contention that we are dealing with "the normal exuberance of childhood" or that we are employing drugs "to induce conformity" or "to stifle rebelliousness."

This is not the place to review in extenso the reports from our own laboratory on the repeated demonstration of beneficial effects from stimulant drugs in the treatment of children with hyperkinetic behavior and school learning problems (Conners et al., 1967, 1969; Eisenberg, 1966; Eisenberg et al., 1963; Eisenberg and Connors, 1963). Suffice it to say that these agents have the unique property of diminishing purposeless motor activity and of enhancing attention span with the result of improving learning, all of this at the price of relatively minor side effects. It has been argued recently that, despite these encouraging findings, we may be introducing youngsters to the use of drugs and thus inadvertently making them more vulnerable to drug abuse in adolescence. An unpublished followup of cases treated by Laufer (1970) of youngsters put on medication in childhood but surveyed in late adolescence or early adulthood revealed no known drug abusers. These findings are not surprising. I am aware of no evidence that epileptics who, of necessity, are long-term drug users are thereby at risk for drug abuse with other substances. No such evidence exists for diabetics, for individuals with hypothyroidism, or any of the myriad chronic conditions that require prolonged drug use. What accounts for this phenomenon, I suggest, is that none of these drugs produces a euphoric affect in the pre-adolescent child and thus there is no subjective experience that leads the patient to seek the drug deliberately. Those alarmed by the abuse potential of amphetamines in adolescence, a real and frightening phenomenon, assume that the subjective effect in the child taking amphetamines resembles that in the older user. But the clinical facts are otherwise. Most often, if the child comments at all about subjective effects, it is to complain of dysphoria or sleepiness; some even are subject to unprovoked episodes of crying. The child may feel positive about the social consequences of the effect of the drug on his own behavior; that is he may feel better about himself because his teacher compliments him for learning or his mother no longer complains about his misbehaving, but he obtains no direct "high" from the drug itself.

Any potent drug may be abused—and that includes stimulants. But should we deny diabetics insulin because insulin can be (and has been) used to commit suicide? Should we deny schizophrenics phenothiazines because overworked housewives can be drugged into insensibility instead of being helped to find a more meaningful life role? Should we deny distractible children stimulants that can enhance their ability to succeed at learning because incompetent or even malicious teachers, doctors or parents may mistreat nonconforming or underfed children? The possibility of abuse is an argument for better medical practice, not a return to astrology. Perhaps the greatest source of confusion with stimulant drugs is the use of the descriptive adjective "stimulant" which, while it may accurately reflect drug action in the adolescent or adult, hardly categorizes its effect in children. If we believe words have power, perhaps we should return to the use of the term sympathomimetic. Would that our social problems could be solved so easily!

Principles of Drug Treatment

No drug should be employed without firm indication for its use, without careful supervision of the patient to be treated, and without due precautions for the recognition and control of toxicity. If a drug is to be used, the severity of the presenting condition and the likelihood of benefit must outweigh the risk of toxicity. If the patients to be treated are children, clinical decisions must be based upon data from pediatric studies; we cannot safely extrapolate from adults to children. Surveillance for toxicity must consider long-term as well as immediate consequences.

The second principle might be labelled pharmacologic conservatism: an old and familiar drug is to be preferred to a new drug unless there is preponderant evidence for superiority of the latter. Unexpected toxicity from a new agent may become apparent only after prolonged experience with its use; we should therefore be cautious in using a new agent except when its benefit is so superior as to warrant the putative risk.

Drugs can be useful agents in the management of pediatric psychiatric disorders when chosen appropriately and applied with discrimination. They can control symptoms not readily managed by other means and can facilitate other methods of psychiatric treatment by allaying symptoms that disrupt learning.

Every study reveals the potency of placebo effects; that is, benefits occurring from expectation in physician and patient. These expectations can be used to potentiate drug effects by recognizing that the prescription of medicine is an important communication both to the child and to his family. Drugs can have negative effects if the physician regards them solely as weapons to impose control or as measures of desperation. The meaning of the transaction is determined by the attitudes of all participants: the patient, his family and his physician. Skill in the use of drugs requires, in addition to detailed knowledge of their pharmacologic properties, sensitivity to their psychologic implications.

Drugs should be used no longer than necessary. Dosage should be reduced periodically with the goal of ceasing treatment if symptoms do not return on a lower dosage or after the drug has been discontinued. This applies with particular force to drugs used over long periods in treating chronic conditions. In the case of stimulant drug treatment of hyperkinesis, it has been our practice to discontinue medication at the end of the school term and to allow a child a trial return to school without medication, the drug to be resumed only if it proves to be necessary. Dosage must be individualized. Each patient is metabolically unique. Under-treatment, as well as over-treatment, can result from rigid use of medication without appropriate sensitivity to manipulation of dosage.

Medication should not be used to relieve the physician of the responsibility for seeking to identify and eliminate factors causing or aggravating the underlying disorder. Stimulant drugs treat symptoms, not diseases. Symptomatic relief is not to be disparaged; often, it is the most the physician can offer. However, since symptom suppression can delay appropriate intervention, treatment should follow, not precede, thorough diagnostic evaluation.

With no intent to minimize the importance of alertness to drug toxicity, it is necessary to balance this risk against the cost of doing nothing as well as the cost of alternative treatments. We, then, must ask: what is the natural history of the disorder in the absence of treatment? The greater the immediate and the long-term morbidity, the readier the justification for heroic interventions. We must ask, also: what is the "toxicity" of alternative non-drug treatments? Psychotherapy is not necessarily benign; it can foster dependency, increase self-preoccupation, and produce feelings of futility and hopelessness when used to "treat" a condition for which it is inappropriate.

Our goal is the healthy development of children. Stimulant drugs may be helpful in suppressing symptoms that interfere with learning. But these agents do no more than make it possible for the child to learn; in themselves, they teach him nothing. To the extent that he has failed to learn or has developed faulty learning habits, he will require remedial educational measures. Thus, the administration of drugs, an important part of the therapeutic plan when they are given appropriately, constitutes only one part of the total treatment program. They must be accompanied by appropriate school plans, parent counseling, recreational programs and other growth-promoting activities that encourage personal development. Pharmacologic methods provide neither the passport to a brave new world nor the gateway to the inferno. With thoughtful selection, careful regulation of dosage and close scrutiny for toxicity, they can add a significant component to total patient care. For all of this, the physician bears a major responsibility as the patient's advocate. To be successful, he will need to enlist the cooperation of teachers, psychologists, parents, and the community as a political body, if he is to create a climate within which each child can attain his human potential.

Drugs in Management of Minimal Brain Dysfunction

J. GORDON MILLICHAP, M.D.

*This paper attempts to condense a very complex and contro-
versial subject into a succinct overview, as well as to provide some
practical guidelines for the clinician. This is an ambitious
undertaking and understandably incorporates some flaws. For
example, the author states that the best responses to treatment
were seen in children with the greatest number of "neurological
abnormalities" which indicates the "degree of brain damage."
"Neurological abnormalities" are not defined, but they refer to
"soft signs"; no one has yet convincingly established that the
latter indicate or represent brain damage.*

*The suggestion for periodic reassessment of children being
treated with psychotropic drugs is well taken. The author does
not define, however, what a "neuropsychological battery"
consists of and one wonders about the clinical practicality and the
expense. Still, standardized rating forms for evaluation and
reassessment of drug efficacy are being recommended with
increasing frequency. Examples are the Werry-Weiss-Peters
Activity Scale to be used by parents and the Conners Rating Scale
for Teachers.*

*Finally, it should be noted that caffeine has been reported as
being a potential substitute for the stimulant drugs (Schnacken-*

berg, 1973). Some clinicians have informally speculated that if this proved to be the case, commercial cola drinks could be used as well. However, the average cup of coffee contains between 100 and 150 mg. of caffeine, while cola drinks average around 30 mg. Having a child consume three to five cola drinks before school might have some drawbacks (Editorial, 1972).

The ideal drug for the treatment of children with minimal brain dysfunction (MBD) should control hyperactivity, increase the span of attention, reduce impulsive and aggressive behavior, and have measurable beneficial effects on visual and auditory perception, reading ability, and coordination, without inducing insomnia, anorexia, drowsiness, or other more serious toxic effects. Central nervous system stimulants are the agents of choice, and the antianxiety and antipsychotic compounds are recommended as alternative therapies in patients who fail to respond to methylphenidate or dextroamphetamine. The antidepressant, imipramine, and the anticonvulsant, diphenylhydantoin, are also beneficial in some cases, whereas barbiturates, such as phenobarbital, are contraindicated, because they usually exacerbate hyperactivity.

The amphetamines were introduced for the treatment of hyperkinesia more than 30 years ago by Bradley (1937), who discovered their paradoxical calming effects in hyperactive patients. Controlled studies are limited, however, and reports conflict as to the type of hyperkinetic child likely to respond favorably. In a recent review (Millichap and Fowler, 1967), the drug therapy for MBD was analyzed, and the agents were listed in order of choice according to effectiveness and toxicity. The designs and the methods of the reported studies were evaluated, so that those lacking in controls and employing subjective assessments of behavior could be compared with the relatively small number of well-controlled investigations in which objective measurements were the rule. Table 1 lists the drugs used in treatment of MBD, the doses given, and the principal side effects associated with each.

Reprinted from *Annals of the New York Academy of Science*, 1973, pp. 321-334.

Central Nervous System Stimulants

Methylphenidate (Ritalin®)

Methylphenidate is the treatment of choice, and amphetamine sulfate is the second most successful drug in the control of hyperactive behavior. The properties of these two agents are similar, but methylphenidate has less tendency to produce anorexia. The results of trials in a total of 337 children with hyperactive behavior were reviewed. The dosage of methylphenidate ranged from 5 to 200 mg daily, and the maximum duration of treatment was four years. Improvement in behavior was reported in an average of 83% of patients. An increased degree of motor activity was observed in only four children, although uncontrolled reports have alluded to an exacerbation of the hyperactivity in approximately 5% of patients treated.

In one well-controlled investigation, Conners and Eisenberg (1963) examined the effects of methylphenidate administered double-blind over a ten-day period to two groups of emotionally disturbed children. Total symptom ratings and objective measurements of learning and maze performance were significantly improved in the drug-treated group, but wide individual variation in response was mentioned. In studies by Knobel, Lytton, and associates and Nichamin and Comly (Knobel, 1962; Lytton and Knobel, 1958; Nichamin and Comly, 1964), the response to methylphenidate was evaluated by reports of teachers and parents and by clinical observations. A beneficial effect was obtained in 70-90% of the patients, and reduction in activity was associated with improvements in attention span and coordination, lessening of impulsivity, and as increase of useful productivity. The response was equally good in patients with hyperactivity resulting from organic or psychogenic factors. Objective tests and placebo controls were not employed; moreover, the authors admitted both that some parents' reports were distorted and that their own expectations in regard to therapy could have colored the final result of the studies.

Millichap and colleagues (1968) studied 30 children with MBD, using neuropsychological tests that were principally objective in type, providing quantitative estimations of disabilities. The patients were treated with methylphenidate and placebo in a random cross-over design, and the influence of factors that might vary with the time of admission to the clinical trial was excluded by the system of allocation and balancing of treatment groups. The possible introduction of bias as a result of drug side effects was prevented by an individual method of coding and labeling concealed from the investigators, and parent and investigator expectations and attitudes towards the value of the drug were eliminated by the double-blind control. The initial daily dose was 0.5 mg/kg body weight divided into two equal amounts given after breakfast and lunch. The medication was begun the day following the first record of neuropsychological tests. After one week of treatments, the dose of medication was increased to 1.0 mg/kg a day. A dose of 2.0 mg/kg a day was given during the third and final week, provided that side reactions had not been observed with smaller doses. The patients returned for repeat neuropsychological evaluation on the last day of the three-week course of treatment. The alternated coded medication for each patient was given for a further three-week period, using the same dosage schedule as for the first course of treatment, and a third and final neuropsychological evaluation was made on the last day of treatment.

A bias that might have resulted from knowledge of the point of cross-over or from a sustained effect of the drug was not observed in statistical analyses of patients grouped according to the order of allocation of medication. Furthermore, a statistically significant improvement as a result of practice could not be shown in any of the tests. The necessity for inclusion of a placebo was demonstrated, particularly in the scores recorded for auditory perception and the Frostig test. Significant improvements occurred in response to both placebo and drug, so that the beneficial effect of methylphenidate on auditory perception and on form and spatial perception was nonspecific.

A significantly improved performance during treatment with methylphenidate was observed in six of the seven neuropsychological tests, and the effect of the drug was specific and greater than that of the placebo in the Draw-a-Man and Frostig figure-ground tests. In the parents' subjective evaluations of conduct and immaturity, improvements in scores during treatment with methylphenidate were not different from evaluations based on the placebo response. The value of a battery of objective neuropsychological tests in the measurement of changes in behavior and learning induced by drugs was thus demonstrated by this study.

A subsequent evaluation of measurements of activity (Millichap and Johnson, 1972) before and after treatment with methylphenidate revealed that the patients with the highest levels of motor activity were most likely to respond, whereas those with initially lower levels of activity were sometimes made worse by the drug. In addition, the most active patients had the highest number of neurological abnormalities, and the response to therapy was related to the degree of brain damage. A similar correlation between brain injury, hyperactivity, and response to methylphenidate has been demonstrated in small animals (Millichap and Johnson, 1972).

Methylphenidate is indicated as an adjunct to remedial education in the short-term treatment of children with MBD. It may be expected to induce small, but measurable, improvements in tests of general intelligence and visual-motor perception, control hyperactivity in the more active patients with neurological abnormalities, and reduce impulsive behavior. The use of methylphenidate and other central nervous stimulants in the long-term management of children with learning disorders must await their evaluation by more prolonged controlled studies.

Dextroamphetamine

Amphetamines have been used for 30 years in the management of hyperactive behavior disorders. In a total of 610 patients reported in the literature (Millichap and Fowler, 1967), the dosage ranged from 5-40 mg daily, and the maximum duration of therapy was four years. Improvements in behavior occurred in an average 69% of patients, and the hyperactivity was made worse in 11%. The incidence of side effects was approximately the same as that reported with methylphenidate. Dextroamphetamine is contraindicated in patients with hyperactivity associated with psychotic symptoms.

Deanol (Deaner®)

Deanol, which is converted to acetylcholine within neurons, acts as a central nervous system stimulant. The results of trials in 239 patients with behavior and learning disorders showed 47% with improvements. Three of six reports, however, showed negative results. Doses of 10-1,000 mg daily were administered for 4-36 weeks, and side effects were minimal and infrequent. It is generally considered that deanol is of little, if any, value in the treatment of hyperactive behavior and learning disabilities.

Pemoline (Cylert®)

Pemoline is a weak central nervous system stimulant presently under investigation in the treatment of children with MBD. Controlled studies have shown that pemoline may alleviate hyperactive behavior and increase scores on the performance scale of the Wechsler Intelligence Scale for Children (Millichap and Schrimpf, unpublished). Side effects include insomnia and anorexia. A single dose of 25-100 mg daily may be given each morning, offering an advantage over methylphenidate and dextroamphetamine, which have a shorter duration of action and must be administered twice daily.

Antianxiety and Antipsychotic Agents

Of the antianxiety and antipsychotic agents studied, only chlordiazepoxide, thioridazine, chlorpromazine, and reserpine have been used to treat a sufficient number of hyperkinetic children for adequate comparative evaluation (see Table 1) (Millichap and Fowler, 1967; Millichap, 1968).

Chlordiazepoxide (Librium®)

Chlordiazepoxide, a derivative of benzodiazepine, may relieve anxiety, reduce aggressive tendencies, and relax the muscles. The results of trial in 237 children with hyperactive and other behavior disorders showed improvements in an average of 60% of patients. Side effects were mentioned in only two of the six reports (Millichap and Fowler, 1967).

Thioridazine (Mellaril®)

Thioridazine has been used chiefly in the treatment of mentally retarded children with hyperactivity. Of 308 patients treated, 57% were benefited, and only 2% experienced side effects, drowsiness being the most prominent adverse reaction. Millichap and colleagues studied 15 patients with MBD and found significant improvements in the Jastak reading test, in conduct ratings, in ratings of maturity of behavior, and in finger coordination.

Chlorpromazine (Thorazine®)

Trials in 153 patients demonstrated beneficial effects in an average of 55%. Side effects, however, occurred more frequently with chlorpromazine than with other tranquilizing agents (Millichap and Fowler, 1967).

Reserpine (Serpasil®)

In two studies employing some objective psychological tests, reserpine had no demonstrable effect, whereas in two controlled trials, subjective methods of evaluation appeared to show improvement in behavior. The occurrence of side effects with a dose of 1 mg daily was rare.

Miscellaneous Tranquilizers

The results of trials of hydroxyzine hydrochloride, meprobamate, fluphenazine hydrochloride, and chlorprothixene hydrochloride were inconclusive, and controlled trials in larger numbers of patients are needed before recommendations can be made for general use (Millichap, 1968). Promazine hydrochloride employed in a controlled trial in six mentally retarded children had no significant effect on hyperactivity (Schulman and Clarinda, 1964). The antihistamine diphenhydramine (Benadryl®) is sometimes advocated, but the effectiveness of this compound has not been proven by controlled trial or objective evaluation.

Antidepressants

Imipramine (Tofranil®)

Imipramine was first noted to be of use in the treatment of enuretic children, and in some of these reports behavioral improvement was an incidental finding. Rapoport (1965) reported improvement in alertness, handwriting, reading, and arithmetic in children with varied behavior disorders, from temper tantrums in younger children to delinquency in adolescents. Huessey and Wright (1970) employed imipramine in 52 children, 3-14 years of age, who were referred because of hyperactive behavior and learning disabilities. Children under five, but over three years of age, were started on a dose of 12.5 mg, and those over five years of age, were started on a dose of 25 mg daily. The medication was given in a single dose one hour after the evening meal. The therapeutic effect, characterized by a marked diminution or disappearance of symptoms was evident the following day. The dosage was increased as necessary, and the range was 25-125 mg daily. Marked improvement occurred in 67% of patients on an average dose of 50 mg. These results were similar to those obtained by the authors using dextroamphetamine and methylphenidate. One child developed mild hypertension and a worsening of eczema; one developed thrombocytopenia, recovering without sequelae after withdrawal of the drug; irritability occurred in four children; constipation in one; coldness of hands and feet in two; and a dry mouth in one. Altogether, side effects were observed in a total of ten children, or 10%. Of the 17 children in whom imipramine was not of benefit, 11 improved on methylphenidate and one did well on dextroamphetamine and thioridazine.

Anticonvulsants

Reports of the efficacy of anticonvulsants in the control of hyperactivity are limited and are concerned primarily with trials in children whose behavior and learning problems are complicated by convulsive seizures (Millichap, 1969). Primidone, found effective in seven of ten patients in one study, has been recommended for use in children with major convulsions and hyperactive behavior, whereas phenobarbital has variable effects, often exacerbating the hyperactivity (Millichap and Millichap, 1966). Diphenylhydantoin sodium was relatively ineffective in the control of hyperactive behavior in one study by Pasamanick (1951) and in another by Millichap and colleagues (1969).

Methods of Drug Therapy for MBD

The drugs of reported value for the treatment of hyperkinetic behavior and MBD in children are listed in Table 2 in order of preference on the basis of efficacy and toxicity. Methylphenidate is the treatment of choice, beginning with an initial dosage of .25 mg/kg daily, divided into two doses given at breakfast and lunch. In children who are of average or below average weight, the medication is given after food; in overweight children, mephylphenidate is given before food. The dose is doubled during each successive week of treatment, up to an average optimal level of 2.0 mg/kg of body weight daily, provided that untoward effects are not observed, such as insomnia, anorexia of a severe degree, or depressive reaction. The dosage is monitored on the basis of the responses indicated by reports of parents and school teachers and by reexamination of the child after 2-4 weeks of treatment. The neuropsychological test battery should be repeated at intervals of 3-4 months in order to measure improvements in perception objectively. In view of the absence of controls in long-term therapy, the treatment should be interrupted at intervals and particularly during vacations, and the effect of withdrawal observed. A relapse in behavior and deterioration in school grades following drug withdrawal are indications for repeated short-term trials.

In patients who develop tolerance to the effects of methylphenidate despite doses of 20 mg twice daily or in those whose parents and teachers report no improvement and for whom neuropsychological tests are unchanged, an alternative medication such as dextroamphetamine or imipramine should be substituted. The antianxiety and antipsychotic agents are recommended for patients who fail to respond to the central nervous system stimulants or who develop troublesome adverse reactions. In patients with a history of convulsive seizures or paroxysmal seizure discharges in the electroencephalogram, diphenylhydantoin should be used in combination with methylphenidate or dextroamphetamine in order to prevent any exacerbation of the tendency toward seizures.

In patients with psychotic behavior associated with hyperactivity, the central nervous system stimulants should be avoided and drugs such as thioridazine should be employed, along with psychotherapy. In the treatment of specific perceptual problems, methylphenidate is of proven value in the treatment of visual-perceptual deficits, and diphenylhydantoin is of benefit in patients with auditory imperception associated with paroxysmal abnormalities in the electroencephalogram. Imipramine may be employed in preference to methylphenidate in patients whose hyperactive behavior is complicated by nocturnal enuresis.

The clinical management of the child with hyperactivity and MBD is complex, requiring a multifaceted approach. Pharmacotherapy must be supplemented with remedial education, parent and child counseling, and psychotherapy, if needed. In children with motor incoordination and speech problems, physical therapy and speech therapy must be recommended.

Duration of Therapy

A tendency to improvement with age is generally to be expected. Hyperkinetic behavior is less prevalent in children after 10 or 12 years of age and abnormal neurological signs become more subtle and difficult to recognize in adolescence and young adult life. Treatment with medications is usually not necessary after the age of 12, when any risk of experimentation or misuse of drugs might possibly become more significant.

Risk of Drug Dependency

Several studies have failed to reveal an association between the medical use of stimulants in the preadolescent child and later drug abuse (Freedman, 1971a). The medical supervision appears to teach the child the appropriate use of medicines, and the hazards of later drug abuse is minimal. Safeguards against misuse of drugs should nevertheless be observed by parents. The child should not be given sole responsibility for taking a medication, and no child in the family should have access to medications not prescribed for himself. The advantages of having appropriate medication readily available for the treatment of behavioral disorders must be weighed against the dangers or disadvantages of rigid drug restrictions and the possible withholding of treatment from a child who may clearly benefit from drugs. Provided the medicine is of proven efficacy and is indicated, a child should not be denied a therapy that will control his hyperactivity, increase his attention span, and permit him to achieve to the level of his potential. It is the consensus among physicians that there is a place for central nervous system stimulants in the treatment of hyperkinetic behavioral disorders in children. These medications should be prescribed with suitable controls, under proper medical supervision, and as adjuncts to remedial education. Evaluations of their effects on behavior, coordination, and perception, using a battery of objective tests, as well as subjective evaluations of parents and teachers, should be used to monitor response to treatment at frequent intervals.

Summary

The ideal drug for the treatment of children with MBD should control hyperactivity, increase attention span, reduce impulsive and aggressive behavior, and have measurable beneficial effects on visual and auditory perception, reading ability, and coordination, without inducing insomnia, anorexia, drowsiness, or other, more serious, toxic

| Class of Compound | Name of Drug | | Preparations (mg) |
	Generic	Trade	
Central nervous system stimulants	Methylphenidate	Ritalin	Tabs. 5, 10, 20
	Dextroamphetamine	Dexedrine	Tabs. 5
	Deanol	Deaner	Tabs. 25, 100
Antianxiety and antipsychotic agents	Chlordiazepoxide	Librium	Caps. or Tabs. 5, 10, 25
	Chlorpromazine	Thorazine	Tabs. 10, 25, 50, 100
	Reserpine	Serpasil, var.	Tabs. 0.1, 0.5, 1.0
	Thioridazine	Mellaril	Tabs. 10, 25, 100, 200
	Hydroxyzine	Atarax	Tabs. 10, 25, 50, 100
		Vistaril	Caps. 25, 50, 100
	Promazine	Sparine	Tabs. 10, 25, 50, 100
	Fluphenazine	Prolixin	Tabs. 1, 2.5, 5
		Permitil	Tabs. 0.25, 1, 2.5
	Chlorprothixene	Taractan	Tabs. 10, 25, 50, 100
	Meprobamate	Miltown	Tabs. 200, 400
		Equanil	Tabs. 200, 400
Antidepressants	Imipramine	Tofranil	Tabs. 10, 25
Antihistamines	Diphenhydramine	Benadryl	Elix. 10 mg / 4 ml
Anticonvulsants ‡	Diphenylhydantoin	Dilantin	Tabs. 50
			Caps. 30, 100
	Primidone	Mysoline	Tabs. 50, 250

*Modified from Millichap (1969).
‡Suggested doses for children aged 5-15 years.
‡Advised in hyperkinetic children with seizure susceptibility.

Table 1. Drugs Used in the Treatment

| Daily Dose (mg) | Principal Side Effects | |
Average Range ‡	Benign	More Serious
10-30	nervousness, insomnia anorexia, stomachache, skin rash	
5-15	anorexia, nervousness, insomnia	
50-100	nervousness, headache, insomnia	
10-30	nausea, drowsiness	ataxia, syncope, leukopenia
10-30	drowsiness, dry mouth, nasal congestion	leukopenia, jaundice, dystonia, skin rash
0.1-0.5	drowsiness, nasal congestion, loose stools	
20-100	anorexia, miosis, urinary retention or incontinence	skin rash, leukopenia, jaundice, dystonia
20-100	drowsiness, dry mouth	
20-50	drowsiness, dry mouth	leukopenia, jaundice, dystonia
1-3	drowsiness, dry mouth	leukopenia, jaundice, dystonia
0.25-0.5	nervousness, dry mouth	leukopenia, jaundice, dystonia
20-50	drowsiness, nervousness, dry mouth	leukopenia, dystonia
200-600	abdominal pain, drowsiness, fever	skin rash, leukopenia
10-50	insomnia, perspiration, dizziness, urticaria, dry mouth	leukopenia, jaundice, hypertension
25-50	drowsiness	
50-200	anorexia, nausea, epigastric pain, gum hyperplasia, hirsutism	ataxia, skin rash, lymphadenopathy
100-500	anorexia, drowsiness	ataxia, skin rash

of Minimal Brain Dysfunction in Children*

Table 2. Order of Selection of Drugs in Control of Hyperkinetic Behavior*

Name of Drug Generic	Trade	Total Patients Tested	Expected Incidence of Control %	Expected Incidence of Control %
Methylphenidate	Ritalin	367	84	14
Amphetamine	Dexedrine	610	69	12
Chlordiazepoxide	Librium	237	60	18
Thioridazine	Mellaril	308	55	2
Chlorpromazine	Thorazine	153	55	25
Deanol	Deaner	239	47	7
Reserpine	Serpasil	165	34	1

*Modified from Millichap (1969).

effects. Central nervous system stimulants, methylphenidate anc dextroamphetamine, are the agents of choice, and short-term trials are justified as an adjunct to remedial education; effective response is related to the severity of the hyperkinesia and the frequency of neurological abnormalities. Antianxiety and antipsychotic agents, thioridazine, chlordiazepoxide, and chlorpromazine, and the antidepressant, imipramine, are recommended as alternative agents in patients who fail to respond to the stimulants. Diphenylhydantoin may improve auditory perception and control behavior and personality disorders and is indicated especially in patients with electroencephalographic abnormalities. Phenobarbital is contraindicated, because it usually exacerbates hyperactivity. Magnesium pemoline (Cylert), a new investigational compound, often controlled hyperactivity and improved IQ performance scale scores in the WISC.

Treating Problem Children
with Stimulant Drugs

L. ALAN SROUFE, Ph.D.

MARK A. STEWART, M.D.

*This report is a thoughtful, critical review of the use of stimu-
lant drugs. By raising several important questions the authors
offer a penetrating, fresh look at some issues which many
clinicians and researchers appear to take for granted. Their
arguments questioning the concept of minimal brain dysfunction,
the need for long-term studies, the importance of placebo effect,
and the possible negative effects of drug treatment are cogent and
well developed.*

*One particularly interesting question is that of whether the
response of problem children to stimulants is "paradoxical" or
whether it is essentially the same as that seen in "normal" adults
and children. If problem children have qualitatively the same
response as adults, the implications are quite serious. We would,
in essence, be putting children on "speed," and the charge of
"drugging" children (Hentoff, 1970; Maynard, 1970) could be
considered valid, even if well intentioned.*

More than 150,000 children with behavior or learning problems are
now being treated with stimulant drugs, with the number apparently

Reprinted from *New England Journal of Medicine,* Vol. 289 (1973), pp. 407-411. Reprinted with
permission.

increasing rapidly as proposals for massive screening begin to appear (Richard, 1972; Safer, 1971; Sroufe, in press; Steinberg, 1971; Wender, 1971). Since the prevalence of hyperactivity is about 5 per cent of children in elementary school (Werner, Bierman, French et al., 1968), and that of specific reading disability 3 per cent (Rutter, Tizard, and Whitmore, 1970), there is a very large population of children who might be treated in this way. We believe that the use of stimulant drugs should be critically appraised before society moves farther in this direction.

The literature on the short-term effects of stimulant medication with problem children can be summarized briefly. Controlled studies employing ratings by parents, teachers and medical or psychologic professionals consistently suggest that stimulant drugs improve both behavior and performance (Conners, 1971; Knights and Hinton 1969). Though the results may have been influenced by rater subjectivity and halo effects, these studies are supported by a growing number of experiments using standardized tests, laboratory tasks and objective measurements of activity level and motor performance, which are less vulnerable to such difficulties. These experimental studies show that drug-treated children perform better than placebo-treated controls on certain subscales of standard intelligence tests (e.g., WISC digit symbol), maze tracing and figure drawing, achievement tests, paired associate learning tasks, and portions of the Frostig Developmental Test of Visual Perception (Conners, 1971; Knights and Hinton, 1969; Conners, Eisenberg, and Barcai, 1967).

Definite drug-placebo differences on various laboratory tasks and reaction time have also been found. On vigilance tasks, such as detecting the appearance of certain letters in a lengthy series of presentations, fewer errors of omission and commission occur in the stimulant-drug groups, and response time is faster (Sykes, Douglas, and Morgenstern, 1972). Matching to standard and delayed recognition performance are also improved (Sprague, Barnes, and Werry, 1970). Finally, reaction time and reaction-time variability are reduced by stimulant drugs (Cohen, Douglas, and Morgenstern, 1971; Sroufe, Sonies, West et al., in press). As with studies on learning paired associates, these effects are enhanced as the experiments proceed, suggesting strongly that motivation or attention is the factor primarily influenced by drugs.

This is an impressive array of experimental findings. Stimulant drugs seem to be effective in altering the behavior and performance of children labeled as hyperactive, learning disabled or having minimal brain dysfunction. However, a number of questions arise that are crucial for the evaluation of these effects and for the management of children. Are the reported effects paradoxical or atypical—that is, are the effects the reverse of what one would expect for normal children and adults, characteristic of these problem children, and thus signs of underlying dysfunction in the brain? Is there an established relation between neurologic or biochemical abnormality and behavioral problems, and are such organic deviations predictive of drug response? Finally, do the positive effects reported in the short-term studies persist, and what is the evidence concerning short-term and long-term negative consequences of drug treatment?

The Question of the Atypical
Drug Response

For years, clinicians and researchers have spoken of a paradoxical drug effect—that is, drugs that stimulate adults seemingly calm hyperactive children. This notion is no longer given credence, since hyperactive children are not sedated by stimulant drugs. Vigilance, persistence, and the level of free-field activity are increased by stimulant drugs (Conners, 1971; Millichap and Boldrey, 1967). Also, whereas a reduction in motor activity has been reported in the context of task performance, this is probably an indirect effect of increased concentration (Sprague, Barnes, and Werry, 1970; Sroufe, Sonies, West et al., in press).

More recently, it has been argued that these children are unusually responsive to stimulant drugs, rather than responding atypically. This argument still implies abnormal function of the brain, but since the studies reviewed above did not include normal control groups, this conclusion is not justified. The only study that has included normal children showed no differences in the response to drugs (Shetty, 1971). Other studies have concerned responses of children who have been simply referred by teachers for "problem behavior" and have not had medical or psychologic evaluations (Steinberg, Troshinsky, and Steinberg, 1971; Conners, Eisenberg, and Barcai, 1967). The uniformly positive drug effects in such loosely defined samples raise obvious questions about "normal" or atypical responses to drugs in children.

Finally, the literature shows striking parallels between the effects of stimulant drugs on normal adults and on problem children. In adult subjects reaction times are decreased, and vigilance, tracking skills and performance in simple arithmetic problems and other tasks requiring attentiveness (e.g., typing) are enhanced. The effects are greater over time and more pronounced in fatigued or hypoxic subjects (Weiss and Laties, 1962). Thus, performance is improved on repetitive, routinized tasks that require sustained attention, and these are exactly the findings with problem children. Reasoning, problem solving and learning do not seem to be affected in adults or children. Both groups seem to have similar patterns of tolerance and withdrawal reactions— for example, maintenance dosages can be easily established with careful monitoring, and neither group has physical withdrawal symptoms after stopping stimulant drugs (United States Department of Health, Education and Welfare, 1971). Adults and problem children may have difficulty getting to sleep on stimulants, and lethargy and increased need for sleep when withdrawn (Small, Hibi, and Feinberg, 1971).

The Hyperactive-Child Syndrome and Brain Dysfunction

Hyperactivity was described first as occurring with various kinds of brain injury or disease (Ebaugh, 1923; Strauss and Lehtinen, 1947). Having undoubtedly seen many children with both hyperactivity and neurologic dysfunction, clinicians have tended to generalize this association (Paine, 1962) and some writers have emphasized the etiologic role of organic factors in reaction to the view that these problems were always due to emotional conflicts (Clements and Peters, 1962).

The concept of "minimal brain dysfunction" has now become widely accepted, even though the reasoning behind it is often circular—that is, authors have assumed that behaviors such as hyperactivity were signs of brain damage independent of neurologic indexes, and, therefore, that many behavior problem children had brain damage. Moreover, a positive response to stimulant drugs has been used as confirmation of the diagnosis of organicity. However, when hyperactivity and minimal brain dysfunction are defined simply as clusters of difficult behaviors, only a small minority of such children seem to have had brain damage (Chess, 1960; Stewart, Pitts, Craig et al., 1966; Werry, Weiss, and Douglass, 1964). Likewise, studies on the frequency of neurologic soft signs or minor electroencephalographic dysrhythmias have produced inconsistent results, with poorly standardized criteria or a lack of control groups often characterizing studies with positive findings (Werry, 1972). To date, no neurologic signs or test or combination of tests has been established through cross-validation to differentiate hyperactive children or those with minimal brain dysfunction from normal control subjects.

Furthermore, the existence of a unitary syndrome of minimal brain dysfunction has not been established. The problems subsumed by the definition of minimal brain dysfunction (Wender, 1971) include hyperactivity, distractibility, incoordination, short attention span, underachievement and "perceptual" difficulties. These behaviors have not been shown to intercorrelate, and the presence of one or more of them does not predict the others (Sroufe, in press; Palkes and Stewart, 1972). Factor analytic studies yield numerous orthogonal factors, each of which accounts for only a small percentage of the variance (Werry, 1968), and generally great heterogeneity among samples is reported (Conners, 1972c; Knights and Hinton, 1969). Conners, for example, distinguished seven discrete groups of problem children, each showing a different pattern of change scores after stimulant drugs (Conners, 1972c). Further research is, of course, required to cross-validate Conners's findings and to determine whether any of these "subsyndromes" can be tied to neurologic dysfunction.

The concept of "minimal brain dysfunction" was nurtured in part by the theory of a continuum of reproductive casualty that was put forward by Pasamanick and his colleagues in the late 1950s and was based on retrospective studies of perinatal morbidity related to neurologic and psychologic problems in children (Kawi and Pasamanick, 1959; Pasamanick and Lilienfeld, 1955). Retrospective studies based on actual medical records (Minde, Webb, and Sykes, 1968) and the prospective follow-up studies of perinatal stress carried out by Graham (Graham, Ernhart, Thurston et al., 1962) and Werner (Werner, Bierman, French et al., 1968) and their colleagues show that stresses of this kind may lead to lower intelligence, but are not associated with later behavior problems or hyperactivity. Werner's study also suggested that there is a threshold of severity at which perinatal stress affects children's development, rather than a continuous relation between stress and its consequences, an observation that contradicts a major premise of the concept of "minimal brain dysfunction."

Looking for associations between specific kinds of assaults on the nervous system and the later development of behavior or learning problems is likely to be more productive than the study of general stresses. For example, Drillien (1964) reported that premature infants are more likely to acquire behavior problems, including hyperactivity, as they grew older; more recently she had found this sequence most likely to occur in a specific subgroup of infants with low birth weights (1972). Other lines of research suggest that specific reading disability and hyperactivity have important genetic determinants (Hallgren, 1950; Morrison and Stewart, 1971; Cantwell, 1972; Morrison and Stewart, in press).

Physiologic and Biochemical
Predictors of Drug Response

Although neurologic indexes of organic deviation have failed to yield consistent results, there has been growing interest in biochemical measures and indicators of arousal level as predictors of stimulant-drug response. Successful prediction of drug reaction would have both practical and heuristic implications.

Some investigators have suggested that hyperactive children are over-aroused, and that amphetamines reduce arousal (Laufer, Denhoff, and Solomons, 1957); others postulate low arousal (Satterfield and Dawson, 1971). Similarly, both low (Wender, 1971) and high (Kornetsky, 1970) levels of norepinephrine in the brain have been hypothesized. Evidence to support each of these positions can be found in the literature, and therefore no definite conclusions can be reached. For example, Rapoport et al. observed that low urinary norepinephrine levels before treatment predicted positve response to amphetamine (Rapoport, Lott, Alexander et al., 1970). However, predrug scores on activity level, the dependent measure, were not controlled in this study, and the relation between levels of norepinephrine in urine and those in the brain is tenuous. Wender failed to find such differences between control children and those with minimal brain dysfunction (1971). Satterfield and Dawson report lower skin conductance in hyperactive children, which is interpreted as low arousal (1971). But others, including Satterfield himself, report either no difference in autonomic indexes of arousal or greater arousal in hyperactive children (Cohen, Douglas, and Morgenstern, 1971; Stevens, Boydstun, Ackerman et al., 1968). Some central-nervous-system measures (evoked potentials, power-spectrum analyses of the electroencephalogram) have yielded important results, but again there is an absence of replication and also uncertainty whether the measures are indicative of high or low arousal (Conners, 1971b; Satterfield, Cantwell, Lesser et al., 1972). In addition, such differences might reflect a psychophysiologic reaction to the testing rather than underlying neuropathy.

A way out of the dilemma posed by these contradictory theories and findings is to assume that some problem children are under-aroused (hyper-reactive) and others are over-aroused (hyperactive). However, if greater variability in arousal is consistently demonstrated in hyperactive groups, this finding may only reflect heterogeneity due to varied sampling procedures. Consistent inter-correlations across studies must be obtained to establish that such high variability is due to the presence of two or more types of hyperactive children, rather than to the disparate makeup of the referred clinic sample as compared to volunteer control subjects. Likewise, differential drug response by high or low aroused subjects must be established through cross-validation.

Need for Long-Term Drug Evaluation

Persistence of Stimulant-Drug Effects

Typical drug experiments are brief, lasting only a few weeks. Therefore, it is not known at present whether the performance effects persist, yielding actual differences in school achievement, for example, or whether drug effects disappear over longer treatment periods. There are a few relevant studies, each of which raises questions about the persistence of drug effects. Conrad et al., for example, did not find a drug advantage over four to six months for a large number of clinical and cognitive measures, including arithmetic and reading achievement, but only for some rating data and certain Frostig subtests (Conrad, Dworkin, Shai et al., 1971). The results of drug treatment were not much better than tutoring by semitrained volunteers. Other studies have also failed to find much evidence for drug effects on measures taken across a long period (Knights and Hinton, 1969; Zimmerman and Burgemeister, 1958).

The deterioration of performance reported when children are temporarily withdrawn from medication may be interpreted as evidence of behavioral dependence rather than persistence of positive drug effects. Work with animals also suggests a deterioration in performance after withdrawal of amphetamine, even when a maintenance dosage has been achieved (Thompson and Pickens, 1971). In addition to long-term evaluation, studies are needed in which subjects are gradually shifted from drug to placebo, to minimize such withdrawal effects.

The only available studies in which hyperactive children have been followed from the time that they entered a psychiatric clinic, usually between the ages of eight and eleven, to when they are in junior high or high school suggest that the outlook for children treated primarily with drugs is relatively poor (Weiss, Minde, Werry et al., 1971; Mendelson, Johnson, and Stewart, 1971). In their teens these children were still having trouble in their families, often behaving antisocially, and presenting academic and behavior problems in school. The last result is particularly disappointing since drug treatments have generally been aimed specifically at helping problem children do better in school. However, neither of these studies included groups of hyperactive children who had no treatment or who were treated primarily in some psychologic way. We can only conclude that the long-range effects of drug treatment are generally modest.

Physicians and parents commonly assume that a hyperactive child who is "successfully" treated with stimulant drugs over a period of months or years will acquire good habits because of the reinforcements he is given for his good behavior while on the drug. The follow-up studies cited above do not seem to support this idea, but we simply do not know whether this crucial assumption is valid. Current research on "state dependent learning" suggests that some habits learned while the subject is under the influence of drugs or alcohol do not carry over into the subject's behavior while he is sober or undrugged (Overton, 1970).

Another common assumption about the use of drugs is that they will "help the child do better in school." Successfully treated children do more of their assigned work in class, but one may question whether this is a truly important goal; doing assigned work is not the same as learning. Palkes and Stewart have shown that the school achievement levels of hyperactive children match those of their normal classmates when differences of intelligence level are taken into account—a finding that suggests that they do not have a deficit in actual learning.

The Placebo Effect: Problems of Set and Expectation

The absence of data on the persistence of drug effects is particularly bothersome because of the well known influence of subject and evaluator set and expectations concerning drug outcome. Both the range and the extent of placebo effects are well known in psychopharmacology. Practically any effect can be obtained with a placebo, and estimates of placebo responders average about 35 per cent, but range up to 70 per cent, apparently depending on the subjectivity of the instrument and the degree of blindness of evaluators (Sroufe, in press; DeLong, 1972). Placebo effects are likely to be greater with active drugs than inert substances—that is, if the active drug produces some clear side effect, the subject's belief in drug potency is enhanced (Cole, 1968). Also, the particular placebo effect obtained will depend to a large extent on the expectation of the child (or parent) concerning the drug. For example, in a study with adults, Schachter found that subjects became either euphoric or angry after administration of epinephrine, depending on the cognitive set created (1964). The effect of set was greater for active drug than for placebo, probably because drug subjects experienced actual physiologic changes, which bolstered their belief that the expected drug effect was going to occur.[1]

These considerations of the power of set and expectation raise important questions concerning clinical reports of the long-term effectiveness of stimulant medication. Placebo effects probably do not account for the array of experimental results reported earlier. However, in the absence of long-term controlled experiments, we do not know to what extent genuine drug effects fade, with persistent improvement being based on the expectations of child, parent and teacher. McDermott reports a case in which the child's parents discontinued stimulant-drug treatment, having misinterpreted a doctor's instructions; yet the dramatic improvement in behavior and school performance that they expected from short-term drug treatment persisted for six months (1965).

Negative Drug Effects

There is little information concerning the detrimental behavioral effects of stimulant drugs or the physical consequences of prolonged medical treatment. From the existing literature one might conclude that stimulant drugs only influence behavior and performance in a positive way. In fact, only one unpublished report could be found in

[1] Such expectation effects may explain why children are not reported to experience euphoria after stimulant drug administration. Like Schachter's "anger" subjects, children in drug studies are not set to experience a "high"; rather, they are persuaded that the drugs will help them control their behavior and improve school performance. These are the effects that occur. Children in Bradley's (1937) early study, not set to be calmed by stimulants, did report euphoric experiences (e.g., "I have joy in my stomach").

which negative as well as positive behavioral effects were predicted (Sprague, Werry, and Davis, 1969); yet an adequate model of drug effects should predict both positive and negative results. For example, if stimulant drugs increase focused attention in a discrimination learning task, drug subjects should show poorer performance on the transfer task when the previously irrelevant dimension becomes relevant. We need to isolate conditions in which hyperactive children do not exhibit a performance deficit, and to gather information on possible detrimental effects of stimulant drugs on incidental learning, for example, to evaluate the treatment fully.

Although the immediate side effects of stimulant drugs—sleeplessness, loss of appetite, irritability and crying without provocation (Conners, Eisenberg, and Barcai, 1967; Epstein, Lasagna, Conners and Rothschild, 1968)—seem to be only of temporary concern, little is known about the long-term effects of these medications. Short-term studies finding negative results and parent questionnaire data (Comly, 1971) are not a sufficient basis for concluding that these drugs are without risk. Recently, Safer et al. reported that relatively high doses of amphetamine or methylphenidate continued over months may significantly reduce weight gain and growth in stature (Safer, Allen, and Barr, 1972). These effects may have reflected the drug's influence on appetite, but it is also likely that they were central effects; amphetamines have been reported to affect the release of growth hormone (Rees, Butler, Gosling et al., 1970). The latter possibility raises the disturbing thought that stimulants might affect the rate of sexual development as well as growth in general. Safer's work points up the aptness of recent remarks by Eisenberg (1971): "... what is given even briefly at a particular developmental period may have unforeseen long-term consequences," and "the available data urge caution upon us."

Potential Consequences of the Drug Solution

In addition to possible consequences for physical development, we believe that there are other potential dangers in the widespread use of stimulant drugs with problem children. The most obvious of these is that the use of the drugs lowers the motivation of parents and teachers to take other steps to help the child. Thoughtful physicians have stressed the point that drug treatment, when employed at all, must be the beginning of a total treatment program for the child that includes parent counseling, special educational techniques and the like (Eisenberg, 1971; Solomons, 1972). Yet there is reason to suspect that drugs are the only treatment offered to many hyperactive children. Using a criterion of two telephone contacts within six months, Solomons (1972) reported that only about one-half of the children in his survey were being monitored adequately, and Browder (1972) reported that children are sometimes put on medication without a single contact with a physician.

It is often argued that drugs may break up a vicious circle of unhappiness, but negative consequences for the child's self-concept may be equally important. The child can conclude that he is not responsible for his behavior: "I can't help being bad today. I haven't had my pill." The child comes to believe not in the soundness of his own brain and body, not in his own growing ability to learn and to control his behavior, but in "my magic pills that make me into a good boy and make everybody like me" (Wender, 1971). When the parent turns to the drug solution child-rearing responsibility is avoided, and when the teacher does the same thing, the development of effective teaching for problem children is less likely.

Drug treatment may also provide an inappropriate solution to what are basically sociologic problems. It has been suggested that delinquency and the problems of impoverished children may derive from "minimal brain dysfunction" (Wender, 1971). Drugs would merely mask the problems of such children, however. Eisenberg (1971), for example, has pointed out the inappropriateness of using stimulant drugs rather than food to treat hypoglycemia. The performance of poorly rested, malnourished children can probably be improved by stimulant drugs, just as occurs with hypoxic or overly fatigued adults (Weiss and Laties, 1962).

In addition, one must be concerned about a possible influence of expanding drug treatment on drug abuse by youth. Most children of elementary-school age are reluctant to take their pills, and seem to be relatively unaware of the ways in which stimulants affect their behavior. When children continue to take stimulants during junior high and high school, however, there may be problems. One of us (M.A.S.) has known patients to take extra doses to do better on tests, and to sell pills. In spite of the obvious possibility that such abuse would occur, no systematic studies have been published on whether hyperactive or other problem children treated with stimulants are more likely to abuse drugs than other children, or corresponding hyperactive children who have not received drugs. Laufer (1971) presented a study that seems reassuring, but his data were based on questionnaires sent to parents, who might well have been unaware of their children's use of drugs (median age, 20), and an appreciable number of parents involved in the study did not return questionnaires.

Finally, it seems that physicians and teachers may be propagating a confusing and ambivalent attitude toward psychotropic drugs when they advise the use of stimulants for problem children. In educational programs designed to counteract drug abuse young people are told that drugs are a "chemical cop-out," and that if they have personal difficulties, they should work on them rather than try to solve them with drugs. They are also warned not to experiment with drugs because of potential dangers from chronic use. On the other hand, the use of stimulants for children with learning and behavior problems is widely advocated as a quick and practical solution, even when the long-term use of such drugs has not been proved to be harmless.

Alternative Ways of
Managing Problem Children

Several authors have reported successful reduction of overactivity in the classroom through "behavior modification" (Patterson, Jones, Whittier et al., 1965; Doubros and Daniels, 1966), and other specific patterns of behavior such as tantrums and disruption have been treated in the same way (Carlson, Arnold, Becker et al., 1968; Thomas, Becker, and Armstrong, 1968). Another psychologic approach to a specific behavior problem is training in self-directed verbal commands as a means of controlling impulsiveness (Palkes, Steward and Kahana, 1968). Both parents and teachers can be taught to manage their difficult children's behavior with operant principles (Madsen, Becker and Thomas, 1968; Berkowitz and Graziano, 1972) or video-tape feedback of interactions between parents and their children (Furman and Feighner, in press). Finally, Schaefer et al. found that bringing groups of parents together to discuss ways of handling specific problems in child management enhances their ability to cope with difficult children, builds their self-confidence, and improves the relations between parents and their children (Schaefer, Palkes and Steward, in press). In this technique, parents read a book on child management (Smith and Smith, 1966) before they attend the sessions, so that they have a base of knowledge from which to work.

These various reports suggest that there are alternative ways of managing the difficulties of hyperactive and other problem children at home and in the classroom. However, the persistent effectiveness of these methods has not yet been demonstrated by follow-up studies. It also remains to be seen whether a combination of these techniques would be as successful and practical a way of managing problem children as the use of stimulants. Finally, as with drugs, behavior modification should be used only after careful examination reveals that the problem resides in the child rather than in deficient curricula, ineffective teaching, or problems within the family.

Discussion

There are surely some children for whom treatment with stimulants or other drugs is essential because they cannot be managed outside an institution without such treatment. These tend to be children whose serious behavior and learning problems are associated with a history of brain disorder such as encephalitis, or an ongoing brain dysfunction like epilepsy.

On the other hand, it seems from reports by Solomons (1972) and others and from complaints in the lay press that drugs are given to many children without real justification, or under inadequate supervision. Frequently, children who are brought to a physician because their teachers find them difficult are given a trial on stimulant medicine with the assumption that improvement will indicate that they truly have "minimal brain dysfunction." This reasoning seems completely unwarranted.

In the middle ground there are very large numbers of children who are genuinely hyperactive or who have specific reading disability or some other learning problem; there may be between two and four million children with such problems in the United States. Some physicians have publicly advocated that such children be identified and given stimulant drugs to maintain their interest in school work and their general self-esteem. We do not question the fact that some of these children, not to mention their families and teachers, benefit from treatment with stimulants. However, we urge greater skepticism about the immediate effects on children's self-esteem and their learning, and even more about the effects of long-term treatment with these drugs. There are promising alternative approaches to the management of children with these problems, all of which involve the child's learning control of his own behavior. The basic flaw of drug treatment is that it cannot teach a child anything, and it is not yet established that drug treatment makes the child more accessible to other intervention techniques.

A few physicians have suggested that the treatment of problem children with stimulants is analogous to the treatment of diabetic patients with insulin. Admitting that the characteristic behavior of a hyperactive child may continue into adulthood, they argue that it is logical to maintain such patients on stimulants indefinitely. The lack of data demonstrating the persistence of drug effects and the failure to establish an organic origin for the majority of these children underscore the presumptive nature of this position. In addition, such a hypothesis raises broad social and ethical questions that must be dealt with before such a practice is considered.

Effects of Psychopharmacologic Agents on Learning Disorders

ROBERT L. SPRAGUE, Ph.D.

ESTHER K. SLEATOR, M.D.

This is a succinct, yet comprehensive, overview of the treatment of learning disorders with drugs. It concludes with some specific clinical recommendations. One of the major points stressed is dosage, particularly in reference to methylphenidate. In their own studies the authors used dosages from 0.2 to 0.3 mg/kg which yielded significantly better performances on short-term memory tasks and increased appropriate social behavior in the classroom compared to placebo. They further report that higher dosages resulted in fewer correct responses. This contrasts to other studies using 1.2-1.9 mg/kg, which also report improved performance. These larger dosages are more in line with those commonly recommended for use in clinical practice (Wender, 1971; Millichap, 1973). To carry the point further, the authors describe a study (unfortunately not referenced) in which subjects being treated with methylphenidate displayed a gradual decline in performance on a short-term memory task as dosages were increased from 0.3 to 0.7 mg/kg, while they correspondingly showed a steep drop in seat activity. This leads the authors to conclude that in using dosages above 0.3 mg/kg we may be purchasing less hyperactivity at the price of decreased learning efficiency. Obviously in a situation with frustrated teachers, discouraged parents, and ostracizing peers, this may be clinically indicated.

The authors propose other reasons for concern with dosage: Safer's work provides strong evidence of decreased growth in children treated with stimulants. Other studies have reported that heart rate in children who received methylphenidate increased an average of 15 beats per minute. It may be that clinicians can achieve desired results with dosages lower than those generally used at present.

Learning disorder implies: (1) school problems which are manifested in the form of deficiencies in academic performance and (2) behavioral problems in the classroom typified by poor attention, impulsivity, poor social behavior, and hyperactivity (Clements, 1966). In this article we will deal with the effects of psychopharmacologic agents in children of school age, primarily those in the middle childhood years. In our survey of drugs, the stimulants are emphasized because far more research has been done with them than with other categories of psychotropic drugs. No attempt has been made to cover anticonvulsant medication.

This article is not a comprehensive and complete review of the voluminous literature in pediatric psychopharmacology. Many of the studies reported in the pediatric psychopharmacology literature simply do not meet minimum scientific standards for acceptability (Freeman, 1966; Sprague and Werry, 1971). In a previous article (Sprague and Werry, 1971) we have listed six criteria as minimum standards for psychotropic drug investigations, and generally these criteria have been followed in evaluating studies for inclusion in this review.

Investigations which have studied the combined effects of psychotropic drugs and other treatment techniques, particularly treatment associated with school programs, have been given strong emphasis. The authors feel strongly that psychotropic drugs have all too frequently been prescribed and used without proper consideration of

Reprinted from *Pediatric Clinics of North America*, Vol. 20 (1973), pp. 719-735.

the viewpoints and information from the school system, the parents, and the child. In the area of learning disorders where the child is encountering school problems, the primary difficulty, thus defined, is school related. If the target problem is school related, then the primary criteria for improvement should be derived from the school, and not necessarily from measures that are only remotely, if at all, related to the child's behavior at school (for example, electroencephalography) (Freeman, 1967).

Review of the Literature

In the summer and fall of 1970 the term "behavior-modifying drug" was thrust upon the general public awareness via television and the front pages of the newspapers, when there was sensational news coverage of a program in the schools of Omaha, Nebraska, in which methylphenidate was used rather extensively (Hentoff, 1970; Maynard, 1970). The "Omaha incident" brought a spate of alarmist journalism in which the writers seemed more interested in a sensational story than substantiating the facts and underlying problems as indicated by some of the titles used: "Pills for Learning" (Dupree, 1971), "Drug Abuse—Just What the Doctor Ordered" (Rogers, 1971), and "Drugging and Schooling" (Witter, 1971).

The public clamor over these stories and news releases resulted in a congressional inquiry by Congressman Gallagher late in 1970 before the fall elections.

Panels formed by professional organization and governmental agencies during this time issued statements on the problem. The Committee of Drugs of the American Academy of Pediatrics issued a statement (Yaffe, 1970), and a "Blue Ribbon Panel" (sponsored by the Office of Child Development) wrote a report which was given wide publicity (Bazell, 1971; Freedman, 1971). Both panels produced reasoned and succinct statements of the problem, which should be required reading for anyone seriously interested in this issue.

The intense public interest in pediatric psychopharmacology can be viewed as only the culmination of a long trend in the treatment of mental health problems in the general population which had been termed a "pharmaceutical revolution" by Lasagna (1969). Concurrent with this trend in psychiatry, scientists interested in learning were producing considerable evidence that numerous drugs and biochemicals influenced learning and memory. Some of these scientists made sweeping extrapolations from their animal data to children and painted illusions about the possibility of "psychoneurobiochemeducation" and "chemical memory pellets" (Krech, 1969). This trend for increased drug usage has been seriously questioned (Lennard, 1970), and the medical system for delivering such treatment has been cogently and severely criticized (Muller, 1972). The facts show clearly that there has been dramatic increase in the use of psychotropic drugs during the 1960's (Balter, 1969) and that physicians who see children, particularly hyperactive children, tend to use psychotropic drugs extensively; Greenberg and Lipman (1971) reported that 91 per cent of the physicians surveyed who treated hyperactive children prescribed such drugs. A colleague of ours, Dr. Karen Stephen, in a survey of 284 pediatricians, 244 psychiatrists and neurologists, and 172 general practitioners (total of 700) in the greater metropolitan Chicago area found that 2 to 4 per cent of the school age children in that area are treated with psychotropic drugs for an average duration of 9 months.

Effects of Drugs on Learning, Retention, and School Behavior

Learning Performance and Laboratory Tests

Even though the target behavior is that of school performance or learning performance, there has been surprisingly little investigation of the effects of psychotropic drugs on learning in children, as a recent review indicates (Conners, 1972b). Most of the limited data come from the three laboratories of Conners in Boston, Douglas in Montreal, and our laboratory in Illinois. Generally the other laboratories do not state their dosage in terms of mg. per kg. but we have estimated below a mg. per kg. ratio on the basis of the mean dosage per day and the mean age of the children.

Conners and his colleagues (Conners, Eisenberg and Sharpe, 1964) have found that methylphenidate enhances learning as measured by paired-associate maze learning and Porteus performance at about 1.4 mg. per kg. (60 mg. per day for a mean age of 12 at about 43 kg.), and that dextroamphetamine at about 0.7 mg. per kg. (25 mg. per day for a mean age of 10 at about 35 kg.) increased visual paired-associate learning and Porteus maze performance (Conners, Rothschild, Eisenberg et al., 1969), and particularly on the Continuous Performance Test. The Continuous Performance Test is a laboratory measure of sustained attention or vigilance to rather monotonous stimulation, usually visual. There are several variations of the test, but essentially the child is required to monitor a visual display and pick out the infrequent targets (for example, the letter A following X in a series of single letters). These stimuli are presented for very brief intervals (1 second or 2) for a large number of trials (usually 200 to 300). Errors and latencies are typically measured, and Conners (1968) has found that dextroamphetamine reduces the impulsively fast response when errors are made and reduces errors of omission.

In a very fine summary of several years of systematic work comparing the behavior of hyperactive and learning disordered children with normal controls, Douglas (1972) has said that sustained attention seems to be the particular impairment of hyperactive children and that stimulants improve attention as measured by the Continuous Performance Test. The view that the basic problem is that of attention has been supported by others (Dykman, Ackerman, Clements et al., 1971).

Two recent informative studies have appeared from the Montreal laboratory. Hyperactive and control children were given the Continuous Performance Tests (Sykes, Douglas, Weiss et al., 1971) and their activity was monitored by a stabilimetric cushion which measures the amount of wiggling the child engages in while seated (Sprague and Toppe, 1966). When the interval between the target presentations was increased from 1 second to 1.5 seconds, the control subjects were able to do better and reduce their number of errors, whereas the hyperactive children maintained the same error rate. However, when methylphenidate in dosages of about 1.2 mg. per kg. (35 mg. per day for a mean age of 8 years or about 28 kg.) was administered to these hyperactive children, they were able to significantly reduce their errors as the pace became slower in comparison with the placebo condition. Moreover, the hyperactive children were more fidgety in this test situation than the controls, and their restlessness increased more on the second testing session than the controls.

In another very similar study hyperactive children and normal children were compared on similar tasks, but only the hyperactive children received methylphenidate and placebo (Sykes, Douglas and Morgenstern, 1972). Dosage was about 1.9 mg. per kg. (57 mg. per day for a mean age of 8.4 years or about 30 kg.). As before, they found that methylphenidate produced a large number of correct responses on the Continuous Performance Test and that it led to less deterioration in the number of correct responses over three test periods in comparison with placebo. On tasks that required sustained attention which the experimenter paced, the hyperactive children were considerably more impaired than normal children in comparison with tasks which were subject paced. This difference noted between experimenter-paced tasks and subject-paced tasks contributes support to the speculation that there is an attention deficit in hyperactive children and that this impairment is decreased by the administration of stimulants.

A study from our laboratory obtained data both from the experimental laboratory and from the classroom (Sprague, Barnes, and Werry, 1970). This is one of the few studies which integrate both classroom observational data and experimental learning data. Thus, it adds some information to the question of whether the experimental laboratory data, although interesting in its own right, are predictive of what happens in the real world of the classroom. A short-term memory task was used which requires the subject to look at a matrix of stimuli (in this study either 1, 2 or 3 pictures presented simultaneously), remember these pictures for a few seconds, and then subsequently indicate on a test trial whether the presented test stimulus was or was not seen before in the previous matrix. In our laboratory dosage is manipulated on a mg. per kg. basis to the nearest 2.5 mg. per child. Methylphenidate (0.25 and 0.35 mg. per kg.) significantly increased the number of correct responses and increased the speed of responding in comparison with placebo, whereas thioridazine (0.75 and 1.0 mg. per kg.) had just the opposite effect in comparison with placebo—reduced the correct responses and reduced the speed. Observations on a standardized scale indicated that methylphenidate increased the child's attention to the school task in comparison with placebo and increased appropriate social behavior in the classroom (Werry and Quay, 1969).

Using a similar short-term memory task, another study from our laboratory indicated an inverted "U" dose-response curve (Sprague and Werry, 1971). Placebo significantly increased the number of correct responses in comparison with no drug, and 0.2 and 0.3 mg. per kg. of methylphenidate increased correct responding in comparison with placebo, but further increases in the dosages up to 0.4 mg. per kg. actually reduced correct responses.

Retention of Learned Material

State-dependent learning or dissociation are the terms applied to a reduction or failure to transfer a habit learned under a drug state to a non-drug state or vice versa. This phenomenon has been extensively investigated by Overton (1966, 1968). Although the phenomenon has been well studied in animals, it is quite surprising that state-dependent learning has received little investigation in children, especially considering the fact that children who take psychotropic drugs are usually actively engaged in learning academic material. There are a few studies pertinent to this problem as we have recently reviewed (Sprague, 1972; Sprague and Werry, 1971). Some of our early studies indicated that there might be differentially more forgetting of material learned under a drug state when tested under a no drug state, but a series of subsequent investigations has not supported the original trends.

Using mentally retarded boys, and the short-term memory task, Hallsten (1970) found no evidence for state-dependent learning over 24 hours under methylphenidate (0.35 mg. per kg.) or thioridazine (1.0 mg. per kg.). In an extensive study of state-dependent learning effects, Aman (1972) did not find any evidence to support state-dependent learning in a group of hyperactive, learning disordered children utilizing methylphenidate (0.5 or 1.0 mg. per kg.) and dextroamphetamine (0.2 mg. per kg.) on three different laboratory tasks: short-term memory, a paired associate learning task, and a motor performance task involving learning a finger maze.

Classroom Behavior

Relatively few investigations have looked at classroom performance mainly because a satisfactory measuring technique was not available. Conners (1969) has developed one of the most widely used and best studied scales which is a Teacher Rating Scale of 39 items that has been factor analyzed to give four factors. Although Conners did not give normative data in his original study, comparative data have been subsequently developed (Kupietz, Bialer and Winsbert, 1972; Sprague, Christensen and Werry, in press). Conners (1972; Conners, Taylor, Meo et al., 1972) has shortened this rating scale to 10 items which makes it very simple and easy to use even by the practicing physician who does not have access to an experimental laboratory. The teacher is instructed to observe the child for some period of time (typically either 1 week or 4 weeks), remember these observations, and then fill out the form at the end of the period, basing her ratings on that child for that period. There are 10 questions, each of which can be marked as either applying not at all (0), just a little (1), pretty much (2), or very much (3). The total score is then averaged, and a mean score is obtained.

A representative study utilizing the Connors' Abbreviated Teacher Rating Scale will be described. A total of 25 hyperactive, learning-disordered children were selected to participate in a methylphenidate dosage study which lasted 16 weeks. Each subject served as his own control; that is, he received for 4 weeks each of the dosage conditions which were: placebo, 0.1 mg., 0.3 mg., and 0.7 mg. per kg. The order of the dosage conditions over time was varied according to a Latin Square design. Because of missing data and a change of teacher raters, two subjects were dropped from the final pool leaving a total of 23 subjects. The mothers were instructed to give the medication to the child on school mornings just before he left for school. Each mother received a file with a month's supply of dated envelopes containing the tablets and was instructed to return the file with both the opened and unopened (when she forgot to give the capsule) envelopes. In order to vary the dose depending upon the weight of the subject, a pharmacist placed tablets of active drug and tablets of placebo (the appropriate number depending upon the weight of the child and the dosage condition) in a number 0 orange gelatin opaque capsule. Thus, all of the capsules looked exactly alike. The numerous assessments were taken at the end of each 4 week dosage. Again, as reported above, the peak effect of methylphenidate on this learning task is at the dosage level of 0.3 mg. per kg. Second, various laboratory indicators of drug effect do not always agree; e.g., the greatest reduction in seat activity is at 0.7 mg. per kg. In contrast to the data from Connors' laboratory and the Montreal laboratory, no statistically significant effect was found on the Continuous Performance Test. But remember that the mg. per kg. dosage used here was less than used in those laboratories.

Even more important than trying to determine which measure of drug can be used efficiently is the problem of coordinating psycho-pharmacological treatment with other important and effective treatments of the child such as special education programs, prescriptive tutoring, and behavior modification programs which have recently gained widespread attention (Graziano, 1971). It is most unfortunate that there is practically no information available on the interactive effects of psychotropic drug treatment and these other very common treatment procedures. The urgent need for such information has been pointed out previously (Brady, 1968; Brady, 1971; Sprague, 1972; Sprague and Werry, 1971). Data from the area of the treatment of enuresis indicate that there are significantly better results if a combination of psychotropic drug therapy and behavior modification procedures (the buzzer blanket) are used together rather than separately (Young and Turner, 1965).

Conrad et al. (1971) studied the effects of dextroamphetamine and prescriptive tutoring consisting of about 40 sessions (2 sessions per week) on a variety of measures including both parent and teacher ratings and laboratory measures. A number of statistically significant differences were found on the gain scores (difference between the pre- and post-scores) between the group receiving placebo and no tutoring and the combined group (receiving dextroamphetamine and tutoring).

These differences included the combined group showing more improvement on repeating a motor pattern, better control of motor activity, and greater improvement in behavior as rated by both teacher and parent. These differences were noted in spite of attenuation of drug effect owing to the fact that 50 per cent of the 16 children in the combined group were receiving the medication erratically.

Using stabilimetric cushions and a procedure that had previously been shown to produce either increases or decreases in activity level depending upon the reinforcement (reward) procedures (Sprague, 1973), Christensen (Christensen and Sprague, in press) conducted a study in an experimental classroom with a placebo group and a methylphenidate group (0.3 mg. per kg.). During the initial period of the study when both drug and placebo were first introduced, methylphenidate significantly reduced the number of seat movements, and after a behavior modification procedure was introduced in combination with placebo and drug, methylphenidate led to significantly lower seat movements than the behavior modification procedure itself.

The two studies above certainly show promise and should be encouraging to those who are interested in drug treatment in combination with other school programs for the child, a combination which almost always occurs in real life.

Effects of Drugs on Behavior at Home, Social Behavior, and Play

Behavior at Home

The Conners' Parent Questionnaire (1970) contains 93 items and has been factor-analyzed into 8 major factors. More important, it has been used in a number of studies and found to be sensitive to psychotropic drug effects. The major difficulty in using this measuring instrument is its length, the inability of some parents to fully understand and comprehend the items, and the length of time it takes to score the questionnaire. Another rating scale developed by Werry and his coworkers is aimed at assessing hyperactive behavior at home (Werry and Sprague, 1970; Werry, Weiss, Douglas et al., 1966) and has the advantage of being shorter (31 items).

Using an actometer (a modified self-winding wrist watch which detects movement), evidence has been collected that methylphenidate increases activity at home but that phenobarbital did not result in any activity change (Millichap and Boldrey, 1967). In a study of children with learning disorders, dextroamphetamine at about 0.7 mg. per kg. (25 mg. per day for a mean age of 10 years at about 35 kg.) was evaluated by a number of laboratory tests and rating scales including the Conners' Parent Questionnaire and the Werry-Weiss-Peters Activity Scale (Conners, Rothschild, Eisenberg et al., 1969). The parents were able to detect a statistically significant reduction in the hyperactive factor of the Conners' Parent Questionnaire under dextroamphetamine in comparison with placebo and also a statistical effect on the Werry-Weiss-Peters Activity Scale. In a study using hyperactive children from both the United States and New Zealand, very few effects were seen on the Conners' Parent Questionnaire when dosage of methylphenidate was systematically varied (placebo, 0.1 mg. per kg., 0.3 mg. per kg., 0.5 mg. per kg. and 1.0 mg. per kg.) administered in a single dose in the morning (Werry and Sprague, in press). Moreover, this study found practice effects (a change in the parents' rating over time not attributable to drug administration) on the Conners' Parent Questionnaire which makes its interpretation more difficult.

Play

Very little study has been made of the effects of psychotropic drugs on play behavior of hyperactive and learning-disordered children. In an experiment utilizing dextroamphetamine at about 0.35 mg. per kg. (10 mg. per day for mean age of 8 at about 28 kg.) and chlorpromazine at about 2.7 mg. per kg. (75 mg. per day), Rapoport et al. (1971) found that dextroamphetamine statistically significantly reduced the activity of the child in the playroom, as measured by the number of times he crossed a grid pattern and reduced global ratings of overall activity in the playroom. In a series of studies in our laboratory, we have generally found that methylphenidate does not influence playroom behavior as measured by observational ratings and analysis of the position and movement of the children on photographs taken every 4 seconds of the playroom (Ellis, Witt, Reynolds et al., 1974). Witt (1971) found no relationship between methylphenidate administration (no drug, placebo, 0.15 mg. per kg., 0.30 mg. per kg., and 0.45 mg. per kg.) on a number of measures, total distance moved, number of visits to play equipment, average visit length, etc. (derived from the repeated photographs of the playroom). Nevertheless, the same subjects showed differences in the short-term memory task previously described immediately after leaving the playroom. There were some statistically significant correlations, between playroom behavior and stabilimetric cushion activity in the laboratory test of short-term memory over some of the drug dosages. These correlations were negative; i.e., the more the child moved in the playroom, the less he moved in the laboratory.

Combining the results obtained from studies of the behavior of children at home and the studies of play behavior indicates that parents may not be a reliable source of information as to the effects of the psychotropic drug on the behavior of their children. This statement is not meant to question the observation of parents in general, but it is meant to point out that in many cases the parents are observing the child under exceptionally difficult circumstances as indicated by the following points. (1) It seems likely that stimulant medication influences attention mechanisms and that these effects are best seen when the child is in a structured situation which demands that he pay close attention to the task at hand. Thus, when the child is at home in a free-field situation or at play, the effects may not be readily detectable. This is further substantiated by the results in the learning tests from the Montreal laboratory which suggest that the basic problem with such children is their inability to pay attention when their task is paced or its speed determined by another person in contrast to when their task is paced by themselves. (2) Although the data are very limited, our results indicate that the effect of methylphenidate lasts only 4 to 5 hours (Sprague, 1972). If only a single dosage is administered in the morning, as we recommended, then the effects will probably be worn off by the time the child returns home from school in the afternoon; thus the parents even though astute observers, would not see any effects of the psychotropic medication.

Clinical Recommendations

How to Evaluate Drug Effects

There is no single measure which is universally appropriate for evaluating psychotropic drug effects. Even the best measures that have currently been devised do not necessarily agree on the behavioral effects of psychotropic drugs. But there are available simple, brief measuring instruments which have repeatedly been shown sensitive to the psychotropic drug effects in school programs which, as we have repeated many times, should be the target of psychotropic medicine for learning disorders. It is suggested that the practicing physician utilize the Conners' Abbreviated Teacher Rating Scale on a regular basis to evaluate school performance. The same scale can be used by parents, but it must be kept in mind that parents may be unreliable observers because of the points indicated above. In our research work, we have always found the school system cooperative in filling out such questionnaires if they are convinced that this aids the treatment of the child involved. It is suggested that the Conners' Abbreviated Teacher Rating Scale be obtained from teachers and parents on a monthly basis as long as the child is on psychotropic medication and is in school.

Appropriate dosage is a matter of contention. Most experimental investigations have used individual titration with very few attempts at standardized dosages. Our emphasis on standardized dosage is in disagreement with other writers in this area (Conners, 1971a; Freeman, 1970).

The controversy should be answered on the basis of experimental manipulation of dosage and measures of its influence on behavior. Repeatedly, we have found that a methylphenidate dosage of 0.3 mg. per kg. produces the greatest increment in our short-term memory task and also produces statistically significant improvement on clinical measures such as teacher ratings and physician ratings (Sprague, 1972; Sprague and Werry, 1971; Werry and Sprague, in press). In fact, we have found effects with methylphenidate at dosages as low as 0.1 mg. per kg. on teacher ratings and physician ratings (Werry and Sprague, in press). A very few writers concur in emphasizing lower dosages of methylphenidate (Comly, 1970), but most recommend large dosages, up to 2.0 mg. per kg.

Considering the generally cautious and sometimes suspicious attitude of the general public about psychotropic drug medication for chidren in general, and increasing governmental scrutiny and regulations, the above recommendations for dosages should be given serious consideration, we think, especially when some evidence indicates the possibility of growth suppression at dosages above our recommendations (Safer, Allen and Barr, 1972).

Side Effects

The most comprehensive coverage of side effects is in a book by Shader and DiMascio (1970), and one chapter in that book is devoted to children (DiMascio, Soltys and Shader, 1970).

The side effects of methylphenidate seem to increase proportionately to the increase of the dosage (Werry and Sprague, in press). Another side effect, the long range implications of which are not clear, is the increase in heart rate under methylphenidate which has been noted in several different studies (Cohen, Douglas and Morgenstern, 1971; Knights and Hinton, 1969; Sprague, 1972). But the evidence indicates dextroamphetamine produces more side effects than methylphenidate (Conners, 1972).

School Phobia: Diagnostic Considerations in the Light of Imipramine Effects

R. GITTELMAN-KLEIN, M.D.

D. F. KLEIN, M.D.

This study is refreshing, since it provides a clinical depth and richness not often found in drug studies. The authors consider the underlying dynamics in school phobia to be of great importance and devote considerable discussion to it. It is interesting that the rationale for using imipramine came from the success the authors experienced in treating panic attacks in adult phobic patients and to learn that about 50 per cent of such patients experienced separation anxiety and often school phobia as children. The authors do not disregard the real differences between child and adult psychopathology. While making interesting comparisons between school phobia and adult depression and phobia, they are not considered equivalent. The interesting and controversial issue of what constitutes depression in children is also discussed.

Again, in contrast to many drug studies where other treatment conditions are held constant or do not exist, the results reflect a combination of treatment, including persuasion and desensitization, which is individually designed to meet patient needs. This variation may elicit remarks critical of methodology; however, it would seem quite relevant and appropriate from a clinical viewpoint. It seems likely that much of the impressive placebo effect noted can be attributed to the broad therapeutic approach.

The authors conclude that the effect of imipramine is to reduce the child's anticipatory separation anxiety, but that the actual return to school is complex and multidetermined.

Typically, the school phobia child has marked distress both during the approach to school and while in school. The anxiety is reduced drastically by avoidance of school. Difficulties comprise various degrees of psychophysiological upset such as malaise, nausea, stomach pains, and pallor. In addition, besides the school situation, most of the children experience various degrees of anxiety from mild discomfort to outright panic, while away from their mothers or from home, e.g., at camp, friends' homes, etc. It has been consistently observed that separation anxiety is a central issue among school phobic children.

Separation anxiety takes various forms. For instance, some children are able to go out freely, provided the mother remains at home accessible to their erratic wishes. However, the children do not tolerate the mother's absence if they themselves remain at home. Here, the child's comfortable adaptation depends on always being able to find his mother should he feel anxious and want to be with her.

Exactly the opposite pattern may occur; the child displays separation anxiety from the home rather than the mother per se. As long as he remains at home, the child does not experience anxiety when separated from the mother. However, he feels anxious away from home, more so if alone, but even in his mother's presence.

A yet further pattern is that of the child who defines a circumscribed area within which he feels comfortable, i.e., a home base. This may consist of a one-block area, or, infrequently, a much larger radius. Outside the extended home base, the child experiences anxiety, sometimes even if accompanied by a parent. The anxiety may engender the fear of being lost, with the fantasy that he will never find his parents.

Other children do not accept any separation and must be in the mother's presence at all times. In one such extreme case, the child accompanied his mother to her part-time job.

In addition to the primary anxiety occasioned by separation, the child also develops marked anticipatory anxiety and refuses to go to school. The anticipatory fear has a gradient of severity so that some children will refuse to get dressed for school; others will do so easily, but will refuse to go to school; others will walk to school with their parents and then refuse separation. This school refusal is labeled school phobia; however, the diagnostic emphasis should be upon the separation anxiety and secondary anticipatory anxiety, rather than upon the school as a specific phobic object, since these children react negatively to all occasions of separation or inaccessibility to their mother.

Study Background

Our experience in the treatment of phobic children follows practice previously established with adults. In studies at Hillside Hospital, imipramine was regularly effective in the treatment of agoraphobic adults (Klein, 1964; Klein and Fink, 1962). These patients have been given a number of diagnoses, such as phobic anxiety syndrome, phobic anxiety depersonalization syndrome, or anxiety neurosis, as well as less justified sobriquets, i.e., pseudoneurotic, schizophrenia, borderline syndrome, etc. These patients suffer from inexplicable panic attacks, accompanied by hot and cold flashes, rapid breathing, palpitations, weakness, unsteadiness, a feeling of impending death, and occasional depersonalization. They progressively constrict their activities until they are unable to leave the house independently for fear of being suddenly rendered helpless while isolated from help. Phenothiazine treatment not only does not alleviate this anxiety, but frequently exacerbates it. However, imipramine is remarkably effective in blocking the onset of panic attacks. Detailed investigation revealed that within a group of phobic-anxious adults, two developmental courses were observable. About 50 per cent of the patients had been fearful, dependent children, with marked separation anxiety and difficulty in adjusting to school, often consisting of a phobic reaction. Such patients' adult onset of phobic anxiety was frequently precipitated by bereavement, separation, or loss of love object.

Procedure

The study presented below is ongoing and expected to continue for another year. At this point, we are presenting findings of 35 patients who have completed a 6-week treatment period of either placebo or imipramine.

Clinical Criteria

Children aged 6 to 14 years inclusive, classified as follows, were accepted for study. 1) The child is afraid to attend school and completely refuses to go to school, has been absent for 2 weeks, and displays manifest separation anxiety, 2) The child is similar to type 1, but less severe. He may be able to go to school intermittently, or go under great duress and experience severe discomfort while in school. He displays manifest separation anxiety, 3) The third type consists of children who have refused to go to school for at least 2 weeks; they are afraid of school and clearly phobic. However, they display no separation anxiety.

The inclusion of the third group of children without separation anxiety stemmed from the fact that, while screening, an occasional child showed clear-cut phobic reactions to school, characterized by severe anxiety leading to avoidance behavior, but no reports of separation anxiety could be elicited from the mother or the child. We included these children to determine whether imipramine was effective only when separation anxiety was present, or whether its clinical action was independent of this factor. Parenthetically, since we added this third clinical category, we have had practically no suitable children. Therefore, our hopes of analyzing imipramine effect along the separation-anxiety dimension will probably not materialize.

Treatment Program

Children accepted for study were randomly assigned to matching imipramine or placebo pills. The drug assignment was stratified by age and sex so that the drug and placebo groups should not differ with regard to these two variables. At baseline the child was rated on a number of measures; these were repeated after 6 weeks of treatment. In addition, school attendance and global improvement were rated after 3 and 6 weeks of treatment. A complete blood count, urine analysis, and liver profile was obtained before giving medication and after a 6-week interval.

The treatment program consisted of giving the child medication with dose ranges from 25 to 200 mg/day. Dosage was fixed for the first 2 weeks: 25 mg for the first 3 days, 50 mg for the next 4 days; 75 mg/day during the second week. Thereafter dosage was adjusted weekly. The medication was given in two daily doses: one in the morning and the other in the evening. At the end of 6 weeks, dosage ranged from 100 to 200 mg/day (mean = 152 mg/day).

The patient and family were seen weekly. At the beginning of treatment they were told to expect an abatement of fear. The case worker instructed the family to maintain a firm attitude promoting school attendance. The treatment program was also explained to the school personnel with whom the social worker maintained continuous contact so that no discrepancies occurred between our instructions and the school's expectations. In most cases, a family member was advised to accompany the child to school and maintain the child's presence there until there was reduction of the child's anticipatory anxiety that severe discomfort might recur while he was in school, and the child could attend school alone. The treatment recommendations varied depending upon the severity of the anticipatory anxiety and upon the mother's ability to set and enforce limits.

To give an example, upon screening one child was refusing to get dressed in the morning; if the mother dressed him, he ran out of the house. The mother was felt to be anxious, distraught, and confused in the face of her child's behavior. Therefore, for the first week, the child and mother were instructed that the child was to get ready for school, but no attempt was made to take him to school. The second week he was to get ready and go to school, without entering the building; this process (essentially one of desensitization) continued until the child eventually went to school on his own. The steps selected reflect a hierarchy of approach to school, each step causing some anxiety, but a degree tolerable to both child and mother. Therefore, the overall results of our study represent the effect of a combination of treatments; persuasive and desensitization techniques coupled with either an active drug or a placebo.

Sample

A total of 35 children completed the 6-week study, 19 on placebo, 16 on imipramine. There were 19 girls and 16 boys with a mean age of 10.8, ranging from 6 to 14 years old. The group is not racially typical of the clinic population; only one (3 per cent) was Negro, whereas 50 per cent of the referrals at the clinic consist of Negro children. The reasons for this discrepancy are not clear.

All except one child were at least within the normal range of intellectual functioning as estimated by school performance. One girl was attending a class for mentally retarded children.

The distribution of school phobia types was as follows: type 1, $N = 23$ (11 on placebo, 12 on imipramine); type $N = 6$ (5 on placebo, 1 on imipramine); type 3, $N = 5$ (3 on placebo, 2 on imipramine). One child was rated as type 1 and 3 simultaneously.

Measures

School attendance. Return to school was the major criterion of change. It was rated by the mother on a scale from 1 to 7 from complete refusal to regular asymptomatic attendance. After 6 weeks of treatments, only one child received a score reflecting intermittent school attendance; the others either attended regularly or not at all, an outcome distribution that calls for appropriate statistical analysis.

Therefore, for analysis, the scores were dichotomized between "not back to school" and "back to school."

Global improvement. The children's overall improvement was evaluated by the psychiatrist, mother, and child, after 3 and 6 weeks of treatment. This rating reflects a global impression of the degree of change which has taken place. It is recorded on a seven-point scale from "Very much Worse" to "Completely Well." When a therapist makes the judgment, considerations such as level of anxiety, mood state, interpersonal functioning, and target symptom changes all enter into consideration.

Mothers asked to evaluate their children's improvement are more likely to take into consideration the child's tractability and manageability in the home both in the process of sending him to school and in situations not related to school. When a mother felt her child was better, she almost invariably reported that he was no longer "nervous," that he was calmer and more relaxed.

When the child rates his own improvement, he is communicating his subjective sense of well-being, and it is difficult to say what accounts for his judgment. When asked why they were better, children, depending on their age, would generally reply that they no longer had "bad feelings," were not scared, were able to go to school, or just felt good.

The manner in which a child's self-rating was obtained varied with the child's level of comprehension. Among older children, the form is shown and read to them to insure that they know its entire contents, and they are asked to fill it out. Younger children are also shown the form; in addition they are interviewed so that the therapist may fill out the form for them. There is no leading of the witness. Statements such as, "I think you're much better, don't you think so?" are never used, nor are the converse. Rather, questioning goes approximately as follows: "Can you remember how you felt when you first came to the clinic?" "Do you feel the same, better, or worse?" If the child says better, further questioning determines how much better.

Psychiatric ratings of symptomatology. In addition to global ratings of school attendance and improvement, children were rated on three instruments by the psychiatrist: a modified version of the Lorr IMPS, where items are scored from 1 to 9; Rutter's Children's Behavior Questionnaire (CBQ) (16) in which items are on a four-point scale; and our own Psychiatric Interview Rating Form (PIRF) which has been devised to record the specific characteristics of this population, but which was not intended as a measure of change, and therefore items are marked present or absent only.

Results

School Attendance

As may be observed in Table 1, imipramine was significantly superior to placebo in effectuating a return to school. It is interesting to note that a period of placebo treatment leads to school return in almost 50 per cent of the cases. Therefore, using school attendance as a criterion of drug effect, any psychoactive medication would have to be extremely effective to exceed placebo, using samples of 15 to 20 patients.

The school attendance data were further examined to see whether, among the school returns, those treated with imipramine returned to school sooner than those treated with placebo. Of the nine placebo patients who were in school after 6 weeks, seven (77 per cent) were back in school after the 3-week treatment period. Therefore, it would appear that if parental pressure and a placebo are going to be effective, they will be so relatively quickly. A different pattern emerges among the 12 imipramine-treated children who were in school after a 6-week treatment period. Among them only six (50 per cent) were in school after 3 weeks of treatment. It appears, therefore, that a 3-week treatment period of imipramine is not distinguishable from placebo as far as school attendance is concerned, and that a 6-week period of active drug treatment is necessary for the child's school attendance to be effected by the drug.

In the school phobia literature much has been said regarding the different psychological meaning of the disturbance in prepuberty vs. puberty years. It is generally stated that school phobia is more pathological if it occurs in the later years. On the basis of this assumption, it could be anticipated that older children should be refractory to treatment. To test this possibility, we examined the relationship between age and the rate of school return. There was no significant difference in the proportion of children 11 years and less and those above the age of 11 who returned to school after 6 weeks of placebo treatment. A relationship might be observed between school return and age given larger samples. It may be that the relationship between school return and age is further limited in this study by the fact that we did not include children of 15 years and above. However, it must be noted that if age is somewhat related to school attendance it is completely unrelated to global improvement on imipramine treatment.

Global treatment. The psychiatrists, mothers, and children all reported significantly greater improvement among the imipramine group. The degree of perceived improvement, however, varies among raters, the children on imipramine all reporting they had been much improved.

Among the placebo-treated children, a few felt they had remained the same, most felt slightly better, few felt much better.

Table 1. School Attendance After 6 Weeks of Treatment (Mother's Report)*

Drug	Back to School	Not Back to School
Placebo	9 (47%)	10 (53%)
Imipramine	13 (81%)	3 (19%)

*$N =$; $p < 0.05$, Fisher-Exact, one tailed.

To see to what extent return to school is associated with the children's reports of feeling better, the school attendance and the self-ratings of improvement were jointly examined revealing interesting patterns of improvement. Although children receiving imipramine all reported feeling better, this improvement was not always associated with school return.

The picture presented by the placebo-treated children is markedly different. Relatively few reported feeling better (four, 21 per cent), but a larger proportion (nine, 47 per cent) went back to school. Therefore, feeling better is not a necessary condition for school return since five

(26 per cent) of the children went back to school in spite of the fact that they reported no overall improvement. The small number of subjects within each type does not allow for statistical analyses.

Self-Ratings of Improvement After 3 and 6 Weeks of Treatment

Having established that after a 6-week period imipramine is significantly superior to placebo, the question arises as to whether imipramine has similar therapeutic efficacy after a 3-week period. The 3-week self-ratings of children who rated themselves as "Much Improved" after 6 weeks of treatment were examined regardless of which treatment they had received. Of the four patients on placebo who felt much better at the 6-week point, two already felt much better at 3 weeks, one felt slightly better. Among the 11 patients on imipramine who felt much better after 6 weeks of treatment, only three reported feeling much better after 3 weeks of drug intake. Therefore, drug and placebo are indistinguishable after 3 weeks, and a 6-week treatment period seems necessary to elicit the drug's true effect.

The difference between 3 and 6 weeks of treatment may be similar to that in depression where frequently improvement requires several weeks from the beginning of drug intake. On the other hand, the difference might be dosage-related rather than time-related, since patients were taking less medication at 3 weeks (mean daily dose = 107 mg; range = 75 to 125 mg/day) compared to 6 weeks (mean daily dose = 152 mg; range = 100 to 200 mg/day). This difference in dosage is unavoidable since careful medical practice prevents the prescription of sudden high doses of imipramine, because some patients may be sensitive to the drug and have behavioral side effects such as motor restlessness, jitteriness, flight of ideas, etc., on too rapid drug initiation. As described in the study procedure, to prevent the occurrence of too rapid over-prescription, the dosage prescribed cannot exceed 75 mg/day over the first 2-week period. It is only during the third week of treatment that the psychiatrist is free to prescribe as much as he wants, up to a maximum of 200 mg/day. However, he is unlikely to increase the dose suddenly within a one-week period. Interestingly, the cautionary guidelines are derived from data on imipramine treatment of adults. None of the children in the study displayed drug sensitivity, and our procedures may be over-conservative for this population.

In conclusion, given the usual precautions necessary in dosage increments, an imipramine effect in self-perceived overall improvement cannot be detected after 3 weeks of treatment, but is clearly present after 6 weeks.

Side Effects

Side effects were recorded on a standard form at every visit. Of the 16 patients on double blind imipramine treatment, 3 (19 per cent) had no side effects during the 6-week treatment period. Among the 10 placebo patients, 10 (53 per cent) reported no side effects.

The difference between the number of patients with side effects differs significantly between the placebo and drug-treated groups (p — 0.025). Further, when placebo-treated children report side effects, they report fewer than children treated with imipramine.

A total of 33 side effects were elicited; 8 of these were found in the placebo group only. Some of them may reflect complaints associated with the patient's presenting problems that may be interpreted as side effects. It might therefore be useful to obtain a list of complaints at baseline, recorded on a side-effects form, to see whether the so-called treatment emergent symptoms are being accurately evaluated.

It appears that complaints of dry mouth, constipation, dizziness, and tremor are more prevalent among the imipramine subjects. Sixty-two per cent of the imipramine children reported feeling drowsy, but so did 31 per cent of the placebo-treated children. The side effect of dry mouth is the only one which is found significantly more often in the drug group (p — 0.005). The difference between placebo and imipramine for the other three side effects just misses significance. A side effect found in one subject only deserves mention. Orthostatic hypotension was significant in a girl treated with 125 mg/day of imipramine; it subsided when the dose was reduced to 100 mg. After a few days the drug dosage was raised to 150 mg without any further hypotension. This is the only double blind imipramine case which required dosage adjustment because of interfering side effects; other side effects disappeared without any dose alterations. On the whole, our experience indicates remarkably little difficulty due to side effects in using relatively large doses of imipramine in an outpatient group of children.

Blood Tests

Blood tests and urinalyses were performed before drug administration and after 6 weeks of treatment. Blood analyses included CBC and liver profiles. In addition, we obtained positional blood pressures and electrocardiograms. The exact values of the above procedures have not been analyzed; however, a perusal of the data reveals no abnormality using generally applied clinical guidelines.

Comment

This study establishes that imipramine is superior to placebo in the treatment of school phobic children between the ages of 6 to 14 years. Using school return as a measure of drug effect, the superiority of the drug just achieves statistical significance ($p - 0.05$). However, this does not indicate a minor drug effect, but rather the fact that with a major placebo effect, only large drug effects can be detected in samples of 15 to 20 subjects. Imipramine induced school return in 81 per cent of the children, placebo in 47 per cent. If a 34 per cent difference in efficacy truly exists between the two treatments, 7 out of 10 study replications would detect it even using our small sample sizes.

By using global ratings of improvement, especially the children's self-ratings, the superiority of imipramine is marked. In view of our findings, the drug's action cannot be viewed as one which automatically leads to renewed school attendance. Rather, it has to be seen as modifying the child's self-perception probably because of an alteration of mood state and experience of panic attacks. This change may enable the child to return to the classroom; however, the maintenance of strong anticipatory anxiety may block this action. The case of one child who was much improved on imipramine but refused to go to school is given illustratively. Mark had separation anxiety, morbid concern about his mother, numerous compulsive habits, and had had difficulty attending school throughout his school career. Absences had been frequent, but the child had never refused to go to school over any length of time. In September 1969, Mark entered Junior High School. He was beaten up twice on his way to school for no apparent reason by unknown groups of older children. Mark developed an obsessive preoccupation with the possibility of violence and completely refused to go to school. When he entered the study, he was rated as type 1 (separation anxiety) as well as thpe 3 (school phobia independent of separation anxiety).

During the course of study treatment, Mark received imipramine and became completely free of separation anxiety, felt much less anxious in general, but retained a morbid obsessional fear of the possibility of being beaten up in school and was unable to return to school. He was eventually hospitalized in an effort to mobilize him.

Therefore, return to school is a complex behavior related to factors independent of drug effect. Some of these factors probably consist of anticipatory anxiety, the school's attitude toward the child, the parents' management of the child, the nature of the psychotherapeutic contact, etc.

In addition to the controlled report by Frommer (1968), a recent clinical report of antidepressants among phobic depressive children by the same author corroborates the usefulness of this drug type (Frommer, 1968). Frommer favors monoamine oxidase (MAO) inhibitors vs. tricyclics. However, the dosages reported for the two drugs are not equivalent. Regular adult doses of MAO inhibitor (phenelzine, 45 mg/day) were used, but imipramine dosage was far below that which we found effective. Thus, the effects of 60 mg/day for children of at least 10 years of age are reported, with lower doses among younger children; our lowest dose was 10 mg/day. In view of the greater risk involved in the use of MAO inhibitors, these could only be useful in the rare exception of the patient who might not respond adequately to imipramine treatment.

A recent British article (Kelly, Guirguis, Frommer, Mitchell-Heggs, and Sargant, 1970) reports uncontrolled results of MAO inhibitors among a large group of adult phobic patients. The rate of improvement falls far below that found by Klein in a placebo-controlled double blind study of imipramine in the same population (Klein, 1964). The discrepancy in therapeutic effectiveness between imipramine and the MAO inhibitors is further support for recommending the former. Frommer's viewpoint regarding dosage reflects the persisting notion that age should be a guide to dose levels in child psychopharmacology. There is no evidence to support such an assumption. Although we have found no child who responded to doses of less than 75 mg/day, children vary widely in their response to imipramine beyond this level. In one instance, during drug follow-up, dosage had to be increased from 200 to 300 mg/day in a 12-year-old child who had been stabilized, but was relapsing. The effect of the added dosage was dramatic; medication was later reduced to 200 mg again, but had to be raised to 250 mg. In this case, 250 mg appeared to be the minimum stabilizing dose. Age has not been one of our useful criteria for determining dosage level. As a matter of fact, no criterion seems to be clearly relevant.

In the same article referred to above (Frommer, 1968) recent onset and early morning awakening are positive prognostic signs; in our work, length of illness is not related to treatment response, and only one child had early awakening. It must be noted that only 3 of 16 children did not return to school on imipramine. Further, all of these children reported being much improved. In dealing with so few treatment failures, it is unlikely that reliable criteria of variation in treatment response will be found. More relevant is a study of treatment response to placebo since greater variation in outcome was observed in this group.

The return to school of placebo-treated children who feel better is easily understood. However, it is difficult to identify the causes of school return among children who do not feel improved. Here again, a number of variables are probably involved. Our assessment of parent attitudes made by the social worker at the beginning of treatment is not helpful, since, except for one exception, all parents were rated as wanting the child back in school. This is hardly surprising since the treatment program is voluntary, and no external threats exist, such as court actions, as is often the case in truancy or other antisocial behvavior.

In the age range studied, age was not a statistically significant factor, although it might be so if children 15 years and above were included. The fact that older children tend to remain out of school, but that they improve just as much as younger children is further indication that school return partly depends upon non-drug factors. In the case of the older children, the parent cannot be used as forcefully in getting the child to school. As a result, successful treatment depends to a larger degree upon the patient's cooperation, rather than the parents'. Therefore, the tendency for older children to fail in a treatment program does not necessarily indicate greater psychopathology. Length of illness was not contributory in predicting return to school. We plan to examine other familial and patient characteristics, such as child's motivation and parents' marital accord, to search for clues as to what factors may play a role in school return among placebo-treated patients.

Using essentially the same therapeutic procedures without pharmacological treatment, Eisenberg (1959) reports a greater rate of success in return to school than was found in this study (72 per cent vs. 47 per cent). However, a large group of the children were preschoolers; comparing this study's 10 placebo patients who received weekly individual psychotherapy, parental counseling, and school casework, to Eisenberg's 15 children above the age of 6 years, it appears that we were less successful than Eisenberg in getting the elementary school age children back in school. The success rates of both studies are equivalent for the older age group.

The results obtained in the placebo group of this study are consonant with those reported by Hersov (1960) in 50 youngsters between the ages of 7 to 16. Forty-eight per cent returned to school within 6 months of treatment comparable to ours and Eisenberg's; another 20 per cent resumed school attendance between 7 to 12 months of therapy. No age-outcome relationship was found. In the absence of restrictions due to research designs, school phobic children are treated for much longer periods of time. Obviously, rates of success derived from 6 weeks vs. months or years of treatment are not comparable.

Frommer refers to children such as the ones described in this study as phobic depressives, since they show "typical" depressive symptoms of weepiness, tension, explosiveness, and instability. However, she goes on to point out that to the lay observers and to themselves, the children do not appear depressed (Frommer, 1967, 1968). Why Frommer considers the above symptoms more characteristic of depression than of other psychiatric syndromes such as tension states, hysterical epidodes, emotional instability, etc., is not clear.

We have found that, as a group, the children are not depressed in terms of a definition of depression which emphasizes inability to experience pleasure and a sense of incompetence (Klein and Davis, 1969). Many of the children do weep easily, and they may be explosive and irritable, but only in the context of threatened or actual separation. When no demands for independent functioning are exerted, they can enjoy themselves and may be active, capable, and gregarious. Many children restrict their peer interaction and seem "withdrawn." However, for the most part, retreat from peer groups is manifest during the school year only. During summer months the children are active and show no aversion to being with their peers. Our impression is that the children are concerned about having to justify their school absences, and therefore they avoid being with their friends to avoid possible embarrassment. Thus, the social withdrawal of phobic children, when it occurs, appears to be largely an attitudinal change due to the anxiety-producing qualities of the peer situation, rather than the secondary manifestations of a depressed mood state.

Of the 34 children rated by the psychiatrist, 12 were rated as quite depressed. Yet, a crucial distinction between this sample of phobic children and depressed adults is that none of the children had lost the capacity to anticipate pleasure, or lost all sense of competence. Remarkably, almost all children had the conviction that somehow, at some point in the future, the next day or next week, they would miraculously be able to attend school without any difficulty. The conviction that everything will turn out well (often referred to as magical thinking in children) is singularly lacking among depressed adults; for that matter, its presence would preclude a psychiatric diagnosis of depression.

Therefore, although depression appears in a good proportion of phobic children (about 30 per cent in our sample), the characteristic pessimism and anhedonia of the adult depressive is not a predominant clinical factor. Therefore, it seems erroneous to us to equate these children's disorder with that of the adult depressions.

Our treatment of school phobia was prompted by the knowledge that imipramine was useful to adult agoraphobes, whose retrospective histories revealed a high prevalence of childhood phobic disorders. The clinical picture of the phobic children resembles that of the adult agoraphobes, but also differs from it in important ways. Like the adults with a history of childhood separation anxiety, almost all the children's onsets (28/35) could be related to bereavement, illness, or some object losses. However, unexplained, out of the blue, sudden panic attacks do not seem to occur in children as they do in adults. Thus, the child may become panicky if separation is attempted; however, panic never occurs outside the context of separation. Among adult agoraphobes, panics are markedly reduced by the presence of a companion or by being at home, but they are not eliminated.

The constant possibility of a panic episode regardless of the external circumstances is clearly not true for the children. We have seen only one child, aged 14, who seems identical to adult agoraphobes. Further, the panic experienced by the phobic children seems physiologically different from that reported by adult agoraphobes. The children do not report getting dizzy, faint, or depersonalized; there are no palpitations with a feeling of impending death. On the other hand the children frequently experience stomachaches, which are not reported by adults. It may be that children and adults are undergoing the same initial stages of their disorder, but that the children's physiological make-up has not matured to a point which allows the adult process to take place and leads to a different phenomenological experience.

In any case, just as school phobias cannot be conceived of as miniature depressions, they cannot be viewed as miniature phobic anxiety states. Their symptomatology and treatment responses are related to the adult depressive states and obviously to adult phobic states, but they do not appear to be identical phenomenologically or psychophysiologically. From cross-sectional evaluation it is impossible to obtain conclusive evidence regarding the significance of a disorder. Only long-term studies of phobic children can elucidate to what degree this childhood disorder is a precursor to adult depressive disorders, or adult anxiety syndromes.

The fact that only one child was Negro, given that 50 per cent of the clinic population is Negro, is puzzling. Marks (1969) reports that adult agoraphobes come from stable families. Others have also commented on the fact that phobic children come from close-knit homes. This has certainly been our observation as well. It might be argued that the sociofamilial environment among lower class Negroes who form the bulk of the clinic patient population does not provide the type of setting which favors the development of pathological attachment to the parent or the home. This possibility might deserve examination if it had been clearly demonstrated that, compared to other groups, families of phobic children are more child-oriented, that they foster to a greater degree the child's dependence on the family, and that the mothers or fathers of phobic children experience greater anxiety at separation from their offsprings.

One study (Hersov, 1960) compared various parental and familial characteristics of three patient groups: two groups of school refusers who had been out of school for at least 2 months (one group showed a preference for staying home, and the other consisted of truants) and a control group of random clinic cases without school refusal and gross brain damage. The first group is equated with school phobia. The results support the hypothesis that the families of phobic children are most stable in that the children in this group experienced less extended separation from their parents. Further, the mothers of the phobic children were rated as being less rejecting and more overprotective. However, the groups were not equivalent for social class, the phobic group being significantly superior. The phobic children also had higher IQ scores and had fewer siblings compared to the truant group. In addition, the ratings were not made without the knowledge of the child's group membership possibly leading to bias, especially with regard to ratings of parental attitudes. Child-rearing practices differ in various social classes. Therefore, it is conceivable that much of the variance observed among the groups could be due to this factor. In a further controlled study, Hersov (1960) describes three patterns of parental management: 1) overindulgent mother and an inadequate passive father, 2) a severe controlling mother and a passive father, and 3) a firm controlling father and an overindulgent mother.

In the absence of adequate controlled comparisons, impressions, although they may eventually prove of scientific value, remain only interesting anecdotal evidence. Thus, our observations of the family were consonant with those of others regarding the fact that a large proportion of the families functioned as a total unit. The parents rarely went out without their children, and only if necessary. If the mother worked, most often she did so during school hours only and had stopped working when the child started having difficulties. On the whole, the feeling was that the children were included in all of the family's social activities and that much of the parents' satisfaction was derived from being with their children. However, one of us spent 3 years working with outpatient psychotic children of similar ages, and exactly the same impression had been noted at the time. The groups are not strictly comparable since it can be argued that, in the psychotic group, families need to be extremely attached to their offspring to tolerate the severely disruptive influence of the psychotic member. In any case, the experience of working intensively with such differing pathological groups has led to a skeptical attitude toward conclusions regarding parental characteristics based upon uncontrolled, biased observations. The limited number of controlled studies dealing with this issue in children with a variety of characteristics certainly underlines the need for avoiding premature closure concerning what type of parent is associated with what type of child.

Another possible hypothesis regarding the low prevalence of Negroes in our sample is that schools may not respond to a Negro child's refusal in the same manner as to that of a white child. A nonwhite child who is not in school may be stereotyped as a truant by the school personnel and may never come to the attention of psychiatric clinics. We know of no epidemiological surveys conducted through bureaus of attendance investigating this problem.

Several theories of the mechanisms underlying separation anxiety and phobic behavior have been postulated. Therapeutic interventions are bound to be determined by the theoretical model adhered to. A large body of psychoanalytic writing traces the dynamic origin of phobic symptoms and separation anxiety to such concepts as the sexual significance of the school due to symbolic displacement of libidinal impulses, or the destructive hostile fantasies harbored toward the parents (Prince, 1968). Such a model calls for treatment of the child with the goal of resolving intrapsychic conflicts. Another formulation is that the mother transmits to the child her own anxiety about separation and individuation. Eisenberg (1958), who is closely associated with this view, recommends, therefore, that the child be separated immediately from the mother since the origin of the conflict does not lie in the child, but in the parent. In addition, he recommends parental counseling to alter the families' attitudes and anxieties regarding separation.

On the other hand, it has also been suggested that separation anxiety is a biological phenomenon whose evolutionary significance lies in eliciting care and retrieval from the mothering figure (Bowlby, 1960; Klein and Davis, 1969). It might be argued that wide constitutional variations can occur in the threshold of such a biological mechanism. In this context, severe separation anxiety may be seen as a pathological manifestation of a normal biological developmental process, around which secondary anxieties may be learned. If such were the case, one would expect relatively little alteration of the biological anxiety threshold via verbal or management therapeutic efforts, although the adaptive mechanisms used by the child to cope with the anxiety could be expected to change as a result of various external interventions.

Our design does not allow for clarification of the issues suggested by the psychoanalytic models since no attempt was made to deal with the children's unconscious fantasies. However, our results challenge the model which posits an extrinsic source of anxiety, i.e., it is not the child's anxiety but his family's which is at the root of his refusal to separate from his mother. If parental handling were the crucial variable, no significant difference in improvement between the placebo and imipramine should have been noted since parents in both groups received identical counseling. This counseling was effective in getting almost 50 per cent of the placebo-treated children back to school, but if one considers the children's feelings of well-being, it did not "work."

   Therefore, our results give support to the notion of the presence of a pathological process intrinsic to the child. Whether this process represents a variant of normal biological separation anxiety, or a specific mood disorder coupled with anxiety, is unknown. It could be that the genesis lies in the parental relationship and that the disorder develops functional autonomy.

   In our study, all parents received counseling; therefore, we do not know what the value of imipramine would be in treating school phobia without this ancillary treatment. Our impression is that parental cooperation is essential; with imipramine alone, we might have many happy stay-at-home children since anticipatory anxiety might continue to prevent the children from returning to school. Therefore, we see imipramine as instrumental in reducing the primary anxiety, and the parental pressure as forcing the child to venture into danger and by extinction obtain relief from the secondary to anticipatory anxiety. It has become a platitude to state that both nature and nurture are important in mental illness; this patient group does not escape this truism.

Biological Interventions in Psychoses of Childhood

In recent years there has been increasing interest in and emphasis on biological factors in general psychiatry. The author provides an interesting introduction to biological child psychiatry as well as a summary of the literature on drug treatment of psychosis in children.

As Campbell points out in her concluding remarks, there are still no clear guidelines as to which is indicated for which child. She feels that drug treatment should generally be part of the treatment of the preschool psychotic child and postulates that at a later developmental stage the child may no longer be as responsive.

Although antipsychotic medications obviously have important therapeutic value, the clinician should be aware of recently reported consequences of long-term use. One study reports weight changes, tardive dyskinesias, impaired learning and ocular changes (McAndrew, 1972). A more recent report describes the appearance of neurological signs in 14 of 34 schizophrenic children after withdrawal of antipsychotic medication. Although they do not designate them as such, the authors compare these signs to adult tardive dyskinesias (Polizos, 1973).

All psychiatric disturbances in early childhood can be viewed as delays, exaggerations or distortions of development which yield fixations and regressions. The most severe distortions are seen in the childhood psychoses involving major behavioral disturbances and overall retardation.

The promotion of development and maturation constitutes the essence of psychiatric treatment of young children. Age is an important factor. The younger child is more globally affected by the psychosis and requires more intensive treatment. Total treatment comprising a well structured clinical residential or day program with individual planning and highly individualized therapeutic objectives is essential for each psychotic child of preschool age. Thus, the promotion of development in psychotic children usually calls for a multidisciplinary approach intended to include special education, individual and speech therapy and also work with parents. All such forms of treatment represent an attempt to manipulate the environment so as to evoke a therapeutic change in the child. Biological therapies, on the other hand, are in a more immediate manner directed toward the organism or the central nervous system.

Biological interventions in the treatment of psychotic conditions in childhood are largely confined to the use of a variety of drugs. Psychosurgery and convulsive therapies have been replaced by psychopharmacology, a rapidly developing specialization which appears to have made some inroads into the rather conservative field of child psychiatry. After a brief mention of earlier forms of biological-organic treatment, this presentation will focus on drug therapy. It is intended to provide an up-to-date review of principal drug agents with occasional comments on efficacy based on the author's experience in the treatment of psychotic children.

Physical Therapies

Psychosurgery

Brain surgery in the form of lobotomy was developed by Egas Moniz (1936) and first performed by Almeida Lima. Modified in this country

Reprinted from *Journal of Autism and Childhood Schizophrenia*, Vol. 4 (1973), pp. 347-373.

by Freeman, it was found unsatisfactory in operations involving children (Williams and Freeman, 1953; Freeman, 1959). Lobotomy and also topectomy, intended to eliminate symptoms of aggressiveness in children, are no longer in use in North America and Western Europe (Ajuriaguerra, 1971).

Insulin Shock Therapy

This form of treatment, introduced by Sakel (1938), had been applied to schizophrenic children in Europe (Annell, 1955; Heuyer, Lang, and Rivaille, 1956), reportedly with satisfactory results with respect to promotion of maturation.

Electroconvulsive Therapy

In this country, convulsive therapy, as first described by Cerletti and Bini in 1938 (Cerletti, 1950), was used extensively in the treatment of young schizophrenic children (without ill effects on development) by Lauretta Bender. The children were said to tolerate shock treatment better than adults. Although the schizophrenic process did not seem to be modified, certain symptoms decreased and the children were "better able to accept teaching or psychotherapy in groups or individually" (Bender, 1947). There was an indication that shock therapy prompted a reorganization, resulting in a more integrated body image (Bender and Keeler, 1952). Intellectual functioning also improved in some children, although not statistically significantly (Gurewitz and Helme, 1954).

Electroconvulsive therapy has also been used to treat manic-depressive and other depressive conditions (Campbell, 1955; Frommer, 1968). In this author's limited experience with two preschool schizophrenic children who failed to respond to other treatment modalities (including drug therapy), shock treatment yielded some positive though transient behavioral changes. Of note were gains in the children's weight and height.

Other Convulsive Agents

In adult schizophrenics, pharmacological convulsive agents were reported to be more effective than electroshock. Hexafluorodiethyl ether (Indoklon®) was described by Krantz, Truitt, Speers, and Ling (1957). Indoklon was administered (i. v.) by this author to a four-year-old schizophrenic child with resulting therapeutic changes such as decreases in irritability and certain compulsive mannerisms.

At present, convulsive therapies have practically disappeared from practice, mainly due to the discovery of major tranquilizers. The use of electroshock treatment in catatonic states in adolescence constitutes about the sole remaining exception in child psychiatry.

Drug Therapy

Experience has shown that drug treatment is frequently a valuable component of the total treatment of the psychotic child. Certain psychoactive agents can make such a child more amenable to educational and play therapies. Even when a comprehensive treatment program is not available, drug induced therapeutic changes can make the psychotic child more manageable and easier to live with in the community.

Hypnotics, Anticonvulsants and Sedatives

Hypnotics and anticonvulsants have been in use for a long time. However, due to the advent of major tranquilizers, they no longer have a place in the therapeutic arsenal. Actually, barbiturates may increase disorganization in the severely disturbed child.

Diphenhydramine (Benadryl®) was found effective even in some schizophrenic children particularly in those with higher IQs (Effron and Freedman, 1953; Fish, 1963; Silver, 1955). It appears that Benadryl has not been sufficiently explored in severe behavioral disorders of childhood and that the cause of such failure may be traced to doses, usually neither individualized nor sufficiently high. Prior to placing a schizophrenic child on a major tranquilizer, it is worthwhile to try Benadryl as a first stage of drug therapy. It is a safe drug, easy to regulate and potentially useful to merit exploration.

Stimulant and Antidepressant Drugs

The psychomotor stimulants, Benzedrine and *d*-amphetamine (Dexedrine®) have been in use in child psychiatry since the 1930's (Bradley, 1937; Bradley and Bowen, 1941; Bender and Cottington, 1942; Bender and Nichtern, 1956; Fish, 1971). Therapeutic results in psychotic children were minimal, absent, or more frequently poor. In our experience, nonpsychotic children tolerate higher doses of *d*-amphetamine than the schizophrenic and autistic who often become more psychotic and disorganized, even on very low doses, regardless of hyperactivity (Campbell, Fish, David, Shapiro, Collins, and Koh, 1972a; Campbell, Fish, Shapiro, and Floyd, 1972). The psychotic child who shows some overall improvement on *d*-amphetamine with decrease in hyperactivity and increase in attention span may at the same time become more withdrawn and less verbal.

More recently, *l*-amphetamine (Cydril®) has been found effective in some disturbed children, particularly in reference to decreasing hyperactivity and aggressiveness (Arnold, Wender, McCloskey, and Snyder, 1972; Arnold, Kirilcuk, Corson, and Corson, 1973). It was hypothesized that *l*-amphetamine via dopaminergic mechanism, may equal dextroamphetamine in benefiting the subgroup of hyperkinetic children who could be diagnosed as unsocialized aggressive by Fish's criteria. If so, this might eventually make levoroamphetamine, with its lower anorexogenic potency and lower potential for abuse, the drug of choice for this subgroup (Arnold and Wender, 1973). Since a great number of young psychotic children is not only hyperactive but also quite aggressive (aggressiveness manifested toward others or in the form of self-mutilating behavior), which interferes with social life and learning (Campbell and Hersh, 1971c), we hoped that by controlling aggressiveness with *l*-amphetamine the child would be able to develop positive and adaptive social interactions which in turn will improve learning (Corson, Corson, Kirilcuk, Knopp, and Arnold, 1972). We also hoped that *l*-amphetamine, because its effects are mediated via dopaminergic neurons (Snyder, Taylor, Coyle, and Meyerhoff, 1970; Taylor and Snyder, 1970) may have less untoward effects on psychotic children than *d*-amphetamine which, in our experience, was a poor drug for both hyperkinetic and hypoactive patients.

Our experiences with *l*-amphetamine in psychotic children is very limited. Preliminary data indicate that it may have fewer disorganizing effects in psychotic children than *d*-amphetamine and that it is effective in decreasing hyperactivity and aggressiveness, thus making the child more manageable. Although increases in attention span were noted, the child frequently also became less verbal and more stereotyped.

Both the tricyclic antidepressants (amitryptyline and imipramine) and the monoamine oxidase inhibitors (phenelzine and isocarboxazid) were used extensively by Frommer (1968) in an outpatient population of childhood depressives as young as 2½ years of age.

Kurtis (1966) treated 16 autistic children, 4 to 15 years of age, with nortriptyline, an imipramine-like antidepressant. These children were mute or had only psychotic speech. Their symptoms, quite difficult to manage, had been refractory to previously applied medication, "particularly to tranquilizers." Among other symptoms, nortriptyline proved instrumental in influencing hyperactivity, aggressivity and destructiveness.

In our pilot study of imipramine in 10 schizophrenic and autistic children, 2 to 6 years of age, the overall effect of the drug was infrequently therapeutic and usually outweighed by toxic effects, showing a mixture of stimulating, tranquilizing, and disorganizing actions. We suggested that imipramine merits further exploration in the most retarded, mute, anergic psychotics, and in children with only borderline or little psychotic symptomatology (Campbell, Fish, Shapiro, and Floyd, 1971b). Our findings were similar to those of Gershon, Holmberg, Mattson, and Marshall (1962), Klein and Fink (1962) and also of Pollack, Klein, Willner, Blumberg, and Fink (1965), in relation to adult schizophrenics. Frommer (1968) also suggested that the "same contraindications as for adults apply" to the treatment of children with antidepressants, and that monoamine oxidase inhibitors may cause disorganization of behavior. One must conclude that well controlled studies with monogeneous populations are needed in this area.

Major Tranquilizers

While the role of barbiturates and other sedatives was only to facilitate management of the agitated and acutely disturbed child, the advent of major tranquilizers created hope that these agents may also be of therapeutic value. It is hoped that these agents would achieve (1) an antipsychotic effect so that the psychotic process would be arrested or decreased and the child, initially in a state of withdrawal and/or apathy, would become less resistant to educational and other therapies; and (2) a symptomatic effect to decrease anxiety, hyperactivity or aggressiveness, such as that expressed in the form of self-mutilation, that would permit the child to develop more adaptive and socially acceptable patterns of behavior which facilitate learning.

Phenothiazines. Although chlorpromazine (Thorazine®) proved to be of inestimable value for psychotic children of school age, and particularly for adolescents with acute symptomatology (where its effect and the results were similar to those in adults) the young psychotic child is often excessively sedated at doses which control certain psychotic symptoms, and thus not amenable to educational therapy. In our experience, many young psychotic children exhibit sleepiness and psychomotor retardation even at very low doses of chlorpromazine, irrespective of body weight and either presence or absence of hyperactivity and aggressiveness (Fish, Campbell, Shapiro, and Floyd, 1969a; Campbell, Fish, Korein, Shapiro, and Collins, 1972b; Campbell, Fish, Shapiro, and Floyd, 1972). Thus, an extremely hyperactive and aggressive schizophrenic boy, 5 years and 8 months of age and weighing 57 lbs., was sleepy on 20 mg per day; a 3-year-old, retarded, hypoactive and irritable girl, weighing 29 lbs., fell asleep on 10 mg per day within less than 20 minutes after administration.

Clinical experience prompted Fish to suggest that very young autistic children, often apathetic and anergic, resemble chronic adult schizophrenics in their response to drugs (Fish, 1960, 1970). It was thus expected that they will respond better to the more potent and less sedative phenothiazines than chlorpromazine. Trifluoperazine (Stelazine®), a piperazine derivative, proved to be somewhat better than chlorpromazine (Fish, 1960; Fish, 1968; Fish, Shapiro, and Campbell, 1966). Even with the high doses, this drug only seldom produced dystonic reactions in this young age group, while in older children such extrapyramidal side effects often limit its use. Fluphenazine (Prolixin®, Permitil®), another compound with a piperazine sidechain, was found to be highly effective in prepubertal severely disturbed schizophrenic and autistic children (Engelhardt, Polizos, and Margolis, 1972; Engelhardt, Polizos, Waizer, and Hoffman, 1973).

Butyrophenones. This class of major tranquilizers proved to be particularly useful in chronic schizophrenic adults, whose predominant symptoms were autism, apathy and inertia (Gallant, Bishop, Nesselhoff, and Sprehe, 1965; Fox, Gobble, Clos, and Denison, 1964).

The combination of excitatory psychomotor and antipsychotic properties of trifluperidol, prompted us to explore its effects in preschool age, retarded schizophrenic and autistic children. It proved to be an antipsychotic agent with stimulant qualities, significantly more effective in the same subjects than chlorpromazine or trifluoperazine (Fish et al., 1969a; Campbell et al., 1972). The most responsive symptoms were psychotic speech, underproductive speech, withdrawal, and apathy. However, the relatively narrow therapeutic index, with extrapyramidal symptoms at doses 1.3 and 2 times higher than the optimal, limited trifluperidol to investigational use and even resulted in its subsequent withdrawal.

Haloperidol (Haldol®), also a butyrophenone, has been demonstrated as a potent antipsychotic agent in schizophrenic (Engelhardt et al., 1973) and mentally retarded children with severe "emotional disturbance." According to Burk and Menolascino (1968) and also LeVann (1969), it was particularly effective in reducing or controlling hyperactivity, assaultiveness and self-injury, in both retarded and nonretarded children. Haloperidol is now on the market for patients whose age exceeds 12 years; for younger children it is still at the stage of investigational use.

Thioxanthenes. Thiothixene (Navane®) was found to have both stimulating and antipsychotic properties, not unlike trifluperidol, in adult schizophrenics (Gallant, Bishop, and Shelton, 1966; Gallant, Bishop, Timmons, and Gould, 1966; Simpson, and Igbal, 1965; Sugerman, Stolberg, and Herrmann, 1965). Our group investigated the possible beneficial effects of this drug in retarded schizophrenic children of preschool age (Fish, Campbell, Shapiro, and Weinstein, 1969; Campbell, Fish, Shapiro, and Floyd, 1970). Later, other investigators (Simeon, Saletu, Saletu, Itil, and DaSilva, 1973; Waizer, Polizoes, Hoffman, Engelhardt, and Margolis, 1972) confirmed our findings that thiothixene proved in daily doses from 1 to 40 mg with a wide therapeutic margin, an effective, safe therapeutic agent in psychotic children. Again, it is the combination of stimulating and antipsychotic properties which makes this drug superior to phenothiazines in young children.

Indoles. Molindone hydrochloride was found to have antipsychotic and stimulant properties in chronic schizophrenic adults (Gallant and Bishop, 1968; Simpson and Krakov, 1968; Sugerman and Herrmann, 1967). The combination of these two properties prompted us to explore this drug in very young, severely disturbed patients, including some who were apathetic and anergic. Our pilot study involved 10 children (8 schizophrenic and 2 nonpsychotic), whose age ranged from 3 to 5 years. Because molindone had occasionally stimulating as well as sedative therapeutic effects, it was felt that it should be further explored in a larger sample of patients (Campbell, Fish, Shapiro, and Floyd, 1971a). To the best of our knowledge, we were the only ones to study this compound in children.

Minor Tranquilizers

Chlordiazepoxide (Librium®) was reported to be helpful in reducing anxiety in inhibited phobic children. It seems to be less effective or even contraindicated in certain diagnostic categories or behavioral profiles. LaVeck and Buckley (1961) reported an increase in "undesirable behavior" and hyperactivity and decreased attention span in a group of 28 retarded and disturbed children. LeVann (1962) while treating 47 mentally retarded children with behavioral disorders, reported an acute paranoid reaction in an epileptic. Skynner (1961) also found a worsening of hyperactivity and aggressiveness in similar children who exhibited these symptoms prior to chlordiazepoxide treatment.

Pilkington (1961a, 1961b) commented on worsening of symptomatology in retarded schizophrenics, while Kraft, Ardali, Duffy, Hart, and Pearce (1965) reported improvement in two schizophrenic children on this drug.

It appears that chlordiazepoxide with its stimulating (mood-elevating, euphoric) actions may worsen the psychosis or even cause a florid psychosis in children with borderline schizophrenic features.

Other minor tranquilizers are usually ineffective in severely disturbed children.

Hallucinogens

The use of these psychoactive agents in the treatment of psychotic children was introduced by Lauretta Bender. She reported that LSD-25 (*d*-lysergic acid diethylamide) administered to 26 schizophrenic children, and methysergide—a methylated derivative of LSD (1-methyl-*d*-lysergic acid butanolamide bimaleate, Sansert®)—given to 28, for a period of up to one year, were effective stimulants leading to improvement in behavior (Bender, Goldschmidt, and Sankar, 1962; Bender, Faretra, and Cobrinik, 1963; Bender, Cobrinik, Faretra, and Sankar, 1966). Bender's patients were 6 to 12 years of age. Therapeutic changes included increases in motor initiation and alertness, and decreases in stereotypy and psychotic speech. However, there was an increase in anxiety and disorganization in some older, more verbal schizophrenic children exposed to these hallucinogens. Clinical trials with LSD-25 in autistic and schizophrenic children were also reported by Freedman, Ebin, and Wilson (1962), and Simmons, Leiken, Lovaas, Schaeffer, and Perloff (1966). The results reported by Rolo, Krinsky, Abramson, and Goldfarb (1965) were inconclusive.

Fish, Campbell, Shapiro, and Floyd (1969b) carried out a pilot study of methysergide on 11 retarded schizophrenic children, 2 to 5 years of age, over a period of 3 to 11 weeks. Most patients manifested a mixed reduction and worsening of symptoms, similar to those observed by Freedman et al. (1962) in the acute study of LSD-25 in older schizophrenic children. Only the two most retarded, mute psychotic children improved, exhibiting increased alertness, affective responsiveness, and goal directedness.

Lithium

In adults, this ion has a well established role in the treatment of the manic phase of recurrent manic-depressive illness, which probably does not exist under 10 years of age. It also appears to be of value as a prophylactic agent for recurrent manic-depressive illness and periodic endogenous depressions. There are some indications in the literature that lithium maintenance may have "a stabilizing and normalizing action" in children and adolescents with "undulating or period disturbances of mood and behavior" (Schou, 1972).

Frommer (1968) treated hypomanic and depressed children, 4 to 14 years of age, with small doses of lithium, (50 to 250 mg per day), either alone or together with antidepressants. Annell (1969a, 1969b) administered lithium to older children, in daily doses from 900 to 1800 mg (serum lithium level of 0.6 to 1.2 mg/ 1). The patients were reported to manifest typical manic conditions, periodic conditions other than mania (with a high incidence of periodic psychoses, including manic depressive illness in relatives), and even schizophrenia. Most of Annell's patients responded favorably. Dyson and Barcai (1970) found lithium effective while treating two boys whose parents were lithium responders suffering from manic-depressive illness. However, the diagnoses of these young patients were unclear.

Whitehead and Clark (1970) found no difference between the effect of lithium and placebo on hyperactivity, while noting a slight decrease in this symptom on thioridazine. In this pilot study of 7 prepubertal children, one psychotic patient showed an overall improvement, while the condition of others remained unchanged. Gram and Rafaelsen (1972) in their controlled clinical trial of lithium in 18 psychotic subjects (8 to 22 years of age) reported a decrease in hyperactivity, aggressiveness, stereotypies, and psychotic speech.

The effects of lithium in counteracting aggression were established in animal work (Weischer, 1969; Sheard, 1970a, 1970b) and noted in adult human subjects (Sheard, 1971a, 1971b; Tupin and Smith, 1972). Dostal (1972) found that lithium had a significant "affect-damping and antiaggressive" effect in treating 14 mentally retarded, aggressive and hyperactive phenothiazine-resistant boys. However, the antiaggressive effects of lithium were seen only when aggressiveness was associated with excitability and explosiveness.

The action of lithium on hyperexcitability suggested that we should investigate its possible therapeutic effects in hyperactive psychotic and nonpsychotic children and compare such effects with those of chlorpromazine (Campbell et al., 1972b). The 10 children involved in this controlled crossover study were 3 to 6 years of age. While more individual symptoms diminished on chlorpromazine than on lithium, improvements were only slight on both drugs, except in one schizophrenic child whose self-mutilating behavior and explosiveness practically ceased on lithium.

A most interesting finding in that study was the role of the child's EEG as a predictor of "lithium responders"; if the drug accentuated the focal abnormality, behavior either deteriorated or remained unchanged. Behavioral improvement usually occurred when the focal abnormality was decreased by the drug, or when the drug caused increases in diffuse slow activity and a slowing of alpha in normal EEGs (rather than no changes in EEG). Such relationship between EEG and clinical responses applied in lithium as well as to chlorpromazine.

We believe that lithium merits further exploration in psychotic and retarded children whose aggressive or self-mutilating behavioral manifestations with excitability represent prominent symptoms, and when such symptoms prove to be refractory to standard drugs (Campbell, 1973).

L-dopa

Psychiatry's interest in L-dopa can be traced to reports of many behavioral side effects which this compound produced in patients with Parkinson's disease. Psychomotor activation, awakening-alerting effect, improvement in cognitive function, elation and depression were reliably observed in Parkinsonian patients receiving L-dopa by various investigators (Arbit, Boshes, and Blonsky, 1970; Loranger, Goodell, Lee, and McDowell, 1972; O'Brien, DiGiacomo, Fahn, and Schwarz, 1971). The antidepressant effect of L-dopa was reported in some adults with retarded depression, and it was noted that this drug enhanced learning and memory in depressed patients (Goodwin, Murphy, Brodie, and Bunney, 1970; Murphy, 1972a).

L-dopa's biochemical effects on the brain include the evaluation of dopamine which may be related to its behavioral effects. In experimental mice, it produces a marked decrease in brain serotonin (Everett and Borcherding, 1970); it may enter central serotonin terminals with ensuing displacement of the endogenous serotonin from vesicular stores (Butcher, Engel, and Fuxe, 1970; Ny, Chase, Colburn, and Kopin, 1970).

Since serotonin abnormalities were found in the blood of some autistic, schizophrenic and other retarded children (Schain and Freedman, 1961; Ritvo, Yuwiler, Geller, Ornitz, Saeger, and Plotkin, 1970; Coleman, 1970, 1973) and in the platelets of children with a diagnosis of infantile autism (Boullin, Coleman, and O'Brien, 1970; Boullin, Coleman, O'Brien, and Rimland, 1971), Ritvo and his associates carried out a study in order to determine whether clinical and biochemical changes might occur in autistic children if their blood serotonin was lowered. Four autistic children were placed on L-dopa maintenance for 6 months. Although a significant decrease of blood serotonin concentration was noted in 3 children, this was not accompanied by clinical changes (Ritvo, Yuwiler, Geller, Kales, Rashkis, Schicor, Plotkin, Axelrod, and Howard, 1971). Children who showed a lowering of blood serotonin were 3 to 9 years of age. The child who failed to follow the pattern was 13 years old. One can speculate that the patient's age or stage of illness was possibly the factor responsible for the failure to elicit a therapeutic response.

We initiated a study of L-dopa in severely disturbed preschool children (most were schizophrenic), even though we knew that L-dopa was reported to produce exacerbation of psychosis in schizophrenic adults (Angrist, Sathananthan, and Gershon, 1973). Our experience with some very young retarded schizophrenic and autistic children indicated that certain drugs which may produce excessive excitement and/or deterioration in acute schizophrenic adults, proved to be therapeutic when administered to such children (Campbell et al., 1971b, 1972b). On daily doses of 900 to 2250 mg therapeutic changes such as gain in social initiation, verbal production and play, and decreases in withdrawal and psychotic speech were in evidence. Also, hypoactive and apathetic children demonstrated increases in motor initiation and affective responsiveness.

Hormones

Endocrine systems and psychoneuroendocrine interrelations in adult depressives as well as in schizophrenic adults and adolescents were studied for some time (Anderson and Dawson, 1965; Brambilla and Penati, 1971; Durell, Libow, Kellam, and Shader, 1963; Gjessing, 1938, 1953; Hoskins, 1946; Persky, Zuckerman, and Curtis, 1968; Reiss, 1954, 1958; Prange and Lipton, 1972; Sachar, 1963; Sachar, Harmatz, Bergen, and Cohler, 1966; Sachar, Hellman, Roffwarg, Halpern, Fukushima, and Gallagher, 1973). The variations of behavioral and endocrine parameters with various biological treatments were also investigated, suggesting possible correlations between endocrine and behavioral characteristics, and implying that simultaneous treatment of both parameters may yield better and more lasting results (Brambilla and Penati, 1971; Reiss, 1954).

Although various endocrine anomalies were found in psychiatric patients, hormones were usually adminministered not as replacements but as drugs (Hoskins, 1946; Reiss, 1954, 1958, 1971). Long term daily administration of human chorionic gonadotropin (HCG) to children from socially deprived homes with stunted longitudinal and mental growth and retarded gonadal development produced an increase in 17-ketosteroid excretion rate and also progress in the rate of growth. This was accompanied by behavioral and academic improvement with increased IQ. Increase in growth hormone content of the blood was found on the first day of treatment, and the increased growth rate did not cease even long after discontinuation of the treatment with HCG. Previously, these children failed to improve in an enriched therapeutic environment (Reiss, 1971).

Thyroid anomalies were found by several investigators in some adult schizophrenics, especially in those with periodic manifestations of the psychosis (Durell et al., 1963; Gjessing, 1938, 1953; Hoskins, 1946; Simpson, Cranswick, and Blair, 1963, 1964). Although behavioral improvements in schizophrenics (with or without thyroid dysfunction) treated with dessicated thyroid or triiodothyronine (T3) were reported (Danziger, 1958; Danziger and Kindwall, 1953; Hoskins, 1946), the most impressive results with these hormones were obtained by Gjessing (1932, 1938, 1953) who managed to prevent the reoccurrence of periodic psychosis.

T3 was effective in the treatment of depressions in adults, either alone (Feldmesser-Reiss, 1958; Wilson, Prange, and Lara, 1972) or in conjunction with imipramine (Prange, Wilson, Rabon, and Lipton, 1969; Wilson, Prange, McClane, Rabon, and Lipton, 1970). To the best of our knowledge, thyroid hormones were not used in the treatment of depressive conditions in childhood.

Sherwin, Flach, and Stokes (1958) used T3 in the treatment of two 6-year-old autistic "euthyroid" boys. Their encouraging results included increases in alertness, social and affective contact, and speech, as well as decreases in stereotypy on 50 mcg or higher daily doses. The clinical trial was followed by our controlled study involving a relatively large number of preschool schizophrenic and other severely disturbed patients and intended to examine the parameters of thyroid functions in greater detail (Campbell et al., 1972a; Campbell, Fish, David, Shapiro, Collins, and Koh, 1973).

Blind ratings on optimal daily doses ranging from 12.5 to 75 mcg ($M = 46.25$) indicated statistically significant improvement in overall symptomatology. Due to its antipsychotic and stimulating effects, T3 is viewed as an agent that is potentially effective in the treatment of childhood schizophrenia and autism.

It is difficult to explain the therapeutic effects of T3 in the psychotic group, since hypo- and hyperactive children responded equally well, and since four of the improved schizophrenic children had somewhat elevated baseline T4 levels (thyroxine iodine by column chromatography and "free" thyroxine). A review of pertinent literature shows that while many schizophrenic adults treated with thyroid hormone were euthyroid by ordinary standards, some were also found to be hypothyroid. However, in adults with periodic catatonia a shift from the euthyroid toward a relatively hyperthyroid state was said to have taken place immediately before, or roughly at the time of the psychotic episode (Gjessing, 1932, 1938, 1953; Durell et al., 1963).

Gjessing, as well as some other investigators (Durell, et al., 1963; Hoskins, 1946) hypothesized that diencephalic (hypothalamic) mechanisms involved in schizophrenia result in a general lack of integration and that the same mechanisms are responsible for dysthyroidal states. The therapeutic effect of T3 in a subgroup of our schizophrenic children (with somewhat elevated baseline T4) might be related to its stabilizing effect on the hypothalamic-pituitary axis and more immediate effects on its interaction with biogenic amines (serotonin and dopamine). Careful clinical studies with detailed workup are needed to evaluate the relevance of biochemical and neuroendocrine changes in response to T3 and correlate such changes with behavioral manifestations and therapeutic response. Until the results of such studies are available the use of T3 should be limited to investigative objectives.

Monamine neurotransmitters are said to control the secretion of hypothalmic releasing factors, including the thyrotropin releasing factor (TRH), and of anterior pituitary hormones (thyrotropin, TSH) which in turn control the secretion of thyroid hormones (Anton-Tay and Wurtman, 1971; McCann, 1971). Serotonin, one of such neurotransmitters implicated in affecting behavior, was found to be elevated in the blood of some retarded and psychotic children (Ritvo et al., 1970; Schain and Freedman, 1961), and its efflux from platelets was reportedly increased in autistic children compared to normal (Boullin et al., 1970, 1971). Thus, alterations in neuronal transmission of serotonergic and other neuronal systems (dopaminergic and noradrenergic) could lead to, or be associated with, thyroidal as well as behavioral changes. Central nervous system dysfunction responsible for a general lack of integration or adaptive inefficiency may be reflected at all levels.

The thyroid hormone plays an important role in the maturation and development of the CNS (Eayrs, 1968; Sokoloff and Roberts, 1971), and animal studies have demonstrated that the long-term effects of dysthyroidal states (both hypo- and hyperthyroid) are deleterious to cerebral development during the early stages of life (Balazs, Kovacs, Cocks, Johnson, and Eayrs, 1971; Eayrs, 1968; Schapiro, 1971).

Some of the developmental lags or defects in childhood schizophrenia and other severe disturbances of early childhood (of unknown origin) might be altered or replaced by biological substances including hormones (such as T3) or even neurohormones (such as TRH). Our limited experience with T3 supports this.

Orthomolecular Psychiatry

The concept of "orthomolecular" treatment in psychiatry was introduced by Linus Pauling in an article published in 1968. Pauling suggested that this method constituted the "treatment of mental disease by the provision of the optimum molecular environment for the mind, especially the optimum concentration of substances normally present in the human body." Deficiencies of certain vital substance(s) in the brain may lead to mental illness. These deficiencies may not exist in the peripheral blood and lymph; they may be "localized cerebral deficiency diseases." Pauling believes that the brain is probably more sensitive to changes in concentrations of these vital substances than any other organ, and that there could be a decreased permeability of the blood-brain barrier or an increased rate of metabolism of the vital substance(s) in the brain of certain individuals, including schizophrenic patients, on a genetic basis.

Ascorbic acid, thiamine, pyridoxine, folic acid and other substances (normally present in the organism), such as L(+)-glutamic acid, were investigated as a therapeutic substance in animal work and in psychiatric patients.

Successful treatment of adult stuporous psychiatric patients (most were elderly with arteriosclerosis) with moderately large doses of nicotinic acid was reported prior to World War II by Cleckley, Sydenstricker, and Geeslin (1939). Hoffer and Osmond, who used large doses of nicotinic acid or nicotinamide in the treatment of schizophrenia (Osmond and Hoffer, 1962; Hoffer, 1973; Osmond, 1973), reported good results. Some of these studies with large numbers of newly admitted as well as chronic schizophrenic adults did not substantiate Hoffer's and Osmond's findings. Clinical trials with nicotinic acid yielded either no therapeutic effect or even negative effects (Ban, 1971; Ban and Lehmann, 1970; McGrath, O'Brien, Power, and Shea, 1972; Mosher, 1970; Ramsey, Ban, Lehmann, Saxena, and Bennett, 1970; Wittenborn, Weber, and Brown, 1973).

While Hoffer reported that niacinamide and ascorbic acid proved superior to placebo in children (1970), Greenbaum (1970) could not confirm these findings in a double blind study of 17 children receiving niacinamide and 24 placebo. Even Rimland, a strong advocate of megavitamin therapy, calls the results of this treatment only "encouraging." In a preliminary report he detailed the results of a study of 190 outpatient psychotic children receiving megadoses of vitamins over a period of 24 weeks with a month-long vitamin-free period at the end of that study (Rimland, 1973). The vitamin regime consisted of increasing doses of niacinamide, ascorbic acid, pyridoxine and pantothenic acid, in addition to multiple B tablets, following a certain schedule. Parents were to record their observations semimonthly and the physicians each month rating behaviors such as "change in speech, alertness, irritability, understanding, eating, sleeping, social responsiveness, tantrums, and overall behavior." Criteria of vitamin efficacy were the reports of parents and physicians during the vitamin therapy period, during the nonvitamin treatment period, and also whether or not the vitamins were reordered. All data were subjected to statistical analysis. The subgroup of 37 children identified as having "classicial infantile autism" showed the greatest improvement on the regime, particularly the six who were receiving Dilantin together with vitamins. Among "specific" vitamin effects, increases in alertness, social awareness and sociability were reported with vitamin C. Niacinamide "appeared" to have an antipsychotic effect, while pantothenic acid made some children more alert, calmer and more accessible. The most obvious changes were attributed to vitamin B6, particularly in increasing the initiation of speech and verbal production. However, some children showed a worsening of behavior, including hyperactivity and irritability, among other side effects. According to the "overall improvement" ratings, 45.3% of the group showed definite improvement, 41.0% possible improvement, 10.5% no improvement and only 3.1% of the children in the group manifested adverse effects. It is not clear how many children were on psychoactive drugs (other than Dilantin and Mellaril) concomitantly with vitamins and whether any differential response to megavitamin treatment was in evidence. It is also not clear what diagnostic categories other than early infantile autism were involved in the study (although presumably some children were schizophrenic). One might also mention the absence of data pertaining to the age of children or treatment program (other than megavitamin therapy) to which some, if not most, must have been exposed.

An APA task force, after an impressively thorough investigation, came to the conclusion that megavitamin therapy does not meet the "test of scientific validity" and has no value in the treatment of schizophrenia (Lipton, Ban, Kane, Levine, Mosher, and Wittenborn, 1973).

Concluding Note

This presentation represents an attempt to outline various biological-organic interventions in childhood psychoses without due effort to evaluate the methodology employed by other investigators or consideration for the possible long-term hazards of drug therapy.

Therapeutic efforts and speculative attempts have been made for some time to find more rational modes of treatment for the psychoses. Since the late 1920's, our libraries have been accumulating volumes devoted to research studies of biochemical, hormonal and physiological deviations and their behavioral correlates in adults. During the past decade, many interesting hypotheses have implicated biogenic amines in depression and schizophrenia in adults, suggesting that clinical distinctions could be correlated with various biochemical criteria. It is believed that neuropharmacology of effective psychoactive drugs may facilitate insight not only into the biochemical mechanisms which serve in conjunction with certain drugs to decrease the symptoms, but also into the biology of the mental illness itself (Himwich, Kety, and Smythies, 1967; Lapin and Oxenkrug, 1969; Kety, 1972; Murphy, 1972b; Schildkraut and Kety, 1967). More recently, such investigations have also been directed toward issues more closely related to the psychoses of early childhood (Campbell, Friedman, DeVito, Greenspan, and Collins, 1973; Coleman, 1973; Coleman, Campbell, Freedman, Roffman, Ebstein, and Goldstein, 1974).

At our present state of knowledge, no specific drug is available for reliable treatment of any diagnostic categories of psychoses in early life. Currently used drugs are most effective in reducing symptoms such as insomnia, hyperactivity, impulsivity, irritability, disorganized behavior, psychotic thought disorder, and certain types of aggressivity. Thus far, lithium appears to represent the first psychoactive agent which is specific in the treatment of a well-defined condition such as the manic phase of the manic-depressive illness. It should be noted, however, that psychotic children do not necessarily respond to lithium or to the other drugs in the same manner as psychotic adults.

Experience indicates that drug treatment is an essential component of the total treatment of the psychotic child of preschool age. Such child may no longer be as responsible to the same drug treatment at a later age as during the course of his first years of life. The severity of illness and generally poor prognosis appear to warrant the risks related to psychoactive agents. Hopefully, a more rational psychopharmacologic approach, which would consider the entire developing organism of the individual child, will lead us to more effective therapies for psychotic children.

Finally, the basic need for uniformity in the classification of child psychoses is still with us. We suggest that certain biochemical and neuroendocrine parameters will facilitate the delineation of categories in the mixed population of psychotic children. There are reasons to hope that this would be of considerable value in predicting whether a child can benefit from a specific drug.

Psychological Effects of Stimulant Drugs in Children with Minimal Brain Dysfunction

C. KEITH CONNERS, Ph.D.

Conners does not believe that the hyperkinetic child represents a distinct clinical entity. He has previously stated that in order to use rational drug therapy the "underlying variables" determining the child's clinical picture must be discovered and used (Conners, 1972b). Elsewhere he has stated, "Perhaps differences between and within studies are due to different kinds of changes in different kinds of patients" (Conners, 1971).

Toward this end Conners combined subjects from three drug studies and through elaborate statistical analysis defined seven distinct patterns of performance and behavior. Each of these groups shows distinctly different changes with drug treatment as measured by six standardized change factors.

Conners' work is important since he provides convincing evidence that "minimal brain dysfunction" is a heterogeneous disorder, that children so diagnosed do not respond in the same manner to drug treatment and that the kind of response depends upon a "profile of abilities."

Although there are no distinct clinical guidelines which can be presently derived from this, it would appear that this is a valuable preliminary contribution to the goal of establishing relevant, reliable and pragmatic clinical guidelines in the drug treatment of children.

> *This subject is explored in greater depth elsewhere by the same*
> *author (Conners, 1973).*

A number of myths have grown up regarding the behavioral effects and use of stimulant medications with children. The first is that there is a type of child uniquely responsive to stimulant compounds, namely, the hyperkinetic child. The second is that the hyperkinetic child is any child who is sufficiently overactive to be considered a menace by adults. The third is that the stimulant medications act primarily to reduce motor activity in a paradoxical "sedative" fashion; and finally, that the drugs do not influence cognitive and perceptual functioning in these children. I belived that these myths are due partly to the historical accident of the manner in which they were first studied, partly to the imprecision in diagnosis and terminology of classification of patients, and partly to the paucity of systematic data on sufficiently large samples under sufficiently varied experimental conditions. I would like to present the results of studies which bear on these issues, and try to draw some general conclusions regarding the present state of knowledge with regard to the use of the various psychostimulants. In this paper I will deal with dextroamphetamine, methylphenidate, and magnesium pemoline.

I. Methylphenidate and Dextroamphetamine

The children for this study were referred from schools, pediatricians, and social agencies for either academic or behavioral difficulties, or both. The subjects retained for the drug study comprised about 2/3 of the original referral sample. They were selected to fit the description of the child with "minimal brain dysfunction" as defined by the National Institute of Neurological Diseases and Stroke (NINDS) Task Force I report. Specifically excluded were children with psychosis, gross neuropathy, delinquency, primary emotional disorders, or mental retardation. Ages ranged from 74 months to 154 months, with a median of 112 months (9.3 years). Seventy subjects (Ss) were male and five were female; 73 were white. About 9% of the sample fell into Class

Reprinted from *Pediatrics*, Vol. 49 (1972), pp. 702-708.

I of the Hollingshead social class index (low), with 34% in Class II, 26% in Class III, 20% in Class IV, and 11% in Class V.

A detailed social and medical history, neurologic and physical examination, parent and teacher symptom ratings, and a battery of neuropsychological tests were obtained. The psychological tests included: Wechsler Intelligence Scale for Children (WISC), Frostig Test of Visual Perception, a measure of verbal fluency, Wide Range Achievement Test (WRAT), Bender Gestalt Test, Draw-A-Man, Porteus Mazes, children's Embedded Figures Test, speech discrimination in background noise, auditory synthesis, vigilance, and rote learning.

The patients are randomly assigned to the three treatment groups by a random code devised and kept by the hospital pharmacy, which supplied medication in identical matched capsules. The assignment resulted in 29 Ss assigned to methylphenidate, 24 to dextroamphetamine, and 22 to placebo. Dosage was increased once weekly. Each capsule contained either 5 mg dextroamphetamine (DA) or 10 mg methylphenidate (MP), or placebo. Dosage was gradually increased to a maximum daily dosage of 15 mg DA or 30 mg MP in divided doses given 20 minutes before breakfast and lunch.

All tests and ratings were scored and administered without knowledge of the treatment condition, before treatment and after 6 weeks on treatment. Results were analyzed by a one-way analysis of covariance for each variable separately. Individual comparisons were made between treatments by t-tests. The results showed the following significant ($p < .05$) treatment effects: WISC Full Scale IQ, WISC Verbal IQ, similarities, digit span, object assembly. Frostig perceptual quotient (eye-motor coordination, figure-ground, form constancy), verbal fluency, teacher symptom ratings, Bender Gestalt, Draw-A-Man, Porteus Mazes, speech-noise test, continuous vigilance test (omissions and commissions). Rote learning and embedded figures showed effects significant at the 10% level. All differences were in favor of the drug-treated Ss. Only two measures, WISC arithmetic and similarities, were significantly different between the two active drugs, both in favor of Ritalin. Analysis of side effect reports showed that both drugs produced significantly more insomnia and anorexia than placebo controls, and DA produced significantly more of these side effects than MP. This was especially true for the side effects rated as moderate to severe, although the percentage of subjects receiving those ratings was quite small.

II. Magnesium Pemoline (P)
and Dextroamphetamine (DA)

This study involved a similar population of children as in the previous study. The same parent and teacher rating scales, a global improvement rating, and the following psychological tests were employed: WISC, Draw-A-Man, Bender Gestalt, Porteus Mazes, Illinois Test of Psycholinguistic Abilities, Frostig, WRAT, Gray Oral Reading, vigilance, Gates Reading Survey, and visual evoked response under attending and nonattending conditions. In addition, the following laboratory measures were collected at baseline, 4 weeks, and 8 weeks during the 8-week study: complete blood count (CBC), hematocrit, hemoglobin, platelets, blood urea nitrogen (BUN), alkaline phosphatase, spectrophotometric method (SGOT), lactic acid dehydrogenase (LDH), bilirubin, and complete urinalysis. Of 132 patients examined, 84 were admitted to drug study, and 81 completed the 8 weeks of treatment. There were 74 males and 10 females; all Caucasian except for one Negro. Fifty-nine children had both behavior and academic problems, 19 had behavior problems only, and six had academic problems only. The age was 6 to 12 years, with a mean age of 8.24 years. Social class distribution was almost identical to the previous study.

Patients were randomly assigned, double-blind, to the three treatments, with P administered in tablets containing 25 mg magnesium pemoline Cylert (18.75 mg pemoline) and DA in 5 mg matched tablets. P was given only in the morning with equivalent numbers of placebos administered in the afternoon to match the schedule of the DA group. Dosage was adjusted twice weekly to a maximum dose for Cylert of 125 mg, with a mean resulting dose of 82 mg. The number of dosage adjustments during the study were 6.2, 6.7, and 7.3 for Cylert, DA, and placebo respectively. Weight, pulse, and blood pressure were obtained with a physical examination at 2, 4, 6, and 8 weeks. Abbreviated parent and teacher ratings on a 10-item scale were obtained at weekly intervals, and all psychological tests were administered at baseline and then at 8 weeks.

Rating Results

A global clinical rating by the staff showed highly significant treatment effects due to drugs. At both 4 and 8 weeks both drugs were superior to placebo. By the end of treatment 96% of the DA and 77% of the P subjects were rated as improved or much improved, with 30% of the placebo patients rated as improved, and none much improved. Similar results were obtained from the teacher's global ratings of academic progress.

The teacher symptom rating was factor analyzed, and the results analyzed by multivariate analysis of variance. Significant treatment effects were found for the defiance, inattentiveness, and hyperactivity factors for both drugs. Although DA showed an earlier effect than Cylert, by the end of 8 weeks the two treatments were indistinguishable on these factored measures. Identical results were found for the abbreviated teacher ratings.

DA showed significant effects by 2 weeks, whereas Cylert showed clear differences from placebo only at 6 weeks and afterwards.

The 93-item parent symptom list was also factor analyzed, and of the eight factor scores, four showed significant treatment effects: conduct disturbance, impulsivity, immaturity, and antisocial behavior. Not affected by treatments were anxiety, somatic complaints, obsessional traits, and hyperactivity. The abbreviated parent rating showed a highly significant treatment effect similar to that found with the teacher ratings. In most of the effects an early DA response is seen by 2 weeks, but there are no drug-drug differences by 8 weeks.

The psychological test battery was first tested for a drug effect by a multivariate analysis of variance, producing a highly significant effect ($p < .004$). Individual analysis of variance showed that spelling, reading, Porteus Mazes, Frostig perceptual quotient, eye-motor coordination, and figure-ground scores were significantly different from placebo, with no drug-drug differences.

Laboratory studies showed no children experiencing abnormal changes over the course of treatment, and analyses of variance indicated no group changes attributable to the treatments. Systolic, diastolic, and pulse-pressure were unchanged for all three groups in the study. Weight changes were +.5 kg, +1.1 kg, and +.9 kg for DA, P, and placebo groups respectively. These changes were nonsignificant between groups.

The major side effects of both drugs were insomnia and anorexia. By the end of the treatment period fewer than 5% of patients were experiencing moderate or severe insomnia, and all of these were on DA. Both drugs produced most insomnia between the seventeenth and twenty-eighth day of treatment, but only at day 28 were there actually drug-placebo significant differences.

In summary, both of these studies provide unequivocal evidence of improved behavior as judged by clinicians, parents, and teachers, and both studies show significant drug effects on some cognitive, perceptual, and achievement measures. However, some inconsistencies are rather striking. Some of the most drug sensitive measures, such as the vigilance task, did not show effects found in the earlier study, and indeed, in several other previous studies. Secondly, the effects on achievement were more striking in the Cylert Study than in the DA-MP Study. In the earlier study, on the other hand, the Draw-A-Man and Bender showed striking and highly significant improvement in the drug treated Ss, but failed to do so in the more recent pemoline study, and failed to do so in two earlier DA studies. It seems unlikely that these differences reflect the difference in length of treatment or dosage schedules; rather, we suspect that they are likely to be fortuitous results of the sample composition. Such inconsistencies led us to analyze the predictive value of various measures, and attempt to achieve diagnostic homogeneity by profile analysis. From several studies in which common pre- and post-drug measuring instruments were used, we were able to obtain 178 previously treated subjects (100 on drugs, 78 on placebo). The various psychological tests were converted to change scores and intercorrelated. This showed that the changes tended to be largely independent of one another, with relatively little communality among tests. However, by factor analysis of the change measures we were able to arrive at six standardized change factors, which we labelled academic performance, attention, perceptual, reading, impulsiveness, and classroom disturbance. These change scores were then predicted from stepwise multiple regression equations, with correlations of .73, .82, .63, .58, .70, and . 57 respectively. Clearly there are a number of rather different types of response to the drugs, and these are predicted by different patterns of baseline performance on psychological tests.

This result is further clarified by subjecting the baseline measures to a computer profile analysis, which reveals at least seven somewhat distinct patterns of performance in our already selected population. When these separate groups are analyzed for drug placebo differences, it is found that the groups have highly significant drug-treatment effects but for somewhat different measures. Group I is characterized by very poor eye-motor coordination and attention. They show significant drug effects on the perceptual-motor factor. This group also shows a very large hemispheric asymmetry on visual evoked responses, with the left side smaller than the right. Group II is very poor on perceptual integration and spatial orientation, and tend to show improvement primarily in attention-related tests and academic ratings. Group III is quite poor in spatial orientation but good in eye-motor coordination. They show improvement similar to Group II in attention but in contrast to Group II do not show a related degree of improvement in academic ratings by teachers. Group IV is low in perceptual integration but good in spatial orientation, and tend to show improvement only on tests such as the Bender Gestalt. This group also has marked hemispheric evoked response asymmetry, but with a markedly larger left- than right-sided amplitude. Group V constitutes about 20% of the sample and show no drug treatment effects whatsoever. Their baseline profile is essentially flat, with some report of conduct and classroom disturbance asymmetry (small left-sided amplitudes) of the evoked response, are low in achievement, and rated poorly by teachers for classroom conduct. This group shows significant drug effects on academic performance, and spelling and arithmetic. Group VII is low in Verbal IQ but very good in parent ratings. They are also markedly asymmetric in the evoked response, with smaller left-sided amplitudes. They show changes due to drugs mainly in reading tasks.

Thus, it is apparent that there is both physiological and psychological heterogeneity in this group of children with presumed "minimal brain dysfunction." All children with this diagnosis do not respond in the same way to drug therapy, and the type of response appears to depend on the profile of abilities, and possibly on underlying physiological responsiveness in the cerebral cortex. Clearly, whether a child should receive this form of therapy depends on a careful assessment of the probability that he will respond for the target symptom or deficit of most concern. Some poor readers do indeed show remarkable progress with adjunctive analeptic therapy, but many more do not; some behavior problem children show improvement in behavior but not in learning, and vice-versa. While the present studies are preliminary, and do not as yet offer useful diagnostic tools for the physician, they appear to dispel some of the myths surrounding this treatment. No single syndrome of hyperkinesis is uniquely responsive to therapy, motor activity itself is not among the more important types of changes found with these children, and several patterns of change of perceptual and cognitive abilities may result from drug therapy.

Group and Milieu Therapy

Introduction

At first glance, it may seem paradoxical to combine group and milieu therapies in a single section. However, this was done with forethought; milieu settings (residential, full hospital, partial hospital, and day programs) have provided much of the impetus for an expanding application of group therapy for children and adolescents with a variety of clinical diagnoses. Indeed, Bettelheim and Sylvester (1948) utilized a fusion of psychotherapy and milieu management in one process, called milieu therapy, in which insight could be translated into uninterrupted action over twenty-four hours a day.

Early writers, including Slavson (1950, 1964) in the mid-thirties and later Axline (1969), described primarily activity group models for latency and younger children usually with neurotic conflicts, and on an outpatient basis. Indeed, the long list of contraindications for group therapy compiled by Ginott (1961) excluded the vast majority of children referred with serious psychopathology. These contraindications often included the precise sorts of children who needed an intensive milieu experience.

Foulkes and Anthony (1965) were among the first child group therapists to question the use of activity (or play) as a sole medium of therapy; they underscored the necessity for verbal and secondary process techniques. They reported techniques for assisting the development from an activity group level to a therapeutic group characterized by secondary process.

However, the major phase in the development of group therapy came from the residential treatment of children. Redl and Wineman (1957) pioneered the application of milieu therapy to those children considered by many workers to be "untreatable." Their work extended through the late 1940s into the 1950s and initiated the greatly expanded use of group therapy in milieu settings. Their book, *The Aggressive Child*, describes with many clinical examples their group techniques. They varied from free activity to more structured activity to serious verbal techniques. Thus, the milieu approach expanded the applicability of group therapy to a wider range of childhood disturbances, including predelinquent, characterologically disturbed, and borderline youngsters.

Subsequently, others began to work with such children in less intensive settings such as drop-in centers, day programs, and outpatient clinics. *Retrieval from Limbo* (1967), published by the Child Welfare League, reports long experience in outpatient group therapy with a group of delinquent children who were on a waiting list for residential treatment. Significant gains were reported for many of these difficult children, but other intensive collaborative work was proceeding with the parents and schools at the same time.

In recent years, newer psychotherapeutic movements have added other techniques to group therapy with children; notable among these influences has been behavior therapy with its systematic observations and interventions. Encounter, gestalt, and transactional analysis have all found their way into adolescent groups and even occasionally into latency groups. In addition, increasing understanding of child development, especially cognitive development, has allowed for more appropriate grouping. Finally, the continuing improvements in videotape equipment (particularly portability and ease of playback) have greatly increased the possibilities for using the equipment in groups for psychodrama, instant playback, and improved training and supervision of cotherapist teams. The software industry and educators have begun to capitalize on children's infatuation with media, particularly film and video, with the introduction of affectively charged material for therapeutic group discussion such as the Inside-Out Series.

The selections presented in this section are an attempt to present a limited cross-section of some of these developments. The articles are less numerous than those of other sections representing exploding fields such as family and behavior therapy (each of which incorporate group therapy articles themselves). This, we believe, represents the current state and level of sophistication of the group therapy literature pertaining to children. Recent books on group therapy with children, including those by Rose (1973) and Berkowitz and Graziano (1972), are recommended for further reading.

The Group in Residential Treatment of Adolescents

MORRIS F. MAYER, M.S.W.

The gradation that exists in residential settings between group living and activity groups and therapeutic groups with their secondary process orientation contributes to the difficulty in defining a clear boundary between milieu therapy and group therapy. Mayer develops the position that the whole living arrangement is therapeutic and structured to develop ego functions. He explores the therapeutic function of rules, structure, daily meetings of living units, staff and institutional attitudes, the development of rituals, and the attempts to change the "crowd" into a cohesive "groups." However, his orientation is that of the traditional residential group specialist who views groups as constantly changing, short-lived, goal-focused, and ad hoc in their make up. Others, in different settings may, on the other hand, emphasize the development of longer term or open ended groups, with either stable or changing group composition. Often such groups take on the characteristics of "clubs," with their structure, rules, and ritual; when such groups are heterogeneous diagnostically, the very dissimilarity in the youngster's personality structures may permit much healthy peer modeling, cohesiveness, and constructive peer confrontation.

The literature on residential treatment for adolescents is full of recommendations for "group" living and "group" work. In practice, however, the implementation of these recommendations leaves much to be desired. Often there is no clinical concept as to what the group is and what part of the treatment it should fulfill. Not infrequently the practice of group living is left to the resourcefulness, initiative and spontaneity of the untrained child care staff rather than being based on the clinical philosophy and planfulness of the total treatment program.

Psychoanalysis has made the most profound contribution to the understanding of the adolescent of his efforts to control his new and powerful drives, of his identity conflict, of his struggle for his own values. Yet these psychoanalytic theories of adolescence have failed to promote a theory on group interaction equally clinical and profound—one that could be applied to the central experience of group living in residential treatment. The psychoanalytic concept of the group has regarded the peer group mainly in terms of the family group (leader equals father, peers equal siblings) and thereby may have minimized the group identity as a whole, even while it has sharpened the awareness of the psychodynamics operating in each of its members.

Group work in a psychoanalytically oriented residential treatment center has suffered from this underemphasis on the group experience itself. Group work has been on the defensive. This becomes noticeable in the discussions in Maier's (1965) monograph on group work in residential treatment which makes a most valuable contribution to the understanding of the role of the group in residential treatment. In his introduction, Maier sees a group as having many essential functions in the provision of dependency, privacy, belonging, individualization and identification. He does not, however, relate the group experience closely enough to the other therapeutic inputs in the treatment. Despite this limitation, his contribution must be regarded as an essential step toward understanding of the group in residential treatment. Similarly, Polsky and Claster's (1968) brilliant work suffers from disregard of the therapeutic tasks of the total institution, and becomes at times too much the champion of one particular group, the child care workers.

Reprinted from *Child Welfare*, Vol. 51, No. 8 (October 1972), pp. 482-493.

What is a group? Perhaps the definition by Catell is most useful. "A group is a collection of organisms in which the existence of all . . . is necessary to the satisfaction of certain individual needs in each. That is to say, the group is an instrument for the satisfaction of needs in the individual" (1953, p. 20). I would add to this definition that not only is the group fulfilling the need of each individual but each individual should feel needed for the survival of the group.

Residential treatment therefore has to establish groups in which each individual finds a place. Adolescents in these groups may be able to identify with each other and develop a better self-image, a greater feeling of hope and optimism, a new, more constructive form of identity. The interpersonal support of their joint ego can develop into an intrapersonal support.

This, however, is not necessarily the case. Many conditions must be met in order to develop the group as a therapeutic instrument. It is indeed possible that the coming together of a number of unhappy, unsettled, aggressive adolescents reinforces their regression rather than their progress. Greenacre, in describing violence, speaks of the "crowd" as a number of people accidentally thrown together like a mob in the street, and says "the crowd not only attracts a great variety of poorly integrated people; it tends to bring out regressive behavior" (1970, p. 350). If group structures are not set up with great care, adolescents may well unite for unlimited freedom, for defiance, for destruction. The youngsters may bring out in each other the desire for regression to an infantile, libidinal behavior pattern, with even more primitive behavior patterns than they showed prior to their coming to the center. The population in an institutional cottage is not a "group." It may well remain a "crowd" if nothing is done to develop a group.

From the Crowd to the Group

Changing the "crowd" into a "group" is perhaps the most important assignment of the professional who works with adolescents in residential treatment. In the following we give some practical suggestions as to how this can be done. This change depends on a number of factors: A) the orientation and organization of the institution; B) authority and rules; and C) the balances (including groups, tasks, rituals).

A. *The Orientation and Organization of the Institution*

Although we cannot here discuss administration of a treatment center, it must be said that a clear purpose of the organization has to be known not only to board and administration but all staff and to the children. There must be a clear line of communication from administration to staff and from staff to administration. Everybody must know what his job is, what decisions he can make, what decisions he cannot make, and where to turn for other decisions. It is sound that there be wide participation in decisions, but it is crucial that decisions be made quickly and according to the purpose of the center, and not be delayed in a bureaucratic network of hierarchy, autocracy or would-be democracy. There must be a unity of command despite the many variations and differentiations necessary for treatment. Above all, there must always be an awareness that the goal of the institution is the treatment of the child.

The spirit that moved people to create institutions for human betterment, to develop treatment, to wrestle with the despairing and the wayward, can easily be lost in an organization's professional and administrative apparatus. To help adolescents it is necessary that this initial spirit, this faith, is in some form communicated to them. This communication is perhaps the most important assignment of any administration. It must be sensed by the youngster who enters the center. He may not be able to accept it and to abide by its values; he must, however, unobtrusively be enveloped by it, even if he resists it.

B. *Authority and Rules*

Maier (1965) finds that the use of the group compensates for three inherent liabilities of institutional living that he calls "authoritarianism, standardization and anonymity." Adolescents have always been particularly sensitive about "authority." What has made the handling of adolescents so complicated in our time is not that today's adolescents are so much more opposed than in the past to the use of authority (Socrates complained about the unruliness and rebellious-ness of the young), but rather that adults have become so much more uncertain and guilt-stricken about using authority. It is understood that punitive, cruel, degrading, sadistic forms of authority are damaging and harmful. Constructive authority, however, is a most essential ingredient in the treatment of the adolescent.

We agree with Aarons that "the so-called enlightened parent adheres to a befuddled logic, by which to understand the reasons for a misbehavior warrants a permissive attitude toward it. What is required instead is that the adolescent know that the parent does not sanction it. ... For the superego to wage a successful struggle against regressive drive forces, parents and surrogates must remain constant and firm in maintaining ego ideals both by espousal and example" (1970, p. 334).

The administration of authority is a major problem for adolescents in group care and for the people in charge of them. The fear of losing the affection of the adolescent, the desire to "reach" him, may distort the staff's concept of their authority role. The joint pressures of the adolescent group on the staff may weaken the counselor's ability to implement this authority role. The adolescents may develop a distorted assessment of reality, since each may receive confirmation of his own distortion by similar distortions of others. Blos's (1962) observation that the adolescent's "self-image formation," with a "paranoid" reaction, is caused by a "hostile identification with a degraded parent image" can easily be amplified to include the identification of disturbed adolescents with each other. There develops what one might term a group-validated distortion.

The child care worker, educator, supervisor and administrator who have to use authority see themselves confronted with a hostile crowd whenever they must limit the adolescent, and they see themselves pushed into the roles of "arbitrary dictators," nontrusting, nonunder-standing martinets. The younger counselor who has not worked through his own aggression, his own feeling about the "establishment," his own conflict with authority will perhaps be overwhelmed by the onslaught of the "crowd." He may confuse authority and punitiveness, fluctuate between intransigence and surrender, and project his own role conflict (in almost the same "paranoid" fashion) onto his superiors, the system, the administration. The older and "established" counselor, on the other hand, may not have to use this kind of defense but may still find it difficult to use authority therapeutically. He may regard the established authority role as so final that the adolescent's attack upon him will seem a personal challenge to his own competence, indeed to society. Any concession to the adolescent will then appear as a surrender not only of personal strength but of the total social value system.

Perhaps the most serious handicap to the implementation of authority is the adult's fear of the adolescent. Often this is a fear of physical violence, of being attacked. Sometimes it is also the adult's unconscious fear of his own counteraggression. Any adult working with adolescents needs to be helped to recognize these fears and anxieties. For treatment to be possible, the group care setting must protect not only the adolescent from physical attacks by the adult, but the adult from physical attacks by the adolescent.

Another confusion about the use of authority in residential treatment is caused by a misunderstood concept of individualization. Individualization is the single most important ingredient necessary for the growth, education and treatment of any child, any adolescent or any adult in any setting. Individualization means flexible adaptation of a general principle, policy or practice to the individual. It means being able to make an exception from general guidelines in order to meet the needs of each child. It doesn't mean, however, the absence of rules, policies and guidelines. Not having rules can mean only chaos, disorder and insecurity. Within such chaos the unpredictable, unmanageable aspects of adolescence become even more disrupting and frightening. The paranoid fears become more overwhelming. The "standardization" to which Maier refers is therefore, not only a "necessary evil," it is an important instrument in the handling of the adolescent.

Similarly, the concept of "causation of behavior" must not become a handicap but instead a helpful instrument in handling of authority. There is no doubt that the psychological cause for any action must be considered in the establishment of sanctions, be they rewards or punishment. The adolescent who breaks a neighbor's window because he wants to burglarize his apartment and the one who breaks that window because he wants to use a piece of glass to cut his wrist certainly require different handling—in the immediate and in the long-range disposition. Nevertheless, in both cases the window was broken, and the neighbor wants some form of restitution. The policeman who is sent to the institution to establish the facts of the offense, even if he is understanding of its cause, will want the evidence and data, and the other neighbors, even if sympathetic, will want protection from similar assaults.

Authority, therefore, has to be based on a logical set of implementable regulations, flexibly applied by nonpunitive and noncorruptible adults. Here are a few guidelines for establishment of such rules:

1) A set of basic rules must uniformly cover the major events of daily living. These rules have to be founded on the developmental and therapeutic needs of the children, and be valid for the whole institution.

2) Rules cannot cover all the minute eventualities of life. These details have to handled specifically within the spirit of the overall rules.

3) If there is more than one living unit within the center, an additional set of specific rules must be established for each unit within the spirit and framework of the general rules.

4) Each staff member responsible for the handling of adolescents must know the rules and be willing to carry them out within the general orientation of the center.

5) Deviations from rules have to be planned ahead of time by the clinical team, rather than on the spur of the moment by one staff member. If these deviations occur without planning—as they on occasion necessarily will—they must be discussed immediately thereafter with the other members of the team.

6) Any individual staff member who cannot accept a rule, and cannot in good conscience carry it out properly, has to discuss his inability with his supervisor and with the administration of the institution, so that his personal incapacity does not interfere with the organization of the unit and the planned order of living.

7) Every adolescent should be acquainted with the basic rules of the institution. The more he recognizes that rules are not arbitrarily set by each individual adult but are responsibly planned, the better he will be able to accept them.

8) All rules are subject to change and should be frequently reviewed. Changes should be made in an orderly fashion with the participation of all staff involved. Similarly, adolescents should be invited to participate in a change of rules. Although it is damaging for children to be used by adults in imposing punishments on other youngsters (kangaroo courts), they can contribute in an advisory capacity to the establishment of rules. They can be better legislators than judges.

9) Frequent changes in rules may be necessary but should not be made in response to dissatisfaction with a specific decision. Otherwise, the respect for and the value of the rules will be undermined. Rather, a clear and acknowledged procedure that includes the administration, the staff and the children should be established for enactment, change and abolishment of rules.

10) Any rule that has not been abolished must be respected. The adolescent who comes to group care must, therefore, find a functioning system of authority with clear rules and with adults ready to carry them out. He must also sense that the system provides for rules to be changed in orderly fashion and for his participation in such changes.

The Balances

A. *The Groups*

Authority can easily become authoritarianism. The adolescents may see themselves as the prisoners of an authoritarian structure that, although fair and humane, does not give them the opportunity for self-expression and identity formation. Authority alone cannot be therapeutic. It must be balanced. The major balances are the group experiences for which there is such ample opportunity in group care.

Group experience offers: a) joint pleasure experiences within a basically painful structure; b) manageable and common experiences; c) identification with society through the medium of identification with peers; and d) voluntarism within a compulsory system.

The most basic group is the living group itself. This group is neither voluntary nor for most parts of the day particularly pleasurable. Because of this, the development of many other group interactions is necessary.

For adolescents, there should be a short daily, compulsory group meeting of the living group for task assignment and review and preview of activities. This meeting is part of the authority structure of the center. It is a transition from authority to the balances, from adult administration to group participation. However, precisely for this reason it is valuable and unexpendable. It serves to clarify reality authority structure lines of communication and rules. It may develop—in spite of its compulsory nature—into an important therapeutic tool. It can become the matrix from which many other group experiences can generate. But this is not necessarily the case. It may be wiser not to try too hard to make cottage meetings group "experiences." They should be short, to the point, task-oriented, daily and regular. Many of the derivative topics stimulated by the cottage meetings should be referred to special groups or subgroups. The leader will have to decide this on the basis of the actual situation, the mood of the children, the climate of the group.

The dynamics of group living are expressed by the optimal movement of the isolate and the follower toward the ingroup. The living group alone does not offer enough opportunities for such movement to all youngsters and must, therefore, be augmented by many other group formations. Ideally, each youngster should find at least one group where he belongs in the ingroup. The creation of such subgroups is one of the major duties, and perhaps the most difficult one, of the group care specialist. He has to be alert to a number of signs in order to fulfill this duty. He has to be aware of the desirable skills and interests each youngster possesses, and know which youngster wants to participate in which activity. He has to have a whole bag of suggestions up his sleeve—and yet he must utilize the initiative of the children to evolve and formulate these suggestions. He has, above all, to be aware of the great desire of the youngsters for fun and excitement and has to identify with this desire. Each evening a child care worker, group worker, unit head should ask himself: What fun and excitement did I provide today for every child? This may at times seem to interfere with his authority function. In reality this is not the case. The two roles, representative of authority and provider of fun, do not conflict with each other but support each other. The group leader must know that group excitement is the culmination point of an intensive group process that entails setting of goals preparation, role assignments, supervision and—yes—rules of the game.

This is where group participation is of utmost importance. Whether it concerns moving a television set into the playroom (Why should that job be done by the maintenance man?), the development of a photography club, a special project (There should be many), the launching of a food committee, the acquisition of a dog, the preparation for a newcomer, the production of a new song—all can become group activities. Of particular interest to the adolescent can be activity around big political issues such as ecology, peace, an election, poverty. Adolescents can organize around issues such as these and feel that they can participate in the major questions confronting society. The adult's commitment to cases that are close to the adolescent can become an important tie between the adult and the adolescent. Then, there are all the parties, birthdays, holidays—legal, religious and homemade ones. Such activities can work only if they are group-initiated, albeit with the discreet assistance prodding and plotting of the adult. Again there are the games, the plays, the evenings around the campfire, the fireplace or the kitchen stove. There are the songs with or without guitar, recordings or popular and not so popular music.

Many of these activities are unorganized and spontaneous, but they can lend themselves to group awareness and subgroup and group discussions. It would be foolish to try to make a group activity out of everything. It is equally foolish, however, not to use these activities for the purpose of group formation. The highet form of group activity is the organized, task-oriented, formal group. Fant (1971) aptly divides such groups into management groups, developmental groups and clinical groups. The management groups include the cottage meeting, the "campus council" and formal short-term groups. The developmental groups include the developmental crisis group to help a group of children master a common developmental task, such as transition from campus school to community school or problems around dating. The clinical groups are psychotherapy groups, partly in lieu of and partly in addition to individual psychotherapy.

I wish to emphasize particularly the role the management group can play in helping the adolescent to participate in the administration of the center through formulation and presentation of grievances and suggestions regarding the issues and tasks of institutional living. These may range from scheduling problems to clothing allowances and food gripes. One must, however, be aware of a number of possible problems and pitfalls in the development of creative group interaction.

1) The life expectancy of a group is usually short. Most successful groups are task-oriented ad hoc groups. The task has to be set in accordance with the ability of the participants to stick to it and to succeed. It is better to plant a small flowerbed successfully than to plan for a whole garden that cannot be cultivated by the group. The initial enthusiasm of adolescents for big projects will often give way to depression and frustration when the task becomes too big.

2) The individual members of the group cannot always participate in the group activity. Their interest spans vary, their moods shift. What they adored yesterday, they may condemn today. In these critical moments of the group, the adult becomes an alter ego. From the more or less passive leader he changes into the more or less active participant. He may play the pitcher in the seventh inning of a ball game. He may take a part in a play, or be one of the waiters during a party. It may be necessary at times to bring such alter-ego help in from the outside. In fact, the more important such an outsider is, the more inspiration he can offer to the children and the more he enhances the status and the pride of the group.

3) Many interactions among adolescents occur without adult support or against the adult's wishes. Although it is necessary to maintain control over the youngsters and to be consistent in the direction of the group one has to be aware that cliques and extragroup activities are natural for all adolescents. One has even to make

provision for these outlets, take calculated risks, perhaps, though always short of losing control. If one can show appreciation, rather than anger, for the youngsters' desire to do things without the adult, one may at times be able to bring those clandestine cliques back into the controllable group structure. One must, however, constantly be aware of the existence of these secretive programs, and at times one may have to intervene or even actively to disband them. This is itself a difficult process and may affect the total group structure and group relationships.

4) Above all, one needs to be aware of the adolescent's need for privacy. Living in a group setting is an almost superhuman assignment for the adolescent. In adolescence seclusiveness and gregariousness rapidly alternate with each other. The disturbed adolescent can experience severe setbacks if his need for withdrawal is not met on occasion. This we have especially found in adolescent girls, whose group potentialities and grouping modes seem sharply different from those of boys. Any group care setting, therefore, needs to make allowances for this need for retreat from the group.

B. *The Tasks (the Need to Be Needed)*

The feeling of not being needed is perhaps the most frustrating and depressing one for an adolescent; his search for relevancy may indeed be the search for a place where he is needed. The adolescent who comes to group care is sensing that nobody really needs him, that his problems, incapacities, failures are a burden to society. Therefore, he not only should know what the group and the agency can do for him, but what he is expected to do for the group. The first task is, of course, the need to be treated. All his assignments, from getting up in the morning, to attending school, his psychotherapy sessions and going back to bed at night, must be related to his cure and improvement. His work on his problems must be the major assignment.

It is interesting that the word "work" is used in the English language not only in the sense of making, doing, producing, but also as a "working through," meaning resolving, evolving, clarifying. Schwartz (1971) regards work as one of the major functions of group interaction.

Communal tasks and individual tasks are the centripetal and centrifugal forces that make the group "work." The adolescent, therefore, must know that he came to the treatment center for work. What is expected of him in psychotherapy, in school, in the cottage, on the campus must be clearly outlined, reviewed, evaluated and redefined and reassigned, at frequent intervals. His participation in the group, in the chores, in recreational activities must similarly be related to this "work." The youngster may not always see the connection between "work" and therapy. It has to be interpreted to him again and again. What is more important, there must be clarity in the mind of the staff as to how chores relate to the treatment of the adolescent. One aspect of this treatment is the development of social awareness and of participation in a social process. The role of work for the community is a substantial ingredient of this process. The maintenance of the group is therefore the second most important task the youngster must participate in.

The tasks can be divided into two parts—communal tasks and projects. Communal tasks are chores that must be done to maintain the orderly operation of the living units and the campus. Projects are especially selected chores that individual children or groups of youngsters set for themselves. Communal tasks are more or less compulsory. Projects are more or less voluntary. Communal tasks are more or less initiated by staff; projects are more or less initiated by the children. Communal tasks are more or less essential to the operation of the center; projects are more or less expendable.

Every youngster in a cottage group and every adult should participate in communal tasks, in the spirit of all having to do their share, each in accordance with his ability. This should not be done under the cloak of a quasi-freedom of choice. Such a requirement should be clearly compulsory. The community needs you—do your share! In this area some of the mechanistic methods of operant conditioning can be applied successfully. Work can be measured and can be rewarded. The unit of work to be done within a given time can be set for every adolescent in accordance with his abilities. His readiness or unreadiness to do his share is a measure for himself, as to his progress. It is here that the adult's role as an alter ego can become important in discreetly assisting one or another youngster to fulfill his task.

As a group becomes more organized and secure, the assignment of communal tasks to children and adults may be carried out by youngsters with the advice of an adult. Disagreements about what needs to be done, why, when and by whom may lend themselves to vital and helpful group discussions. Although adolescent participation in the tasks of daily life is an important socioeducational tool, and "hard physical activities" have been recognized as helpful to him, it would be erroneous to rely on "child labor" for all the work that needs to be done within the institution. The work must be assigned solely in accordance with the psychological capacities of the adolescents. The resistance of the group can become explosive if its members feel they are being exploited by the adults.

Staff must always explain to youngsters the reason for work assigned, its values for them and for the institution. Again and again one must handle their resistance to work. I have always been impressed with the expression of elation and pride after the much-disdained job was completed. "Our cottage is the cleanest on campus." "Our room is the nicest." "We won't let anybody mess up our garden." The "we" feeling achieved by the completion of a task compensates in full measure for the gripes and complaints aired during its execution.

Work projects lend themselves even more to the achievement of such "we" feeling and positive group identification. Work projects are useful tasks chosen by the youngsters in order to improve their surroundings, their living quarters, their own mode of living. They usually require a good amount of imagination, planning, enthusiasm, perseverance and skill. There are long-term and short-term projects, projects for individuals, for small groups and for larger ones.

Every child in a group setting should at all times be active in a project. The "loner" can have projects that he can do himself, such as preparation of a flowerbed, building a footstool or a radio or a bookshelf, making Christmas cards, house numbers, signs. The group can develop joint projects such as bike repairs, gardening, car washing, painting, cooking or baking. There is no end to the list. Although the projects must be initiated by the children, the original stimulus can come from the adult, particularly if he can do this discreetly. There should be some personal advantage to the adolescent in a project, such as status, recognition, excitement or money. With adolescents the utility of this project must be measured in their own value system. Planting a flowerbed may not mean anything to them, but fixing a motor may mean a lot.

There are many ego-guilding elements in the successful achievement of work projects:

1) The feeling of doing something useful brings adolescents closer to society, albeit their own society.

2) The feeling of having created "something" brings about a sense of uniqueness and of identity.

3) The feeling of having produced something on one's own brings the development of self-confidence.

4) The feeling of having done something together with others brings a sense of belonging and respect for each other—helps to satisfy the adolescent's great need to be needed.

C. *Rituals*

Every organization develops its own rituals as it develops its own identity and pride. Certain rituals have come down through generations and have become the symbols of tradition and establishment. As such, they are unacceptable to many adolescents. However, adolescents do need symbols and rituals. They create their own symbols at the time whether it is in the length of their hair, their dress, their language.

Similarly, rituals are significant expressions of the feeling of belonging. Although we cannot and should not impose on young people rituals that they will not accept, we can help them develop rituals on their own—singing a song after a meal, playing a guitar around the table, sitting on the front steps or the back porch before retiring. When we observe the adolescent group closely we find that they have developed the beginnings of certain rituals. A clever child care worker can fortify such beginnings and bring them to group consciousness.

Once the rituals are created and accepted, they will be transmitted to newcomers and to the next generation of youngsters. These new youngsters will then find the forms and rituals that symbolize the spirit of a vital group. Although they will modify and adapt these rituals to their own style, they will serve as a useful bridge from one generation of youngsters to the next, a bridge they themselves have built.

Activity Group Therapy:
A Bridge Between
Play and Work

HOLLY VAN SCOY, M.S.W.

This description of an activity group is quite different from Slavson's earlier latency groups. Van Scoy emphasizes a somewhat simplified Eriksonian-derived developmental task of latency, i.e., mastery, with work being the endpoint of a metamorphosis from play. While the process of change in this "activity" group is not detailed in the paper, one might view one aspect of it as follows: These children, who appeared incapable of handling abstractions and formal insights, were repeatedly exposed to "themselves as others see them" with the videotape recorder (VTR) functioning much as the "observing ego" traditionally developed by patients in therapy; perhaps the equipment functioned to develop an ego split, a vehicle leading to meaningful insights and subsequent behavior change.

Children in the midstage of development, between the ages of 6 and the onset of puberty, present interesting challenges for the clinician. Though they may be "latent" in terms of dormant sexual drives, this is an age of excitement, activity and constant inquiry. Therapists who devote much time to patients in this "lull before the storm of puberty"

Reprinted from *Child Welfare*, Vol. 11, No. 8 (October 1972), pp. 528-534.

soon become aware of the unique difficulties and demands latent children present.

One underlying problem at this stage is that serious difficulties are not so obvious as in infancy, early childhood or adolescence. The activity orientation of these youngsters frequently masks or obscures emotional turmoil; the range of normal behavior is wide and includes much that later becomes unacceptable or problematic. Therapists as well as parents constantly struggle to distinguish between what is merely boyish or tomboyish immaturity and what is disturbed acting out.

Still another formidable consideration is the selection of treatment methods appropriate to the unique developmental needs of this period Erikson calls "the age of mastery." As all children in midchildhood must invest much energy in peer relationships, the task of the child therapist is to promote growth within a maturational process that necessarily involves partial exclusion of the adult world. Traditional psychotherapy is frequently nonproductive and its limited effectiveness is probably related to a need not only to deny the specific doubts, fears and tensions that are experienced with a therapist, but to prove to themselves that they achieved the norms of peer trust as a defense against infantile dependence on the adult world.

As others have noted, activity group therapy is frequently an acceptable alternative, particularly if "activity" is defined broadly enough to include any number of ventures children and their therapists find mutually stimulating and satisfying.

The Group

This paper deals with an activity group of four boys in the midstage of childhood. Three boys were 11, one was 12. All four were patients of The Oaks, a residential treatment center of the Brown Schools, Austin, Texas.

Pete, at 12, had been in treatment for 18 months. Although his IQ was high-average, he consistently underachieved in school, particularly in mathematics. He received weekly individual therapy and had been a member of an earlier activity group, but appeared to be making little progress. Pete was extremely passive-aggressive, at one point refusing to leave his bed for several days.

Butch, 11, was outgoing and likable, but for more than 18 months had shown little growth in academic skills. The alphabet was a continuing mystery to him, as were many mathematical computations, despite his average IQ. By the time the group was formed, Butch appeared to be ready for a return home, with outpatient therapy and special academic tutoring.

Harry, 11, had been a patient for 4 months when the group began. He was depressed and morose much of the time, but interrupted this with periods of destruction and assaults. Harry had broken eight chairs and four windows in 15 weeks; his school work was erratic, but satisfactory. His IQ was average, and achievement test scores showed him to be working at grade level.

Donald, 11, was also nearing the end of inpatient treatment when the group began. After almost 2 years of care, his symptoms of encompresis and extreme stubbornness were no longer seriously disabling. Enrolled in a nearby public school on the fourth-grade level, Donald was doing class work, but was one grade level behind despite average intelligence.

The four boys lived together in a single residence with eight others. They were markedly different from one another except for repeated observations by teachers, child care staff and therapists that each consistently acted "silly," "immature," "showoffish," "dumb," or "babyish," and had done so since admission. Specific actions mentioned frequently ranged from simple face contortions and noises to gross acting out in the community. For example, Harry stood on his head in a movie theater on a dare and was irate when reprimanded. "I was just playing," he complained.

Overall in behavior, all four expressed a commitment to play rather than to work and a general reluctance to assume any responsibility for their actions, much less to change them. Lacking was Erikson's sense of industry, the bringing of a productive situation to completion that gradually supersedes the whims and wishes of play" (1963, 259).

Because this sense of industry seems critical to eventual functioning as a productive adult, these boys were selected for an experience that gave special emphasis to its development.

The Project

Twice weekly for 5 months Harry, Pete, Butch and Donald met with two leaders, a male child care worker and a female psychiatric social worker, for activity group therapy. Since all four felt most comfortable "at play," the group was loosely organized around an activity that ostensibly was merely "fun," the making of a videotape movie. In this way, the boys were encouraged to use their highly developed abilities to act silly and show off to produce a worthwhile product. Several goals were set by the leaders within this framework: 1) that the boys would be introduced to the pleasures of the "tool world" in which objects can be comfortably manipulated toward a specified end; 2) that the boys would recognize a larger task as composed of smaller operations; 3) that the boys would have enhanced self-esteem as a consequence of knowing how to operate the complex videotape equipment; 4) that the boys would become more aware of their personality assets and liabilities by seeing them recorded and replayed; and 5) that the boys would learn to work together as a unit, sharing the leaders and the equipment, in order to complete the task.

The group, then, was constructed to help bridge the considerable distance between play-oriented childhood and work-oriented adulthood, with care given to the concept that work is not drudgery but can, in its own way, be as enjoyable and satisfying as play.

Group Sessions

During all group sessions the videotape recorder (VTR) was used, except for three meetings that took place off the residential campus. Literature dealing with videotape techniques in similar situations is scarce but the leaders familiarized themselves with the equipment and were able to improvise a basic format from the beginning session.

One boy was responsible for the operation of the camera at each meeting. This included selection of the lens, as well as positioning and wiring the machine. Because the machines were expensive as well as complex the boys were encouraged to read the VTR manual thoroughly before attempting to record a session. At first this advice was ignored, but when Butch came to the second session ready to film but unable to connect the wires correctly, fit the lens or thread the VTR, this reluctance was overcome. The leaders operated the camera for the first four meetings as the boys became progressively more knowledgeable about the procedures. At the fifth session Butch was able to assume his duties with minimal supervision from the leaders; thereafter each boy took his turn.

Equipment utilized included the camera, three lenses, a microphone, the VTR and a monitor. The VTR allows for instant replays in addition to slow-motion viewing. Both of these processes provided novel ways of giving the boys immediate visual and audio feedback from a neutral source. The first 25 to 30 minutes of each session were taped and the final 30 minutes were spent viewing the film, allowing stopping and rerunning at members' discretion. Not surprisingly, the boys themselves soon tired of constant stillness when they had to sit through replayed sessions.

Early in the third meeting, Pete announced, "Hey, guys, let's get down to business. I'm tired of watching you all goof off and then having to watch it all over again."

During the initial meetings, all four boys were eager to begin the actual filming of a movie. Because it was apparent that they had little concept of the sequence of preparatory activities, the leaders during the fifth session permitted the boys to proceed as they wished.

By this time the members had loosely agreed to a Western theme and had a few vague ideas for the plot; however, two boys wanted to work with a gold miner as the central character; the other two wanted a cowboy.

The fifth session was predictably chaotic. With Butch as cameraman, the other three earnestly began the movie. Some problems were immediately evident. There were no props, no costumes, no scenery and, most of all, there was no script. Within a half an hour, the boys were angry at the leaders, projecting their feelings of inadequacy on them. Donald, Pete and Harry angrily accused Carl, the male leader, of being "stupid." Donald was the most verbal of all, "Don't you know we have to have costumes and stuff to make a movie?" he demanded.

The leaders permitted the boys to ventilate some of their frustrations, but encouraged them to make a plan for the remaining sessions. This planning took two meetings, since they had difficulty defining the necessary steps and setting them out in order. Each time a member verbalized his impulsive desire to skip a step or to go on to a less demanding task, the leaders agreed. After two or three disastrous false starts of this type, the boys gradually began to check on one another's impulsivity and to follow their plans, step by step.

As drawn up by the group, production plans were: 1) write a script, 2) get costumes, 3) make scenery and get props, 4) practice makeup, 5) draw titles and credits, 6) rehearse, and 7) film. The first task proved to be the most complex, but also the most satisfying. At least six sessions were spent writing the seven-act skit that when typed by the secretarial staff, covered four and a half pages triple-spaced. After the boys decided on the gold miner theme, a plot was discussed and characters took shape. The actual writing was tedious and interspersed with periods of "trying out the words," which afforded an opportunity to release the pent-up energy inactivity produced in young boys. All group members, including the two leaders, took turns recording the collective contributions. With four sessions, the boys became accustomed to the format. Donald was early for the sixth session and was seen in the waiting room busily sketching on a note pad. When the others arrived he noted that they were "two minutes late." "We can't waste time," he said, "I've already been planning the bar scene."

By the fifth session there was much more discussion of "getting down to work" and less random activity. At some point the boys also became able to visualize mentally the activity described in the script without resorting to acting in order to, as Pete put it, "see what the words looked like."

Once the script was written, the rest of the steps were quickly completed. A scant 3 weeks, or six sessions, were needed for steps 2 through 6. The actual filming, including numerous retakes, required four more sessions.

The final meeting was spent viewing the completed product, a 12-minute videotape "masterpiece."

Outcome

It is difficult to assess the contribution any single aspect of the therapeutic milieu makes to an individual patient. Jumping to cause-and-effect conclusions based on one therapeutic effort such as group or individual therapy is improvident and obscures the critical relationship among efforts that itself constitutes the real strength of the residential environment. Even so, it is equally unwise not to attempt to isolate single endeavors for evaluation especially when a new method is being tried in the midst of an otherwise constant, relatively unchanging institution, as was the case with the present project.

Returning to the theoretical formulations of Erikson cited earlier, retrospective analysis hinges at least partly on this group's contribution to the "real mastery" of members. Because all four boys, after varying periods of intensive individual therapy, appeared ready to grapple at last with "industry versus inferiority," outcome must be considered in terms of the five goals set to aid in that struggle. In addition, an evaluation requires some brief comments on the effectiveness of the use of the VTR and the methodology employed.

In selecting group members, the leaders had chosen boys who were "gradually developing a sense of responsibility and gaining some simple feelings for the institutions, functions and roles that would permit them to anticipate responsible participation as an adult[so that they could] soon find pleasurable accomplishment in wielding tools and weapons, in manipulating meaningful toys and in taking care of themselves." That is, they were reasonably well-organized children with intact egos who demonstrated consistent reality orientation. None was psychotic, but they were immature, emotionally in the earliest stages of childhood, while physically nearing puberty.

At the completion of the group sessions 4 months later, some noticeable changes had occurred. For all four boys there was considerable decrease in silly behavior, both at the residence and in school. They also enjoyed enhanced status among peers from mastery of the VTR equipment. And of the four, three were discharged within 2 weeks of the final session. Movement toward goals 2 and 5 could be seen most clearly: At termination, the four functioned well as a single unit and appeared to be well aware of the smaller operations involved in larger undertakings. Moreover, there was a general feeling of pride that they were able to verbalize and relate to the completed project.

At the 15th meeting Pete and Harry talked at length about the "good job" they felt the group had done. "It was hard work," Pete commented to the accompaniment of the group's laughter, for he had been the most vociferous member in complaining that the project was too much work.

Carryover to the residence and school was striking. Once the four boys began to make a concerted, united effort in group sessions they began to work together at the residence as well. In weekly meetings with peers in the dormitory they gradually introduced much group learning to others. For example, Butch was instrumental in making up a schedule for dormitory cleanup that divided the work into smaller jobs; Donald suggested and organized a softball team; and Harry suggested that the dormitory plant a small garden that "would be fun to work in."

Daily observational notes recorded "silly behavior" less and less frequently. Apparently seeing their antics on film, in possible combination with the scheduling of a regular time for acting, helped the boys repress and sublimate these impulses. As the immature behavior decreased there was almost simultaneously an increase in positive feedback, not only from the inanimate VTR, but from peers and staff as well. The self-defeating cycle of silliness, negative feedback, and low self-image was broken and a more positive cycle established.

In addition, the experience of participating in a unique and greatly admired group project contributed to their newly developed sense of importance. It was critical to the outcome that others viewed their work as exciting and worthwhile and did not devalue it as merely "play therapy." The leaders were careful to speak of the project in terms that helped convey its work-orientation. The cooperation of other staff members who were willing to discuss the boys' work seriously was essential.

It is probably necessary to add a few brief comments on the VTR and its part in the process. As has been previously noted:

> The videotape is a new tool. In itself it is not a method of therapy but only takes on value as it is used in an important way to make implementation of any particular therapy approach more effective.

In this particular project, the VTR was an indispensable aid in providing instantaneous feedback from a source that had no emotional investment in the situation. Denials or avoidance techniques that previously had taken the form of argumentative struggling or sullen withdrawal were overcome as each child saw with his own eyes and heard with his own ears his actions and reactions. As Alger and Hogan noted in videotaped marital sessions:

> Not only does the patient more easily become aware of his own behavior and feelings, and the behavior and feelings of others, but he tends to remember the new insight. In addition, he is more able to hold onto it and he feels more like acting on it, since he feels he arrived at it through his own observation and is not making a change under another person's orders.

This seems especially true in the case of children who are struggling with the critical theme of independence, either in the latent period or adolescence that soon follows.

Encounter Techniques in Analytic Group Psychotherapy with Adolescents

ARNOLD W. RACHMAN, Ph.D.

Olsson and Myers (1972) were among the first who described the use of some modified sensitivity techniques with adolescents. The encounter movement, so enormously popular in the 1960s, has somewhat faded, leaving a most useful residue in the form of interpersonal maneuvers, which can now be applied to work with youngsters when appropriate in group work.

In this excerpt, Rachman presents several encounter techniques he has found helpful in group therapy; his experience found role-playing to be most valuable. He concludes with some thoughtful comments on motivations for using such techniques, resistances, timing, and the kinds of techniques. It is of some interest to note that this author, as Van Scoy in the previous article, utilizes an Eriksonian framework, in this case formation of the inner continuity or ego identity as a developmental objective to be aided by group psychotherapy in which the adolescent is encouraged to experiment with feelings and explore identity problems within a group. The combination of techniques derived from the encounter movement of the 1960s, with the social developmental dimension Erikson has contributed to psychoanalytic theory, is not surprising, since together they provide an interpersonal theory and a technique which can be seen as fitting together.

The purpose of this paper is to outline some theoretical and clinical considerations relevant to the use of "encounter" techniques in analytic psychotherapy with adolescents. The word encounter is used to denote a meaningful emotional interaction between two or more people in a group psychotherapy setting. The purpose of the encounter is to heighten the emotional experience of the moment. It is felt that the analysis of emotional conflicts and the development of insight is best accomplished during periods of heightened emotional experiencing, when feelings are "more available" for cognitive examination by the ego.

Divergent schools of psychotherapy seem to agree that successful therapy is related to some operative emotional component.

Encounter Techniques in
Adolescent Group Therapy

Role Playing

Role playing, a traditional concept and technique of sociometry, is admirably suited for adolescent group therapy since it allows the adolescent to experiment with a variety of roles within a meaningful social context and thus fulfills Erikson's theoretical notion of role experimentation as a therapeutic necessity for ego identity formation.

A role-playing encounter was employed during an adolescent group therapy session (a group of neurotic and borderline adolescents in private practice) to highlight the experiencing of an intrapsychic and interpersonal distancing maneuver between two adolescents. Both Stan and Dave had joined the group because they acknowledged having serious difficulties in peer relationships. They had no friends of either sex; led lonely, socially isolated lives; had serious difficulty separating from their mothers; projected their own intrapsychic and interpersonal avoidance of peers outwardly onto the environment and other people. They had developed compulsive mechanisms to defend

Reprinted from *International Journal of Group Psychotherapy*, Vol. 21, No. 3 (July 1971), pp. 319-329.

against the awareness that their difficulty in forming relationships with peers was an intrapersonal problem rather than an interpersonal one.

In one group session, Dave began with his usual repetitive lament: "I'm so lonely. No one wants to be friends with me; no one ever calls me on the phone." Stan joined in the lament, by saying: "I know just how you feel. No one ever calls me up either." Since the group therapist and the group had been unsuccessful in previous attempts to help Dave and Stan gain awareness of their feelings and behavior by the traditional techniques of interpretation and development of insight, the group therapist suggested a role-playing situation in which Dave and Stan would call each other to make a social appointment. A portion of this interchange vividly illustrated for the group, the group therapist, and the two boys themselves the underlying intrapsychic conflict.

Dave: How about going to the movies with me on Saturday?
Stan: Well . . . I don't know what I'll be doing on Saturday; it's only Wednesday now. I might have a cold on Saturday. What about Saturday in two weeks?
Dave: I might not be home on Saturday. Well, see you. Goodbye.
Stan: Goodbye!

For the first time, in the history of their participation in the group, Dave and Stan acknowledged that, while they both desired relations with others, they pushed others away. Immediately after the encounter, it was apparent that both Dave and Stan, as well as the group, were more related to the conflict and had a heightened sense of experiencing it in the "here and now." With the help of the group therapist, the group explored what they had witnessed in terms of the psychodynamics of the two role-playing participants, launching into a lively, active, meaningful confrontation with the two role players. The first level of dynamic exploration centered around the group's interpretation of Dave and Stan's mutual, interlocking avoidance, distancing, and rejection of each other. Both Dave and Stan related positively to this interpretation by citing other examples of rejecting others in social situations at school.

Then the group focused on Dave and Stan's primary social relationship, their symbiotic relationships with their mothers. On target, Chuck offered the following: "You guys can't make it with anyone 'cause you're too interested in making it with your mother." The group was able to "back up" this interpretation with a live example witnessed in the group setting, and Dave and Stan, when confronted in this way, recognized that they were actively doing things to prevent closeness with a peer. On the basis of this new awareness, they began active attempts at forming relationships with peers outside the group therapy setting.

The Greek Chorus

The writer has used a verbal encounter technique called "The Greek Chorus." This method is helpful in challenging repetitive defensive stances in the group. During a group session (a group of neurotic and borderline adolescents in private practice), Alan, a passive, compliant, and ingratiating adolescent, allowed himself to be interrupted by Mal, the most aggressive, domineering, and verbal adolescent in the group. This kind of interruption had occurred on several occasions, and the group therapist began this encounter by observing that Alan had again allowed himself to be interrupted by Mal. Alan attempted to resume the conversation by trying to engage the group therapist in a dyadic interaction. The therapist then began to reiterate, in a louder voice, that Alan should tell Mal to "shut up" and not interrupt him. Alan again tried to re-establish their dyadic interaction with the therapist by insisting he had something important to say, ignoring Mal's continued interruptions. By now the group picked up on the intent of the encounter. As Alan tried to continue the conversation, the group, following the lead of the therapist, began to chant in unison, "I can't hear what you're saying, Alan, because Mal keeps interrupting you." Alan finally got the message and shouted to Mal and the group: "Shut up, damn it! I've got something important to say and I'm not going to let you interrupt me!"

The group, including Mal, broke into applause and congratulated Alan for standing up to Mal. Alan continued this new way of being assertive in the group, and from then on, he was able to challenge other group members. Eventually, he was able to change even further by beginning to challenge and interrupt the group therapist, and eventually he became more assertive with peers outside of the therapy group.

The Split Ego Technique

The "split ego" technique, derived from Gestalt psychotherapy practice, was utilized to help an adolescent group member encounter a repressed portion of his ego. Tom started to complain in a group session that he was failing physical education in high school. This led into his usual complaint: "I am not an athlete. I am not physically coordinated. I never have been. I will never be able to play ball or athletics."

Eli challenged Tom's self-image by saying he was "coping out," "putting himself down," and didn't want to try to change. The group picked up on this, forcing Tom to defend himself against the onslaught. During one portion of the interchange, Tom admitted that he did have some desire to participate in athletics, and the therapist decided to employ the split ego encounter technique to help Tom own the portion of his ego that wanted to become athletic. Tom was instructed in the following way:

I want you to talk to the two parts of you, the one part that doesn't want to be athletic and the part that does want to try something athletic. When you are sitting on the couch, you'll be the part of you that doesn't want to be athletic. When you move into the empty chair across from you, you'll be the part of you that wants to be an athlete. While you move back and forth between the two chairs, keep talking to both parts of you.

In the encounter and in the analysis that followed, Tom revealed and began to understand that he didn't want to be athletic because it was associated with being more independent and mature; being athletic would force him to relate to and play with peers; it would mean being responsible to peers; therefore, being athletic would mean growing up, moving away from mother. In later group sessions, this dynamic material continued to be analyzed, and several sessions after the encounter, Tom reported that he took and passed the physical education examination. In addition, Tom arranged to play baseball with several group members after school.

Discussion

The use of encounter techniques in group psychotherapy raises several important issues: the motivation for encountering; the timing of an encounter; resistance and encountering; and the nature and variety of encounters employed.

It is helpful to consider the motivation of the therapist in the employment of encounter techniques. Is the therapist expressing a need for novelty and stimulation in the use of encounter techniques? Does the therapist feel stale, tired, unsuccessful, or angry with himself or his group? Ideally, encounter techniques should be used only when there is a meaningful theoretical or clinical rationale for intervening to heighten emotional engagement within the group.

The timing of encounter techniques is important. Adolescents usually need some time at the beginning of a session to reorient themselves to the therapy situation after a week's absence, and introducing an encounter situation immediately could produce confusion and increased anxiety. Encounter techniques should be used when the feelings to be encountered are near the intrapsychic surface of the individual(s) and the group. In addition, there should be some indication of a willingness to work on the difficulty. The therapist should not pull encounters "out of the air" in order to perform some magic on the group. Such attempts are more likely to produce confusion and resistance than insight.

Concerning the utilization of encounter techniques, there has been created an aura of excitement, novelty, and positive anticipation about employing these methods. When a therapist first anticipates using them, he is not likely to envision that they may fail or produce negative results, but this can happen, as witness the following example.

Kyle was a particularly difficult adolescent patient who rarely spoke in the group (a group of neurotic and borderline adolescents in a clinic setting). Both the therapist and the group had unsuccessfully attempted to engage him in sustained conversation on any level. During a particular session in which the group was again attempting to help Kyle to have a conversation, he admitted that he talked more freely with his neighborhood friends while they were smoking marijuana. The group therapist was delighted with his apparent disclosure as he had been waiting for months for some revelation which could be employed to help Kyle open up.

The therapist decided to employ an encounter technique predicated on the "re-creation of a real life experience." The attempt would be to stimulate the atmosphere and interaction of Kyle talking to a group of friends while smoking marijuana. The scene was set: the room was darkened; Kyle and two other group members (who had smoked marijuana) were seated together; Kyle had a cigarette which was to be smoked as if it was a joint; the instructions were: "You're all in the park at night, seated behind some trees. Kyle takes out a joint, lights it, and passes it on to the next person. Then you guys begin to rap to each other."

In the scene that followed the other two boys attempted to engage Kyle in a discussion about smoking marijuana: how they felt; the quality of the goods; whether the quantity was adequate; etc. Kyle's response was minimal. The interaction was very much akin to the stiff, inhibited interchange during a regular group session. The therapist and the group felt the encounter was unsuccessful.

An important theoretical issue is raised when a group member refuses to participate in an encounter situation. Traditionally, refusal to cooperate in the therapy relationship has been looked upon as a form of resistance. Is refusal to encounter a resistance? It is possible that not wishing to participate in an encounter situation is a defensive maneuver by the individual, and the therapeutic handling of such a refusal should follow traditional lines, that is, it should be handled by observing the resistance and exploring its underlying dynamic meaning. A cautionary note should be sounded, however. There appears to be a tendency to employ encounter methods in an atmosphere of "total push" for change. This type of "forced encountering" resembles a totalitarian method, while psychotherapy should be based on democratic and humanistic principles. Therefore, a person or a group must be granted the freedom not to encounter.

Concerning the kinds of encounter situations to be employed in adolescent group psychotherapy, this writer has found it most helpful to employ role-playing encounters. Originally, the writer initiated these encounters in the group sessions, but role playing has become so meaningful to the adolescent group participants that they now initiate such encounter situations with one another.

Breaking the Bonds of Tradition: A Reassessment of Group Treatment of Latency-Age Children

ROSALIND M. SANDS, M.S.

SHELDON GOLUB, M.D.

Sands and Golub found the traditional activity group lacking in many respects for the variety of problems of latency. While in their article they indicate their theoretical approach and technique were only recently discovered and put into action, they probably accurately represent the current thinking of most group therapists today. The focus around a club to provide rules, interpersonal roles, attachment behaviors, etc., is now widely used. But their renunciation of the passive, mainly interpretive role of the therapist for a much more active one probably represents one reason for the long delay in the general acceptance and development of effective group techniques with children, i.e., the inappropriate transfer of the traditional role of the individual therapist to group work, and Slavson's model of activity group as the primary model to follow.

We had experienced in our groups the failures reported by others or had been unable to sustain the groups for a meaningful experience. For many in our clinic population—children with behavior disorders and fragile ego functioning—there was not sufficient material for

Reprinted from *American Journal of Psychiatry*, Vol. 131, No. 6 (June 1974), pp. 662-665.

interpretation, and the catharsis experienced in free play exacerbated the problems of children with poor internal controls. We began, therefore, to alter the traditional forms of activity group therapy.

Our initial changes concerned the actual setting of the treatment. We found that the usual large playrooms filled with a variety of equipment and play materials were too stimulating. A shift was made from the large room to a small one and from much play material to little or none. But, we had not sufficiently analyzed our methods and clarified our theoretical position first, and therefore we met with many difficulties. To reach a compromise of play and talk we decided to use the talk time to discuss the play period. Some materials stimulated the request for more materials. The use of food often could not be controlled. Our expectations of verbal productions were not realized; these were not sufficient or consistent enough to enable us to rally around a theme, as one could with adults, or to delineate a conflict. The long-cherished neutrality of the therapist was not a viable therapeutic tool; adherence to such a position promoted disorder. Our results in this transitional period were thus disappointing. We realized that we could not use the usual techniques of group therapy. We needed to conceptualize a new form of treatment, and we began to consider what was available to us.

Conceptualizing a New Form of Treatment

Upon assessing our working tools and our theoretical base, we delineated several major premises. The first of these was the need for a developmental position. In a departure from the labeling of the standard nomenclature we gave renewed recognition to the special characteristic of childhood—the process of development. Neubauer (1963) viewed "the capacity to develop progressively [as] the most significant factor in determining the child's future." Such a view leads to a different conceptualization of disorder and consequent methods of intervention. The determining criteria in the application of treatment are not the child's difficulties and problems alone, but whether or not the child is moving toward his developmental responsibilities, even though he may retain residues of unresolved struggles.

For example, Katherine, aged eight, was striving for satisfactory peer relationships and adequate socialization skills but was not meeting with success; she clowned and was boisterous and loud. Although she displayed regressive behavior at home, she also took pride in growing up and being like her mother. She had had a stormy life, but the environment had stabilized and there were presages of maturity and growth. Viewed in traditional terms she could be labeled neurotic or as having an adjustment reaction of childhood or a behavior disorder—all terms that do not clarify precise methods of intervention. Seen more dynamically, however, we could understand how the thrust toward latency-age development needed to be supported.

With such a formulation there is a departure from global terminology and renewed emphasis on health, the use of resources, both familial and environmental, and on coping, mastery, and the idiosyncratic factors of child development.

A second premise was that these are specific tasks of latency. The postoedipal lessening of drive urgency and the transfer of libido from parental figures to peers, teachers, leaders, and impersonal ideals must be fostered so that there are appropriate defenses against oedipal fantasies. In the transition from the pleasure principle to the reality principle, the ability to control, modify, or inhibit impulses and to delay gratification needs strengthening. The child's psychic responsibility to become part of a peer group, to move away from primary objects, and to prepare himself for the separation-individuation tasks of the adolescent is aided by ready availability for new attachments and interest in joining clubs or peer groups. Behavior control and sublimation are abetted by cognitive growth (entry into school), physical mastery (taking part in teams, games, sports), and encompassment of the "realness" of the world (interest in collecting, hobbies, crafts, science, and nature).

The third premise we delineated was the latency-age child's potential for investment in groups, the lines of development described above indicate the particular need of the latency-age child for entry into various forms of group life.

And last, we saw the need for a holistic view of the latency child. Such a perspective precludes viewing the treatment hour as either the primary or only treatment tool and points to a multifaceted form of therapy, with special use of groups, specific approaches to the familial environment, the use of community resources that fit into the psychic economy of the latency phase, awareness of the child's body, and concern with his entire life space.

Putting Our Premises and Tools to Work

We have set up groups in which talking, not activity, is the medium. The evolution of the group process—each child finding his place among his peers and becoming part of the group—is the basic group intervention. There is no longer concern with obtaining fantasies, with pressure for material—whatever is offered, from quarreling over where to sit to reports of daily activities, is used in molding a collection of individuals into a group or club. The group process itself is used as the material of therapy.

The neutrality of the therapist is abandoned. He must actively promote the formation of the group and serve as an adult model of social behavior and social relatedness. He outlines procedures for group work, such as choosing a name, and discusses the goal. With such a role he can demand, insist, limit, and always stand for the reality of the group situation. The therapist does not encourage regression or interpret it but instead identifies himself with the wish to grow up. He allies himself with the maturing forces rather than the regressive ones and gives underpinnings to these through the group process. He is not committed to an abstract concept of confidentiality but rather meets regularly with the parent or parents individually or in a group and uses the information they give him or the understanding he has gained of the child. He is in contact with school personnel for information and can report this back to the group. Thus distortions and fabrications are immediately dealt with.

The power of the group is a collective tool arrived at as the group exerts its influence and does not arise from the dominance of the adult, as it does in a classroom situation. The group is actively encouraged to form its own rules. The group is expanded in size—from three or four to eight—to permit use of the strength of the group. The sexes are mixed; we no longer see any reason for segregation according to sex and think that the group is a more realistic situation when it involves both boys and girls.

Vis-à-vis the family environment, work is aligned with parents within the context of the tasks of latency. There is definition of phase needs, such as longing to be accepted by peers and belonging, and parents are encouraged to stimulate such links. Lessening of environmental stress in school or home is abetted by counseling, problem solving, and guidance. Even when the parents' own problems demand therapy for themselves, the focus is on the child and his life-phase and the parents' responsibilities in light of them.

Such environmental resources as Boy and Girl Scouts, Little League, Big Brother, church groups, and available recreational facilities are looked upon as sources for corrective experiences and are actively encouraged.

Physical problems are evaluated to ensure that even if concessions are necessary the child may carry on with his developmental tasks. In relation to a child's total life space, there is sensitivity to the problems of minority children in a hostile community, the placement of single black children in a white class, the ambience of a school. Ways are sought to provide a more tolerable atmosphere for the child, with intervention in the school directly or through the parent.

The Talking Club

We will briefly describe one group of eight boys and girls, approximately eight years old, that met once a week for 16 sessions. During the same period their mothers met for five sessions on a bimonthly basis. It was not possible to form a group of the fathers, but they were included in the total treatment plan as fully as could be arranged.

The children were directly involved in the formation of their club, from choosing its name to delineating the rules. Enhancement of belonging was promoted by putting each child's name on his chair and by letting the group decide on the placement of the chairs. Initial difficulty in behaving was discussed as a group problem, with the group deciding whether certain children should be separated to lessen the amount of contamination and disruption. There were no materials. Topics had a wide range, from what to tell friends about the absence of a father recently separated to making friends in school. True to the latency phase, discussion was short-lived, but the ability to hear each other out, to compare one's strength with others, to take turns in speaking, gradually drew the group into a sense of belonging. When a child was absent his chair was immediately removed by the group in order to avoid the temptation to move around.

There was insistent work with the family on what we considered the primary conflict within each child that impeded developmental thrust. Thus with Peter, outshined by his younger brother, increasingly shy and withdrawn, the parents learned what sibling rivalry is in day-to-day terms, of Peter's need to define his own boundaries and to find his own satisfactions. With Katherine, prone to regression in the group, the emphasis was placed on helping her grow up, on fostering identification with the mother who had been missing in her life for several years, on finding her place in a family in which there was rampant jealousy of the children who belonged to the new father.

With Arnie, whose mother had deprived him of his past in relation to his father, who did not permit pictures, letters, or remembrances, and who infantilized him, there was emphasis on restoring his past to the point where the mother permitted the father to communicate with him again. With Betty, whose father had deserted and whose mother seesawed between divorce and reconciliation, the child's turmoil was brought into focus, as was the need for her mother to be more empathetic with her and to be careful not to foster too much renunciation. We encouraged this mother to find therapy for herself but did not lose sight of Betty's struggles and what her mother needed to do in relation to her. In the case of Mattie, who had a beginning school phobia, whose father's death had not been revealed to her for months, the mother realized the widening areas of constriction and inhibition, understood in greater depth the sources of Mattie's fears, and was able to move toward countering them. Cecil's parents became aware of how overpowering for him were his brother's bullying tactics and could see how he blossomed as he assumed an active role in the group and a less passive one with friends in school. The tentativeness of Robert, afraid to commit himself to new relationships after abandonment and neglect by his father, was apparent as he stood on the periphery of the group. This situation was duplicated at home, where he was fearful of committing himself to a new stepfather, and his mother recognized the need to tune in to the sources of this indecision.

The children's attachment to the *Talking Club* was solid, and its influence apparently helped promote changes in the world outside. Each child showed improvement in school behavior, school work, relationships with friends, and behavior at home. Although we had chosen 16 weeks rather arbitrarily, this seemed to be the limit of the children's tolerance; we believe that latency-age children are too restless, particularly after the long confinement of the school day, to have a talking group that can continue indefinitely. Moreover since we do not see the group as the only means of achieving progress, we can make an assessment at the end of the experience and formulate additional recommendations. This was done with each of the children; for example Arnie and his mother were briefly seen individually until the father's return was stabilized.

A Developmental Model

We wish to emphasize that what we have attempted to do is a beginning. In a field so committed to long-term treatment, in which individual therapy is often considered the only "real" therapy, in which play and therapy are used concomitantly and play is considered a form of treatment and not simply another tool, in which activity and latency are equated in the prevailing mode of group treatment, much more stirring of ideas, introspection, and evaluation are necessary. Our approach emphasized a developmental-environmental model in which the child's life stage, the continuous interactive influence of development and environment, and the thrust to health are underscored. The goal is not to resolve conflict but to make possible a developmental progression. Treatment is multifaceted, directed toward sufficiently freeing the child to be able to assume (as much as possible) the tasks of his appropriate phase. There is emphasis on the power of the group and its evolution as an arm of treatment, with the child finding his place in it and modifying his behavior to achieve this. In yet another departure from tradition we experimented with predetermined limitations of time, an experiment that deserves further study if we are to find other ways than the "therapy terminable and interminable" of traditional treatment.

A new era of mental health calls for reexamination of past practice and reconceptualization as the basis for more relevant and broader practice. We have already delineated the conflicts of the preschool child and the adolescent so that we can accept difficulties and problems, even turmoil at times, if these are part of "normal" struggles. The same delineation has not—but needs to be—applied to latency.

Structuring the Early Phase of Group Psychotherapy with Adolescents

JOHN E. MEEKS, M.D.

Meeks provides support for those of us who have hesitated to deal with adolescents in groups, feeling they are formidable enough individually. Yet it is precisely through peer group support that teenagers, so often threatened by individual therapy, may become seriously engaged in real therapeutic work. Meeks describes the criteria he has found useful in his own experience for successful "grouping," and illustrates the maneuvers he uses, especially early in therapy, that make the process gel. Yet he cautions that the techniques and maneuvers he has as aids are not as important as the underlying process and the therapist's personality, i.e., the willingness to be open and free with his own expression of feelings. Indeed, this free expression of affect is a primary technique in getting a group started.

The idea of rules and regulations to provide the structure which many argue is so vital to work with adolescents is depreciated as a rationalization for the therapist's own anxiety. The "contract," however, can be redefined to an identification and acceptance of goals and objectives, especially useful in engaging the adolescent in the therapeutic process in a mutual sense. Yet specific "do's and don'ts," while helpful as guidelines from an experienced clinician, are debatable.

> *Meeks's central theme in the seeking of mutually acceptable goals between therapist and patient is the essence of the treatment and provides the solution to his theory of one core adolescent problem to be dealt with, the power and control conflicts between adolescents and parent-adults.*
>
> *This article was selected to show how an experienced therapist approaches group work with adolescents, incorporating facilitating techniques from recent years introduced by encounter, gestalt, and psychodrama movements. The synthesis and combination of these approaches, rather than their polarization, is the central theme of this volume.*

Several features of adolescence make it difficult to foster therapeutic group cohesion (Meeks, 1973). The group leader must actively pursue a therapeutic alliance with group members and foster therapeutic group cohesion; they rarely evolve spontaneously, yet both are prerequisite to dynamic psychotherapy.

Some basics of structure can be disposed of quickly. The group experiences described below occurred in private and clinic outpatient co-ed groups with age ranges of thirteen to seventeen (usually fourteen to seventeen), which met weekly for one hour and fifteen minutes in large, pleasant, carpeted offices. Food was not routinely offered, although the youngsters knew that soft drinks and candy were available. No significant differences in the problems of achieving cohesion were observed between the clinic and private patients. All groups were conducted by male-female cotherapy teams.

This paper will explore in greater detail other structuring techniques and devices, unblushingly purloined from a variety of origins, that are more directly related to achieving therapeutic cohesion in adolescent groups. Basically, they are ways for the therapist to assume active group leadership without being inappropriately directive or suppressive. In the final analysis, the direction of any group will be determined mainly by its constituency and the therapist's comfort with the open

Reprinted from *International Journal of Child Psychotherapy*, Vol. 2, No. 4 (October 1973), pp. 391-405.

and free expression of feelings. Technical maneuvers are valuable only because they represent concrete ways to convey the therapist's willingness to interact freely, and because they may help the adolescent to deal with his anxiety and inhibitions.

Expression of Therapist's Feelings

When the therapist reveals his own anxieties, affects, and vulnerabilities, he makes his interest in promoting free emotional interaction more compellingly clear than he can by any amount of exhortation (Anderson, 1972). This openness not only helps to undercut generational formality but provides a model for self-revelation without loss of self-esteem. Since many of these feelings represent the therapist's tactful but frank reaction to behavior in the group, his example encourages similar interactional freedom between the group members and provides a model for nondestructive confrontation.

Certainly a group should not be overwhelmed with premature discussions of strong intimate affect, but even in the initial session the therapist can begin his demonstration that the group is a place to discuss feelings.

The opening moments of a new adolescent group were tense and largely silent except for occasional embarrassed giggles. The therapist looked around the group and became aware of his own anxiety. "I don't know how the rest of you are feeling, but I'm very nervous."

A fourteen-year-old boy, who had seen the therapist for some time in individual treatment and who had been encouraged to join the group because of a chronic, painful sense of social isolation, looked at the therapist with intense relief. "*You're* nervous? Well, I'm, terrified!"

The group responded with cathartic laughter, and then several members talked about their fears on coming to the first group meeting.

Later in the group work, subjective statements of affect are valuable in other ways. For example, they provide ways to question behavior and to elicit group support in setting appropriate limits.

A fifteen-year-old boy bragged about his prodigious drug intake during the first two months of a group. He often cast sidelong glances at the therapist as though inviting him to censure his behavior. The group members were reluctant to sound "square," although they seemed to regard the boy's indiscriminate drug intake as foolish and dangerous.

In the ninth group session the therapist said, "You know, if you are trying to scare me, it's working. I am worried about all these drugs you take, and it does seem to me that your thinking is getting confused."

The boy looked at the therapist quizzically. An aggressive seventeen-year-old boy who used some drugs himself said, "I don't think he really got that, Doctor." He turned to the fifteen-year-old: "What the doctor is trying to tell you is that you're gulping too much shit and it's fucking up your head. You're already a little bit spaced out."

The next two sessions the group became very active in questioning the boy's motives and in limiting his self-destructive drug usage. Although he became anxious and angry at the time, later he was able to voice his appreciation for the group's concern.

The therapist must use caution and careful clinical judgment in utilizing this style of intervention in interpersonal interactions between members. Individuals may feel that the therapist is showing preference or taking sides. For example, if one adolescent consistently attacks or belittles another, or if the entire group scapegoats a member, the therapist must avoid the position of "taking up" for the weak member. A comment such as, "I'm getting uncomfortable with the way Bill just sits there and takes it when Joe puts him down or tries to tell him how angry he is," invites the group to consider both aspects of the interaction. Generally speaking, emphasis is placed on the behavior that poses the greatest obstacle to group work.

Mickey, a shy, schizoid sixteen-year-old boy, discovered the pleasures of interpersonal interaction for the first time in his life in group psychotherapy. In response to his exuberance he became almost hypomanic, interrupting others and applying almost everything anyone said to himself in such a way as to demand constant attention. The group showed their discomfort with this behavior by teasing him about how much he talked, but they were reluctant to be firm with him since they recognized that this was mainly an exaggerated improvement. Of course, the teasing only fueled the fire since it continued to keep Mickey at the center of the group's attention.

The therapist had a good personal relationship with Mickey, based on previous individual treatment. This made it possible for him to turn to the group with an appeal: "I need your help. I have watched Mickey sweat through a lot of individual sessions, and for a while here in the group, without being able to say a word. He has been down since I've known him until the last month or so. Now he is up, but he is overdoing it in such a way that he is going to get himself put down again. How can we slow him down without pushing him into depression?"

The group accepted this invitation to deal with Mickey in a more direct way. The group members whom he interrupted began to explain to him that this was annoying and that they wanted him to listen to their ideas and feelings at times. They were always careful to point out to him that they did like and accept him even though they were irritated by some of his behavior. "You only ask to get kicked two or three times a session," one grinned.

Mickey initially reacted in a martyred way, grumbling, "You guys are just trying to pull me down again." However, he gradually accepted the confrontations and became more appropriate and sharing with other group members.

This kind of personal statement can also be useful between cotherapists.

Late in an excellent adolescent group the male and female cotherapists confronted one another rather directly. The discussion grew out of comments in the group about the dangers of intimacy and the fear of being hurt by other people, but it was also an expression of interpersonal strife between the cotherapists.

Two of the group members were talking of their idealization of the male therapist. He commented that he did not like this role; he felt it kept him from being emotionally close to this boy and girl, since they insisted on keeping him on a pedestal, ignoring his faults but also refusing to recognize his human needs. Another older male group member commented that there were advantages to being viewed as godlike, such as an immunity against getting "hit" (meaning criticized, insulted, etc.). The male therapist responded to his competitive tone and defensively said that he would like to feel that he was available to be touched as a human being, but that he did not particularly like to be hit.

The female cotherapist said flatly that she did not think it was possible to be open to touching without being open to being hit. She stated that she felt the male therapist contributed to the transference adulation that he received. The male therapist argued and the disagreement was spirited, though not hostile. A very shy and retiring boy supported the female therapist and said he found her confessed vulnerability touching. She elicited in him a warm, protective feeling that he could not recall experiencing toward any other adult. There was also an obvious increase in openness between group members over the next few weeks. In the termination phase of the group, two members mentioned the open conflict between the cotherapists and its friendly resolution as the most meaningful occurrence during the year and a half of the group's life.

Group Selection and Preparation

Group selection and preparation are important factors in structuring a group that can tolerate the anxiety of honest emotional interaction. Many criteria for selection of successful group members have been described (see, for example, Kraft, 1968, and Geller, 1972), but the author has confidence in only three. It seems necessary for the adolescent's parents to have an essentially unambivalent commitment to group treatment. If this requirement is waived because a youngster wants to join a group despite parental opposition, group leaders may find themselves unsupported when resistances appear later. The parents utilize these crisis times to undercut the therapy, often withdrawing the child. Secondly, the youngster should be willing— preferably eager—to come into the group for a two- to three-month trial at least. It may not be reasonable to require the adolescent to make an unambivalent commitment. It is also important, although not essential, to select group members who attract one another socially. This is primarily important in the initial phases of group formation.

Individual sessions with potential group members prior to beginning the group and during the early phases of group formation help to cushion the anxiety arising from group therapy. The therapeutic alliance with the individual therapist is a great asset that is usually transferable to the group setting. Individual sessions are also used to explore anticipatory fears of group therapy. The youngster is encouraged to accept and to verbalize any uncomfortable reactions to other group members. If members of the group make him angry or anxious, he is told this is a desirable stimulus for self-exploration.

We have also found an initial group meeting with the parents valuable. In this meeting the dual purpose of the group is explained. The parents are told the group will deal with individual problems primarily by serving as a microcosm of social interaction in the here and now. Care is taken to illustrate, with concrete examples, how this can be a valuable learning experience for the adolescent, especially developing capacity for self-observation and fairness in relations with other people.

The parents are also told that group therapy is an anxiety-producing experience that their youngster may wish to flee at times. Some of the common manipulations that may be used to enlist parental support for quitting the group are mentioned. They include suddenly behaving like "a perfect child" and claiming that all problems are solved, complaining that the other group members are drug addicts or worse, and criticizing the therapists directly or indirectly, along with many others. The therapists tell the parents that the wish to withdraw may be appropriate, and in any case it would be unwise to force the child to stay if he is really determined to drop out. However, the parents are asked to refer the adolescent's complaints back to the group and also to encourage the adolescent to return for at least one session to discuss fully any thoughts of dropping out. It is explained that the purpose of this suggestion is to prevent impulsive bolting based on anxiety or tension that might be resolved by discussion.

The need for confidentiality is explained. The parents are encouraged to call if they have information or questions. They are requested to tell their youngster of their intention to call, and they are told that the therapists cannot promise to keep their statements from the adolescent patient. Airing these matters with parents in a group setting seems to produce a more cooperative attitude than do similar discussions held individually. Perhaps this is because the parents have the opportunity to get acquainted and to gain together a sense of involvement with the group, with the therapists, and with each other. This may be less secretive and more supportive than individual reassurances from the therapists. Of course, observing the parents in a group setting may also provide the therapists with diagnostic data as well as providing a background for any necessary contacts during the group.

Rules and Contracts

In our early experience with adolescent groups we placed great emphasis on rules. We have had rules against contact between members outside the group session, against smoking during group sessions, against coming to the group intoxicated on any chemical agent, and against quitting the group without prior discussion—to mention those that aren't too embarrassing to recall. In retrospect, these prohibitions—and others even more petty—probably were established primarily in an attempt to contain our adolescents without "strict limits."

Without exception we have found that arbitrary rules interfere with the establishment of a therapeutic alliance. The adolescent has an infinite capacity to externalize a variety of internal miseries in a power struggle if given half a chance. In group psychotherapy, as in family life, the angry adolescent holds all the cards if interaction degenerates into a battle. What sanctions can the group therapist possibly apply? He cannot go to the youngster's parents and "tell on" him without forfeiting all hope for therapeutic leverage. The only power he has is to exclude the youngster from therapy, rarely a corrective emotional experience for the patient.

The adolescent's preference for an alloplastic fight is demonstrated by the events in a recent group that had no "rules."

The male cotherapist entered a group finishing a cigarette. There had been no smoking in the first three group sessions, but neither therapist had thought much about it. One of the group members chided the therapist, "Aha, *you're* smoking!" The therapist was puzzled, and his face showed it. "Well, how come you can smoke if we can't?" the youngster continued.

"I don't remember that we said anything about smoking." The mystery was solved when a thirteen-year-old girl who had seen the therapist individually spoke up. "You never would let *me*."

She was a borderline youngster with a harsh and primitive superego. She had asked the therapist to give her a cigarette and let her smoke it some months earlier in an individual session. He had refused since she was so guilty about smoking that she occasionally had the delusion that she had smoked and would develop lung cancer even though she had never had a cigarette in her mouth. He told her, "I don't think smoking a cigarette with me is going to straighten out your conscience problems. By the way, if your mother doesn't mind you smoking, as you tell me, why don't you have her give me a call to tell me it's okay?"

She had told the group in the waiting room that smoking was not permitted. They believed her without asking the therapists. For the first few sessions they silently and resentfully accepted what they regarded as a pointless, unilateral rule.

We have come to believe that the treatment contract virtually obviates the need for routine rules. In the first session we do mention the advisability of regular attendance, request notification if the patient must miss, announce the planned duration of the group, and discuss the need for confidentiality and the therapists' commitment to confidentiality except in regard to specific actions that threaten immediate danger to the patient or others. More important, however, the therapists begin in the individual sessions that precede participation in the group to insist that every group member commit himself to a clear treatment contract. This contract represents an agreement between the therapists and the adolescent, concerning the adolescent's goals. It is serious, concrete and mutually binding. That is, the adolescent agrees to work as hard as he can to achieve a goal that the therapists accept as reasonable to the group setting. As Dusay and Steiner (1971) have suggested, every effort is made to make the contract specific and behaviorally concrete. However, even general goals, such as "I would like to learn to communicate better" or "I would like to get along better with my family," are acceptable temporary contracts with adolescents. Although it is preferable to define goals more definitely, this may have to await further group work.

One sixteen-year-old girl's contract changed from "I want to learn to say what I mean and to stop doing dumb things," to "I would like to understand why everyone makes me mad inside and why I can't have fun unless I'm doing something dangerous," after her group experience helped her understand her problems more clearly. People are always "misunderstanding" her because she was unaware of her tremendous hostility. She did a lot of "dumb" things (such as becoming illegitimately pregnant) because her conscience denied her any pleasure which was not followed by punishment.

Contract negotiations help establish quickly the therapeutic atmosphere of the group. They also acquaint the group members with each other's difficulties and provide the opportunity for the therapist to clarify that his sincere desire to help is circumscribed. There are no vague promises that the group may somehow enrich life or provide instant happiness.

Since the group member has made a direct request for help with certain problems, the other group members do not feel that they are intruding or "hassling" him by commenting on his behavior or their reactions to it.

Jay, a fifteen-year-old boy, entered the group because he had no friends. Diagnostically he was a borderline youngster with strong paranoid features of suspiciousness and secret grandiosity. When frustrated by his father, teachers, or schoolmates, he would withdraw to his room and indulge in daydreams of masterminding a perfect war against Russia. In the group he first offered a contract of just coming to listen, since he wished to be a "psychoanalyst" some day. The other members simply wouldn't accept this. Since he was hungry for the group's approval, he reluctantly agreed to a contract to "learn how to make friends." Despite the contract, he continued to sit through sessions in absolute silence.

A sixteen-year-old girl said, "It's no wonder you can't make friends. You never say anything, just sit and laugh at people. It makes me want to hit you, not be your friend."

He tried to explain he wasn't laughing at the group, and he just didn't know what to say. The members said they couldn't believe that unless they got to know him. Most of them agreed that he should leave the group if he couldn't reveal himself. They felt they could not open up about themselves in the presence of someone so secretive.

The therapist intervened to say that he could understand the group's feelings, but that he thought Jay was telling the truth about not knowing what to say. He suggested that they make Jay "patient for the day" and interview him. They accepted the idea and took turns asking Jay questions. Finally one of them asked, "Do you feel on the spot?"

"Not as much as when I wasn't talking. I knew all of you were mad at me."

A few sessions later cookies were brought to a pre-holiday meeting. The group made Jay say at least one sentence before he could have a cookie. Jay obviously enjoyed the game, making pantomimes of great distress when he could not get the floor to say his sentence and have another cookie. The group thought this was funny and were no longer threatened by his pretended superiority.

Of course, the group may also use permission for confrontation as license to scapegoat; this is especially likely to occur when new members are added.

A boy and a girl were added to a very active and open adolescent group. Adele, the sixteen-year-old girl, had identified with her extraordinarily masochistic mother and was determined to be rejected by the group. They soon caught on to her techniques of denying anger, provoking guilt in others, and help-rejecting complaint. Louise, a very aggressive seventeen-year-old who was battling similar problems, began to attack her viciously and soon had the group totally behind her.

When the therapists tried to interrupt this assault, they were accused of protecting Adele. "I thought we were supposed to be emotionally honest in this group," Louise griped.

"Louise, I don't think you are being emotionally honest. For example, I don't think you're telling Adele why she annoys you so much, that she reminds you too much of yourself. In fact, I think the whole group is hiding behind Adele's problems right now. I certainly don't think you're doing all this to help her. On the contrary, all of you have let her use you to repeat her pattern of being rejected without really understanding why."

One of the group members spoke up. "I wonder if we're not trying to get rid of her. Remember we weren't too sure we wanted a new member anyway."

The observation was correct. The therapists had hurried Adele and the other new member into the group in the face of open ambivalence. Some of the displaced anger was soon directed toward the therapists.

Finally, as was mentioned earlier, the greatest advantage of therapy contracts is their removal of the adolescent fantasy of being helplessly controlled by adults. This "knee-jerk" response to adult therapists is largely a defense against the fear of independence and autonomy. The adolescent does not have to be ashamed of his anxiety about self-reliance if he can point with pride to his brave struggle against the adults who are trying to mold him.

Requiring a contract forces a mutuality of aims that simply will not accept a "cop-out" of passive resistance. Most adolescents who are treatable as out-patients can accommodate to this pressure for active involvement in their own therapy, especially with the support of the group. Occasionally a group is unable to come together around therapeutic goals, but more often this is a threat and a testing maneuver.

Three members of an adolescent group refused to commit themselves to a contract, insisting they didn't know why they were there except that their parents seemed to think they had a problem. The therapists insisted that this was not an acceptable reason for coming to group and asked what could be done about it. "Why don't we just forget the whole thing?" one of them said sarcastically.

The therapist ignored the provocative hostility. "That may be our only choice, if it's what everyone wants. We realize that groups don't always work out. Some of them just can't get off the ground."

Another member said, "We could just let those who don't want to have group quit and get some new members who want to do something."

"Yes, we could do that, too. I would suggest we give ourselves a little time. It may be that some of the members are so angry at their parents that they don't realize yet that the group isn't interested in bossing anyone or changing them to suit their parents."

One member who had been in a group with the therapists earlier said, "It's true. I think my parents feel deep down that the group has made me worse because I stand up to them more. They'd probably make me quit except they're afraid I'd get depressed again and make another suicide attempt."

Two of the boys made a contract and stayed in the group, the third dropped out.

The therapist must insist on mutuality even if it eventuates in the "therapeutic failure" of group dissolution, with its narcissistically damaging implication of personal and professional failure. The timid therapist may remind himself that a quick, clean group death may be preferable to the lingering, wasting illness of an uncommitted group.

Through the persistent search for mutually acceptable goals, the therapist is transformed from the "powerless parent" (Brackelmanns and Berkovitz, 1972) to an ally whose authority rightly derives from expert knowledge and emotional honesty. Limits may be set on behavior, but the reasons for the limitations derive logically from the mutually undertaken therapeutic task. Coming to group "stoned," threatening to strike another group member, missing group, and so forth, are not personal affronts to the authoritarian therapist but are revealed in their true light as resistances against experiencing and exploring inner conflicts, pains, and confusions. Naturally, this does not magically stop acting-out, but there is greater potential for learning from it. There is also less tendency for group therapy to deteriorate into a caricature of the "generation gap," with therapists and adolescents hiding their real difficulties in relating behind age labels. It may even be necessary to exclude an occasional youngster from group, but the exclusion must be due to his inability to work on his contract, not that he irritates the therapist or challenges his adult authority.

Of course, not all limits are set for therapeutic reasons. For example, therapists may refuse to answer intimate questions or prohibit specific behaviors because of purely personal discomfort. As long as one is candid about it, this rarely creates difficulties. Naturally if one is irritated or shaken by too many adolescent behaviors, it is probably better to avoid treating adolescents.

Tools and Gimmicks

The basic instruments in dynamic group psychotherapy with adolescents are the same as in all dynamic psychotherapy. They include the creation of an exploratory, nonjudgemental, and permissive atmosphere and the recognition of emotionally important themes and defensive maneuvers. These emotions are identified and clarified through confrontation and interpretation. As in all dynamic therapy, the timing of therapeutic intervention is crucial. The therapist must be especially careful that his comments are closely related to content. They should make sense and not sound farfetched or stereotyped and "textbook."

An adolescent group was laughing and joking about sex transformation operations and a movie in which a man masqueraded as a woman. The therapist commented that it seemed safer to talk about these extreme, distant examples of sex role confusion rather than one girl's comment in the previous session that she thought boys "had it made." The group quickly settled into a serious and intense discussion of boy-girl relationships and gender role anxieties and jealousies.

In addition to traditional verbal interventions in response to spontaneous group interactions, there are other methods of eliciting important material. Group therapy, in its various forms, has historically had less of a taboo against active structuring than has dynamic individual psychotherapy. A variety of artificial devices have been used to supplement and even provoke spontaneous interchange between group members. In recent years psychodrama, gestalt therapy, and the encounter movement have produced a fascinating variety of techniques for encouraging rapid, undefensive emotional interaction. Many of these, especially the less threatening "warming-up" exercises, have great merit in adolescent group work if used judiciously (see Rachman, 1971, and Olsson and Myers, 1972). Timing is important, both for the group and for the individual who is the focus of the exercise. Generally speaking, the group is ready when it perceives a problem that does not yield to verbal interaction.

Mark, a fifteen-year-old boy who had difficulties making friends ("I seem to come on either too strong or not strong enough") was referred to group by his parents who recognized that he was overly dependent on them. The parent-child relationship had been relatively healthy, but Mark had required multiple plastic surgery procedures for correction of hare-lip and cleft palate. The procedures were successful, but the overall effect of the deformity and the surgery was to intensify a closeness with the parents, especially with the mother that interfered with the development of peer relations.

In the group Mark was quiet for the most part. When he did make a comment it was usually stammered awkwardly and somehow inappropriate. He seemed to lack real empathy for the concerns of others his age. Occasionally he talked of antisocial escapades, trying to present himself as a daring, "regular guy." The group commented from time to time that Mark didn't really seem like a member. He responded mechanically to the complaints they offered, talking more, mentioning his problems or commenting on theirs, but remained somehow detached and outside the group. He was only animated when speaking directly to the male cotherapist.

One day the group was asked to join hands in a circle, with Mark outside. He was told to "try to get into the circle." He grew visibly anxious, walked around the group uncertainly and made desultory efforts to wedge his way in. After a few minutes he walked over and sat on the couch, defeated.

The group then sat down to explore his reaction. He was blank at first, stating there wasn't any way he could have gotten in "without hurting somebody." The group members pointed out that he didn't try asking, threatening, bribing or any of several maneuvers that might have gotten him in. He could only consider brute force or passive withdrawal.

The therapist asked him how he felt when he sat down on the couch. Mark replied that by then he had convinced himself that he didn't really care whether he was in the group or not. He recognized that this was his usual reaction in social situations and in the group. He was also able to admit, "I'd rather be sitting in your chair, be the leader. It seems like I can't do that if I become a group member."

The other boys in the group joined in, discussing their competitive feelings toward the therapist. Translating Mark's symbolic stance into a physical reality seemed to help him and the group to grasp it as a psychological reality and explore its origins.

This dual effect of permitting the individual to get in touch with his feelings and helping the group to empathize with his dilemma is also striking in the following example:

> Sean, a seventeen-year-old high school senior, had been very withdrawn for the first two-and-a-half months of the therapy group. He also consistently denied having strong feelings about any of the other group members.
>
> He was asked to hold each member of the group in a way that would express his attitude toward them. With great anxiety and considerable reluctance, he agreed to do this. The subtle and careful way that he thought through the embrace that he would use with each group member helped him to understand how frightened he was of getting involved with people, but also showed the group that rather than dismissing them he was giving them a great deal of thought. Although they were bothered by his "frightened fawn" poses, they no longer saw him as merely uninterested, self-contained and aloof.

Adolescents respond well to the kind of emotional structuring described above. Therapists must insure that such emotionally laden interactions are properly digested and absorbed by the group. It is exciting and fun to interact so directly, but without proper reflection and analysis it becomes little more than sophisticated acting-out. Verbal interaction and thorough discussion are necessary to assure constructive utilization of the emotions stirred and revealed in nonverbal interactions. In fact, in the absence of a therapeutic alliance that permits and encourages open verbal expression of feelings for their therapeutic utilization, it is unwise to unleash strong emotional currents in the group.

SECTION V

Family Therapy

Introduction

Growth

In recent decades there probably have been few areas in the field of mental health that have grown more explosively, or for that matter more creatively, than the area of family therapy. Indeed, as a realm of clinical endeavor it is generally credited with an official history that is scarcely twenty years old. This compact history serves to highlight the energy underlying its emergence. During the 1950s there were but thirteen published articles that had to do with family therapy, its theory or technique. The first five years of the 1960s saw the publication of more than a hundred papers on the topic, and in the ensuing five years (1965-1969) well over two hundred papers appeared in anthologies and journals (Glick and Haley, 1971). Books devoted to the clinical study of the family have increased in near-parallel, almost geometic progression from two in the first five years of the 1950s to forty in the last half of the 1960s (ibid.). The early 1970s provide ample evidence that the literature on family therapy continues to expand without deceleration (witness the books by Bloch, 1973; Ackerman, 1970a, 1970b; Ferber, 1972; Haley, 1971; Howells, 1971; Skolnick and Skolnick, 1971; Skolnick, 1973; Sager and Kaplan, 1972; Minuchin, 1974; Bermann, 1973; Zuk, 1971; Speck and Attneave, 1973; Satir, 1964; Anthony and Koupernik, 1970, 1973, 1974; Framo, 1972; Boszormenyi-Nagy and Spark, 1973; Glasser and Glasser, 1970; Group for the Advancement of Psychiatry, 1970; Rabkin, 1970).

One can only speculate that the number of therapists utilizing some form of family therapy has increased commensurate with the growth in publications. There is as yet no handy way of making such an assessment, since there exists no national association of family therapists. Yet, the speculation that the growth has kept pace with publication rate seems warranted, in view of (1) the rise in subscriptions to the journal *Family Process* (Bloch, 1973, reports increments of 15 percent each year), (2) the increasing numbers attending "family therapy conferences" (ibid.), and (3) the proliferation of "family institutes" for training and treatment (ibid.).

Some Cautions

While the foregoing indices certainly substantiate the initial assertion regarding the explosive emergence of the family therapy field, they do not speak for the claim of creativity. There is no pretense, nor even realistic expectation, that the nine papers that follow this introduction will suffice in any way to convince a reader that the field of family study is richly creative of quality and substance. Reading in and of itself can hardly decide the issue. Indeed, it would be fair to say that most family therapists (Beels and Ferber, 1973) would claim "reading about" to be the least efficacious means of learning about or assessing the creative potentialities of family therapy. For these purposes they would recommend, in ascending order: (1) listening to audiotapes of family therapy; (2) watching family treatment done via videotapes or movies; (3) direct observation of family treatment over time; and, of course, most preferably, (4) doing family therapy oneself. And, as will be evident from the readings, it is the claim of at least one family therapist (Haley, 1971) that only extensive firsthand experience in doing family work (with perhaps 200 families) can ultimately make the difference for a practitioner coming to the field from more traditional training.

Hence, the papers that follow were not selected with any intention of persuading the reader that family therapy should become his way. Rather, they were selected with an eye toward introducing and informing. They make it clear, first of all, that the field of family therapy is alive; that it is conceptually vital, if unsettled, searching, and moving, at times contentiously electric and attacking. Second, the readings were selected so as to introduce the reader to some of the past and present shape of the family therapy domain, and to some of the ways in which it promises to evolve or reshape itself in the future. Third, while the articles were picked because they discuss issues relevant to technique, they do not constitute a "how to do it" guide. (Readers seeking a basic introductory guidebook to family therapy technique are referred to Donald Bloch's 1973 primer). It is hoped however that the papers reprinted here will convey some of what family therapists do and what they think about what it is they do. Further, it is anticipated that the nine selections in this section will highlight significant theoretical issues bearing on method: that at one level they will serve to call attention to some shared and disputed premises among family therapists, displaying the variegated texture that exists within the field itself. At another level, these selections will make apparent some important linkages as well as some fundamental conceptual tensions that obtain between the working assumptions of family therapists and those assumptions made by therapists without a primarily family orientation to child treatment. This last suggests that it is *not* simply a benign matter when therapists maintain somewhat different vantage points (e.g., intrapsychic versus interpersonal) regarding the same clinical phenomenon (e.g., treatment of childhood phobia) but that crucially different consequences can flow from the adoption of one orientation at the conceptual expense, or exclusion, of another.

A second caution is in order regarding these articles. The reader should not only ready himself to be unconvinced as to the creative aspects of the family field—that is, be prepared to suspend positive assessments—but a second caveat suggests that he ought, as well, be prepared to suspend negative valuations. For, despite its obvious achievements, its considerable appeal, its growing numbers of adherents, and its undeniable significance (virtually everyone recognizes the family unit to be a ubiquitous phenomenon, and who would deny that it influences the mental health of its members)— indeed, despite its not infrequent attempts at persuading, cajoling, proselytizing—the family field is simply not easy to embrace. While many may approach it with curiosity or are even initially drawn to it with some enthusiasm, not a few turn away bewildered and dismayed. Others, perhaps possessing greater tolerance for ambiguity, stay on, lingering at its periphery in a state of fascinated skepticism. Still others, more and more in fact, plunge in, though even then one wonders with what comfort they do so. The reasons for the sometimes tentative quality of these reactions to family therapy are likely manifold. They are worth trying to fathom in order that persons not turn away from the area prematurely. They can, perhaps, best be understood by taking the field of family therapy, quite literally, on its own terms. Doing so promises to help with the recognition that one does not easily join another person's "family system," not without running the risk of misunderstood communications and rules, or the perils of violated norms, or the inadvertent overstepping of boundaries. To join an ongoing group invites the creation of improprieties, not stemming from malice, but from ignorance of unspoken, informal assumptions. Ultimately, there may be anxiety about rejection and concern about inheriting the label of deviant. Comprehension of the field of family therapy on its own terms might well, at a minimum, forestall these potentialities. At best, it promises to shed light on the substance, contours, and strains on family therapy as a movement in mental health.

The Field of Family Therapy as "Family"

Presuming that any attempt to characterize the field of family therapy in its own conceptual language is not too farfetched an enterprise, one may proceed to raise a series of family-oriented questions. For example, is the field of family treatment really comprehensible as a "social system"? Is it truly a "field" with an identity of its own and attendant social system characteristics? If so, what are its parameters? What are the sources of its bondings, its homeostatic mechanisms? How does it go about defining its boundaries? Indeed, how permeable are those boundaries? Are its internal aspects differentiated? Undifferentiated? Amorphous? Fragmented? Integrated? How does the field structure its psychological space? What of power struggles? Are there internal splits and alignments that are recognizable? Sibling rivalry? What family myths does it perpetuate, promote? Are there family secrets that it harbors? Does it maintain parenting functions? Manifest concern for generativity? And, what of its genealogy, its history, its extended kin?

Is the Family Therapy Field Truly a "Field"?
Does It Have Defining Characteristics? A Family "Identity"?

First and foremost, it must be recognized that the field itself is a hybrid—an amalgam of disparate theoretic sources and disciplinary offshoots, variously interwoven, seldom coherent. To the outsider, to the onlooker, to the traditionalist, to the newcomer, to the would-be convert, the entire arena can have a dizzying, kaleidoscopic impact. The conglomerate of viewpoints, each exciting, exasperating, heretical, and conceptually contradictory or mutually exclusive in its own way, may genuinely give one pause to question whether something so variegated could be dignified with the term "field." Two considerations, however, encourage an affirmative response.

One factor that seems to lend coherence to the area is the view that now imbues all its proponents—theorists, practitioners, clinicians, researchers alike—namely, that the family, rather than the individual, is the appropriate unit of study or treatment. This credo, so deceptively simple in its reading that it is frequently misunderstood, is nonetheless a view qualitatively different from any that had preceded it in the field of mental health. It alone suffices to give family therapy its recognizable identity. The most frequent misinterpretation of its meaning is that family treatment requires the presence of all members at therapy hours. Anything less than total family involvement therefore would not be deemed family treatment. This view once prevailed among some family therapists (Framo, 1965) and still finds expression on occasion (Zilbach, Bergel, and Gass, 1972). However, as will be evident from the reading of Haley's article on "Beginning and

Experienced Family Therapists" (1972) in this volume, the physical presence of all family members is not a criterion of family treatment. Family therapy, then, has become less defined by technique than by an orientation construing emotional disturbance in systematic terms, transactionally in the context of family dynamics, and without regard to family members actually on location.

The second defining characteristic of the family therapy field, qua "field," is its frequently militant and occasionally petulant insistence on what it is not. This insistence is tantamount to boundary maintenance, asserting that family therapy is *not* traditional psychiatry with an individualistic orientation, *not* psychoanalysis with its emphasis on intrapsychic events and introjects, owing nothing to disease concepts of emotional disturbance or to the medical model. Contrary to the integrationist aims to which this volume is dedicated, the family therapy field assumes the segregationist posture that it is not another form of treatment that a therapist can tuck into his armamentarium of therapeutic strategies. It is, according to its own claims, a totally different orientation to human circumstance, and thereby not exchangeable with other treatment methods. This probably represents an insufficient distinction between the *study* of family processes and the *treatment* of them. Like a university's departmental structure, a field of study generally is enhanced by segregation, while therapy and the people it is designed to help differ from university departments in that they benefit more from integration. Nevertheless, the family therapy field eschews personality theory, partakes little of psychological testing, and rejects traditional diagnostic categories and procedures. Not infrequently it conscientiously condemns inference and theorizing about activities internal to the "black box" and thereby dismisses with vehemence the better part of what mental health professionals have spent a lifetime in learning.

To the extent that it does these things in order to define itself, the family field may be characterized as possessing a negative, or at least reactive, identity. This would not be an unusual circumstance for a movement that proclaims itself revolutionary and prides itself on its maverick qualities. Nonetheless, it runs the risk of discouraging onlookers who might be prone to experience its negative segregating identity as its most prominent defining characteristic. Hopefully, this will not prevent clinicians dealing with children from learning from the fruitful efforts of the family therapy field, some of which are reprinted

What Family Therapists Do

C. BEELS, M.D.
A. FERBER, M.D.

This paper by Beels and Ferber presents what is probably as broad and compact an overview of various family treatment styles as currently exists in the literature. The authors, who describe themselves as "second generation family therapists," seek to initiate their readers to the nature of family treatment through characterizations—some might, and others have, argued "caricaturizations" (Zuk, 1973)—of the working identities and behavioral styles of several pioneering, "first-generation," family therapists. Their account is lively, challenging, provocative, informative, understandably nonconceptual, and eminently readable. It effectively conveys the flavor of the family therapy movement by allowing the reader to "feel his way into" a new therapeutic orientation. With the articles that follow, the point of view that family therapy is more of an outlook and orientation than a method or specific technique becomes clear. Concomitantly, the myth that family therapy requires the presence of the entire family is dismissed—indeed, some highly renowned family therapists prefer to work almost exclusively with individuals. Illustrated also and often in dramatic fashion are the varieties of data family therapists find most useful, and how such data may be put to therapeutic use.

It is interesting that the paper, first published in 1969, then updated and republished in 1972, is not the first of its genre in the family therapy field. As such, it is a time-limited, temporary guide to the area—one that bears historical comparison with its earliest antecedent, Jay Haley's "Whither Family Therapy?" published in 1962. Haley's comparative review of family therapies was prepared for the initial issue of the journal Family Process. *In the introductory paragraphs of that paper Haley noted that the treatment of families had been largely an underground movement before 1962. Fearful of being labeled theoretical or methodological heretics, and concerned lest they commit themselves in print to uncertain techniques, family therapists had whispered furtively about their "experiments" in backrooms, but seldom, if ever, in print.*

The founding of Family Process *heralded their "coming out," and Haley as its editor toured the country talking with and observing practitioners of family therapy in order to learn about their methods and describe them. The resultant paper contained no references to published articles, but provided a "humorful" characterization of eight or so "schools" of family treatment. Significantly enough, Haley chose to maintain the anonymity of the trailblazers, naming the "schools" of family treatment somewhat facetiously, but not the protagonists (though a curious reader might decipher who they are easily enough). Haley forecasted, however, that a deluge of published papers on family therapy would follow, implying that anonymity would cease to be the order of the day.*

The Beels and Ferber article reprinted here demonstrates how accurate Haley's predictions were. Less than ten years after the Haley paper, Beels and Ferber describe more than twice the number of family therapy schools. Moreover, these are now full-blown "schools," many of them replete with masters and disciples. Also, a total of eighty-one published articles about family therapy are cited by the authors. And, perhaps most significantly, the brash, trumpeting, confident, muscle-flexing tones that permeate both the therapeutic work and written style of family therapists finds full expression in the Beels and Ferber paper.

As a matter of fact a virtue of the paper that follows is that it typifies the field, embodying many of its abuses as well as its delights. It seeks to delineate styles of treatment, for it accurately states that there is no single mode of family therapy, but instead a variety of family therapies. It is unapologetically atheoretical, for it realistically reflects a field in which family therapies have been methods in search of theories. To the extent that theories have been advanced they served as explanation for established practices.

Impudent, clever, adventuresome, by turn, the paper is at the same time graciously humanizing of its subject matter. Smugly accusing of traditionalists, it pays no attention to aspects of its own conventionality and stereotypy. While calling attention to the achievements of family therapists—emphasizing the significance of action as opposed to insight, the import of nonverbal communication as opposed to words, the emphasis on "change" and "effect" rather than the search for ultimate "truth" or historical causation—the paper neglects to note deficits within the family movement, e.g., its asociological character, and so its emphases are consonant with those of the approaches it reviews. Though it is eminently fair in its concerns about certain features of family therapy—the blatant and "chilling" manipulativeness of many family practitioners—it remains relatively unquestioning of the middle-class values that dominate the field, and is almost totally impervious to any consideration of ecological factors that may influence family interaction. And finally, while it lauds family therapists for their innovative concern with the dynamics of the ongoing, natural group, as opposed to a more conventional focus on intrapsychic events and past introjects of the individual, it violates this self-same principle by literally taking the therapist out of the family context and milieu. The paper seriously hazards misleading its readers by describing the style of family therapists in a manner that is totally divorced from any consideration of the families they see.

Nonetheless, the Beels and Ferber paper succeeds because it depicts the field not as it should be but as it actually is.

This personal view of the practice and the literature of family therapy is written to inform those who, like ourselves, are second-generation family therapists, entering a field which began in the early 1950's, and has since developed rapidly. The field has its journals, its books, its GAP committee, its training programs, its internal wars, its multiplying hundreds of practitioners, and, most important for us, its pioneering teachers. In an attempt to bring coherence out of the various teachings and practices of these leaders of the field, we try here to evaluate them by imposing our own order upon them, in the light of our own experience with teaching and practice.

Approaches to Family Therapy

We have looked for systematic efforts to evaluate the results, the outcome, of family therapy, but evaluation has been neglected here as in other therapies. We know of only three aspects of any substance on outcome:

1. The multiple impact (MacGregor et al., 1964) therapists report a favorable result in seventy-five percent of their sixty-two families of disturbed adolescents at one and one-half year follow-up. All their schizophrenics got better.
2. Murray Bowen, looking back over twelve years of practice with five hundred families, feels that in four years' time he can change the dynamics of most families, providing they are not schizophrenics. He feels he has never changed the fundamental dynamics of a schizophrenic family.
3. Langsley in Colorado (Langsley, Pittman, Machotka, and Felder, 1968) has used a family approach to prevent hospitalization in over ninety percent of acute crises judged to require hospitalization in the emergency room.

Reprinted from A. Ferber, M. Mendelsohn, and A. Napier (eds.), *The Book of Family Therapy*, Jason Aronson, Inc., New York, 1972, pp. 662-665.

The main deduction from this is that no one seems to be talking about the same kind of outcome or treatment.

Our second approach to family therapy has been to watch it. We have succeeded in getting some experience, other than reading, with most of the people mentioned in this chapter.[1] The nature and extent of this direct experience varies widely: listening to audiotapes, watching videotapes and movies, directly observing "demonstration" interviews, consultations, and ongoing therapy, and observing continuous therapy for periods of months to years. Clearly, there are some crucial differences between a therapist's behavior during a visit with a strange family in a strange setting, and his behavior in a private session of a long-term therapy in his private practice, and we have often had to compare the observation of one with writing about the other. We have tried not to endanger by over-generalization the great advantage which direct observation has given us: the opportunity of seeing personal and perhaps unwitting styles of work.

Watching family therapy and talking with the therapists about the experience has led us to believe that there is no "right" way to do it. Each man made his own style of work, and from those we got to know best it was clear that each had forged it from a life-long fascination with families, beginning with his own. It was pointless to try to abstract "the technique" from these many approaches, since the personal stamp of the therapist was so clearly the first thing we had to understand.

Many reproductions of interviews are now available. Haley and Hoffman's *Techniques of Family Therapy* (1967), a detailed analysis of taped interviews by distinguished family therapists, with the therapists and Haley as discussants, is especially revealing. Murray Bowen has videotaped some of his work and Ackerman has made movies of his. The Eastern Pennsylvania Psychiatric Institute has films of Ackerman,

---

[1] The following is a list of people with whom we had more than a reading acquaintance: Virginia Satir, Ivan Boszormeny-Nagy and Geraldine Lincoln, James Framo, Murray Bowen, Frank Pittman and Kalman Flomenhaft, Salvador Minuchin, Braulio Montalvo, Gerald Zuk, David Rubenstein, Nathan Ackerman, Normal Paul, Don Jackson, Jay Haley, Jerry Jungreis, Lyman Wynne, Hanna Kwiatkowska, Carl Whitaker, Israel Zwerling, Harold Searles, Roger Shapiro, John Zinner, Gentry Harris, Fred Ford, Ross Speck, Edgar Auerswald, Richard Rabkin, Augustus Napier and Frederick Duhl.

Jackson, Whitaker and Bowen, each interviewing the same family. Minuchin's *Families of the Slums* (Minuchin, Montalvo, Guerney, Rosman and Shumer, 1967), Ackerman's *Treating the Troubled Family* (1966), and the Houston Group's *Multiple Impact Therapy With Families* (MacGregor et al., 1964) all contain extensive transcriptions of interviews, with discussion by the therapists. The spread of this practice would make a new and uniquely valuable kind of library.

The most important approach is to do family therapy oneself. This is the only way to integrate the literature with one's experience. Reading or talking about it from the perspective of other therapies is an empty experience.

As teachers we have had to be explicit about our choice of tactics. We have each watched and discussed several hundred hours of family therapy interviews over the past six years.

We have abstracted from the literature certain themes on the family therapist's use of himself as an agent of influence in interaction with the family. In doing so, we did not discuss in any depth the subject of "family dynamics" or "theory of family pathology"—that is, the family's behavior as it is imagined in the absence of the therapist. That field has, of course, a much larger and older literature, well reviewed by Meissner (1964), by Mischler and Waxler (1966), by Zuk and Rubinstein (1965), and by Frank (1965), and which we put beyond our scope. Nor have we said much about "theories of family therapy."

We avoided the evaluation of theory because we believed that in many cases the theories advanced were a rationalization for the practice of the therapy and not what we thought a real theory in this area should be: an ordering of diverse clinical phenomena to a scheme that would organize their diversity and provide a reason for different therapeutic measures.

There are some outstanding exceptions: Wynne's *Some Indications and Contraindications for Exploratory Family Therapy* (1965), the *Multiple Impact Therapy* by MacGregor et al. (1964) which contains a four-part diagnostic scheme, Tharp's breakdown of types of family contract (Tharp and Otis, 1965), Minuchin and Montalvo's differential descriptions of family types and therapist styles (Minuchin, Montalvo, Guerney, Rosman and Shumer, 1967), and some parts of the work of Bowen (1966), and of Ackerman (Ackerman and Behrens, 1956). Clearly, another paper could be written on systems of diagnosis and therapeutic strategy.

A Definition of Family Therapy

To define family therapy, let us begin by comparing it with individual therapy. Ford and Urban in *Systems of Psychotherapy* (1963) abstract four common elements from all types of individual therapy that they surveyed: 1. There are two people in confidential interaction; 2. the mode of interaction is usually verbal; 3. the interaction is relatively prolonged; and 4. the relationship has for its definite and agreed-upon purpose changes in the behavior of one of the participants.

Applying these considerations to family therapy:

1. There are more than two people, and the interaction between them is to that important extent not confidential. As we shall show later the change of technique in the jump from a dyadic to triadic (or more) interaction is a discontinuous one.
2. Nonverbal interaction assumes a primary importance along with the verbal; manipulation of membership, gesture, seating arrangement and posture, by any and all participants is significant.
3. It is often shorter than individual therapy, but this is enormously variable.
4. The relationship has for its definite and agreed-upon purpose changes in the family system of interaction, not changes in the behavior of individuals. Individual change occurs as a by-product of system change.

This goal of changing the family system of interaction is family therapy's most distinctive feature, its greatest advantage and, especially to those who come to it from other disciplines, its greatest stumbling block.

Critics from the tradition of individual therapy fear that family therapy must be damaging or frightening to the members if it is going to deal effectively with what is "really" going on between them. Handlon and Parloff (1962), comparing family therapy with conventional group therapy, point out that, in attacking the family system, family therapy dispenses with almost all the tactical advantages of group therapy in order to make "an heroic frontal assault on manifestly relevant but securely guarded relationship." The interlocking system of family relationships may be the nub of the problem, but to approach it directly in its natural state seems to group and individual therapists a venture too radical or risky. They prefer to work with individual patients in safer contexts where, they think, it is more possible to enlist the ego functions of the patient in the examination of behavior which is the shadow rather than the substance of family interaction.

In addition to these experimental reasons for avoiding the family system in interaction, there is for all of us a conceptual difficulty with labeling systems. Even if we were able to remove ourselves from it emotionally, which we are not, the problem of accounting intellectually for the interplay of events and sequences in a family session is one for which there is not yet a good language.

In spite of these difficulties, let us look more closely at the family therapist's concern with the system of relationships rather than with the individual. Almost every treatise on family therapy begins with the author's view on this. John E. Bell (1963) states it most succinctly, and most radically:

> Family group treatment takes the family and by professional action tries to help itself into becoming a more perfectly functioning group. The contract with the family specifies this end. To work thus with a group is new in psychotherapy. When we have worked with groups before we have used them instrumentally, as a means to the

cure of individuals. We have not sought the effective functioning of the group as an end goal. Even the professional specialist in social work who calls himself a group worker, and who knows more than most mental health workers about the theory and natural history of groups, has not seen himself working with a group first for its own sake but rather as a means to help the individuals who compose it.

I draw this distinction sharply. Family group treatment is a consulting sociological or socio-psychological technique and as such is unlike psychological treatment methods that aim for the welfare of an individual. Let it be recognized, however, that although family group treatment seeks the well-being of the family, secondarily it has important consequences for the status of the individuals who make up the family. This reminds us of the arbitrariness in our distinctions between the family group and individual members of the family. Both the group and the individual are correlated open systems. To look at one or the other as independent is only a professional choice that later requires us to follow for the limitations imposed by our selective starting position. It is easy to see this in electing to work with the family. What now has become more apparent is that a similar choice process has been in operation in our work with individuals. Culturally we are so biased in favor of the individual that we have tended to ignore the fact that the choice to deal with him could be arbitrary, and that we are prejudiced in favor of seeing him as a closed system. Carelessly we ignored that we had adopted a posture for thinking. We believed that there was some positive objective validity to the individual, and that as a consequence it was our primary obligation in treatment to concern ourselves with his personal progress.

We shall return in our conclusion to some of the consequences of this definition of the family therapist as a professional whose commitment is to make the family "a more perfectly functioning group." Although different therapists might disagree on how to recognize that more perfect function, or what its relation is to the "status of the individuals," the therapists reviewed here would agree that the first purpose of working with the family group is to improve its function as a family. This definition is especially inclusive if one remembers that family therapists regard as one of the family's most important functions the promotion of the differentiation, and in the case of the children, the ultimate separation, of the individual from what Bowen (1966) calls the "undifferentiated family ego mass." The therapist does not simply try to make the family more "groupy," more cohesive, but on the contrary tries to promote its growth and differentiation.

The Relation of the Therapist to the Family Group

The therapist is a new member of the family group. How does he present himself to them? We will take this question and apply it to each of the therapists in turn. In this way we will also be presenting the therapists to the reader as they present themselves to the family.

To organize this catalogue, we begin by dividing conductors from reactors. Since the family is a group with an organization of its own, the therapist can enter it either as its conductor in this special and unfamiliar activity of meeting for therapy, or as a reactor who responds to what the family presents to him. Obviously all therapists do some of both in keeping control of the meeting, but if one thinks of what appears to be their dominant mode of keeping control, then some generalizations might be made concerning a classification of conductors and reactors. In a general way, conductors remain on the dominant side of dominance-submission complementarities or on the senior side of a generation hierarchy. They maintain that position, staying in the group by staying on top of it and leading it. Reactors may shift out to the boundary of the group from time to time, such as when consulting with co-therapists, and they may join in symmetrical same-generation relationships with family members.

Many of the conductors are vigorous personalities who can hold audiences spellbound by their talks and demonstrations. They have a keen, explicit sense of their own values and goals which they, in one way or another, hope to get the families to adopt. Some of them are regarded by their critics as sadistic, manipulative, exhibitionistic, and insensitive.

The reactors have, on the whole, less compelling public personalities. They present themselves to the families not only as themselves but in various roles dictated by the tactics or by the group dynamics of the family. They refer often in their writings to the danger of being swamped, confused, inveigled, or excluded by families. They have goals and values, but they are more likely to be, as Whitaker (1965) says, a secret agenda in the therapy.

The reactors can be further divided into two groups, the analysts and the system purists, depending on what they observe and respond to. The analysts tend to see in the family interaction and in the therapist's behavior things that would be recognizable to the psychoanalytic tradition, and they call them by familiar names such as "transference," "counter-transference," "acting-out," etc. To a variable degree, they are concerned with the internal processes of individuals. The system purists see in the family a system of countervailing power—a network of influence governed by rules that shape and constrain it. They have a minimal "black box" model of the individual psyche and are not concerned about what is happening "inside." They ask few questions about the motives of the power struggle. They see themselves as scientifically parsimonious while their psychoanalytical critics see them as naive.

The Conductors

Let us begin with two of the conductors who might be called respectively the East and West coast charismatic leaders of the field, Nathan Ackerman and Virginia Satir. Both generally made more statements than any family member during the course of a session, and although the aim and effect was to promote interaction between family members, they did it by establishing a star-shaped verbal communication pattern with themselves as the center.

Ackerman mobilized family interaction, watching it for non-verbal gestures and interactional clues to the more primitive relations of sex, aggression, and helpless dependency in the group, and then "tickled" the defenses against these. He cut through denial, hypocrisy, and projection, forcing the members to be more open to him than they were to each other. With his confident manner and his honesty he promised them for the moment a relationship to him in which the defenses could be dispensed with. He opened up a family that was frozen with the fear of aggression, or promoted a sexy interchange in a couple where sex was feared. He broke the family's rules about the unmentionable, because nothing was unmentionable to him, and he went after what people were trying to hide until he got it. When he brought it out, it was under his own sponsorship—he loaned the family his pleasure in life, jokes, good sex, and limited aggression.

Satir presents herself to the family as a teacher and expert in communication. She says of the therapist, "He must concentrate on giving the family confidence, reducing their fears, and making them comfortable and hopeful about the therapy session. He must show that he has direction, that he is going somewhere. His patients come to him because he is an expert, so he must accept the label and be comfortable in his role. Above all, he must show patients that he can structure his questions in order to find out what both he and they need to know" (1964). Satir is determined to teach the family a new language, with which they can resolve the communication problems that she sees as the root of their trouble. To do this, she makes herself the embodiment of clarity and perception in communication, using simple words, keeping up a running explanatory gloss on what she is doing, and arranging encounters between family members according to her rules. She does, of course, much more than this, and her work with family dynamics shows that she translates into her own language the concepts of many more traditional theorists, but basically she is a teacher of a method of communication. The treatment is accomplished when the family has learned it, and the deepening of their relationship is a by-product.

Murray Bowen and Salvador Minuchin, the next two conductors, have as a primary tactic a selective way of arranging the therapist-family interaction—a sort of stage direction which enforces differentiation within the confused relationships of the family. Bowen (1966) retains absolute control of the process of the therapy meeting and refuses all other responsibilities. He even avoids calling himself a therapist and eschews the model of a doctor treating someone with an illness, since that model implies a dependence of one person on another that is part of the family pathology. He presents himself as a researcher teaching the family to be researchers. There, however, the open-endedness ends, and shortly after his initial reconnaissance with the family he begins to work toward his goal. The goal is the differentiation of individuals from what he has called the "undifferentiated family ego-mass." He chooses one part or the other, usually the more mature one who is closest to differentiating to begin with, and through individual sessions or joint sessions works on the marital relationship and the transference to himself. The emphasis is on the futility of trying to influence, change or depend on, the other. Bowen presents himself as uninfluenceable, unchangeable and not to be depended on in this situation—he says what he will do and what he will not do. When he succeeds in getting one spouse to take such an "I stand," the other is shortly motivated to move off in his own direction. The marriage, after a stormy period, reaches a new equilibrium between two more different people who are still relating to each other. The subtlety of the process consists in the fact that only the pathological bonds are broken, and Bowen's trenchant definition of these is his great art.

Minuchin (Minuchin, Montalvo, Guerney, Rosman and Shumer, 1967) is more elaborate in his stage direction. He works with poor families who have little ability to delay impulse or examine processes which are pointed out to them verbally. His interventions are directed to giving the family what he calls an "enactive," or "iconic," rather than a verbal, experience of a new way of operating. For example, he selects a mother and daughter in whose relationship a grandmother cannot avoid interfering. He instructs the mother and daughter to continue their talk while he takes the grandmother behind the one-way screen to observe and tell him her feelings about the other two. He thus gets the grandmother to enact the separation. He talks to a silent child about something unrelated to the family in order to give the family and child the experience of the child's talking. He silences an overbearing wife by talking to the husband about the effect of her tactics on the men in the room, and colludes with the husband to handle her. The emphasis is on breaking patterns of action to produce feelings, and the therapist uses himself as the explicit agent or intermediary in making the break. For both Bowen and Minuchin the pattern of present interaction is manipulated—the unconscious content for the individual. The psychoanalytic theme is secondary if it is noted at all.

The next group of conductors, Roland Tharp and the Multiple Impact group under the leadership of Robert MacGregor, are most explicitly concerned with conventional family roles. Their therapies are brief and action-oriented.

Tharp (1963) makes an acknowledged simplification of family dynamics by examining the functional roles that the family members take in one of four areas: solidarity, sexuality, external relations, and internal instrumentality. He diagnoses the division of responsibility as it is within each of these, picks the area where the most trouble exists, and requires a new contract between the members. They are to work out an explicit contract, which will sometimes take the form of a written budget, or a legal-looking document describing jobs and penalties. The family is taught a technique of negotiating on concrete issues, which they can generalize. It is a secondary by-product that enhanced self-esteem comes to members who are newly seen to have bargaining power and responsibilites, and with this legitimate source of self-regard available, the pathological forms of seeking (the symptoms) will become dysfunctional and disappear.

The next example of the leader approach is the group that practices what they have called Multiple Impact Therapy, or MIT, at the University of Texas in Galveston (MacGregor et al., 1964). They treat families with a disturbed adolescent in crisis. The family comes to Galveston, checks into a motel, and at eight in the morning begins two days of kaleidoscopic interaction with a team at the clinic that includes doctors, a female social worker, psychologists, ministers, and others. The whole team meets with the whole family for an hour, and then they split up into different combinations of interviewers and family members according to a strategy that is worked out during the opening meeting. The team with its leaders and followers, its male and female members, is a model of role differentiation, flexibility, open criticism, and communication, at the same time that it is examining the family's difficulties in this area. During the course of the two days, the marital relationship is examined in individual and conjoint interviews, the appropriate areas of authority and autonomy of mother and father are confirmed, the child's expression of anxiety about the parental relationship is acknowledged, and by the time of the last plenary session at the end of the second day, the family knows that it can be under the leadership of a father whose wife has first place in his heart, and whose children know their place in their developing separateness from the family. They are then told to go out and try it until the first six-month follow-up visit in the home. This is a very intensive, powerful experience—historical, prescriptive, and future-oriented. The team brings to bear the power of their number, the solidarity and depth of their relationships to each other, and their experience with their own and other families. They are explicitly conveying the values of the culture, as well as the understanding of the idiosyncratic position from which the family starts.

Up to this point we have presented our catalogue of conductors in pairs that have implied a similarity, at least for didactic purposes, however different the members of the pair might be to all other intents. We come finally to two at the end of our list for whom no such bracketing is implied—Norman Paul and John Elderkin Bell.

Norman Paul's (1966; 1967; Paul and Grosser, 1965) undertaking with the family, like that of a shaman-healer, is to exorcise the ghost that dominates their lives. He conducts an inquiry, which is in style something like individual therapy, into the present and past of the family. The aim of the inquiry is to disclose the figure from the past, usually a parent of one of the parents, whose influence as an unrelinquished object affects the present relations of the family members. In this inquiry, he is the center and organizer of the communication pattern, and does not spend much time with the analysis of open interaction between family members.

When the unmourned parent of, say, a husband is identified, Paul will interview the husband intensively, bringing out memories and fears, while the wife listens and Paul points out to her, in an aside, whose shoes she was being asked to fill. If the grandparents are still living, all three generations may come together for what is often a very tearful session of recognizing and relinquishing.

Paul tries to present himself, the therapist, as the transference substitute for the lost one, and encourage in the separation at the end of therapy a more open and benign recognition of the realities of parting. He also presents himself as the model of empathy, which is the second cornerstone of his method. When one family member is in the process of re-experiencing the misery of early loss, or another conflictual experience, Paul empathizes deeply and openly with his experience and invites another family member to do the same. One of his goals for the family is that through his example they can discover the rapport with one another that comes from the conscious exercise of empathy.

The point to carry forward is the central position Paul gives to unresolved internal object relations as the key to pathology. We will meet this again when we come to the analysts: Paul's theoretical background is very close to theirs, and indeed he would be classed with them in our scheme if he did not present himself so clearly as a conductor with the definite goal of freeing the family through mourning.

John E. Bell is a lone and original figure in family therapy. He was one of the people who independently began it as a technique in 1951, and he has continued to break new ground in his writing about it, as can be seen from the number of passages in this review where we have felt that the best way to make a point is to quote him. His Public Health Monograph of 1960 is the first handbook of family therapy, and we have taken our picture of his style of leadership from the case report in that publication (Bell, 1961).

The quality of Bell's leadership is rather gentle, sympathetic, and polite, but it is at the same time clear that he knows where the family ought to be going and how to get them there. He proceeds through an orderly and definite set of phases, each one laying the groundwork for the next, and by comparison with many other therapists he works quite rapidly—the treatment reported in the monograph took eleven sessions.

Working with families in which the symptomatic one is the child, he begins by seeing the parents alone in an initial interview. There (as Haley has noted) he makes a paradoxical contract with them: he bears their complaints about the child, thus seeming to accept for the moment the idea of the child as a patient, and then asks them to bring the child and siblings next time, and to agree beforehand to accept a suggestion the child may make in the second interview about a change in the family's way of doing things. This puts the parents in the position of control as co-strategists with the therapist, but paradoxically their first move is to agree to see what happens if the child is put in control of a limited aspect of the family's rules. We shall meet this kind of technique again, more explicitly tied to theory, in the paradoxical instructions of Jackson.

With this unsettling of the usual order, Bell enters a "child-centered phase" where the aim is to encourage the child to state his fears, grievances, and wishes, while the parents listen and react but do not dominate. The key to this phase is the therapist's supervision of the dialogue so that "everyone has a chance to speak." He thus establishes the rule that the family members will be equals in the task of self-expression, and in this way he gets himself benignly but solidly established as the rule-maker.

He next moves to a "parent-child interaction," where the major resistances, tensions, and often denials of difficulty by the whole family occur. The handling of this crisis by sympathetic urging, interpretation of parents' childhood experience, encouraging some resolution outside of sessions, or getting suggestions from the children, leads to a decision by the couple to do something differently.

From here, the therapy moves to a denouement of consideration of sibling relations, roles outside the family and termination. During this phase, the family makes plans for how they are going to continue to manage their affairs by using the techniques they have learned—they discover new potentialities in each other for the resolution of difficulties and thus do not have to depend on the therapist. There is also an increased interest in the success of each member in his role outside the family, which goes with the release from the pathological function each was serving within the family—the differentiation from the family ego-mass of which Bowen speaks.

We have abstracted Bell at such length because in this first paper in the field he brings together so many of the subjects that other therapists have developed over the years. In addition to Jackson's paradoxical instruction, there are: the establishment of communications in the session as the focus of interest and of the therapist as communications expert (Satir, Zuk); the redefinition of the child problem as a parent-conflict problem (Satir most explicitly, but many others as well); the focus on positive interpretation (Haley, MIT); planning for the future (MIT, Tharp); and phase-specific planning of tactics so that the therapy proceeds from one focus to another, from the family's definition of the problem to generation conflict to parental conflict (Framo).

Before we proceed, notice the abundant value-statements of the conductors: Ackerman's writing is replete with statements about what the good life is like. Satir has a remarkable summary where she says: "Everyone must manifest uniqueness in himself and validate it in others, settle differences according to what works rather than who is right, and treat all differentness as an opportunity for growth" (1964). Bowen (1966) has a scale of 100, designating degrees of mental health on which he is confident that he can rate people within five points or so. MacGregor (1967) makes no apology about reinforcing what he refers to as the "middle-class values" of his patients. Bell speaks of establishing "a more perfectly functioning group," though he has in mind that "the value system that should be the family's own system rather than that of the therapist."

We would summarize this section by saying that the conductors conduct a meeting with a very definite end in view. They arrange for the family a new experience in the possibilities of relating to one another, and they are quite direct about setting that experience up.

Reactors-Analysts

The first group of reactors are Carl Whitaker (1958, 1965a, 1965b) whose co-authors in several papers include Warkentin (Warkentin and Whitaker, 1966), Felder and Malone (Malone, Whitaker, Warkentin and Felder, 1961), Lyman Wynne and his colleagues at NIMH, and the group of family therapists in the Philadelphia Family Institute who are best known under the editorial leadership of Alfred Friedman (Friedman et al., 1965), Ivan Boszormenyi-Nagy, and James Framo (Wynne, 1965). The group is distinguished by a terminology and interest more or less similar to that of the psychoanalytic tradition of therapy. They believe that the individual carries within him a non-rational and unconscious truth that, when encountered meaningfully in the therapy, will help to set him free. They are also the leading exponents of the use of co-therapists. Sonne et al. (1965) of the Philadelphia group, for example, prescribe the use of male and female co-therapists for the working through of parental transferences in the family members, and they would agree with Whitaker that having two therapists is essential to the emotional equilibrium of either one. The following quotation from Whitaker (1965) conveys the mood of the co-therapy team in the family:

We have been forced to admit that family psychotherapy can be effectively undertaken only by a team of two therapists. A good surgeon can do a routine appendectomy, but even a good surgeon wouldn't attempt a major abdominal operation without a colleague of equal adequacy across the table. We believe family psychotherapy is a major operation. Moreover, we are convinced that no team is powerful enough to "handle" the family. Manipulative psychotherapy may be sufficient in minor operations, but it does not seem effective in major operations. Although we do manipulate transference feelings, it is impossible to gain "control" of what goes on in a family. Furthermore, it is not possible at this stage of our knowledge to understand the family. We do not know enough, we are not clever enough, and God knows we are not mature enough, to be subjectively involved in a family and still be objectively perceptive of our own subjective involvement and its relationship to the family process. By implication, then, our task in family psychotherapy is to be available as a team to move as participants in the psychological and social patterns of this family, and thereby to aid the family unit in its autopsychological reparative process.

The concern about the dangers, pitfalls, and need for help in the major abdominal operation is something that often seems to distinguish these therapists from the conductors.

Whitaker (1965) describes as the heart of the therapeutic process the periodic almost acting-out by one therapist of the protected wishes of the family, such as their wish for a parent figure. Attention is called to this when he stops himself, or is rescued from it by his co-therapist, and the dynamics of the group that would have induced him to play this role are thus first illuminated and then frustrated. This is similar to a tactic described by Jungreis (1965) in which he threatened to give in and have himself adopted by the family in the place of their schizophrenic son—he considered being taken care of by the father, seduced by the sister. It was too much for them, and they began to change.

Whitaker sees himself as functioning in the role of activator. His intent is to invade the family as a person either by usurping one or another family member's place or by forcing a new mobility of roles within the family. He may link with father to help him become dominant, be seductive of mother and make father jealous, or organize an overt war between the generations. His constant use of co-therapist helps this objective and helps maintain his freedom to deny his involvement and serve as prototype for each member by moving back out of the family at will. He demands an exciting experience for himself to give them the courage to raise the family thermostat.

Wynne's group has written little about treatment other than his excellent paper on "Indications and Contraindications" referred to above, in which he writes about the effort to tailor the approach precisely to the family's problem. This concern does not easily lead to "structured admonitions about method," as Wynne says. Schaffer, Wynne, Day, Ryckoff, and Halperin (1962) described the inevitability of the therapist's becoming disturbingly involved in the family's confusion and distress, and noted that the involvement can be turned to therapeutic account. For the most part this group at the National Institute of Mental Health also prefers to work in co-therapist pairs. From what we have observed of Wynne and Harold Searles working together there, they count on each other very much for support as they register the confusion, blurring of focus, futility, anger, and so on, induced in them by the family system. Their struggle to be empathic with what is happening at the moment in the family, and to talk with family members about it with intuition. Candid self-revelation is followed, sometimes, by a demand that comes from the therapist's involvement: that the family clarify something to help him out of his confusion, for example, or fight openly because the therapist is oppressed by their deviousness.

For Nagy and Framo, the heart of the therapeutic undertaking, after the initial scuffling and settling down, is th uncovering of the distorted internal part-objects of the family members, especially the internalizations and projections of the parents within the current family. This is analyzed by examination of distorted pseudo-involvements between family members and transference projections onto therapists, and especially by the identification of stereotyped phasic interaction patterns (Boszormenyi-Nagy, 1965). Thus, a mother repeatedly provokes her daughter to misbehave and her husband to punish her, so that the mother can then both identify with the punished daughter and attack her husband for being too strict. She later sees the connection between this and her own punishing father, for whom she has not mourned, and when she revives to live again in the play between her husband and daughter. As we saw, this return to an arrested mourning for lost objects is also central in the method of Norman Paul.

One final note about the experience of the Philadelphia group: Jungreis (1965) remarks that in the midst of all the interpretation, most of their therapies with schizophrenics moved forward after the therapists had insisted on a particular strategic change in the family's activity. For example, they insisted that the family have more contact with friends. This is a particularly obvious abandonment of the reactor and commentator role, and there are others of a subtler sort that Jungreis describes. The family therapist, he points out, must be active and insistent, or he will not have an effect.

System Purists

This leads us to the final group of reactors, the system purists: Gerald Zuk, Jay Haley, and Don Jackson.[2] Jay Haley is a far-reaching

[2] A note on our sources for Jackson. There are, unfortunately, only three descriptions written by himself of Don Jackson's work with families (1962; Jackson and Weakland, 1961; Jackson and Yalom, 1963-64). The rest of our acquaintance with him was through lectures in which he presented tape fragments and anecdotes, a movie of a demonstration interview, and the excellent interview in Haley and Hoffman's book (1967). He also discussed two tapes with us during a visit.

student of other therapists' work. He does not call himself a "school" of family therapy, but we include him because his formulations about how family therapists behave have been very influential in the development of the field.

We group Zuk, Haley, and Jackson among the reactors but they are also very conscious activists of a certain kind. They each have a wary regard for the power of the family to maneuver, exclude, and otherwise subdue the therapist, and each is for that very reason interested in devising a strategy by which he can emerge as a covert leader. In this search for the pivot point where the therapist's influence can be applied, they seem sometimes cynical or disingenuously artful, and it is this attitude that offends their critics. They do not think, for example, that the truth of the unconscious shall make the family free. The curative agent is the paradoxical manipulation of power, so that the therapist lets the family seem to define the situation, but in the end it follows his covert lead. There is something chilly about the idea of the therapist as trickster, as presented in their theory, and we have found it hard to recognize in their warm and concerned work with actual families. We shall pay attention to their theories as well, however, because there is a power struggle involved in all therapy, and these workers have made a perspicacious attempt to define what it is.

The general basis for these theories is the communication concept of behavior first described by the group working with Gregory Bateson (Bateson et al.) in California in the 1950's. It has been more recently elaborated in three texts: Waltzlawick, Beavin, and Jackson's *The Pragmatics of Human Communication* (1967), and two papers by Jackson (1965a,b). The reader should really look at these words to see the system in its logical elegance. We present some of it here because the method of therapy is impossible to appreciate without it.

The communication theorists assume that human interaction is like a chess game: although an historical explanation of the position of the pieces can be found by looking at the moves that have been made from the start of the game, the crucial question is, nevertheless, what is the relationship of the pieces at present, what are the rules that govern the players, and what is the next move? They adopt a "black box" model of the mind, comparing it to an electronic instrument so complex that the investigator pragmatically leaves speculation about its inner workings to the psychoanalysts and concentrates instead on its input and output—what it is actually seen to do in response to certain stimuli.

Some axioms that govern the human communication game are, greatly abridged, as follows:

1. All behavior is communicative. It is impossible not to communicate, since even the refusal to send or receive messages is a comment on the relationship between people who are in contact.

2. Messages have "report" and "command" functions. Thus, "It's raining" is a report, but depending on the context, inflection, and relationship of speaker to hearer, it may also be a command to remember an umbrella.

3. Command messages define relationships. The command aspect of communication is the troublesome part, because it is the medium through which relationships are shaped, and in this process, ambiguity, misunderstanding, and duplicity are possible. Communicants are often unaware of commands they are giving, receiving, or obeying.

4. In families, command messages are patterned as rules. If two or more people are in relationship for a long time, the multiplicity of commands they exchange assumes a pattern from which rules for the relationship may be derived. These rules constrain and order the behavior of family members in patterns of mutual influence that have cybernetic properties. When anybody's behavior approaches the established limits (the governor, the setting of the homeostat) sanctions (negative feedback) are dealt out until the behavior is again within the acceptable range.

5. Change and stability. If a family wants to change the relationships, the regulating response of others that stabilizes the system by reducing change makes it appear that the "governor" or conservative element in the system resides in the person or persons resisting change. Children, especially adolescents, are natural initiators of change in families, and mothers in the family literature have acquired a reputation as the guardians of homeostasis. Jackson and others

present good evidence, however, that all members resist change by any of them.

6. Inability to change rules is system pathology. The system is considered pathological when the rules are set in such a way that there is no way of changing them. This happens when there are two rules that paradoxically negate each other: an operating rule and another rule-about-rules that denies it.

Thus, a family has an operating rule that says, "Mother decides when we go to bed" and another that says "None of us believe that anyone sets the rule for bedtime—we need sleep for our health." In such a family it is impossible to negotiate about bedtime without breaking one or both rules. No one can take a position outside the communication (become meta to it) and talk about it with the intent of changing it. Jackson calls attention to the pernicious effect of the invocation of values ("health") to conceal operating rules.

7. The family therapist must install himself as the metacommunicator, or change-maker of the family. He can help them set the stuck family homeostat in a new way. The techniques for this are tricky, and some will be described below. The general form of the process is this: he is the third person to whom two (or more) others present themselves with their "stuck," endlessly cycling system. They are playing a "game without end," and he must intervene to change the rules because they cannot get out of it.

Zuk (1966, 1967) describes a particular kind of change-maker with the phrase, "the go-between." The go-between mediates between two people in conflict, trying to change the relationship by selecting issues for the two to struggle or negotiate about. He sides judiciously with first one and then the other, and finally insists that the conflict have new rules, with himself as the referee.

Zuk says the therapist must take over from "pathological go-betweens" in the family. A pathological go-between is a person who avoids being one of the principals in a conflict by deflecting it to an innocent third party and then assuming the stance of mediator. The therapist must capture this position of go-between, because in any triangle, it is the most powerful spot. The therapist must avoid being the judge, since he is then a principal in a conflict, and the rest of the family who bring him the victim for sentence become pathological go-betweens or mediators.

Haley (1963) notes several strategies therapists use to establish themselves as the family's change-maker.

1. A therapist may engage in alternate siding to force a stalemated conflict to resolution.

2. He comments openly on the way he is being influenced, thus breaking the rule of silence that has maintained the paradoxical bind between the conflicting rules described above.

3. He presents a professional relationship to a conflicting pair, which is outside their rules, since they are unwilling to acknowledge any such complementary relationships between themselves.

4. He gives directives impossible to avoid, such as "express yourself."

5. He accents the positive aspect of otherwise conflictual relations, which presents the family with a paradoxical situation in which their efforts to fight are redefined.

6. He encourages and labels behavior that is already going on at the direction of the family's rule-keepers, thus making the momentary leadership of the group explicit and breaking its power.

A quotation from Haley (1963) on marital therapy will illustrate some of these points.

As an example of a typical problem, a couple can be continually fighting, and if the therapist directs them to go home and keep the peace this will doubtfully happen. However, if he directs the couple to go home and have a fight, the fight will be a different kind when it happens. This difference may reside only in the fact that they are now fighting at the direction of someone else, or the therapist may have relabeled their fighting in such a way that it is a different kind. For example, a husband might say that they fight continually because his wife constantly nags. The wife might say they fight because the husband does not understand her and never does what she asks. The therapist can relabel or redefine their fighting in a variety of ways: he might suggest that they are not fighting effectively because they are not expressing what is really on their minds; he can suggest that their fighting is a way of gaining an emotional response from each other and they both need that response; he might say that when they begin to feel closer to each other they panic and have a fight; or he can suggest that they fight because inside themselves is the feeling that they do deserve a happy marriage. With a new label upon their fighting, and directed to go home and have a fight, the couple will find their conflict redefined in such a way that it is difficult for them to continue in their usual pattern. They are particularly tempted toward more peace at home if the therapist says they must fight, and that they must for certain reasons that they do not like. The couple can only disprove him by fighting less.

Note that in this view, the precision of the explanatory insight is unimportant; it is the precision of the intervention of relabeling the fighting and thus taking control of it that counts.

In the writing and work of Don Jackson, the intervention of the therapist in the family's communication system, its balance of power reaches its most inventive heights. These prescriptions or tasks sometimes have the quality of magic rituals, the carrying out of which seem to deliver the family from a curse; in fact they are carefully tuned to a clinical picture of repetitive interaction patterns, which the therapist sees but keeps to himself. "Our experience with this kind of repetitive pattern is that pointing it out does little good. However its meaning, intent, and focus can be shifted by the therapist's intervention" (Jackson and Weakland, 1961).

Before making his move, however, the therapist constructs his position with the family carefully. He starts with a frame of minimal ground rules that are optimistic, forward-looking, minimizing the "sickness" of the identified patient, and leaving the therapist free to make any response: "Free, to me, is not to give them so much direction that they know how to use it against you" (Haley and Hoffman, 1967). Jackson was particularly expert at increasing this freedom by remaining casually "one-down," avoiding struggles by changing the subject, and emphasizing the positive and appealing aspect of the most disturbing communications. Saying such things as "I can't get too upset about that," he showed himself proof against the family's attempts to bind him and each other with the threat of disaster.

In this context, the intervention is the one requirement he made of them, and it was delivered as a serious prescription that they must follow in order to improve. The instruction, like the pathology it counteracts, has two levels: the obvious one in which it appears to be something not very difficult to do, and the interpersonal one where it shifts the meaning of a symptom, or the balance of power. There is, of course, also the third "meta" feature of the intervention—that it comes from the therapist and therefore cannot be irresponsible or "crazy" like the symptoms.

Though they should be read in the original papers to be appreciated, we present here a few examples of Jackson's interventions.

1. The "well" sibling of a schizophrenic is instructed to be more of a problem to the family. This has the effect of revealing how much of a problem he already is, and changing the "sickness" image of the patient (Jackson and Weakland, 1961).

2. The depressed widow of an alcoholic who has moved in on her married son is instructed to have a drink with him every evening, no matter how much she dislikes it (Jackson, 1962).

3. A family is told to have a fight before they go on vacation so that they can enjoy the trip (Jackson, 1967).

4. A delinquent stepson who will not mind his new stepmother is asked to agree that no matter how angry she gets he will pay no attention to her orders—indeed she is not give any. He will be disciplined only by his father (Films).

Note that in each case the prescription is to continue or exaggerate something already going on—"prescribe the symptom"—so that it comes under therapeutic control. Often the symptom will disappear before the task is carried out—it seems to wilt under intention.

Looking back on the methods of the reactors, it appears that they gain entry and control in a way that is more indirect and complex than that of the conductors. They may, for example, impose the relationship between co-therapists on the family system, and that is a more difficult "foreign object" for the family system to deal with, since the cotherapist's relationship is part of the larger social system, and has some other "incorruptible" qualities, such as freedom to change, or a feedback loop of its own, etc. Or they may, like Jackson, impose their control in such a way that it is "unbeatable" because it is a paradoxical instruction. The point we want to make is that it is, in some crucial sense, control.

Moves and Tactics

Having completed a survey of the various presentations of self with which therapists approach families, let us turn to what happens next— what the therapists attempt to deliver. We will select here some moves and tactics that are of special interest to us, since a comprehensive survey would be much too long.

Membership

As we said in the introduction, one of the most powerful moves the family therapist makes is to concern himself with the family as a group. This concern does not require, however, that everyone in the group participate equally. The extremes of membership policy may be seen by contrasting the work of Ross Speck with that of Murray Bowen (1966). Speck sees "networks"—the extended family and friends of the nuclear family that contained the original patient—about thirty or forty people in the same room. Bowen may see one person at a time, but in this retrospect he is the exception among family therapists, and one which "proves the rule." Even when he is seeing an unmarried person living in a different city from his family, he starts by teaching about the operation of family systems. Then, he says, "time is devoted to the part this one plays in the family system and some fundamentals of 'differentiating an I' out of the 'we-ness' of the family system, and to changing the part that 'self' plays in the system. It is necessary that [he] arrange fairly frequent visits home with [his family]... these [sessions] are similar to supervisory hours with young family therapists. When this 'differentiating one' begins to change, the family will get negative or reject, at which time it is absolutely necessary that [he] keep in contact with the family in spite of the rejection."

The point we want to make is that family therapy's attention is devoted towards a family group, but the whole group does not need to be present at any one time. The interest and allegiance of the therapist is towards the whole family, and this interest and allegiance defines family therapy, not the number of people in the room, or the membership of the meeting. The membership of the meeting is, rather, something that the therapist manipulates for particular ends.

One approach to the problem of membership, prevalent in Philadelphia and in Wynne's group at NIMH, is to set up a fairly inclusive membership of the nuclear family and continue with it for some time. The practice is sometimes not to meet if one member is absent and to treat this as a resistance, called the "absent member phenomenon" by Sonne, Speck, and Jungreis (1965). This is a safe form of projection, resistances being attributed by those present to the absent member. Such meetings of the whole family may represent the first time they have talked together in any healthy self-awareness of themselves as a bounded group with real relationships and responsibility for their feelings toward each other. Thus, the inclusiveness of the membership has a therapeutic value in itself, as well as supplying information to the therapists not obtainable otherwise.

Others, such as Satir and Bowen, deal with only the marital pair in the main part of the therapy, seeing the whole family mainly to get some information about how the children are expressing the marital conflict or attempting to mediate it. Bowen, Jackson, and others have observed that even when the family presents their very disturbed child as their symptom, if the therapist makes it clear that he is going to work with the parents, and the children should go on about their business, the symptoms of the child usually stop at an early stage of the treatment and the trouble in the family does shift to the marital relationship.

There are many rationales for focusing on the marriage, e.g., Bowen's three-generation hypothesis, Shapiro's delineation hypothesis, Bowen's idea of "the triadic one," Satir's child-as-a-messenger, and Tharp's role theories. They might be summarized by the idea that if the illness is in the family group, one should start with the group's leadership, and the parents are, in Satir's phrase, the architects of the family, the place where the main authority ought to be and where the lasting sexual and contractual bond should be cemented. Bowen (1966) and Haley (1967) carry this further in pointing out that the therapist-husband-wife group forms an essential triangle in which the therapist replaces the child or grandparent, and this puts the therapist in the position of the projected external others who have formed pathological triangles with these parents. The ideas of these authors about triangles seem to us of great theoretical importance and practical power, and are worth more attention than we can give them here.

In the remainder of this paper we will compare various approaches to the problem of bringing the family to a new experience of their behavior. Framo describes this as the "middle phase" of family therapy, following the initial phase of confrontation and accommodation between family and therapist. It is the phase during which the essential work is done. For Framo, in the ideal case, that is the "understanding and working through . . . the introjects of the parents, so that the parents can see and experience how those difficulties manifested in the present family system have emerged from their unconscious attempts to perpetuate or master old conflicts arising from their families of origin" (1965). This is often called "insight." We note at the outset, however, that there is an argument about what this means, which turns around some of the most fundamental attitudes in the field.

In its most superficial form, the question is, "Do the family members acquire what a classical psychoanalytic writer could call insight in such forms as, say, a resolution of the Oedipus complex?" In another form the question is the one posed by Ackerman (1965) in answer to the challenge, "Is family therapy a 'deep' therapy or is it merely support, suggestion, and environmental manipulation?" He concluded that family therapy was as "deep" as any other because there are no issues or emotions with which the family therapist does not deal in as intense and decisive a way as a psychoanalyst does.

There is an exchange about this in the pages of *Family Process*, where Haley reviewed Nagy and Framo's book (1966). The book, the review, and Haley's reply to a letter of ours about the review (1967) are worth reading, because they summarize a major division within the field. This is a conflict between the psychoanalytically oriented and the communication theory-oriented partisans, and although much of it is a mere conflict of loyalties, it reflects a genuine dilemma: What should one search for in working with a family? Should one just get them to change what they are doing, on the assumption that a stuck pattern of behavior is the cause of their trouble? Or should one seek a further cause in the subjective experiences of the individual members, which, unchanged, will re-establish the troubled patterns? Haley says the answer to this question lies not in argument but in experience, but there has been no evaluation of our experience that would tell us the answer.

Looking back on it, we think, on the one hand, that the argument was a trade union dispute about whether analysts or non-analysts do better family therapy, with the implied further question of whether classical individual psychodynamics is an important part of the training of family therapists. On the other hand, politics aside, the question is even more critical and more difficult to answer as we now see it: it is not a matter of the family's gaining insight but rather of the therapist's doing so. Understanding what is happening in the family, the therapist may interpret it, or arrange a task in the light of it, or reflect on it to himself in the hope that knowing it he will in some empathic way be more useful to the family. Now the question is, does an understanding of the individual motivations put him in a better position to do any of those things? We think so, but until someone does an outcome study of family therapy with that question in mind, our answer will have to be based on personal experience.

Let us proceed by examining several forms of insight or redefinition of experience as they appear in different schemes of therapy.

Insight: Projective Identification

Let us look first at one kind of insightful formulation that turns up so frequently and in so many forms in the writings of different authors that it is worth our particular attention. There is a whole group of phenomena that Klein (1964, 1963) in individual terms calls projective identification. By this is meant a splitting off of a disavowed part of the self and projecting it onto others. Lyman Wynne points out that in families this results in what he calls a "trading of dissociations . . . there is an intricate network of perceptions about others and dissociations about oneself in which each person 'locates' the totality of a particular quality of feeling in another family member. Each person receives one or more of the others in a starkly negative preambivalent light and experiences himself in a similar but reciprocal fashion, with the same abhorred quality in himself held dissociated out of his awareness. . . . The fixed view that each person has of the other is unconsciously exchanged for a fixed view of himself by the other. The interlocking result is similar to the system of reciprocal role expectations that sociologists have described in intrafamilial relationships. However, here I refer to a system or organization of deeply unconscious processes, an organization that provides a means for each individual to cope with otherwise intolerable ideas and feelings . . ." (Wynne, 1961).

Zinner and Shapiro refer to a "defensive delineation" of the adolescent by his parents so that the adolescent is seen as having qualities that the parent denies in himself. The adolescent, allowing unconsciously for the parents' need to preserve their self-esteem through this denial, shapes his developing identity to fit the parents' delineation.

Nagy (Boszormenyi-Nagy, 1965) locates the prototypes of many such defensively dissociated and projected part-objects in the parents' experience with their own parents, thus completing a three-generation picture of this phenomenon that often results in the illness of the developing adolescent of the third generation. He and Paul describe their versions of the therapeutic working-through of the parents' attachment to or denial of the grandparents' objects as essential to the therapy. Other workers confront the families with these phenomena in other ways, but their importance is widely recognized. Bowen sends his patients on trips to visit their parents and grandparents and in-laws to "establish a person-to-person relationship" with each of them and to interview them about their family tree. We suspect that one of the effects he achieves is the realignment of fundamental-object relations in which those kinfolk serve as distorted part-object representations.

Insight: The Active Experience

We next come to something we think is of central importance in family therapy, not only because it unites so many seemingly disparate practices, but because it is crucial to our own thinking about what we do. This is the idea that the altered perception of family relationships that is the therapeutic sine qua non results from an active or participatory or nonverbally immediate experience within the therapeutic hour.

First, as we have said before, the mere act of getting the family members together for treatment implies that something more immediate is going to happen than would be possible if they met separately to talk about one another. They will have more an encounter than a discussion, more drama than narrative, more theater than literature, and the therapist, to keep himself clear about what is happening, will use more the juxtapositions of the stage director than the explications of the literature. Kantor and Hoffman (1966) have compared family therapy with Brechtian theater, emphasizing in each the liberating effect of seeing an interaction both as a participant and an observer. The whole subject of nonverbal communication in family therapy was also discussed in a symposium of Zwerling, Scheflen, Jackson, Ackerman, Nagy, and others (1967), which is well worth reading.

Having worked with this sort of medium for a while, some family therapists and people allied with them have carried this natural property of the family interview further into an interesting array of practices and conceptions. We will conclude our review by putting this array together before the reader. In several ways, these workers seem to be saying that the words people use—the verbal channel of communication—is at best a recapitulation and affirmation of something primarily experienced in a nonverbal mode, and is at worst a means of disguising what is happening between people. Family therapy provides a means of getting at what is happening, not as in individual therapy, by explicating the contradictions, connotations, and hidden levels of the verbal channel, but by bringing the happening into awareness, manipulating or highlighting its features: seating arrangements, gestures, interruption patterns, tones of voice, laughter, and what Zuk calls "silencing strategies" (1965); and visual (symbolic) artifacts, whether natural (such as clothing and posture), or intentionally unfamiliar (such as pictures drawn by the family or the reviewing of videotapes of the interaction).

Arranging the Experience

We present next, in no particular order, examples of what therapists are doing that seem to come under this heading. These techniques are more fully described in *The Book of Family Therapy* (Bodin and Ferber, 1972; Bodin, 1972).

The Use of Tapes

Norman Paul (1966), Alger and Hogan (1968), and many others have written of the practice of using audio or videotapes of the interaction to give families a chance to observe "from the outside" what is happening. The response to this is often a revelation to the family members because the things attended to are manners of influencing the interaction, especially ones of voice and facial expressions, which are extremely powerful, and of which the members are unaware. These experiences often have the force of an interpretation, without, as Alger points out, the accusatory mode, "Let me tell you what you are doing." Paul uses a videotape from another family to put the family before him in an empathic mood from which he wants them to proceed. This is, literally, the use of theater in therapy.

Role-Playing

We have described the use of role-playing and role-reversal as a means of developing sympathy between family members, but further to our purpose, we notice that it has the effect of making people aware of their nonverbal influencing behavior, since they cannot play the part of another without noticing the discrepancy between what they say as the other person and how they say it.

Family Art Therapy

Gentry Harris and Hanna Yaxa-Kwiatkowska (1967), successfully treated a family with a schizophrenic son by getting them to draw pictures at the beginning of sessions and in connection with impasses. The pictures avoided the level of verbal exchange and mystification that Harris says is the schizophrenic's weakest area, and produced enduring images that the therapists and other members could recognize and validate. In accounting for the importance of the visual iconic level, Harris uses an explanation that is similar to Minuchin's explanation of his own technique.

Tasks

The assignment of tasks, either within the hour or outside it, is a frequent practice in family therapy. We mentioned Jackson's "interventions" above. Any such intervention, if the members agree together to try it, even as an experiment, has the effect of putting them in a new behavior pattern with one another and of shaking up their present methods of mutual control. We mention here several kinds of tasks that seem to have a particular relevance to this.

Virginia Satir assigns tasks that make it impossible to continue the old forms of mutually disturbing action. She has a blaming couple sit for five minutes a day, holding hands, facing each other and talking only of their own feelings, or she has an adolescent daughter communicate with her mother only in writing for a week (1967). Her insistence that the family adopt her own form of completely unambiguous clarity makes it difficult to shade communication with provocative inflection.

Bowen asks a husband to estimate with accuracy, "What percent of the time are you successful in getting your wife to blow up at you?" "How many times in the last two months have you succeeded in turning away when she starts trying to get you worked up? Is that getting better as compared with six months ago?" He carries on a cool, precise, interrogation in these terms, changing from one member of the family to another, asking the next, "What is your reaction to that?" thus keeping the whole communication system under his control. No family member responds directly to another in his interviews. The thing to note here is that it is impossible under these circumstances to perform any of the dramatic projective provocations on which family trouble depends—one is induced by the questions and the format to think of the problems as a rational one, full of percentages and frequencies.

We referred above to Bowen's techniques of sending family members on trips to visit parents and in-laws. He instructs them not to "do the same old two-step that you always did when you visited before, but try to get a real person-to-person relationship with them." He suggests settling disputes that have lain dormant for years, and often assigns the specific task of interviewing the relatives about their kin, to get an accurate family history, and find out what the ancestors were really like. The unaccustomed visit, the unusual task, and the emphasis on changing the old dance-step are all ingredients of an experience designed to put the "patient" in benevolent control of the interaction by which he felt victimized before. The taking of the family history is a task with a surprisingly powerful effect on the mutual understanding of both parties: it must be tried to be appreciated.

The authors (Ferber and Beels, 1970) use an interview format that is the opposite of Bowen's but which has the same objective of changing interaction patterns. We ask the family to interact directly while we observe, and wait until we see a sequence being repeated over again that we recognize clearly. We may play a tape back to demonstrate the general form of the sequence we are referring to. We then show them the gestures and postures they use to keep the sequence going. We ask them to try changing these monitoring signals to see if they can stop the sequence. The kind of sequence we are talking about is very similar to the phasic interaction pattern described by Nagy and we suspect it is what he is interfering with by interpreting that pattern to the family.

Minuchin

Salvador Minuchin's system of treatment is one of the most carefully described in the literature, and we think his description bears a remarkable similarity to what he actually does. He says, in *Families of* the Slums (Minuchin, Montalvo, Guerney, Rosman and Shumer, 1967), that his method is designed especially for lower-class families with an impaired ability to use abstraction and delay: the benefits of the verbal channel of communication. In the light of the comparisons we are making here, it seems to us that his method is not special to that group, but rather describes something of much more general importance.

Minuchin gets the family to talk briefly until he identifies a central theme of concern, and has an impression of who is most involved with it. He also makes a guess at what interrupting, silencing, or diverting maneuvers are keeping the discussion from going further. He then assigns the family the task of continuing with their work on this issue, but he gives them specific stage directions, as described above: he rearranges the seating, blocks an interruption pattern, or takes a family member behind the screen where they can observe but not interfere. He paces the family by adopting their mood and tempo at the beginning and then changes it through his example. His questions are in an enactive mode: not, "Why doesn't your mother talk to you?" but, "See if you can get your mother to talk to you."

Watching Nathan Ackerman interview a family was always a vivid experience, and sometimes a confusing one because of the strong feelings the observers had about what he does. Sometimes he seemed by turns intrusive, insulting, seductive, and autocratic. Families and therapists who consulted with him, however, generally found that he focused on important problems of theirs with speed and accuracy, and with liberating effect. If we examine what he did in terms of the comparisons we have been making, we may understand this discrepancy. Ackerman worked rapidly, paying careful attention from the beginning of the interview to the nonverbal relationship messages of the family members (Sherman, Ackerman, Sherman and Mitchell, 1965). He engaged them directly with his own posture and gaze, and talked to them about the ways in which they were covering themselves from him with their behavior. He spent some time clearing away what he called "hypocrisy" in the verbal channel, and tried to read what the family was telling him directly. He offered himself directly also, not only in the above way, but sometimes as the interview proceeded, his hand, the seat next to him, his lap to the children, his handkerchief to the crying mother, a cigarette to a woman who said, "My husband won't let me smoke," his tie to a young man who felt he was not respectable enough. He worked quite literally as a catalyst. By his availability and what he called "tickling the defenses," he opened interpersonal balances in the family members that then became available for interaction between them. Once that interaction was going, he interpreted it in terms of sex, aggression, dependency, and so on; a language that he then shared with the family.

In addition to the comparison with other forms of nonverbal work, it was almost impossible for an observer listening to the words to be in tune with what was going on in an interview with Ackerman. Later interpretations may sound just intrusive. It is hard to imagine that the family was prepared for it through any change of their defensive position. We suspect also that one of the reasons Ackerman had so few successful imitators was that the personal use he made of the nonverbal material was almost impossible to teach.

Conclusion: Not the Danger but the Dance

Looking back now, we are in a position to see some patterns that have been running through our explorations.

We saw that the family therapist works with the family as a natural group whose members or acts are related to each other in a mutually responsive way so that we may describe them as a system, and that the conceptual difficulties of viewing them so come from our arbitrary (cultural) assumption that the individual is the "natural" unit, rather than the group or system. Once we are committed to the idea that the group is the unit to be addressed, we can ask the following questions:

Is there a way of viewing the individual-in-the-group that bridges the gap in terms of two different approaches? Norman Paul seeks to define a person in the family as suffering unexpressed grief in a way the others have not recognized, and his task is to get everyone to validate that unique experience through empathy, to see the person as a sufferer and not a manipulator of the others. This is the opposite of the position taken by Jay Haley, who would see the family as a group of people trying to influence one another by various means, including suffering.

The group's organization is one level in a hierarchy of open system; the individual's organization is another. Seen this way, the dichotomy between the group and individual foci is a false one, and both are always true: behavior that is expressive for the individual is communicative for the group. For momentary tactical purposes, one may use the approach either of Haley or of Paul, but the richness of the practice of family therapy consists for us in seeing the interlocking of these systems.

The family maintains what Jackson and Haley call its homeostatic organization—and troubled or "stuck" families seem to be particularly concerned with doing so. How does the therapist introduce himself as the new element in the system? He must do so in such a way as to avoid becoming a regulated part of the system, or he will produce no change. The therapists we have called conductors enter with their own values and rules of communication strongly in the fore, and in certain crucial respects they take charge. The reactors are more gradual and indirect, but they also eventually require that a key element in the system move the way they want it to.

How is this done? Our review of the delivery or discovery of the altered sense of family relations suggests that it is somehow encoded in a level of communication or perception other than the verbal-abstract. In fact, one of family therapy's reasons-for-being is the experience of some of the early workers that for some people "understanding" or "insight" did not "take"; it was not acted upon unless it was somehow brought forth in the midst of the family.

This suggests that both the family's regulatory system—benign and pathological—and the experience which is the key to change in that system are embodied in a communication system that is only fully developed and clear when the family are in each other's presence. When they are not present to one another, but represented by verbal or symbolic traces, the system is much more difficult to read, for both them and the therapist. In this way the "conjoint" and "nonverbal" aspects of family therapy are clearly related.

Let us conclude with one scientific and one clinical citation, each of which seems to make this point in a different way.

Albert Scheflen (1964, 1966, 1968), in examining motion pictures of family therapy and other groups, has worked out in some detail a description of repetitive patterns of body positions and shifts, gestures, gazes, paralanguage, etc. These patterns occur in relatively unvarying sequences, enacted over and over again. When the "meaning of these patterns is analyzed by careful recording of their contexts as beginning, ending, or changing other sequences, they reveal a rather simple grammar of command to, or comment on, relationships in the group." Scheflen suggests that this is how, often outside awareness, the relationships in a group are defined and controlled. Further, the sequences are themselves organized into larger sequences he calls "programs." These programs are participated in by several members, as if they were dances, and have a cyclic, automatic quality familiar to both family therapists and watchers of family therapy.

John Bell, in an address we have quoted before (1963), described his experience with trying to provide families with insight into their behavior. He began in the old way, relating history to motivation and thus "interpreting" the motives of family members. He also tried a sort of positive approach to family dynamics, saying they must have "good reasons" for the things they do. All this fell flat. He then turned to making rather neutral observations of nonverbal communications between family members. He found that at last they did not feel he was accusing or taking sides, and that, having noted what was going on, they provided their own "insight." This agrees with our experience.

Bell went on to suggest that his experience tells us something about "emotional insight." He said, "As a consequence of this technique and the reactions that occur, we have revised our theories about the relationship of insight to action. We have concluded that in part we have seen the sequence entirely the wrong way about. Whereas formerly we assumed that insight ultimately led to action by some unknown process, we have now concluded that action may be seen more fruitfully as coming before insight. Action has the primacy rather than insight. That is, insight and action do not take place in some parallel psychological processes, but insight is within the mainstream of action. What is even more important, we have concluded that the action that leads to insight takes place with, for, and because of others—that it is a process of, and in, a social group rather than of and especially within an isolated individual. Insight has the appearance of identity with an individual because it is abstracted from the social action, and, as all thinking, is seen from the point of view of a person who is acting. Thus, to call it intellectual insight is indeed appropriate. But we have traditionally overlooked the social matrix within which this occurs, forgetting that the individual is never independent, a fact that becomes especially obvious when the whole family group is before us."

What interests us is the way in which these observations again suggest that the action in a group is primary, the declarations of the members secondary. Especially in families, we are doing a dance, listening only rarely to what we say to one another. Family therapy is the bringing together of the family and the therapist in order to experience that pattern of action and change it.

Beginning and Experienced Family Therapists

JAY HALEY

Probably no person in the arena of family study is better qualified to attempt an article of the kind that follows than Jay Haley. Haley's career has been practically synonymous with the development of the field of family study. He has been a catalytic agent virtually since its inception. He seems always to have been where the action was, and nearly as often he has created that action.

Originally a member of Gregory Bateson's ethnological research team on communication, Haley began doing therapy with schizophrenics and their families as early as 1953. He was a coauthor of the research group's landmark article on the "double-bind" (Bateson et al., 1956) and subsequently he joined Don Jackson at the Mental Research Institute, where he and Jackson in 1962 founded the journal Family Process *on which Haley served as first editor. The journal has been crucial to the growth of the field of family studies; it provided a much-needed forum for the publication, discussion, and dissemination of materials and ideas in the clinical realm of family studies. Its particular emphasis has been on family mental health and family therapy, but it has been, in addition, the basic cohering and shaping force in the family field. While still editor of* Family Process *Haley moved his base of operations from California to Philadelphia, where in 1967 he joined Salvador Minuchin at the Philadelphia Child Guidance Clinic. There he has been instrumental in transforming a traditional child-clinical setting into a family-oriented treatment facility, a transformation which many expect will set national trends as a model for the updating of child guidance clinics across the country.*

Haley's impact on the entire field of family study has been profound. As editor of Family Process *his functions were broad; as much as anyone he took an active role as historian, shaper, and shepherd for the field, and interpreter of family work to other disciplines, as well as to its own participants. He was politically aware of the fledgling status of the new ideology of family in the field of mental health, and he attempted to nurture it by navigating a course for the area that would allow its aspiring identity to emerge and solidify without its being subsumed into, or co-opted by, more established disciplines or therapeutic outlooks. Thus, more than occasionally he struck a militant posture toward traditional psychiatric positions, eschewing those concepts and terminology that derived from the psychology of individuals emphasizing the internal dynamics of patients. Instead he promoted the search for newer relevant concepts— variables and a language appropriate to small groups. He adopted an environmentalistic approach akin to the "black box" thinking of American behaviorists, and sought to put distance between the Freudianism that dominated the American mental health scene and the new family orientation. While attempting to draw a solid boundary demarcating these two domains, he was at the same time influential in opening new territories and in making more permeable the boundaries with other traditions, encouraging reciprocity between the experimentally oriented research tradition of empirical psychology and family work. Similarly, he invited exchange with social learning theorists, and promoted open and public discussion of various innovative therapies (e.g., Milton Erickson's "uncommon therapy"—see Haley, 1973). Haley has not shied from controversy, and has frequently gener-*

ated active debate, inducing strong emotional reactions in others. Yet, remarkably enough, he has perpetrated all these things with careful and insightful attention to the overriding conceptual and political issues involved. There is possibly no one else with as solid a grasp and as complete an overview of the major influences and determinants in the field.

Haley's paper, which follows, introduces the reader to the field from an entirely different perspective than did the preceding article by Beels and Ferber. While they dealt primarily with personalities and clinical styles, Haley is concerned primarily with issues—with differentiating concepts and perspectives. jhe attempts to delineate those things that are fresh and distinctive about family therapy. He does so by subjectively cross-cutting the sixteen or more schools described by Beels and Ferber, and extracting from them some common outlooks, concerns, and themes. The result is a topic-by-topic comparison of the conceptual premises and operating frames of beginning and experienced family therapists.

His points are made decisively enough. Experienced family clinicians seek "change" not "insight," focus on the "present" not the "past," include themselves in diagnostic formulations and not just the family, assess situations (crises) rather than "types" of families, fit the treatment approach to the problem and not the family to the method. In sum, the comparative method, hinged as it is on pointed contrasts, gives the reader much assistance in assessing where he himself may stand in relation to some of the fundamental parameters of family therapy.

The clinicians who began to do family therapy in the early days were primarily people who had been trained in the ideology and practice of individual therapy. Whatever their professions, their focus had been upon how to change a person. As they began to discover the new problem of how to change a family, each of them developed a unique approach. Often their approaches differed because the therapists were innovating on their own and did not know that other people were doing family therapy. As a result, a number of "schools" of family therapy have developed which

*have their students and their followers. New approaches continue
to develop as clinicians take up family therapy in different parts
of the country and develop unique ways of working.*

Comparing different family therapists is difficult because they differ
markedly in their techniques of intervening into families. However, as
family therapists have gained experience they seem to have developed a
shared body of premises about human problems and the nature of
change, despite working with families in quite different ways. Some
family therapists, particularly those imbedded in academic psychiatry
or the tight professional organizations of a large city, do not seem to
change their views with experience. Yet most family therapists have
gone through a transitional process, sharing now a basic shift in their
ideas which comes about from the experience of working with families.
One can assume that the shift in ideas comes from exposure to families,
since often family therapists shift to a common view even though they
have not been exposed to the work of other family therapists. At about
the time a family therapist passes his two-hundredth family, he usually
changes his perspective markedly and finds himself in a different
conceptual world from the one in which he was trained. One way to
describe this shift in thinking about therapy is to describe where a
family therapist begins and where he ends. Contrasting the premises of
a beginning family therapist with those of a person who has had many
years of experience can help clarify what is new in the family therapy
field.

Method vs. Orientation

The beginning family therapist tends to see family therapy as a
method of treatment—one more procedure in a therapist's armamentarium. As he gains experience, the therapist begins to view family
therapy not as a method but as a new orientation to the arena of human
problems. This conceptual difference has practical results. For
example, when asked what the indications and contraindications for

Reprinted from A. Ferber, M. Mendelsohn, and A. Napier (eds.), *The Book of Family Therapy*,
Jason Aronson, Inc., New York, 1972, pp. 155-167.

family therapy are, the beginning family therapist will attempt to answer the question. The more experienced family therapist will appear puzzled, since he finds himself defining any kind of therapy as a way of intervening into a family. Having shifted his unit of diagnosis and treatment from the single person to the processes between people, he defines psychopathology as a relationship problem. He cannot say this person should receive individual therapy and this person family therapy, because he views individual therapy as one way of intervening into a family. The therapist who treats a wife may be dealing with the woman's fantasies, fears, hopes, and so on, but by seeing the wife and not seeing the husband the therapist is intervening into a marriage in a particular way. While the family therapist might interview only the wife, it would be with the assumption that her problem involves the context in which she lives, and that the treatment must change that context. Even if drugs are given to only one person, the family therapist does not see this as drug therapy in the usual sense; it is the introduction of a drug into a family system with consequent concern about who is being labelled as the patient, or as the one who is at fault.

Whether family therapy is seen as an orientation or a method is similar to the contrasting approaches in psychiatry forty years ago when psychodynamic theory developed. It was not a question of deciding whether the neurological method of treatment or the psychodynamic method of treatment was indicated; the issue was the difference in conceptual framework between the two approaches, because they each represented a different way of thinking about the psychiatric problem. Similarly, one cannot contrast individual and family therapy as two different methods; they are not comparable at that level.

Color the Patient Dark

The beginning family therapist tends to emphasize the individual patient as the focus of treatment, seeing the remainder of the family as a stress factor. He may even do a style of family treatment which is called interviewing the patient in the presence of his family. The more experienced family therapist gives family members more equal weight, and struggles to find a better term than "patient" for the family member who is chosen to be it. Terms are used such as "the identified patient," or "the supposed patient," or the "person in pain," or the "person expressing the symptom," and so on. While the beginner tends to see a particular individual as a container of psychopathology or a person with a low stress threshold, the more experienced therapist sees the family system as needing some individual to express the psychopathology of the system. For example, if a child is agitated and is quieted, the mother will become agitated, and if mother and child are quieted, then the father or a sibling will become agitated because the system is such that this is necessary.

In a similar way, the beginner tends to see the family as a collection of persons who are describable with the past language about individuals. He sees relationships as a product, a projection, of intrapsychic life. For example, he will emphasize how a wife is being mistreated by a sadistic husband: the husband is expressing his aggression and the wife is satisfying her masochistic needs. The more experienced family therapist sees intrapsychic process as a product of the relationship situation. He will describe such a couple as involved in a game in which they must both contribute behavior which keeps the distressing sequence going. In a similar manner the beginner often sees the child as a victim of the parents' strife or as a scapegoat, while the more experienced therapist will view the child as a contributor and an essential part of a continuing sequence of events among all the people involved. As a result of this difference, the beginning therapist tends to intervene to get a person to shift his ideas or behavior, while the more experienced therapist intervenes to change a sequence of behavior involving several people. For example, in an interview the father might interrogate the child, while the child weakly protests. At a certain point the mother will come to the support of the child and attack the father. The father will back down and apologize. After a while, the sequence will begin again and repeat itself. The more experienced family therapist will see the sequence occur, and when it starts again he will intervene. He might do so while the father is interrogating the child, just before the mother comes in to attack the father, or just before the father backs down when the mother attacks. His goal is to give the sequence a different outcome, and he may or may not point out to the family the nature of the sequence. The beginning family therapist will tend to see the behavior in smaller units, and he will usually intervene to interpret to the father that he should not behave as he is doing, or to help him understand why. He will be thinking about the father's motivations and possibly his history with his own father, rather than about the current sequence that is happening in the family.

Where Is History?

The beginner at work seems much more interested in history than is the experienced family therapist. The beginner tends to see the family as a collection of individuals who have introjected their pasts, and the therapeutic problem is lifting the weight of this "programming" out of their inner space. The more experienced family therapist learns to see the present situation as the major causal factor and the process which must be changed. He inquires about the past only when he cannot understand the present, and thinks the family can discuss the present more easily if it is framed as something from the past. Assuming that what is happening now has been happening for a long time, the therapeutic problem is what is happening now. At times a therapist may emphasize the past when he is trying to define a time when the family members were enjoying each other more; that is a way of labeling the current problem as a temporary upset as well as clarifying a goal of the therapy. In general, the more experienced the family therapist, the more he assumes that a current problem must be currently reinforced if it is continuing to exist.

What Is Diagnosis?

The beginner tends to put more emphasis upon diagnosing and evaluating the family problem. He prefers to gather information before intervening. He tends to use diagnostic ideas in an individual language, and tries to define, in as much detail as possible, the family dynamics. The more experienced family therapists frequently work with minimal information. Since they view the opening session as important to the ultimate therapeutic outcome, particularly when it is time of family crisis, they wish to intervene as rapidly as possible to bring about change. Therefore they intervene as soon as they have some grasp of what is going on. Many think careful diagnosis helps the therapist more than the family. Such therapists spend much less time talking about differences in family dynamics than they do in talking about ways they have intervened to bring about changes. Generally they like to end the first therapy session with some therapeutic aim accomplished so that the family has gained something from the immediate encounter and knows what the therapeutic experience will be like. This more action-oriented point of view does not mean that family therapy is always brief therapy.

Whether treatment is short or long term, most experienced therapists share an awareness of how much can be accomplished with active intervention at a time a family is in crisis and unstable. Some experienced family therapists say that if adolescent schizophrenia is not resolved with family treatment, the case has been mishandled. However, they are referring to family treatment at the time of acute onset of the family crisis and not after the adolescent has been hospitalized and the family has been stabilized. When hospitalization is involved, family treatment can become interminable because each improvement leads to renewed hospitalization.

The more experienced therapist looks upon long-term therapy as necessary to accomplish particular ends, rather than as meritorious in itself. It is also typical of more experienced therapists to see change as occurring in discontinuous steps, and they "peg" a change when they get one so that the family continues to the next stage of development and does not slip back. Instead of the desultory movement one sees in the beginner's family treatment, the more experienced therapists tend toward a developmental improvement in the family.

Is the Therapist Part of the Diagnosis?

A major difference between the beginner and the more advanced family therapist is the beginner tends to leave himself out of the diagnosis. He describes the family as a set of problems independent of him, much as the individual therapist used to describe the patient's production in therapy as if they were independent of the therapist. The more experienced therapist includes himself in the description of a family. For example, the beginner will say that the family members are hostile to each other; the more experienced therapist will say the family members are showing me how hostile they are to each other. This is not a minor distinction. As a consequence, the more experienced person does not think of the family as separate from the context of treatment, and he includes himself in that context. He will consider, for example, whether the particular difficulty he sees between a husband and wife is created by the way he is dealing with the couple. A vignette can illustrate this: An experienced therapist was supervising a beginner by listening to a tape recording, and after five minutes of the first session with a family the supervisor said that several minutes had passed and the therapist had not yet made a therapeutic intervention. The beginner replied that it was an evaluation interview and he was gathering information about the family problem. The experienced supervisor replied, "Evaluation of a family is how the family responds to your therapeutic interventions." This example illustrates how much more rapidly the experienced person prefers to work, and how he sees the family problem in terms of how the family responds to him. With such a view there are not different diagnostic categories of families, but different families in different treatment contexts. An important aspect of this more contextual view is the realization by experienced therapists that they must take not only the family into account, including the extended kin who always influence a problem, but also the other helping professionals who might be involved. In some cases, a family has been divided, with each fragmented part being treated by some professional, often without knowledge of each other. The record might be a family in California which had fourteen professional helpers involved. To deal with the family unit, the experienced therapist finds he must also deal with the wider treatment morass, or the total ecological system. The beginner tends to see the other helpers as irrelevant until he gains experience.

In relation to diagnosis, a sharp difference between the beginner and the experienced therapist is the concern with using a diagnosis that defines a solvable problem. Unless the diagnosis indicates a program for bringing about change, it is considered irrelevant by the more experienced therapist. The usual psychiatric categories are seldom used—not only because they apply only to individuals but because they have nothing to do with therapy. The beginner tends to think of diagnosis as something that exists independent of him, and he must adapt to it. For example, a family therapist who was both a beginner and worked in the conservative network of a large city posed a question to a more experienced family therapist from the provinces. She said she was working with a family, and after three diagnostic sessions she concluded with the family that the problem was a symbiotic tie between the mother and her daughter that was unresolvable. She asked, "What would you do with this problem?" The experienced therapist replied that he would never let that be the problem, and she did not understand what he meant. She saw the problem not as one which she defined but one which was independent of her and she must struggle with it even though she had defined it as unsolvable. Given the same family, the experienced therapist might have concluded with the family that when the daughter began to move toward independence the mother became upset and there was open conflict between mother and father. This diagnosis indicates ways of bringing about change, and by the third session an experienced therapist would already have begun a change.

The Positive View

Beginning family therapists tend to feel that it is helpful to the family to bring out their underlying feelings and attitudes no matter how destructive these might be. He interprets to family members how they are responding to each other and expressing their hostility through body movement, and so on. The more experienced family therapist has less enthusiasm for the idea that interpreting feelings and attitudes brings about change. In particular, he does not feel it is helpful to confront family members with how much they hate one another. Instead, he tends to interpret destructive behavior in some positive way—as a protective act, for example. His premise is that the problem is not to make explicit underlying hostility, but to resolve the difficulties that are causing the hostility. Therefore, the more experienced therapist is less free with his interpretations, except when using them tactically to persuade family members to behave differently. At times the beginner can seem to be torturing a family by forcing them to concede their unsavory feelings about each other. The more experienced therapist feels this is a waste of time and not therapeutic. For example, a beginning family therapist working with the family of a schizophrenic saw the mother pat her son on the behind. He could not overlook this opportunity to help her by interpreting this behavior as the product of an incestuous desire, with the result that mother and son avoided each other even more than previously. A more experienced family therapist would probably have congratulated the mother on being able to show some affection toward her son. Although more experienced family therapists do not emphasize negative aspects of family living, they are quite willing to bring out conflicts if they are necessary to break up a particular pattern.

The Problem Is the Method

The beginning family therapist, like the beginner in any field, would like to have a method that fits everyone who comes in the door. Being uncertain, he would like to have a set of procedures to follow each time. The more experienced family therapist tends to feel that any set procedure is a handicap; each family is a special problem which might require any one of several different approaches. Instead of fitting the family to a method, the experienced therapist tries to devise a way of working that varies with the particular problem before him. In contrast, the beginning family therapist tends to set rules which include seeing the whole family for a set length of time at regular, set intervals. Most family therapists began by working with whole family groups, but as they gained experience they found this too restricting. With experience, they shifted to seeing the whole group sometimes to get a total portrait of the situation, but then they interviewed people singly, then the marital pair, or the siblings, or any combination that seemed appropriate for the problem involved. Some family therapists are now

trying out multiple family as well as network therapy, where not only
the family but friends and neighbors are brought into treatment
sessions.

Equal Participation

When the experienced family therapist interviews the whole family
group together, he puts special emphasis upon getting all the members
to participate. If a family member is not speaking, the therapist tries to
involve him. Often the experienced family therapist will turn the family
upon each other so they talk together rather than to him, and when he
does this he likes them all to talk. The beginner often focuses upon one
person at a time, and tends to have the family members talk largely to
him rather than to each other.

The Factional Struggles

When a therapist intervenes into a family, whether he interviews one
person or the whole family group, he is caught up in the struggle of
family factions. The beginner tends to side with some part of the
family—often he sides with the child against the victimizing parents,
or, if he is older, he may side with the parents against the child. In
marital struggles, the beginner is likely to find himself siding with one
spouse against another. The more experienced family therapist
assumes quite flatly that if he sides with one part of a family against
another there will be a poor therapeutic outcome. This is particularly
so if he joins one faction while denying he is doing so, which often
happens if the therapist still responds to one person as the "patient" but
is trying not to. When experienced therapists take sides, they state this
explicitly and announce that they are doing so, usually defining it as
temporary.

Live Supervision

Since the vital part of bringing about change is the way the therapist
behaves in a session, the experienced person wants to know what is

happening when he is supervising a trainee. The beginner tends to think in terms of traditional supervision, where he makes notes about what happened and carries them to his supervisor for discussion. This kind of delayed, content-oriented conversation arouses little enthusiasm in the experienced family therapist. He prefers to watch the trainee in a session through a one-way mirror or on a videotape replay, so he can give instructions in the technique of interviewing, which is the essence of therapy. More commonly, the experienced family therapist does live supervision by watching a session and calling in on the phone to suggest changes, calling the trainee out to discuss what is happening, or entering himself to guide the session. In this way a trainee learns to do what should be done at the moment something happens, not when the opportunity to change his form of intervention is long passed.

Emphasis Upon Outcome

The beginning family therapist tends to emphasize what is going on in the family; the more experienced therapist emphasizes what therapeutic results are happening in terms of quite specific goals. Some beginners become so fascinated with family history, family dynamics, and the complex interchanges in the family that they lose sight of the goals of treatment. Often the beginner will seem to define the goal as proper behavior by the family—if the family members are expressing their feelings, revealing their attitudes, and the therapist is making sound interpretations, then therapy is successful. The more experienced family therapist emphasizes whether the family is changing, and he shifts his approach if it is not. This does not mean that family therapists scientifically evaluate the outcome of their therapy, but it does mean that outcome is a constant focus as well as a subject of conversation among experienced family therapists. They talk about family dynamics largely in relation to family change. The willingness of therapists to shift their approach if it is not working is one of the factors that makes family therapy difficult to describe as a method. Not only will a particular therapist's approach vary from family to family, but his way of working evolves into new innovations from year to year as he attempts to produce better results.

What family therapists most have in common they also share with a number of behavioral scientists in the world today: there is an increasing awareness that psychiatric problems are social problems which involve the total ecological system. There is a concern with, and an attempt to change, what happens with the family, its interlocking systems, and the social institutions in which it is embedded. The fragmentation of the individual, or the family, into parts is being abandoned. There is a growing consensus that a new ecological framework defines problems in new ways, and calls for new ways in

The Open Door: A Structural Approach to a Family with an Anorectic Child

HARRY APONTE, A.C.S.W.

LYNN HOFFMAN, M.S.W.

The article that follows treats the reader to a great many understandings about what family therapists do, how they do it, how they construe their efforts, and the ways in which they seek to teach by presenting a verbatim account of a clinical interview conducted by Salvador Minuchin, with interpretive commentary and analysis supplied by the authors. The paper may be read with various foci in mind and at a number of complementary conceptual levels.

At one level it may be taken as explicit, concrete, clinical documentation for all that the two preceding articles describe. Minuchin employs the tactics of stage direction, fosters inactive modes rather than insight, takes sides in an effort to rearrange familial splits and alignments, challenges by indirection, advances positive constructions and avoids frontal criticism, maintains high levels of therapist activity, redefines problems and symptoms, shows no interest in history, endeavors to manipulate the outcome of typical interaction sequences, and trades on paradox. Of course he does more as well, and the reader might find it of interest to try and trace the ways in which principles described by Beels and Ferber or Haley are translated into action by Minuchin.

At another level the paper is a vivid portrayal of "structural" family therapy in action. This form of family treatment, which has come into being under Minuchin's leadership at the Philadelphia Child Guidance Clinic, is conceptually more articulated than most family approaches described to date (Minuchin, 1974). Its relative maturity may be attributed to the blending of conceptual premises that it has achieved. Elements of ecology, and ethology (territory, private space, geography) are interwoven with the ideational legacies of such family research pioneers as Lidz (notions of generational and sex boundaries, their maintenance and violation), Wynne (notions of pseudo-mutuality, and amorphousness in role definition), Bowen (undifferentiated ego mass), as well as with more recently developed tactical procedures (benevolent manipulation, exaggeration of the symptom, relabeling, prescribing the symptom, etc.).

At a third level, this article may be used as springboard to the burgeoning literature on the effectiveness of family therapy in the treatment of psychophysiological disorders in children—anorexia nervosa, brittle diabetes, intractable asthma (Baker and Barcai, 1970; Combrink-Graham, 1973; Liebman, Minuchin, and Baker, 1974a, 1974b, 1974c; Minuchin, 1970, 1971; Minuchin, Baker, Rosman, Liebman, Milman, and Todd, 1973). In this regard it should be noted that Minuchin's one session involvement with the "C" family described below is but a small piece of an ongoing clinical research project aimed at assisting clinicians in the pursuit of new paradigms for the treatment of these perplexing and all too often fatal syndromes. It is certainly hoped that the detailed accounting of a family therapy session, as given here, will promote that effort.

A fourth level for approaching the paper is to view it as typifying the "systems" orientation to understanding familial events and the role of the "symptom" in family dynamics. This approach is unabashedly "configurational" (Henry, 1971; Lake, 1974; Bermann, 1973)—that is, it employs high-order inferences as a means of unifying diverse observations in many, if not most, areas of a family's life. As will be elaborated later in the editors' introductions to the Weakland, Fisch, Watzlawick, and Bodin, and the Stuart articles in this volume, it is the configurational emphasis that separates most family therapists from behavior modifiers. For the moment, one need merely recognize that Minuchin, Aponte, and Hoffman are, like their colleagues in the field, much given to "configurational" thinking. Thus, in considering the anorectic symptom focal to the session recounted on the pages that follow, they state:

Aponte: *Not eating has been a way of trying to keep some kind of territory for herself, some area she can control.*

Minuchin: *You see . . . there are so few areas in which this family has, um, problems of control, or rules, that it is very difficult for Laura to fight the battle for growing up. She doesn't have—it's almost like if Laura is creating her own arena, at least, around food.*

It is this configurational view that also would appear to underlie the often employed technical intervention of family therapists— namely relabeling the symptom. This tack is legitimized because according to this orientation the "symptom" is at most not all that it seems, and at the least considerably more than it appears to be. The idea of symbolic expression in symptom formation has been transposed from psychoanalytic thinking about the individual to the dynamics of family conflict but with a seminal difference: family clinicians are unconcerned with providing the family "insight" into the "true" meaning of the symptom. Rather, their concern is for "relabeling" it in such a way that behavioral change might result. This relabeling might have nothing to do with "insight."

A fifth level for reading this selection could be that the format of the paper represents an instructional modality frequently employed by family therapists—the use of videotapes of family treatment sessions with step-by-step analyses by family therapy experts and the participation of less experienced family clinicians who are in attendance for learning purposes. As such, it highlights the ready public display that family therapists are willing to make of their work. Concomitantly, it illustrates the openness this group has encouraged since the pre-1962 inhibitions dissipated. The diverse elements combined in Minuchin's "structural" family treatment approach epitomizes one of many potential kinds of payoff this openness can yield. It is worth emphasizing that the field's utilization of audiovisual techniques is not limited to training purposes, but is with increasing frequency being extended to families in treatment. Audiovisual playback aimed at self-confrontation becomes a more and more feasible method as the cost of needed equipment declines (Alger, 1969, 1972, 1974; Bodin, 1972).

This paper is not without its problems. Its authors do tend to treat disconfirming evidence—i.e., evidence not consistent with the "configurational hypothesis"—as annoying variance that can be lightly dismissed or totally ignored. It seems also that Aponte and Hoffman tend to "relabel" the therapist's errors as virtues having intentionality, a procedure that could be viewed as consistent with the family therapist's efforts at avoiding confrontational criticism. Nonetheless, it is a procedure that can promote a view of the family therapist as a godlike, inviolate creature; a vulnerability that is not limited to family therapy.

On balance, the paper that follows remains useful, in numerous ways, for the reader. It not only permits entree to the field of family study at many levels, but additionally lays out all the data for its reader, inviting the reader's participation in meaningful, manifold ways—we are invited to place ourselves, in turn, in the shoes of each family member, of each therapist, of each expert observer, or each "naive" student. Beyond this, the reader is free to do his own post-hoc conjecturing. There is little more one can ask the printed word to do on behalf of informing what family therapy is about at the present time.

The R. Family came to the Philadelphia Child Guidance Clinic after Laura, age 14, was hospitalized for excessive weight loss. She was observed in Children's Hospital of Philadelphia for five days, and nothing was found to be medically wrong with her. During the previous summer she had started dieting, and while away at camp had continued to lose weight. The apparent reason was that she had started camp late and found it hard to get accepted by the other children. Later it turned out that she was also upset because her father had made a financial sacrifice to send her to camp. However, even after she came home, she continued to lose weight, until she got down to 62 pounds. It was at this point that the family became alarmed and sought medical help. After the girl left the hospital, the family was referred to the project on Families of Children with Psychosomatic Problems, a study examining the applicability of family therapy techniques to children with psychosomatic disorders that is being conducted by Dr. Salvador Minuchin and other staff members of the Philadelphia Child Guidance Clinic in conjunction with Dr. Lester Baker of Children's Hospital.

The transcript that follows is an excerpted version of the first videotaped interview with the family after they started treatment at the Clinic. Present were Mr. and Mrs. R.; Laura; Jill, age 12; and Steven, age 10. The therapists were Dr. Minuchin and Dr. Barragan. Dr. Minuchin came in as a consultant for the first interview and did not see the family after that. Dr. Barragan continued to work with them over a period of three months.

The following commentary was made by playing back the video-tape of the condensed family interview to an experienced therapist, Mr. Aponte, in the presence of a group of less experienced therapists and observers. The resulting conversation was then taped and transcribed. The data does not include the afterthoughts of the therapists who conducted the interview. The authors made their own interpretation of the material, though drawing upon a set of concepts shared with the therapists. In the finished version of the commentary, the question-answer form was retained, although edited and condensed, in the interest of retaining some of the flavor of

Reprinted with permission from *Family Process,* Vol. 12, No. 1 (1973), pp. 1-44. Copyright © 1973 by *Family Process.*

puzzlement, inquiry and speculation that even experienced clinicians feel in the presence of such a complex entity as a family with a symptomatic member.

The interview itself was chosen because it possessed intrinsic clarity and interest as a document about a certain kind of family and a certain kind of therapy. The bias of the therapists, as the reader will see, is a structural one. Very little is done with content, only with form. Metaphors of territory—boundaries, fences, walls, doors, chairs, cracks, and windows—come up constantly. The family uses them to express its most characteristic relationship configurations, and the therapist, in attempting to change these configurations, also uses them. Instead of "diagnosing" an "illness" in one family member and attempting to "cure" it, he sees his job as one of discerning the "structure" of the family—its recurrent, systemic patterns of interaction—and finding out how the symptom relates to that structure. His business is then to shift the structure about in such a way that the symptom, which is presumably keeping it together, will not be needed.

For this session, a strategy was planned beforehand: the family was to be served lunch right in the room. Up to the point food was brought in, the therapist was exploring the structure of the family, its most persistent dyads, triads and larger groupings, and at the same time trying to rebuild them. These efforts were directed toward freeing a pathway for the identified patient so that she could eat. How this was accomplished will be described in the commentary.

The transcript begins about twenty minutes after the interview started. The participants were seated in a semi-circle in the following order: Steve, Laura, Jill, Mrs. R., Mr. R., Dr. Minuchin, Dr. Barragan.

The family was first asked about the problem that brought them in. They explained it as Laura's inability to eat and her sudden weight loss. Dr. Minuchin then explored the history of the family. It turned out that when the girls were little, it was Laura who was on the heavy side but otherwise they were so alike they were treated as twins. However, at age six Laura was having school problems and was taken to a psychologist. The psychologist felt that there was nothing basically wrong with her but that her parents were pulling in different directions in regard to the children, and Laura was caught in the middle. In any case, after the one visit to the psychologist, Laura's difficulties disappeared.

Dr. Minuchin then asked the parents what it was about Laura that bothered them most. Mr. R. said it was only the weight loss and her thin appearance. Mrs. R. said she was upset because Laura never seemed happy.

Dr. Minuchin next tried to find out how disagreements were handled in the family. He was told that there were no disagreements. Pursuing the subject, he asked Laura if she had any criticisms, anything she would like changed. She could think of nothing except that it irritated her when her parents urged her to eat. Dr. Minuchin asked Laura and her parents to re-enact the sequence that generally took place when she refused to eat. As the transcript begins, he is requesting Laura to pretend that her father is trying to get her to eat and to answer him the way she would do at home.

Dr. M: (to Laura) When you get annoyed, how do you express your annoyance? What do you say to dad? Say it now, the way you said it then.

Laura: (to father) No I don't want any food. (pause)

Dr. M: What do you do then? (pause) Dad, what do you do then, when she says that?

Mr. R: I naturally insist.

Dr. M: You insist. Insist now. I want to know how it works.

Mr. R: (overlapping) Well, this is more present than recent. This is not. . .

Dr. M: O.K., yeah, O.K. Make believe that it's happening.

Mr. R: O.K. (to Laura) I'm going downstairs, Laura. Do you want something?

Laura: No.

Mr. R: Nothing at all, no snitch, something, a piece of fruit?

Laura: Nothing. I don't want anything.

Mr. R: A little ice cream?

Laura: No.

Mr. R: O.K.

Dr. M: (to Laura) Do the same thing with mom. How does it go? (to Mrs. R) It goes also with you similar?

Laura: Uh . . .

Dr. M: (indicating that Laura should continue) O.K.

Mr. R: (to Laura) Try it at the dinner table with Connie. I think that might be better because (to Mrs. R) you don't go down as often as I do. (laughter)

Laura: (laughs) My mother stops, and she stops after once. My father he keeps going on and on.

Mrs. R: I see it annoys her, so I stop. You know, if I say to her, "Do you want a little broccoli?" or "You want something?" She'll say, "No," and I'll just leave it at that because I know it does irritate her. (pause)

Mr. R: This all took place from the 23rd of August till now—after the camp season.

Dr. M: So we have five weeks that you have been having fasting problems.

Mr. R: I guess if you want to term it as that, yeah, (buzz on intercom) it all is the appearance.

Observers: What is the therapist doing here?

Aponte: He's starting with the struggle over food. First he asks: How does it go between dad and Laura? Then: How does it go between mother and Laura? He finds out that the real struggle is between Laura and her father. Mother insists a little but then stops. So he knows that this father-daughter relationship is a particularly charged one, and he assumes that this must have something to do with the girl's refusal to eat.

O: In other words, it's a way she's fighting the father.

A: Well, that would be simplifying it. Minuchin is trying to find out the ways the relationship in this family are structured. In most families where a child has a symptom, you find that he is in a special kind of triangle with his parents. One parent will be intensely involved with him. The other parent will be more peripheral. This usually happens when the parents are in a conflict but can't openly admit it or resolve it. The child brings them together by giving them a focus for their concern.

O: So the father and daughter are the two who are the most intensely involved.

A: Yes, they are the over-involved dyad. Mother is more peripheral.

O: Was Laura diagnosed as a real anorectic?

A: No, and this is what made it hard for the family to deal with. Laura was an accomplished calorie-counter and she didn't refuse to eat, she just wouldn't eat anything that would put weight on her.

O: So Minuchin interprets this as the family having "fasting problems."

A: Sure. Laura's not eating is a behavior that affects everyone in the family, because eating is a community endeavor.

O: The father seems a little puzzled by this way of putting it. He says, "If you want to call it that."

A: Well, he's not quite ready to accept the symptom as something family-wide.

Dr. M: (alluding to the buzz) I know what this is. Yeah, let me tell what we will do now. We will have lunch.

Dr. B: (speaking on the intercom) All right, wait a minute, let me ask Sal.

Dr. M: Yeah it's my secretary, Joanne. (to Dr. B) She should wait a minute.

Dr. B: She should wait. All right. (over intercom) Joanne, he says for you to wait.

Dr. M: My secretary will come now and we will order lunch and we will have lunch here all together. I want to know how the family eats. O.K.? Joanne, come here. So we will find out—instead of making believe, we'll just make it. (Mrs. C enters) This is Joanne Crooms.

Mrs. C: Hello.

Dr. M: (introducing parents) Mr. R, Mrs. R.

Mrs. C: How do you do.

Mrs. R: Hello.

Dr. M: Jill, Laura, Steve.

Mrs. C: O.K.

Dr. M: O.K. (to Mrs. R) What do you want to eat? You are the one that, ah—(indicating Mrs. C) she will be our waitress.

Mrs. C: All right, we can order sandwiches from Chop. You know, they have the usual hamburgers and things like that. O.K.?

Mr. R: Let's start with Steve here. All right, Steve, what do you want for lunch?

Steve: I don't know what I want.

Mr. R: Want a menu?

Steve: (laughing, shakes head)

Mr. R: Whatever you want to eat is O.K.

Steve: Do they have hot dogs?

Mrs. C: Sure.

Steve: I'll have a hot dog.

Mrs. C: With relish? (Steve shakes head) No, just plain. O.K.?

Mrs. R: Do you want mustard? (Steve nods yes) And a little mustard.

Mrs. C: (to Steve) Want soda or milk?

Steve: Do you have 7-Up?

Mrs. C: Do I have what?

Steve: 7-Up.

Mrs. C: I think we can arrange that.

Mrs. R: That's it?

Mrs. C: Okay. Laura?

Laura: Umm . . . chicken salad on toast and a 7-Up. (laughter, long pause. Mr. R turns to Jill.)

Jill: Umm—hot dogs and 7-Up.

Mrs. C: O.K., same thing on your hot dog? Mustard? Mrs. R?

Mrs. R: I think I'll have the Chop Shop Special.

Mrs. C: O.K.

Mrs. R: And coffee.

Dr. M: What is the Chop Special?

Mrs. R: A cheeseburger with bacon.

Mr. R: Bacon, lettuce, tomato on toast.

Mrs. C: Dr. Minuchin?

Dr. M: The Chop Special.

Mrs. C: How about you, Mariano?

Dr. B: I'll have a steak sandwich.

Mrs. C: And Mr. and Mrs. R, what would you like to drink?
Mr. R: A coke would be fine.
Mrs. C: I beg your pardon?
Mr. R: A coke.
Mrs. C: Mariano?
Dr. B: I'll have a coffee.
Mrs. C: And I know what you take, Dr. Minuchin.
Dr. M: No, I will change. I want 7-Up. I will join the family. (noise and mumbling)
Mrs. R: Regular on the coffee.
Mrs. C: Fine.

A: See, Minuchin is ordering his lunch very selectively. He ordered the sandwich in collaboration with mother.
O: Why is that?
A: Because it's the father who is the aggressive one, the one who handles the controls in the family. So Minuchin backs the weaker party, the mother.
O: He's also pushing out the over-involved parent.
A: Right. And what he does next is to order 7-Up in collaboration with the kids. He's with the mother on the food and with the children on the drinks. The father's really on the outside now.
O: Why does he say, "I will join the family," when he orders the 7-Up? He's only joining a part of the family.
A: Well, he isn't going to say that directly. You see, the family has told him very explicitly that this is a family that agrees, and he doesn't want to contradict them. But by aligning himself with various people in the matter of the food, he is already setting up battle lines. He is splitting the family into camps and setting the stage for disagreement.

Dr. M: O.K., why don't we—it will take us probably fifteen minutes till we get lunch, so let me explore a little more about disagreements in this family. You know what you have told me about the family is that it is a family that agrees, ah, you have ways of agreeing that seem to work. Ah, and apparently (to Laura) you have sometimes—

you are able to disagree with daddy and mommy and it's mostly around food. And then (to parents) it was also you disagreed—ah, father insists a bit, but then he gives in, and mom just gets a little bit scared of you and she agrees also. So—how is it with you and Jill? When you disagree with Dad?

Jill: I—when dad and I disagree, I usually just talk it over with him or something.

A: What Minuchin is doing is to accept that framework of agreement the family offers and within it go to the kids and ask about the disagreements. He repeats what he found out about the disagreement between Laura and her parents, then turns to Jill. He's aligning himself with the children, separating them from the parents. And he's doing another thing. By going to the other daughter, he's lining up an ally for the identified patient. Laura can't openly differ with her father, but Jill can. He's building up the army.

Dr. M: What kind of disagreement do you have with dad?

Jill: I don't know—well—sometimes I will go into his room and he will ask me to comb his hair or something (Mrs. R laughs), and he asks me to, and I'll say, "No, I'm tired," and he'll say, "Oh, just a little bit," or something like that, and I'll say, "No," and . . .

Dr. M: And then what happens?

Jill: Nothing. I don't get that mad, but . . .

Dr. M: You leave?

Jill: Well, no—well, I don't know, can't think of anything right now (inaudible words) if he asks me something like that, I just say, "No, I'm too tired."

Dr. M: And what happens then?

Jill: Nothing.

Dr. M: Is it about the hair that he's talking? (crosses the room and musses up Jill's hair so that it covers her face). Is it like that it happens? (everybody laughing) Let's see if we can do something. (continuing to muss up Jill's hair, Mrs. R and Jill still laughing) O.K. Now what happens? Is like that, um . . .?

Jill: But, ah, he tells me to get the hair out of my face.

Dr. M: (to Mr. R) Can you do it, Dave?

Mr. R: What's that? (Dr. M points to Jill.)

Jill: No, he doesn't do anything, just says, "Get the hair out of your face."

Mr. R: (to Dr. M) You misunderstand. Ah, we have a thing in the family that . . .

Dr. M: Do—act this thing now with her.

Mr. R: Ah, well, I think you misunderstood originally about the hair. We will be in my bedroom, which we all congregate in . . .

Jill: (laughing) Oh, no!

Mr. R: . . . and I have a robe on and we're all—before bedtime—and we're watching TV, and all the kids will come into our room, and on the bed, and so on, and we're watching TV. Even though they have TV's in their rooms, we all congregate in our bedroom.

Dr. M: How many TV's do you have in the house?

Jill: Six.

Dr. M: (astounded) Six TV's! (Jill laughs) (to Dr. B) That's the new model of the American family, one TV more than the number of people. (everybody laughs, Dr. B and Mr. R both talking, inaudible)

Dr. M: So what happens then?

Mr. R: We congregate in our bedroom and, ah, Steve he will cuddle and scratch my back, and I'll scratch his back (Jill laughs), and, ah, mommy, she'll be doing something—ah, Laura, she'll be . . .

Dr. M: Do you scratch her back also?

Mr. R: Whose?

Dr. M: Mom's.

Mr. R: Mommy? No. (laughter and more talking)

Mrs. R: (laughing) I don't like my back scratched.

Mr. R: So, ah, I'll maybe massage the girls, their legs, and Laura—I haven't done too much for Laura lately. You see, it's been reversed, ah, Laura always enjoyed combing my hair, or if I get dandruff and don't have time to wash my head, some of the girls will take the comb or brush and brush my hair out . . .

Jill: That's what I was talking about.

Mr. R: . . . and, ah, like last night, ah, I guess my head itched or something and I was too lazy to wash my head at that time so I'd say, "Jill, comb my hair out because I think I have a little dandruff. . ."

Dr. M.: (pointing to Jill) She's . . . ?

Jill: Yes.

Mrs. R: (simultaneously) Yes.

Dr. M: Oh!

Mr. R: (to Dr. M) That's why I thought you misunderstood. So we were cuddling, we always seem to cuddle, and so on, in our room, or I'll go to their room and cuddle, or what have you . . .

Dr. M: Oh.

Mr. R: . . . so, ah, we're always—sombody doing something for one another; yet in their minds, they're always doing for me. I'm not doing for them, they're always doing for me. If daddy will get a cramp in his left leg, "Ooh, Jill, I got a cramp in my left leg, ah, work it out for me." So Jill will put a little alcohol on it, or hot cloth, and she'll massage me, so on and so forth. And I'll do it for Steve, I'll do a little something for Jill. Laura—in the last year or so, ah, we seem not to have done too much for one another, have we? (Jill turns and looks at Laura, who does not respond.)

Dr. M: (to Laura) No?

Laura: (softly) No.

Mr. R: Laura used to comb my hair, rub my back, and so on.

Dr. M: Ah, dad is describing a lot of nurturance going between him and the kids. (to Mrs. R) Where are you when all that happens.

Mrs. R: Well, sometimes I'm just laying on the bed, you know, watching TV with them. Ah, sometimes she'll just want her back rubbed, I'll rub her back—he'll want his back rubbed. Other times I'll just be sitting on the bed, either doing needlepoint, or maybe I'll be going down to the kitchen and emptying the dishwasher, or heating up coffee or . . .

Dr. M: Daddy's a cuddler, he likes to cuddle, he likes the children to cuddle with him . . .

Mrs. R: Yeah, he enjoys that at night.

Dr. M: (to Mrs. R) What about you, are you a cuddler?

Mrs R: Am I? Ah, not as much as him I guess. Ah—I don't know, I'm always busy in the house it seems. I don't know, I'm folding clothes and putting them away, or . . .

Dr. M: Do you like to cuddle with him?

Mrs. R: Yeah. (laughing)

Dr. M: But he likes to cuddle with the kids?

Mr. R: Yeah.

Dr. M: Sometimes would you like him to drop the kids, and be with you alone?

Mrs. R: No! No, absolutely not. (shaking her head)

Dr. M: There are times in which you say to the kids, O.K. kids, it's the end of—you leave because it is now time for . . .

Mrs. R: No.

Dr. M: . . . time for me and daddy alone?

Mrs. R: Never! Never!

Dr. M: The door of your room, do you leave it open during the evening?

Mrs. R: Always.

Dr. M: Always open. (to Dr. B) I would expect that.

Mrs. R: In fact, I don't even like the children to close theirs, which they very rarely do for sleeping—they do for (inaudible words).

A: This is a revealing scene. Minuchin asks about the disagreements, Jill starts to tell him, and what he gets is a complete denial from the father that there are any. Or not a denial, but the father turns it around so that what comes out is a narration about family closeness. At the same time, all the information about the relationships spills out.

O: At the beginning, why did Minuchin go over to rumple Jill's hair?

A: He thought she meant father criticized her for having messy hair. This is a technique Minuchin often uses. He will ask people to re-enact an issue: "Play it back for me."

O: The father says Minuchin doesn't understand.

A: That's true, he didn't. Jill meant that sometimes father asks her to comb his hair, and she doesn't want to. But the father, in setting Minuchin straight, takes the issue of disagreement and buries it. Instead, you get this idyllic picture of how everybody cuddles on the bed before bedtime, and father gets the children to comb his hair, and look for dandruff in it, and massage his legs.

O: You could interpret this as a symbolic statement about incest. Apparently Laura and her father did this a lot before she began to mature. He says now they don't do it so much, so it has turned into a kind of avoidance. But he is still very involved with her.

O: You could also interpret it structurally. There is no boundary between this father and his kids. Family therapists who think along structural lines see a "healthy" family as one where there are clear demarcations between the generations. Within each generation level, there will be strong ties, as well as adequate differentiation between individuals. The pair that is the governing unit, the parents, have to have a particularly strong alliance and clearly worked-out areas of functioning special to each. The same is true of children, except that differentiation with them should be appropriate to age. Of course, much of this will be defined by the culture, but the general rule of clear generation lines and adequate differentiation will hold. In an "unhealthy" family, or what Minuchin sometimes calls an "enmeshed" family, there is a blurring of the generation lines and a lack of differentiation. So this is what the therapist goes for. Here Minuchin has been working to get the two girls in an alliance against the father, so he gets them separated off from dad. Now dad has brought them back to cuddle with him again.

O: Why does Minuchin then turn to the mother?

A: It's another attempt to differentiate. He asks her, "Where are you when all this happens?" And she admits she doesn't take part. She isn't a cuddler.

O: The tone of that "Never," when Minuchin asks whether she ever tries to be alone with her husband, is so final, so sharp.

A: Sure. She's an accomplice in this. You see, what you often find in these enmeshed families is that there is a hiatus between mother and father but it isn't openly expressed. Mother depends on the kids to console dad for the fact that she isn't very interested in him. In asking the two parents whether they ever get to be alone together, Minuchin is putting a circle around the dyad. At the same time, he finds out about the hidden crack between husband and wife.

O: He uses a very concrete image: "Do you keep your bedroom door open?"

A: You'll see that this is no empty metaphor. One of the big issues that comes out in this session is the family's use of household space to express relationships. Nobody is allowed to shut his door. But this is really an issue about intangible borders between people.

Dr. M: Laura do you close the door of your bedroom?
Laura: No.
Dr. M: Don't you want sometimes . . .
Laura: No.
Dr. M: . . . to close—don't you want some privacy sometimes?
Laura: No—yeah, I do, but I get enough leaving the door open.
Dr. M: And are there some times when you want the door closed?
Laura: Yeah, when I do my homework.
Dr. M: And then you do close it?
Laura: Yeah, I close it when I do my homework.
Dr. M: And then if Jill wants to enter into your room, does she knock?
Laura: Sometimes she does, and sometimes she doesn't.
Dr. M: If mom wants to enter your room, does she knock?
Laura: Yes.
Dr. M: What about dad?
Laura: Yeah. (pause) Yes, he knocks.
Dr. M: You are doubting.
Laura: Sometimes he does, and sometimes he doesn't.
Dr. M: Do you like him to knock at your door before he enters?
Laura: (softly) Yes.
Dr. M: Hm?
Laura: (louder) Yes.
Dr. M: Hm?
Laura: (louder) Yes.
Dr. M: When daddy enters without knocking, do you tell him that you would like him to knock?
Laura: No.
Dr. M: Why not?
Laura: I don't know.
Dr. M: Hm?
Laura: Sometimes I do, and sometimes I don't.

Dr. M: Would it bother him if you tell him that you would like him to knock?

Laura: Pardon?

Dr. M: Would it bother dad to tell him that you want the door closed, and you want him to knock at the door?

Laura: I don't think so.

Dr. M: Are you certain of that? Hm?

Laura: (laughing) I don't know.

Dr. M: I have the feeling that it would bother dad because he is a very loving kind of dad that likes always to have people respond to him and he responds to people—to the children certainly. That's my hunch—ask him. Ask dad if it will bother him if you asked him to knock at your door instead of entering. (Mrs. R and Jill both look sharply at Laura, then look back at Mr. R.)

Laura: (to Mr. R) Would it bother you if I asked you to knock at my door?

Mr. R: Probably so (Laura laughs), because I like to have all the doors open. (Jill and Mrs. R exchange looks.)

Dr. M: (to Jill, who is trying to break in) Hm?

Mr. R: I'm always hollering about keeping the doors open.

Dr. M: (mixing up Laura with Jill) What did you say Laura?

Jill: I was gonna say that he usually doesn't knock because he has just opened the door because he doesn't like the doors closed.

Dr. M: (to Jill) And do you want sometimes for your door to be closed?

Jill: Yes.

Dr. M: And do you close it?

Jill: Yes, and then he tells me to keep it open.

Dr. M: And what do you say then?

Jill: I say, "Well, I'm changing."

Mr. R: Fine, then the door can be closed.

Dr. M: (to Jill) You want to have some—do you have a room of your own?

Jill: Yes.

Dr. M: (to Laura) And You?

Laura: Yes.

Dr. M: (to Steve) And you?

Steve: Yes.

Dr. M: Do you have your door closed sometime?

Steve: (nods yes)

Dr. M: When?

Steve: Well, when I'm getting undressed.

Dr. M: Does mom enter into your room without knocking?

Steve: (long pause) Sometimes.

Dr. M: And what do you say to her?

Steve: I don't know.

A: You notice that Minuchin makes a switch here. He goes from the parents shutting their door against the kids, to Laura shutting her door against her father. And what he is doing here is to facilitate her claim for privacy.

O: Is that why he moves so carefully?

A: Sure. First he gets an admission from the girl that she sometimes does like her door closed. Then he asks if at those times her sister and mother respect her privacy enough to knock, and she says yes. Only then does he ask her about her father: "Do you ask him to knock?"

O: He gets a very doubtful answer.

A: And he respects her reasons. He's trying to help her to challenge her father, but he sees that she can't because she knows her father would oppose her. So then he says, "Well, I think it would hurt him because your father is a very loving father." He makes the father's opposition a positive rather than a negative thing. So he has diluted what could have been a very stressful transaction. It's though he were saying, "We can talk about boundaries in terms of flower hedges; it doesn't have to be guns."

O: At Minuchin's suggestion, Laura gives her father the option of refusing her. And he does refuse her.

A: Yes, but in a very muffled way. The main thing is that Minuchin did get these two people to oppose each other. He couldn't have done it without softening it.

O: Why does Minuchin now turn to the other girl?

A: This is interesting. She has been trying to interrupt and he lets her.

Now Minuchin hardly ever lets one person break in on another. So you know he has a good reason for this.

O: To cut the father out?

A: Right. He was hoping Jill would come in on Laura's side. She takes the same position as Laura, but she is able to state it more forcefully. Here you notice Minuchin doesn't go into "How loving your father is." He gets Jill to say right out how much she wants privacy and how important this is to her.

O: Instead of challenging the father himself, he's getting the other girl to do it.

A: Yes. There is another thing here. You notice that he moves on to the little boy and gets him to state that he, too, wants his door closed. Structurally, he is again creating an alliance of the children against the father, stressing the generation line. But the purpose of the move is to bolster Laura, who cannot assert herself. Soon, as you will see, Minuchin will attempt to bring mother in on her side, too.

Dr. M: Let me try to explore a little bit that area, because I was sure that this is a family that has their doors open. That's why I followed that line of thinking, because this is a family that likes to be huddled, you see, and so, in families that act like that, to close the doors is, ah, a little bit of an insult, a bit of an attack, because you are a bunched-in family, because . . .

Mr. R: (interrupting) We like to think that.

Dr. M: (placing his hand on Mr. R's shoulder, smiling) You like to think that—don't make it a "we." (smiles at Mrs. R, who laughs back)

Mr. R: (smiling too, Mrs. R still laughing) I like to think that. (Covers face with hand in mock defeat.)

Dr. M: Yeah, dad, you know, maybe Connie also likes to think that—and maybe not so much. (rubbing Mr. R's shoulder) You like your back to be rubbed more than she does—O.K. (to Mrs. R) Isn't that so?

Mrs. R: Yes.

Dr. M: Mom doesn't like her back to be rubbed. What's your thinking, Connie, about this question of the closed doors? For your grown-up—growing up—daughters?

Mrs. R: I don't mind if their doors are closed. I don't like them to lock them, but I don't mind if their doors are closed.

Dr. M: Um hm. So what do you say to Dave when he says that the doors should be open?

Mrs. R: Well, sometimes if he—you know, if he'll hear them shut the door—maybe they'll have a friend over and they'll be up in the bedroom and they'll shut the door—I'd say more times its Jill than Laura, you know has friends up, and they close the door, and Dave will, you know, maybe he'll holler and he'll—they can't hear but he'll holler and say, "No closed doors, tell them to leave the door open," and I'll say, "They're not doing anything, just leave them alone, they want their door closed, she's not doing anything . . ."

Dr. M: And then what happens?

Mrs. R: And that's it, we just leave it at that.

Dr. M: That means—Dave accepts your point of view?

Mrs. R: Yeah, I—I suppose so.

Mr. R: I accept it that she previously knows they're up there in the room and has checked on them to see that everything is O.K. and then I accept it at that point. I don't like it when a friend comes over. . .

Dr. M: (motioning to Jill, whom he again mixes up with Laura) Laura wants to say something.

Jill: Who, me?

Dr. M: Yeah—you raised your hand and you (to Mr. R) didn't see her. (realizing his mistake) Jill, excuse me.

Jill: Well . . .

Dr. M: (to Dr. B) You see, I mix them up.

Dr. B: Yes. (laughing)

Jill: Well, I have a girl friend come over, and we usually like to stay up late, so, like if we're noisy, my father comes in—I go in there or something, then he says, "You'd better be quiet," so I close the door, so—in case we want to watch TV or something.

Dr. M: Will daddy then let you close the door?

Jill: Yeah, because he said to be quiet. (inaudible words)

O: Why did Minuchin say, "I was sure this was a family that had the doors open"?

A: He was speaking out of his experience with enmeshed families. In those families, everybody is in everybody's else's business, there are no clear boundaries. One definition of "enmeshment" is a family where no two persons can get together, either to fight or to be close, without a third person breaking them up. This is true in normal families, too, but not as much as in a family with a symptomatic member.

O: In other words, there's no independence of parts.

A: Right. It's like an error-activated system with extremely high resonance between the elements, so that one part can't move without affecting all the others. Now, here Minuchin is trying to get across the fact that in such a family, there is a penalty for not being bunched-in. Closing the doors will be taken as an insult.

O: He also uses the word "attack." It's a little odd to think of boundaries as an attack. Usually you think of them in defensive terms, as preventing an attack maybe.

A: Well, if you think of boxers, when one boxer doesn't want the other to hit him, he doesn't move away, he clinches with him. That's how he stops the fight, with an embrace. A referee has to separate them to get the fight going again. This is what Minuchin is getting at, the family's very great fear that if they don't huddle, they will start to fight. Or that they will be vulnerable to attack.

O: I notice that this time when the father cuts in to deliver his pronouncement, Minuchin puts him in his place.

A: But not by contradicting him directly. All he says is "Don't speak for your wife." That is the first time he has attempted to differentiate between husband and wife.

O: It's such a quick alternation. Just now, he suggested that the father would be hurt if Laura insisted him to knock, and then got her to ask him if he would mind if she did. Here he says that closing the door is seen as an attack in this family, and then immediately gets the mother to say she doesn't mind closed doors. I should think it would be very hard for the father to handle that kind of thing.

A: Yes, Minuchin is on the offensive with this father. You notice that when the father comes in again, Minuchin stops him. He repeats the maneuver of letting another person cut in. I suspect it for the same reason that he allowed Jill to interrupt the first time. He was hoping to get an ally for the mother, to strengthen her position in relation to the father. He knew that Jill would back the mother because the mother had just defended Jill's right to have the doors closed. It's like a game of chess, surrounding the black king with white players.

O: Apparently he mixed Jill and Laura up again.

A: Yes. It may have been because they are treated so very much alike by the parents. Not only is there no differentiation by space in this family, but there is no differentiation by time, either. Minuchin makes a big point of this latter. But here the main structural action is to draw the mother and the children together and to cut the father out. Minuchin started by making Laura's struggle with her father overt and then expanded that by getting the other children and the mother to join in the alliance against him.

O: Isn't there a danger that this will affront the father?

A: In a way. But here is where a therapist's skill comes in. You notice that at some level he is always maintaining the relationship. When he is talking about how it is a bunched-in family, he puts his hand on the father's shoulder as if to say, "It's okay to be bunched-in. I can bunch with you too."

Mr. R: The only time I accept the doors being closed is in a situation like that. If they have a friend over and they're carrying on that you can hear, beyond the door being closed, I then knock on the door and say, either be quiet, control yourself, ah, open the door—so that I know the noise is . . .

Dr. M: (to Mrs. R) In that situation, Connie, your way of thinking is accepted by Dave. Is that true?

Mrs. R: Yes, I would think so.

Dr. M: But you have a disagreement in this area?

Mrs. R: (nodding) Yes, he prefers the doors being open and I, I— doesn't matter, I mean, if they want their door closed, it's all right with me.

Dr. M: In what other areas do you disagree about raising children?

Mrs. M: Hm. (pause) I don't know. (laughing)

Dr. M: Don't tell me that you are unique also ...

Mrs. R: I—

Dr. M: Don't tell me that you are unique also that way, that you don't have disagreements. Normal families have disagreements.

Mrs. R: (laughing) Maybe that's the problem—that we don't disagree enough. I don't know, we, ah ...

Mr. R: (to Dr. M) We seem to communicate ...

Dr. M: (overlapping) I am talking about disagreements,

Mr. R: (trying to break in) Disagreements ...

Dr. M: If there is communication, there is disagreement.

A: In this second stage of the interview, Minuchin deals with the marital conflict which is the keystone to the father-children intimacy. The mother is submissive in her relationship to the father, but she isn't close to him. That's why he tries to get together with the children. To make the parents closer, what the therapist has to do is first differentiate them, then put them on a more equal footing. The mother has to be able to oppose the father, but she can't do that from a one-down position.

O: Minuchin is really bringing out the split between them.

A: Yes. You notice that a few lines back, he laid the groundwork for this move by telling the husband not to speak for his wife. Here he makes the disagreement explicit, brings it out into the open. And then adds that it's normal to disagree.

O: He is really backing the mother up. She responds by saying that maybe the problem is that they don't disagree enough.

A: You can see what it cost to say that. Both parents laugh so nervously. But it's the first near-admission of a problem between them.

O: Which the father immediately denies when he says, "We seem to communicate."

A: Yes. Mother is beginning to suggest that there is a crack between them; father is saying, "No." Notice how delicately Minuchin phrases his next statement. "If there is communication, there is disagreement."

O: That sounds like a way of contradicting someone without contradicting him.

A: Well, there is a contradiction if you analyze it semantically. The father is obviously interpreting disagreement as disunity, and disunity is a bad thing. Minuchin is implying that disagreement is a good thing since you can't communicate without it.

O: He is also setting it up so that either the father is wrong when he says they communicate, or else he has to admit that they disagree.

A: I think his major point is that people can have boundaries between them and take different viewpoints and not necessarily be enemies. One of the virtues of a structural approach is that it doesn't imply values. If you talk in terms of territory: enlarging estates, or setting up gates or fences, or whatever, it avoids implications of who's right, who's wrong, who's sick, who's bad. Minuchin may be cutting the father down, in one sense, and backing the mother up, but it's more in the interest of changing the structure of the family so that the boundaries necessary for normal family functioning can emerge.

Mrs. R: The only thing that bothers me is the phone calls, like at dinner time. Dave gets a lot of phone calls at dinner time, when we are eating, and we're constantly being disturbed. I would just like to tell them to call back, and he wants to talk to them. You know, the phone is on the wall where I'm sitting, and it goes right across my head for him to talk . . .

Jill: The wire.

Mrs. R: . . . and I find it disturbing, I mean at meal time (pointing to Mr. R, who is sitting with his head down) . . .

Dr. M: Then what do you do? You tell that to Dave.

Mrs. R: Sometimes I get riled up about it, and he knows I'm annoyed—I don't always holler about it. Maybe I'll just say these phone calls, you can go nuts, you know, or something to this effect, but that's the end of it. I mean, I don't make an issue out of it, and, ah, the phone calls keep coming. (laughter) I find it disturbing when you're having dinner to have these kind of phone calls. I mean if he would call their house or their place of business or whatever when they are eating, I know darn well they wouldn't speak.

Dr. M: But why—why doesn't that change? You don't like it.

Mrs R: I don't know, I guess you get—just get into a pattern and—just don't do anything about it.

Dr. M: Yes, but what? Could you talk to Dave about it? How could that be changed?

Mrs R: Yeah, I'm sure . . .

Dr. M: Talk with him now.

Mrs. R: (laughing, leaning toward Mr. R) What do you want . . .

Mr. R: (laughing, leaning away from Mrs. R) Talk with me now . . .

Mrs. R: I don't know (laughing) those damn phone calls are so very important early in the night—I don't know. (pause)

Mr. R: (to Dr. M) Well, sometimes on the phone she will mention that, ah . . .

Dr. M: No, No! Talk with her, because this is a question . . .

Mr. R: (to Mrs. R) Can you call back, we're eating . . .

Mrs. R: Yes.

Mr. R: You've done that—if it's not important, call back (inaudible words) and it's been O.K.—or if it's an important phone call having to do with something that's important, and you realize and give the phone, I talk for a moment or two and get off the phone and we continue eating and I make the phone calls back when (inaudible words). Sometimes I can't call them back because the people are at a particular place, or couldn't call back because of their situation, or I answer them, but Connie feels that certain . . .

Dr. M: No, No! (inaudible words) I want that to remain between you and Connie. (Mrs. R and Dr. M both talking simultaneously, inaudible words.)

Mrs. R: (to Dr. M) I just want you to realize . . .

Dr. M: (to Mrs. R) You talk to him, because I don't like . . .

Mr. R: (to Mrs. R) You realize that certain phone calls are important enough that I have to accept them at that particular time, so, ah, you don't get so upset, because you know they're important. Nothing phone calls, it's just disturbing, it's a phone call that they can call later, but why do they have to, ah, to call now—certain people . . .

Dr. M: (turning to Mrs. R) Connie, I want to tell you that Dave did a much better job of defending his position than you did in defending yours. You were not convincing at all. You apologized for your position, so that I don't think that Dave—if I would be Dave I would not change, because you were rather nice and apologetic and I don't know if that is really so important to you. It seems to me as if it is not important—it just seems to me you are fabricating an issue and it's not an important issue for you. If it is important, you will need to tell Dave in ways that he will think it is important.

Mr. R: (leaning back, arms folded, to Mrs. R) Certain people that call, you'll accept at any time, whether it's dinner, or you're busy or whatever. Other people at the same time, you will not accept— which I accept as the same thing. I say, "Well, fine, have them call back or tell them we're eating," or you'll say it yourself. But other people, you separate that it's important, in your own self, because you know their situation. So you do not say to them, "Well we're eating now, can you call back in an hour?" You don't want to insult them, so you accept it because the party that's calling, you've accepted that that's their way and no matter what you say, you're not going to change it. So it's equally important to you as well as me. So you don't knock them off the hook—but other people do ...

Dr. M: Connie, you seem to be agreeing. You see, what Dave is saying is that his open-door policy is not only at home but is also outside the home. He always maintains his door open. He maintains the door open in his—in your bedroom. Both of you have your door open always so the kids can come in. He maintains the door open to the outside—the telephone is a window—so Dave is saying, "Let's keep always a window of our home open," because dad, he's an open-door man.

Mr. R: With everybody.

Dr. M: Hm?

Mr. R: With everybody and everything.

Dr. M: Yeah, um hm. (Dr. M and Mr. R both talking at once, voices raised, inaudible words)

Dr. M: (to Mrs. R) You're not an open-door person, so explain to your husband.

A: Let's look at the sequence that led up to this exchange about the phone calls. Minuchin started out with disagreements and got nowhere. Father blocked him on every turn. Minuchin went along with this, but he was constantly teasing away at it. When father said, "We like open doors," Minuchin said, "You like open doors." As I said before, this is like a first stage, prying the two people apart. You can't have a disagreement until you have two different people who can take two different sides. Once this is done, you can move to the disagreement stage.

O: He finally gets the mother to come out with something she actively dislikes.

A: Yes. This is the first complaint she's made about something the father does. Phone calls at dinner. And Minuchin tries to get her to talk directly to her husband about this.

O: It doesn't work. He keeps turning back to Minuchin.

A: And Minuchin keeps turning him back to his wife: "Talk to her!" At the same time, you notice he moves his own chair back, as if to shorten the distance between the couple by increasing his distance from each of them.

O: When the father finally does turn to his wife, his whole body expresses disdain. He leans back, gets himself in an imperial position and tells her the way things are. Then when she tries to say something, he ignores her and turns back to Minuchin.

A: He felt he could stop the fight because he had won. But Minuchin keeps it going. He makes the father talk a little more, and then he concedes. Because, actually, the woman had lost. But by this maneuver, Minuchin maintains himself in a position of strength. In effect, he says to the father, "I'm running this show."

O: The way he handles the woman's defeat is very nice. Instead of accusing her husband of pushing her around, he blames it on her: "You didn't fight well enough. Maybe it's not an important issue."

A: Yes, he puts her in a bind. She can't acknowledge publicly that the issue isn't important to her, and yet if she does, she is going to have to speak up against her husband.

O: There's also an element of backing someone's pride. If Minuchin had accused this woman's husband of wiping the floor with her, he would have only pushed her further down. This way, if she has any vanity at all, she would have to show some spirit.

A: I think what is operating here is another example of how to get the family to change without directly attacking the father. As before, Minuchin prefers to go to someone else, rather than engage the father in a debate. This time he goes to the wife.

O: He still makes the point that her husband steps all over her. What is also odd is that he is just as condescending to her as her husband is.

A: I don't think this is coincidental. If you watch a good therapist for a long time, you see that he uses the same pathways that the family uses. This man talks to his wife by talking down to her. Minuchin uses the same slightly insulting style. He's asking for a change in a manner that implies "no change."

O: He doesn't use the same pathway as the family when he deals with the father. He ignores him, contradicts him.

A: Only by supporting someone else. He is very indirect with this man. If he were challenged directly, I think he could get very aggressive, and he would become central to the discussion. So Minuchin simply continues to address the mother. By focusing the conversation on her, he supports her; by refusing to discuss the issue with the man, he weakens him. I think that is the overriding dynamic in the interchange between the man, the woman, and the therapist.

O: I notice that the father comes in with another bombastic speech.

A: Yes, and you see how quickly Minuchin turns the rebuttal over to the wife. Since her husband is an open-door person and she is not, why doesn't she tell him how she feels?

O: Minuchin makes a nice tie between the phone call and the doors. The father maintains an open door not only within the home but with the entire outside world. That's really keeping the metaphors connected.

A: It's also a way of keeping the main point in view, which is always this matter of boundaries and how important they are.

Mrs. R: Well, I like a certain amount of privacy, which I feel I don't get. There are some times that I just want to be lay in bed and watch TV and relax . . .

Dr. M: Tell him, tell Dave. I am not in your home, I don't care.

Mrs. R: Well, I can't only tell him, it's the children too . . .

Dr. M: Tell him.

Mrs. R: (to Mr. R) Sometimes I like to lay in bed and watch TV and I just—you know, maybe the kids have a lot of homework that I've helped them with right after school—and when we finally go up to the room and we lay down and watch TV, sometimes I just like that quiet time—not all the kids piling in on the bed . . .

Mr. R: (interrupting) Well, you spend a lot of time . . .

Mrs. R: . . . and the phone calls, you know. We can get phone calls twelve o'clock at night.

Mr. R: Ah, you're trying to say that from about, uh (to Dr. M) Connie does an awful lot for the children . . .

Dr. M: (to Mr. R) Hear what she has to say and answer to her. (Mrs. R laughs)

Mr. R: (to Dr. M) Well, I hear it.

Dr. M: To her, then . . .

Mr. R: I hear it. (turning to Mrs. R) Ah, a lot of things happen in an afternoon with the children—picking them up from school—when they get home from school, you are with the children from 3:30 until about 6:00 . . . (At this point in the father's speech, Dr. M crosses over to the other side of the room and places his chair next to Steve. Then he goes and gets Jill and places her in that seat. Next he places himself in her seat. It is a long, time-consuming maneuver. The seating order now is: Jill, Steve, Laura, Dr. M, Mrs. R, and Dr. B.)

Mr. R: (cont'd) . . . I then come home. You have then spent about three hours with the children. I now come home and there's about an hour and a half of things that I take care of personally. That makes it to 7:30. In the meantime, we have dinner. Then there's more homework, and, if I am home and there is something for me to do with the children, then we do it. Most of the time you do it. Now at about 8:00 it's finished, unless there's an extra thing with Laura or Steve or Jill. So by the time 10:00 rolls around, at that point, you've had it, you now want to unwind, you want to relax, but now everything is chaos. (momentary break between reels)

O: Why does Minuchin go through that complicated change of seats? It doesn't seem to have any meaning in the context of what is being said.

A: I think he was reacting to the fact that the wife is losing again. He gets her to make an outright request for privacy and the husband starts on a long discussion that confuses the issue completely. By now there's a real struggle going on between Minuchin and the father. Minuchin is asking him to talk to his wife, and he is resisting. So Minuchin challenges the father with what is really an unanswerable move; he goes over and sits next to the wife. He moves to the wife's corner in the ring. He's been bunching with the father, now he gets on the wife's side, literally.

O: He also places himself as a physical boundary between the couple and the children.

A: Well, I think this was more a reaction to the father shutting him out. There's a lot of emotion in this move. I don't think it was just a little strategy on Minuchin's part.

Mr. R: (cont'd) . . . because we were rolling around having a good time, and now that it's time at 10:00 to relax, you're out now and ready for bed. So you don't really relax . . .

Dr. M: (interrupting) Dave, sit here, and you (to Mrs. R) sit in Dave's place. (gets up and motions Mr. R to sit in his chair while he places Mrs. R in her husband's chair. He then sits between them, in the chair vacated by Mr. R. The line-up now is Jill, Steve, Laura, Mr. R, Dr. M, Mrs. R, and R. B.)

Mr. R: O.K. (continuing his speech) So we have this little row. Now Connie doesn't get upset or say too much about this . . .

Dr. M: (leaning towards Mrs. R and away from Mr. R) You see, I want to talk with you because I think Dave is a very good salesman. (Mrs. R laughs.)

Dr. M: And he is selling you the idea that his relationship with the kids is extremely important and that it's more important than what you want at this particular time in your relationship with him—that's why I sat here, because he is bundling there with the kids, having Laura (mixing up the girls again) huh? (correcting himself) having

Jill unknotting his calf and Laura combing his hair (touching Mr.
R's hair) and Steve rubbing his back (placing hand on Mr. R's
shoulder), and you (to Mrs. R) are there kind of unemployed.

Mrs. R: (laughing) Well . . .

Dr. M: Your children are not employing you, and your husband is not
employing you.

Mr. R: She's employed too.

Dr. M: No! (continuing to lean toward Mrs. R) He is really having all
the bunch of kids employed with him. Where are you?

Mrs. R: (laughing) Well . . .

Mr. R: (laughing) She's down heating the . . .

Dr. M: (to Mrs. R) No, no, no, where are you?

Mrs. R: (still laughing) Well, sometimes like I said I'm sitting on the
bed—sometimes I'm laying on the bed, sometimes I'm downstairs. I
don't know, I'm emptying the dishwasher or . . .

Dr. M: But they are bunched together, and you are—well, what kind
of corners are there where you are?

Mr. R: You have a point.

Mrs. R: (inaudible remark)

Dr. M: (to Mrs. R) No, no, you told him something, and he gave you a
long, long spiel about his needs and explaining your needs. You
have told him about some of your needs. He gave you such a lovely,
long spiel that you forgot what it was that you wanted. He is selling
you the idea that his relationship with the kids is very important.
You were telling about some of your needs. (Mr. R is sitting with his
head bowed, body turned away from Dr. M.)

Mrs. R: Well, you know, um . . .

Dr. M: Because what he told me—let me hear what he says—is he
spends time with the kids at a time in which you are most alert and at
a time which you could talk with him. But then you are tired, you
had your day gone, so you go to sleep.

Mrs. R: Well, it's true we don't have too much time together to sit and
talk, that's for sure . . . (laughter)

Mr. R: She likes to talk between 9:00 and 10:00.

Dr. M: (placing hand on Mr. R's shoulder) Wait a moment . . .
(tape cut off about five minutes. Dr. M turns the conversation back
to the wife. She describes how hard it is to get the children to go to

bed. She would like Steve to go to bed at 9:00, but he insists on staying up till 10:00, and somehow she has never been able to force him. Laura goes to bed early, but Jill is a night owl, and she, too, doesn't get to bed till late. The result is that mother has the children on her hands most of the evening.)

Dr. M: (to Mrs. R) . . . and so what also happens is that—so you're telling two things—one is that there are some things you want about the children that they don't want, like if you want Steve to be in bed at 9:00, he does not want. This other thing you are saying is that you and Dave are so busy with the kids that there is very little time that you have together without the children. Is that so?

Mrs. R: Yeah, I would say so.

Dr. M: (touching Mr. R on the knee) Come back, Dave, now—I want you to come with your wife, you belong here. (gets up and exchanges chairs with Mr. R) The kids are going to grow up and some day go away and then you will be alone with your wife and you will not know her. Now what kind of things have you lately done together without the children? (leaning back away from couple)

Mr. R: Well, we have, um, as time has allowed—Wednesday or Thursday nights, we go out to dinner . . .

Dr. M: Without the kids?

Mr. R: Yep.

Dr. M: Good. I just didn't know that.

Mr. R: And Saturday night is our night without the children.

Dr. M: This means every . . .

Mr. R: Every week, two nights a week, we go out socially.

O: What triggered off that second move of Minuchin's, where he, mother and father all switched chairs?

A: I would guess it was that long speech which begins with the father laying out the whole day for this woman. He gives her no room at all. So Minuchin keeps on with this game of chairs. It's something he often does. Sometimes it takes him several different moves to get people positioned where he wants them. This was a three-stage maneuver. You saw how he moved the children and got himself into the chair next to the wife. Now, with one more move, he cut the husband out completely. By placing himself between husband and wife, and turning to the wife, he is saying, "If you're not going to talk to her, I will."

O: Why didn't he just change seats with the wife? He would still have been between the couple and next to the wife. It would have been a much simpler move.

A: I think he wanted to do something stronger, and two chair switches is stronger than one chair switch. Also, what he does points up the father's implicit message that his relationship with the kids is more important than the needs of his wife. By placing the father on the side next to the children, he more or less forces the father to bunch with the children right there in the session.

O: I notice he turns his back on the father completely.

A: Yes. Just before, the father had complete control of the situation. Telling his wife, "At 5:30 you do this and at 6:00 you do that." In one gesture Minuchin has undermined the man's control.

O: And at the same time praises him. "He's such a good salesman, look what he's done to you," he says to his wife.

A: Well, he is a salesman. That's his profession. Now see how uncomfortable he gets. He turns away from Minuchin and starts to talk to Laura. But all the time he has to be affected by the fact that another man is getting cozy with his wife and being sympathetic to her and saying, "You poor thing, your husband amuses himself with the kids and leaves you out in the cold."

O: It could have been done offensively, but Minuchin has a nice way of phrasing things. Sometimes his not-quite-correct English can be an asset. How can you be angry with someone who says to your wife, "What kind of corners are there where you are?"

A: It's also interesting to look at this sequence in terms of body postures. When Minuchin starts to play up to the wife, the father turns away from him, almost in retaliation, and raises his arm in such a way that if forms a barrier between them. But when Minuchin reaches out and touches him, saying, "Come back, Dave," the man veers right in. That's when Minuchin relinquishes the wife. He's been dancing with her; now he turns her around to where her husband can cut in.

O: And sits them together again. What is curious is that the first time he differentiates the couple, it's to promote a disagreement. This time it's to get them closer together.

A: I don't think he could have got them closer if he hadn't engineered the disagreement first. He said before: "If there is communication, there is disagreement." Translated, this could mean: "In a case like yours, you'll never get together until you disagree." The thing is he would never have gotten anywhere just telling them this. He makes them experience it right there.

O: You could look at it this way. If there's a range for the limits of distance and closeness between these two people, as there seems to be with most married couples, you could say that Minuchin is rocking the system. If he pushes them too close, they will have to seek distance; if he pulls them apart, they will move together. That may be what was happening here. First he pushed them to disagree. But it takes closeness to have an argument, and they resisted. So then Minuchin reversed the thing; he split the couple, got between them, and made a grandstand play for the wife. It was like stretching a rubber band. The husband had to come back in.

A: Yes. But I'd like to point out another important thing, which is that by this time, the whole emphasis of the interview has changed. It started with the question of the rights of people in the family to privacy. A territorial-imperative kind of thing. And here, it suddenly becomes a question of the wife being lonely and needing a man. From an issue that had the overtones of a battle or a confrontation, there is a shift to an issue that calls for consideration and concern.

O: Maybe that's what made the husband come back in so nicely. Previously, you see, the wife was very anxious to keep her husband at arms length. It isn't all his fault if he cuddles with the kids and leaves her out. Now the picture is different. Minuchin is paying her all kinds of attention, and her whole manner has changed. She becomes very responsive, and that's when the husband finally concedes to Minuchin: "You have a point."

A: The main thing is that Minuchin gets the two of them together. And then cements it by reminding them that someday they may be sitting without the children between them, facing each other, and then what will they do?

O: He asks what they do without the kids, and when they say they go out at least twice a week, he acknowledges it and then drops it. Why doesn't he push this more?

A: Well, if they had said, "we never go out," he might have made more of an issue of it. But since they do, he approaches and lets it go. He has got them in the same corral and has set up a little fence. Once he has the fence up, he doesn't worry about nailing down all the planks.

O: There's another thing he does, which is to touch on the subject of sex between the parents without ever mentioning sex. You get the message very clearly when he observes that they are so busy with the kids that they have little time to be alone.

A: Yes, but what's different is that some therapists will use other things as metaphors for talking about sex. Minuchin uses sex as a metaphor for talking about boundaries. In this case, it is one more metaphor for the generation boundary.

Dr. M: And what happens with the kids? (turning to Laura) Do you babysit for them Laura?

Laura and Mr. R: (simultaneously) No.

Laura: We usually have somebody to sleep in—our housekeeper— and, if we don't have anybody, I usually stay. (glances at father)

Dr. M: (waving hand in front of Laura's face) Don't look at daddy! Checking—my goodness! (Dr. M throws up his hands in a gesture of mock astonishment; everybody laughs; Mr. R drops his head, smiling.)

(Tape cut of about five minutes. Dr. M turns to Laura and asks her if she considers herself old enough to babysit. She agrees that together she and Jill could take this responsibility. Dr. M asks Jill and Steve to change seats so that Laura and Jill can discuss the issue. While they are talking, he answers a buzz on the intercom; it is evidently Mrs. C announcing that lunch is ready. Dr. M returns to his seat and now asks the girls to discuss the possibility of babysitting for their parents. The parents state that they feel more comfortable if there is an adult in the house when they go out. At this point, Mrs. C looks in the door.)

Dr. M: O.K. Let me—ah, Joanne, can you bring the lunch? (Dr. B places the coffee table in the middle of the room.) There is one way to—Laura, you know one thing that I noticed is that daddy talks with both of you as if you are the same age. So does mother. They don't talk with you as though you are the oldest, they talk as if you are 12 years old, and of course instead of talking with Jill as if she's 14, they talk with you as if you are 12. Did you notice that?

Laura: (very softly) Yes.

Dr. M: You know they kind of lower your age in some way. Both of them do the same thing, and I don't know why. You know, I was talking with you as the babysitter, but the points at which daddy started he immediately, he made both of you the babysitters, immediately lowered your age, and so did mom. Why do they do that?

Laura: I guess they treat us equal.

Dr. M: Why don't you treat her as if she's 14? Why do they treat her— why do they treat you as if are 12?

Laura: I don't know.

Dr. M: But—(to another child who starts to interrupt) No, no, no, I am talking with Laura here. (to Laura) Do you like to be treated as if you are 12?

Laura: No.

Dr. M: Don't you think that you are the oldest? (Laura nods) Do you think your parents know that?

Laura: Yeah.

Dr. M: No, they don't, they don't! If I asked them how old you are, they would say 14. But when they treat you, they treat you as if you are, ah, the same age as Jill. That is strange, because you are not. So something can happen that—or it makes Jill growing too fast or it's making you growing too slow, and I think they don't mean it. (glancing at parents) I don't know why. (to Laura) Probably you are also—maybe you are telling them that you are 12. Are you? Are you . . . (inaudible words)

Laura: (overlapping) Not that I know of.

Dr. M: Look about that, because maybe you are telling them that you are 12, and maybe you are telling them that you are 10, and maybe we are just making a concession in treating you as if you are 12. But something is wrong here. (looking around room questioningly; gestures to Mrs. R) Mom, can you serve the food?

Mrs. R: (getting up to do so) You're right. (inaudible comment; noise from paper bags)

Dr. B: (to Dr. M) Joanne says you have to leave at a quarter to one.

Dr. M: Yeah. (Everybody takes positions around the coffee table.)

A: This is a move to a new stage. Minuchin is ready to come back to the children, but this time he is separating them from mother and putting a clear line between them and the parents. The way he brings them back in is by talking about a way they can help daddy and mommy go out together.

O: Is that why he asks if Laura babysits?

A: Yes. It is also a way of differentiating her from her siblings.

O: What's this business about Laura checking?

A: Laura was looking at her father, to see if he approved. Minuchin has set the couple up as if on a date. They're out of the house, and yet the father keeps peeking back in the window. So Minuchin pulls down the shade.

O: And asks for lunch. Why does he decide to have it brought in now?

A: Because he's finally got the parents together by themselves. He knows that as long as they use the struggle about food to avoid getting together in more personal ways, Laura can't eat.

O: But, instead of talking about food, Minuchin goes off on this age business. What is his purpose here?

A: Well, he has noticed that along with the lack of boundaries between parents and children, there is also no differentiation between the children in terms of age. A clear sign of enmeshment, as I said before, is when the natural hierarchies in the family are blurred. So he points out that the parents treat the two older girls as if they were the same age, or worse, as if they were both the same age as the younger one. He's beginning to establish a boundary between them as older and younger daughters.

O: He seems to be putting responsibility on Laura as much as on the parents. He suggests that maybe she is responsible for this confusion.

A: It's a two-way street, but here Minuchin is emphasizing the daughter's part. If she is letting her parents treat her as younger than she is, she is really choosing it. He makes it voluntary. There's another interesting point. Minuchin caught himself back there, when he started out by pinning the blame on the father. He begins by saying to the girls. "Daddy talks with you as if you were both the same age," and then quickly amends it to, "So does mother." He doesn't want at this point to re-create the covert alliance between mother and the kids. This was useful at the beginning of the session, to help the mother get some strength and give Laura some support, but now it would defeat Minuchin's purpose. Because he had finally got those two adults together. It becomes very clear here that even while he was trying to cement the parents, he began to be sucked back into the family's way of splitting them.

O: It's nice to see a therapist make this kind of mistake. It's an index of the power a family has over the therapist. And it should make beginners feel a little better when they see an experienced therapist feel the undertow and have to pick his feet up out of the waves.

A: No one is immune. But to get back to the previous point, there's another reason to bring up the issue of the girl's independence. This has a direct bearing on her symptom. Not eating has been a way of trying to keep some kind of territory for herself, some area she can control.

O: You mean that by redefining the fight as a struggle with the parents about growing up, he takes it away from the issue of food?

A: Right. He creates a different arena for the girl to fight in, one more appropriate to the normal struggle adolescent kids need to go through with their parents.

O: In preparation for bringing in the lunch.

A: I would think so. He could never have got this girl to eat at the beginning of the interview. But look what has gone on. These steps and stages, marking off boundaries, differentiating between first this group, then that, are all preparations for getting back to the fight over food. You could say there are three different contexts for therapy in this interview. First there is the sequence where the therapist separates the kids from the father and brings out the covert coalition they have with the mother. This makes father odd man out and creates backing for the identified patient. Then, in the second stage, he moves to the marital dyad and puts a circle around that. In the third stage, he deals with a sibling group, differentiating them by age. Only now does he feel it is safe to get back to what the family came in for—because he can finally bring up the unacknowledged disagreement between the parents and Laura about her right to grow up.

O: You don't feel there could have been any short cut? Were all these stages and sub-stages necessary?

A: It's anyone's guess. But I assume that if Minuchin's goal was to get that girl to eat in the room, he would have to go very patiently, very slowly, one step at a time. If he had said to the family in the first five minutes, "You are not allowing your daughter to grow up, so she is fighting you by refusing to eat food," he would have gotten nowhere. It would have been an interruption—a move without influence. It would not have changed the structure of the family in the least.

O: Even here, he is not too explicit. He doesn't connect the symptom with the fact that Laura is not being treated her age.

A: But at some level, people pick the connection up. It's just that if you don't make it explicit, they can't deny it. In the beginning, when Minuchin asked if the family had disagreements, they said, "We have harmony." Father, in particular, said, "We like to cuddle." How could the daughter fight him then? As I said before, you can't fight someone if you are in a clinch with him. Laura could only fight obscurely, through an issue unrelated to the real one. Now, hopefully, she can go another way.

O: So Minuchin says, "Mom, serve the food."

Dr. M: Ah, we have ten minutes (to Dr. B). But we have—look, we have learned something about the family. We have learned some things about this family that if we are working with them, I think would be useful to continue looking at (gesturing toward Mrs. R.

who is giving out the sandwiches). Let's take lunch and not discuss that, but (turning to Laura and shaking his finger at her) I want, Laura, I want you to see that, you know, something wrong, you know, and I don't know who is the one that is doing that.

Mr. R: Do you think, doctor, that we don't realize it ourselves? (everybody talking, rustling of paper bags) I think that probably we wouldn't—on my behalf, Connie's, or Laura's. (Mrs. R makes an inaudible remark.)

Steve: I have something to say.

Dr. M: You have something to say?

Mrs. R: You do? Well let's hear it.

Steve: Well, once when my mother and father went out, um, they were coming home late and my sisters were real tired, and so they went to sleep, and I was still awake and I babysitted for them.

Dr. M: You babysitted for them?

Steve: Yeah, right. I fell asleep, and my father paid me.

Dr. M: Your father paid you?

Mr. R: I paid him for babysitting at 50 cents an hour. (Steve is talking about his babysitting, inaudible. Mrs. R is handing around napkins. Group is now sitting around the coffee table, eating.)

Mrs. R: That's right, we called to see if everything was all right, and he answered the phone.

Mr. R: It was only one time. One time it happened and Steve was a babysitter and he was babysitting for the girls. (pause) This all was very interesting, ah, going back five years ago, the same thing was occurring—lowering one, with closeness—it's difficult to realize.

Dr. M: (to Jill) You see, they are not treating you as if you are 14, Jill—they treat you like if you are 12. So you see, it's very special what they are doing. They are just putting the ceiling on Laura. I'm wondering if daddy doesn't want his big girl to grow up. Laura, you know if you grow up, what will happen?

Mr. R: Maybe I don't want both of you to grow up.

Dr. M: What will happen if you grow up Laura? Huh?

Laura: I don't know . . . get married.

Dr. M: You will then be interested maybe in rubbing the back of

somebody else. Dad, what would happen then? Maybe you will need
to have Connie rubbing your back.

Mr. R: It's very possible.

Dr. M: Connie, do you like to rub Dave's back?

Mrs. R: I don't mind. I do it once in a while.

Steve: I want a straw.

Dr. B: (handling Dr. M a paper bag) Here you are.

Dr. M: What's—is this the special?

Mr. R: Chop Stop—Chop Shop Special.

Dr. M: That's a Chop Special?

Mr. R: Chop Shop—

Mrs. R: It's a tongue twister. (Everybody is now eating and talking.
Laura is seen to be eating for the first time.)

Dr. M: (gesturing toward Dr. B, who sits across the long table opposite him. The table also separates parents and children, with the two
therapists at either end.) Mariano, we are making a perfect wall now
between the parents and the children.

Dr. B: Uh hm.

Dr. M: We are moving them out (pointing to children on his right) and
moving them together (pointing to the parents on his left), but I tell
you something, I think we'll need to push a lot.

O: I gather Minuchin routinely has food brought in during an
interview with an anorectic child. Does he ask the mother to serve it
because that is what mothers in our society do, or does he have some
other reason?

A: It's partly cultural, but I suspect that it also has to do with the fact
that she is less intensely involved in the struggle over food. It's
probably as much a structural thing as a role thing. In another
family, in which the mother was the over-involved parent, Minuchin
might keep the mother out of the picture entirely. In one family with
an anorectic child, he pushed the mother out and took control of the
daughter's eating himself.

O: There's a pause here while people are getting served and the little
boy speaks up. How do you see that?

A: He took the opportunity to say, "Hey, here I am. I babysat for my big sisters, and I got paid for it. Don't forget me." It sort of completes the family. So Minuchin stops what he was beginning to say and draws the boy out.

O: He still comes back to the fact that the family is putting the lid on Laura. In fact, he puts the finger on dad. He doesn't want her to grow up.

A: But he's talking to Laura, not to her father. The father keeps coming in on top of him, and Minuchin ignores him and goes on talking to Laura.

O: It's again as though he's trying to put the father down.

A: No, I think it's more that he is continuing to differentiate, to draw boundaries. Notice how this maneuver gives the girl the freedom to say, "If I grow up, I might get married." This might have been impossible for her to say if Minuchin had not been there, acting as a shield.

O: He's so casual when he asks who is going to rub the father's back after Laura finds someone else. It's so clear he's talking about sex.

A: I don't know if every therapist would be skillful enough to do that and get away with it. Minuchin touches the subject in the lightest possible way, then backs off. But as I said before, you miss the point if you think that he is only talking about sex. By mentioning physical tenderness between husband and wife, he again draws the circle about them. Husband and wife belong together; daughter will eventually grow up and belong to some other man.

O: He makes that goal quite clear when he says to Barragan, "We are making a perfect wall between parents and children." Does the fact that he is going to hand the case over to Barragan have anything to do with his explicitness here?

A: Perhaps, but Minuchin does tend to explain what he is up to more than other therapists. It may have to do with the fact that when he is taping a family, he's always remembering that this will be used for teaching. Also, it's a useful technique to talk to your co-therapist in the presence of the family, especially if you want to make a point, or sum things up, as Minuchin is doing here. They are overhearing it, which makes it a little different than if they were being addressed directly. It's harder for them to object.

Dr. M: I don't think we have any problems with Laura's eating—she will eat. (Laura, watching him, takes a bite.)

Dr. B: Yeah.

Dr. M: (watching Laura eat) At the point at which you are 14, Laura, you will eat without any problems. (Laura finishes her mouthful.) But I think, I think it is good that you are not eating now, because I think that what's happening is that this is the only area in your family, Laura, in which you have a say-so. And at 14 you'll need to have a say-so in another way. And you know, at this point, that's the only way in which you say, "No." (Moves Steve forward, so that he can talk with Laura better.) What about—there are some, some other things, Laura—some other areas about which you have a say-so? What about clothes—do you buy your own clothes?

Laura: No, I don't pay for them.

Dr. M: No, but do you choose them?

Laura: Yes. Most things.

Dr. M: Do you go in and buy by yourself?

Laura: Yes.

Dr. M: What do you buy?

Laura: Pants, skirts, shirts.

Dr. M: And you do that by yourself—your Mom gives you money?

Laura: Yes, the charge.

Dr. M: You have a charge account. (taking a bite in unison with Laura) What about dresses—the way in which you are dressed now. Did you decided the way you are dressed now, or did your mother pick it?

Laura: I did.

Dr. M: Your mother doesn't tell you to do that? You dress the way in which you want? (Laura nods. She is still eating.) What about going to bed, do you go to bed whenever you want?

Laura: Yes, when I'm real tired, I just go to bed, except when there's a favorite TV show, and I'll stay up to watch it.

Dr. M: And nobody tells you when to do that? (Laura nods. She is still eating.)

Dr. M: (to Dr. B) You see, there are, Mariano, so few areas in which this family has, um, problems of control, or rules, that it is very difficult for Laura to fight the battle for growing up. She doesn't have—it's almost like if Laura is creating her own arena, at least, around food. (to Laura) Around food, at least, you can fight. You can say, "That's my body, and that's what I want to eat." Isn't that what you are saying?

Laura: Um hmm. (continues to eat)

Dr. M: Then, then it's O.K.—there—with nobody pushing you.

Mr. R: Is this also a cry for help? As an individual?

Dr. M: All right—you people are really giving Laura everything . . .

Mrs. R: Let me say something, ah . . .

Dr. M: You are treating her as if she is eight—as if she is ten years old. And I think that Laura is acting like as if she is ten. You are acting much younger, Laura, you realize? Jill is acting like if you—like as if she is your older sister, and your parents are treating her like that.

Dr. B: You know Sal, I have the impression that (turning to Mr. R) what you're doing is, you are so used to this very nice way of negotiating things in your family, that everything is open and everything is fine, that maybe you lost track of the fact that the children in order to grow up need to fight, and you are not giving them that opportunity.

Mr. R: Um hm, nothing to fight for . . .

Dr. B: That's right, because everything is going fine, you know . . .

Mr. R: . . . (simultaneously) everything is good; no arguments, no fighting, we don't argue in the house at all.

Mrs. R: Yep, very rarely.

Dr. M: Look what happens with Connie when she doesn't fight. She doesn't get what she wants . . .

Mr. R: (indicating the children) She's got . . .

Dr. M: (pointing to Mrs. R) No, Connie, your wife here—the lovely woman that is sitting near you. She doesn't get results either.

Mr. R: In my own mind I say to myself: "As a provider, as a father, what is it that they want? Individualism?"

Dr. M: (interrupting) Don't talk about "they."

Mr. R: All right, Connie.

Dr. M: Connie, your lovely wife who wants some things from you, and she doesn't have . . .

(Mr. R spills his drink in his lap, says something inaudible.)

Dr. M: Was I too rough, Dave?

Mr. R: Yeah, you were very rough. You just touched a nerve, and I just cracked up.

Dr. M: I am sorry—I will be gentle with you now.

Mr. R: Ah, terrible!

Dr. B: You have to remember that they are used to . . .

Dr. M: To the gentle touch.

Dr. B: Right.

Mr. R: I thought we were used to closeness (Dr. M trying to break in), but evidently it was not as I thought.

Dr. M: (overlapping) Oh no, sir, you are used to closeness, and I don't have anything against closeness, I think it is very nice, but um . . .

Mr. R: Perhaps I've forgotten the little things that are very important.

Dr. M: I just—I just would like that sometimes you should close your doors, so that you and Connie are alone.

Mr. R: I wouldn't have any problem of, ah (Dr. M and Mr. R speaking simultaneously, inaudible words)

Dr. M: That's very good, then . . .

Mr. R: (interrupting) I'm not opposed to love in any form at all. Personally, I don't feel this . . .

Dr. M: (breaking in) I want, Dave, that you should—I will give you a little—some homework, O.K.?

Mr. R.: We have closed our doors.

Dr. M: (trying to make his point) I want, I want . . .

Mrs. R: (to Mr. R) After they are asleep. (short laugh)

Dr. M: (touching Mr. R on the arm) I want you to hear a little. Here and there, Connie says some things that I want you have gotten accustomed not to hear her.

Mr. R: I hear, and I don't think it's important.

Dr. M: Well, that's exactly what I'm saying. That's exactly what I have said. And sometimes this (pointing to Laura) muted voice wants to say something. (to Laura) You had forgotten already that you have a voice to be heard more.

Dr. B: She remembers all the time that she has a voice when she won't eat.

Dr. M: Yes, that's when she has a voice. (to Laura) It's a very narrow area that you have a voice, so I want you to begin to say. (turns to speak to Dr. B)

O: Why does Minuchin now, for the first time, focus on Laura's eating?

A: Well, this is the moment the food is brought in, and Minuchin always likes to deal with a symptom when it is taking place in front of him. But the reason also has to do with the direction he has been going in. All this time, he has been dealing with boundaries, privacy, rights, and privileges. Now he can get to the symptom within this structural framework. When Laura finally gains her independence, when she is really grown up, she will have no trouble eating. It is a prediction.

O: Why does he then say, "It's good that you are not eating"?

A: It puts her in a bind. There's no way she can resist it. If she eats, she's fulfilling his prediction; if she doesn't she's obeying his command.

O: It's interesting. Just as he is saying, "You will eat," she is taking a big bite of her sandwich.

A: Yes. This is a beautifully timed dance-like sequence. At the point where he said, "You're going to be eating when you are 14," Laura was eating from both sides of the sandwich, and she was drinking to get the food down. Then, when she swallowed and stopped chewing, he said, "It's good that you're not eating." And she wasn't eating. There was no food in her mouth, and she wasn't about to take another bite. Now it could have all been an accident, but that's the way it happened.

O: He goes in synchrony with her.

A: Sure, matching her rhythm. It's a subtle, gestural reinforcement of his suggestions to her. In the exchange about clothes and bedtime that follows, you'll notice that he's practically singing a duet with her. They aren't talking about food any more, but you know that Minuchin is monitoring every mouthful. He seems to time his bites with hers.

O: Does Minuchin stress the other areas of choice as a way of suggesting she should be more independent?

A: That, and it also takes the issue away from the symptom, where it can't be dealt with, and puts it into an area that's negotiable. All the things he asks about are age-appropriate: clothes, bedtime. He's saying, "It's important for you to decide about these things."

O: But he also says that when the family is so nice to her about letting her decide, she's being cheated of her right to fight.

A: Well, this is again one of those two-in-one messages. He tells her: "You can use other areas to establish your independence in, like clothes and bedtime." But he also says, "You still have to fight over food, because it is the only way you have to differentiate yourself right now." In other words, give up the symptom, but at the same time don't give it up. It's the same thing as when he said, "Eat" and "Don't eat."

O: I notice that he is again relabeling harmony as a negative thing. By this illogic, the symptom becomes something good, because it's the girl's only weapon against this harmony that is strangling her. Why does the father come in so quickly there?

A: Minuchin has put the finger on the family again for not giving Laura the chance to rebel. So father says, "It's not us, it's Laura's problem as an individual." And you notice that Minuchin does a lot of different things here. First he compliments the family for doing so much for Laura, then he says that they are treating her as if she were 10, then he tells her that she is behaving like a kid anyway. So nobody ends up feeling "It's all my fault." And yet Minuchin hasn't retracted anything he has said, only made it stronger.

O: Barragan comes in here, very straightforward, and says to the parents "You need to let your children fight, otherwise they can't grow up."

A: Yes, and Minuchin takes the point even further, saying that fights are good, but moves it to the husband and wife, "Look what happens to your wife when you never fight. She never gets what she wants either." This shifts the struggle between father and daughter to the one between the parents.

O: Everybody starts to get excited now, and the father spills something.

A: Minuchin has just tried to push the husband toward the wife again, saying "Your lovely wife who wants some things from you." That's when the spill occurs. The father says, "You touched a nerve and I guess I just cracked up." He is joking, but it's clear that this is exactly what happened.

O: It's an acknowledgment of sorts, almost a capitulation.

A: Well, he only appears to give in. This is exactly they way this man fights, by agreeing. He's been totally agreeable all through the interview. It's really a way of avoiding the struggle, by staying in the clinch.

O: He goes on giving in, by suggesting ways in which he's been deficient.

A: Yes, he's defensive now. But Minuchin ignores any implication that the father's at fault and, instead, gives the couple a task: they must close their door and have some time alone together during the week.

O: The father immediately replies, "We have closed our doors." You were right when you said he doesn't really give in.

A: But see how the mother rises to the occasion. She comes right back, "After the children are asleep." So Minuchin says that the father should learn to listen to his wife.

O: And to his daughter, too. He makes an identification between mother and Laura when he talks about Laura's "muted voice." She has something to say, too.

A: But she doesn't say it in an appropriate way. Mariano points this out when he says that the only way she makes her voice heard is when she refuses to eat. Mother is able to attack the open door policy a little bit here. But Laura still can't, except through food. So this is what Minuchin is after: to change her language, if you will, or rather, to change her method of fighting for her rights.

Dr. M: (to Dr. B) We'll need to think, Mariano, about some kind of task that will help these people to train themselves in doing something that they don't do—that is, to give them some time that is theirs. (turning to the group) Now I would like if—for Laura, not for Jill—but I would like, for this week, you should close the door of your bedroom whenever you want—at least it should be two hours a day. And I would like your father, and your mother, when they want to enter, they'll be careful to knock. Just that, that's very simple— but every day you need to have your door—do you think two hours is too much?

Laura: No.

Dr. M: No? You think two hours? O.K., then I want you to close the door for two hours. (to Jill) Now I want you to keep the door like it has always been, O.K.? (to Steve) And I want you to keep the door open. (turning to Mrs. R) Now I want during this week you should close the door of your bedroom from 9:00 to 10:00, whenever it is, and I want you to be with your husband, which is to be alone. That's all. No, I don't want anything else. That's it. (to Mr. R) You, I want you to knock. I am sure that you will be interested in knowing what Laura is doing and talking with Laura because you are this kind of father. So I don't want—notices Laura putting part of her sandwich away) No, Laura, you need to finish that sandwich. (Laura obeys; to Mr. R again) No, I don't want you to stop doing this kind of thing, I want you to do it, but it needs to be in such a way that Laura knows that you are treating her with the respect of her privacy that a 14 year old deserves. Because a 14 year old deserves privacy and I think— now maybe (saying something about Jill, inaudible) maybe next year she will have the right to close her door. Laura has the right to close her door now. (to Laura) What do you think about that, will you do it? (Laura nods.) And then we will be meeting—Dr. Barragan will continue working with you. He has joined me here, and by design I have run this session, but he will continue these sessions. (to Dr. B) And now you will see if these people will, will follow—it will be easy for Laura to do it, and I think, maybe, it will be easier, easy, for Connie, I don't know. It will be very hard for Dave, to keep the doors closed.

Dr. B: I know, yeah.

Dr. M: Now I want Connie, besides—(to Mrs. R) you do some negotiating with this young man. (indicating Steve). I want you to negotiate with him at what time you want him to be in bed. You decide that, and for this week I want you—that he should go to bed whenever you think he needs to go. You do any way you want.

Mrs. R: I'd like to get another thing straight, too, while we're talking. Ah, when we moved to this house, there were four bedrooms. Ah, at that time, Laura and Jill were together in one bedroom and Steve was in the other bedroom and, of course, we were in ours, and we had someone from Jamaica with us who was sleeping in the spare room—they were living with us.

Dr. M: Can you make it snappy?

Mrs. R: Yeah.

Dr. M: I have to run away—I am five minutes late.

Mrs. R: Yeah, all right. Ah, we added onto the house so that Steve would have his own bedroom and the girls would have their own bedrooms. When we added onto the house, Steve never slept in that bedroom that we added on. It was in the back of the house. He felt like it was separated from the rest of the house, and he never wanted to sleep in there; he always slept in Jill's room. Finally, I told him when he started school that he was a big boy and he had to sleep in that bedroom. Well, I had to sit with him for a while until he fell asleep at night, and he finally got used to the idea and he was sleeping in there. Every once in a while he'd want to sleep in Jill's room, and I didn't wish to allow it because I knew what was going to happen—that the one night would lead into going back to Jill's room permanently. But Dave said, "If he'll get to sleep, let him sleep in there." And this is what's happened. He ended up going back into Jill's room.

Mr. R: He's in Jill's room, Laura has her own room, he's in Jill's room, and the other room is empty.

Mrs. R: Now there is a new habit where Jill isn't sleeping in her room, and she and he are sleeping in his room.

Dr. M: Connie, change that for this week.

Mrs. R: O.K.

Dr. M: And we will then see you next week. Make an appointment at the time in which you are (inaudible words). Ah, Laura's problem with food is not a problem . . .

Mr. R: I don't think so.

Dr. M: I think it will disappear just at a time in which she grows up, (to Laura) and that can be very fast if you want to grow up fast, and I am not so certain. I think in some way you still want to be 10, but maybe if you insist, they will let you. O.K.? (getting up to leave, shaking hands with Mr. and Mrs. R)

Dr. B: (to parents) I'll be right with you to get together as a family. (Dr. B and Dr. M go out. Family lingers until Dr. B returns to set the date for the next interview, then leaves. End of tape.)

O: Why does Minuchin tell Laura to close her door for only two hours a day?

A: Because he knows that for her to close it even for a short length of time is tampering with the family's territorial system in a big way. He wants to build in something not too drastic, something that the family can tolerate.

O: Isn't it also a way of prescribing the symptom by default? Laura can go on doing as she has been doing the rest of the time. So the therapist again governs the situation whether she makes the change or whether she doesn't.

A: Right. Now with Jill he says, "You should keep your door open."

O: Is that to individuate her from Laura?

A: Yes, she isn't as old as Laura, so of course she can't have her door closed yet.

O: Could he also be thinking that to leave the father with all doors closed would be too much for him?

A: Sure. He restricts the time husband and wife are to be alone for the same reason. He even puts in the activity they are to share: TV. He knows they are anxious about intimacy, so he orders them to do something together that will make the least demand on either of them. And this sets things up so that, if intimacy does follow, it will come about spontaneously, and not in response to an order.

O: He also tells the father that he knows he will want to check on Laura, and that it's okay to come in if he knocks.

A: That's again going along with the family system. It's like entering a freeway. You start by fitting the position and speed of your vehicle with those already on the road. Then, when you are well established, you can maneuver to go faster, or slower, or jockey about, or even affect the movement of other cars.

O: When Minuchin goes back to Laura and tells her to finish her sandwich, it's so casual. You'd never guess that this was what the family came in about.

A: Well, she smiles and eats. And Minuchin goes on about his real business, which is to continue to differentiate people. Laura can close her door; Jill can close hers next year; Stephen, being younger, has fewer rights; mother and father still have to make decisions about him.

O: Why does mother bring a new topic just as Minuchin is closing?

A: She is asserting herself, I would guess, trying to get one more problem solved before she leaves. She's not a stupid woman, and she has clued in to what Minuchin is trying to do. She mentions that the two younger children are sleeping in the same room, and Minuchin gives the backing to separate them. But he really wants to tie the session up and be done.

O: How would you describe Minuchin's last speech. It seems to contain so much.

A: Minuchin is defusing the problem with food. It's not a problem, it's just a stage that will disappear as Laura grows up. Then he spreads the burden both ways, by saying that the family has to let Laura grow up, but that Laura has to push, too.

O: What happened subsequently with the family?

A: Barragan focused mainly on the relationship between the parents. He found that working directly with the symptom was useless, since Laura was an accomplished dieter, and, even when she did eat, chose food that didn't put any weight on her. What he did was try to get the mother to stand up to the father. As the conflict between the couple came to the fore, the involvement between Laura and her father got less. The father and mother began to have intense quarrels, and the father went to the hospital for two anxiety attacks, which seemed to be caused by a sense of isolation from both his children and his wife. In therapy sessions, he began complaining that he had too much responsibility and his wife was not carrying her share of the load. As a result, the wife became more active. Once the couple had established a better partnership, Barragan gave them the task of making their daughter gain ten pounds in three weeks. The father, now that he had the support of his wife, was able to make the girl eat. For the first two weeks, they didn't get anywhere. But in the third week, Laura gained eight pounds and two weeks later had gained twenty-four. The family has not sought further help, but a follow-up six months later showed that Laura was not only in good physical shape but had a boy friend.

O: In other words, she began to lead an independent existence.

A: Yes. She could finally shut her door.

The Birthday Party: An Experiment in Obtaining Change in One's Own Extended Family

RABBI EDWIN H. FRIEDMAN

The paper that follows is by a student of Murray Bowen, a pioneer family therapist, who was working clinically with "live-in" families having schizophrenic offspring at NIMH more than twenty years ago and has since been described as "the family therapist's family therapist" (Framo, 1972). In more recent times he has evolved a treatment philosophy and method aimed at the induction of change in long-standing patterns of interaction within family systems often by working with an individual. The method has at its centrum a concern for the extended family network and the conception of the "genogram" (a diagram of the entire kinship system with a graphic analysis of interpersonal bondings and divergences). Its goals are to enhance the differentiation of family members through the erasure of stabilized "emotional cutoffs" (alienations) existent between some parties and the diffusion of dysfunctional bondings operative between others. Often enough it seeks to achieve these ends through the "domino effect"—that is, via the deliberate introduction of disequilibrating data and/or events into the system. The resulting disruptions and reverberating, progressive displacements engendered in previously counterbalanced splits and alignments of the extended family network are presumed to now release individual members so they may better extricate themselves from the web of the family's "undifferentiated ego mass." The emphasis placed on transactions between extended family kin is a hallmark of this therapy, and makes it a strong countervailing force to the alienating pressures rampant in our society at large.

With this in mind, the article by Friedman, which follows, is noteworthy on a number of counts:

1. It shares with other family therapies the view of the family as a social system, but by design seems to rely more blatantly on a "cause and effect" model and the presumption of interdependently arranged subsystems within the family. While, in the end, Friedman puts in a disclaimer as to his role in any obtained change in the family, his intent is clear from the outset.

2. Insofar as it describes how to obtain change in one's own family, it implies a model for family therapists to follow. That is, the article may be seen as making the unstated communication that perhaps family therapists ought to attend to their own house before attending to those of others—that in effect, they should attempt to extricate themselves from the emotional complexes of their own family in advance of endeavoring to "differentiate" clients from their emotional embeddedness. The parallels to the "training analysis" for prospective psychoanalysts are obvious, and need no elaboration. It might simply be noted that a substantial number of Bowen's students have followed the examples of Anonymous (1972) and Friedman and published their personal accounts (Colon, 1973; Guerin and Fogarty, 1972; Bradt and Moynihan, 1971).

3. The paper is instructive because it exemplifies in bold form a feature of much family therapy that is roundly attacked by others. It is vulnerable to the accusation of "manipulativeness." Friedman, for example, endeavors to initiate change by concocting the most "unthinkable" event he can conjure for "shocking" his family system. He compounds the procedure by deliberately and selectively divulging family secrets. He "arranges" situations and confrontations without informing the parties involved as to his motives. Friedman, however, is fully aware that others will condemn his actions as manipulative; he is not impervious to the charge that he may be "playing God." And, indeed, he acknowledges trepidations about the fact that he did not forewarn his family of what he was about. Just how satisfactory one finds his defense of his actions to be, or whether, in fact, one believes a defense is even called for, is a personal judgment. Each reader must decide for himself.

5. Like so many articles on family therapy, this one does not speak specifically about children. The systems approach often precludes such a focus. That it does so, however, does not mean that children will not be substantially affected by family interventions, or receive beneficial fallout from changes in other parts of the system. The presumption is that they will. In this connection, though, it must be acknowledged that Friedman's work with his own family seemed to provide most help for the family's older generation. This style of family therapy may have some special significance in this regard. Friedman's interventions not only run counter to the prevailing societal pressures promoting alienation and isolation, but they meet head on those additional forces at work in contemporary youth oriented America which demean the elderly. Inadvertent as Friedman's tampering with cultural forces may have been, one cannot help wondering to what extent his "success" with his family was contingent on his intervention with the older generation. By his actions he attended to them, consulted them, enraged them, embarrassed them, flattered them. Most of all he reincluded them as persons of significance in the family system. How appreciative they must have been.

Friedman's experiment, then, has some decidedly developmental implications. If conscientiously addressed, these might add immeasurably to the potency of his methods. Like all papers out of the Bowen school, his work both exemplifies the phenomenal power that human connectedness can have for all of us, and articulates the sad circumstance of how we may play lightly with, or take for granted, those things we hold most dear.

It is thought by many that anyone who engages in the practice of individual therapy would benefit, both personally and in his work, from experiencing such therapy. Can the same be said for those who practice family therapy? My guess is that, in fact, many who practice family therapy with their patients are often tempted to use their skills and insights to try to obtain change in their own families. Perhaps the family therapist may be said to be in a perpetual multiple family group as he draws parallels and refers insights back and forth between relationships in his own family and those in the families with which he works.

To work therapeutically with one's own family could be concealed expectation of the family, and a major force in drawing the therapist to that kind of professional work. After all, if patients are to be seen as symptoms of their family networks, why not therapists? We talk about identified patients, why not talk about identified therapists? I shall come back to this idea more explicitly later.

This paper will describe a studied, carefully planned attempt to obtain change in my own extended family over a two-year period, the focal point or fulcrum for the whole process being a surprise birthday party for my mother on the occasion of her seventieth birthday. The work was done in consultation with Dr. Murray Bowen under whose supervision I received my general training in working with families.

The format of this paper will be as follows: first, a brief description of the extended network in which I wished to see change occur, pinpointing those areas where I felt dysfunctional symptoms of the network could be identified; second, a description of the way I tried to encourage the process of change with some exposition of the theory on which I based my own actions; and third, some after-thoughts and general conclusions about how the professional person may work within his own extended family to obtain change.

Figure 1 describes my extended family on my mother's side. My mother is represented by the circle which occupies the next to the last position in the third generation (containing the number 70); my own

Reprinted with permission from *Family Process,* Vol. 10 (1971), pp. 345-359. Copyright © 1971 by *Family Process.*

position is represented by the square containing the letter "E." The diagram represents five generations, though only the third and fourth (with one exception) are relevant to the experiment carried out. As the reader can see, the first generation had three children, two girls and a boy. They were born in Europe and came to America where they produced fourteen offspring (all first generation Americans). The sisters each had five children, the brother had four. My mother's generation of fourteen cousins, on the other hand, produced only twelve offspring, primarily in multiples of one! Four of my mother's cousins had no children (one never married), and only two of the remaining had more than one child. In each case, the two cousins who were the only members of their generation to have more than one child were the siblings who became most involved in their spouse's extended family—that is, they were most out of the system.

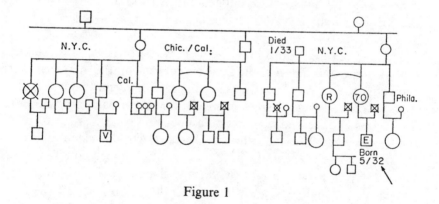

Figure 1

Some other interesting attributes of the system are these: every one of my mother's first cousins at the time of the party (July 1968) was alive and in his seventies except for her younger brother who was sixty-eight, and the woman who had been the oldest. She had committed suicide twenty-five years previously. Secondly, in each of the three sets of siblings that made up my mother's generation, the sisters had stuck together. My mother and her older sister (R) live on the same floor of the same apartment house in New York City. The two sisters in the Chicago group live in the same apartment. All four are widows, having lost their husbands around the age of fifty-five to sixty. None remarried. My mother and aunt, however, have had almost no contact with the Chicago cousins and never met the younger one. The other two sisters from the group on the left lived within walking distance of one another on the northern tip of Manhattan throughout their entire lives. They have never had children, and they have never become widows!

It should be noted also that in the middle set of my mother's cousins, the two boys have always lived together, the youngest of that set living with his married brother in California. In contra-distinction to this pairing off among siblings in my mother's generation, their children live almost totally separate lives from one another. It is true that they are cousins and not siblings, but generally speaking it can be said that the cousins on my level are almost never in communication with one another.

There were three points in the network where I wished to see change; that is, where I felt pathological symptoms of the network were showing up. One was my own relationship with my mother which I felt was distant and rigid despite many efforts on my part to be closer to her. Second concerned my next oldest cousin's son (the male member of the fifth generation indicated on the chart) who started taking drugs at thirteen, was obese and doing poorly in school, in contrast to his older sister, who was bright, witty and charming. The third place I wanted to see change was with regard to the younger of the two New York City cousins (V), who, despite the fact he was an extremely successful professional person, was nearing forty and was unmarried, indeed the only unmarried member of my generation.

At the time of writing this paper, two years and three months after the party, not only has my relationship with my mother changed considerably but my younger cousin has just been enrolled as a freshman at George Washington University and allowed to take honor courses his first year, and my older cousin has been married for more than six months.

The Process

Since my own work with families is at the systems end of the continuum rather than the analytic, I should like to begin this section by indicating my conceptual approach to family systems. By system I mean a set of relationships which, upon achieving homeostasis, functions to maintain that homeostasis through inner-adjusting compensations. Change in one relationship of a system so defined will usually bring about change in another relationship.

When it comes to family systems, I do not equate the degree of physical distance with the degree of emotional distance. People certainly are involved in important non-family relationship systems, but I think those other systems are rarely as intense emotionally as the family system so that a family relationship that is physically distant can be much more influential than a non-family relationship of greater physical proximity. The potential for becoming free from the influence of one's family system, however, is much greater in an approach that brings one towards the family than in an approach that takes one away. I think, therefore, in terms of differentiation of self within the system rather than independence of it, and do not believe it is really possible to become independent of one's family system except by becoming intensely part of another system (and then all one has succeeded in doing is transferring the dependency).

Success at achieving such differentiation of self can be measured, I believe, in the extent to which one can be a part of the family without automatically being one of the "emotional dominoes." The path towards such a goal can be achieved best not by a process of internal analysis of oneself but through a process of external perceptions that analyze the system. In other words, I do not think in terms of a sense of self, which seems too unverifiable, but in terms of a position of self.

In my work with families, therefore, I have been influenced by an approach to general systems thinking known as "black box" theory. As computers and other sophisticated electronics equipment became too complex to take apart when they dysfunctioned, an attempt was made to deal with this by inserting new inputs into the system instead of trying to analyze the dysfunctional elements. The method is not all that hit-or-miss, since one always knows some of the major characteristics of the system (contained, but unseeable) within the "black box." Some of the ramifications of that approach are to see dysfunctional parts as always symptomatic, to define dysfunction always in inter-relational terms, to note that the definition or label of dysfunction also includes a large measure of perspective and to diminish the distinction between essence and function.

One other fact has influenced my decision to apply black box theory to human beings and their family systems. Miniaturization with computers has reached the point that ten thousand elements can be put on a disk one-tenth of an inch square. By the end of the decade that should be increased to one hundred thousand. To achieve the density of cells in the human brain one would need a cubic inch of the latter. Thus I have been asking myself if less complex systems than human relationships are now being considered too complex to change through methods that analyze the components (or even the relationships sometimes), surely a similar approach is worth considering in trying to obtain change in families.

The Birthday Party

Applying black box theory to my own family, I began by asking what seemed most to characterize the program of my own family system's set of relationships. How could I go about changing some of the most significant inputs, at least some of my own most significant inputs?

What struck me most about my mother's extended family was the set pattern of relating; the isolation of the cousins, the closeness among my mother's cousins of the sets of siblings—with little crossing of lines there. Within my mother's sibling group alone I was struck by the fact that my mother herself was like Cinderella before the ball—she had been given the job of taking care of their mother in her seventies, when she was old and feeble and defecating in our bathtub because she was too blind and unaware to know where she was. I also decided that the biggest "no-no" in the family—perhaps because no one was dying—

was age; I took note of my own relative disengagement; I noticed also that I was almost the only member of my family with a "helpful" title.

In these terms the question was, what would be the most "unthinkable" event one could carry out in this family system. Obviously, to give a birthday party—indeed a surprise birthday party—a ball for Cinderella, so to speak, outside of New York City, and given by the last person the family might have expected to throw a ball.

For three months, therefore, I set about calling every one of my mother's cousins and siblings—from the top down, in deference to age. Her sister, as you can imagine, was against it—until I put her in charge of something. Added and unexpected benefits came during this phase, as in conversation with each relative I had to ask information about the others, received the information in the form of opinions I did not expect but made sure to pass on to the others when I called them. It was as though there were little light bulbs connected into each circle and square on the genogram that were either all out or all on (steady state sort of thing); the day I started telephoning those bulbs started flashing—out of phase—for the first time in many, many years. Something dormant (and apparently dead) came to life.

One interesting detail during this part of the process may be mentioned. When I called the oldest group of cousins, living in Manhattan, the brother said they couldn't come because one of his sisters was very, very sick but he would tell his sisters for me and I needn't call. I called the sister who wasn't sick and she said she couldn't come because her sister was very, very sick and she would tell her for me; I needn't call her sister. Now remember it was the brother's son who was unmarried. When I spoke to the sick one, I found her much brighter and much more knowledgeable about the family than the other two—this certainly fit all my ideas about families, namely that it couldn't be clear at all who was sick for whom, that indeed the symptomatic one was often the most aware and responsible one. So I wrote her a short note saying I was sorry they all couldn't come down for the day and I realized that she had a responsibility to keep the family together, but how would we ever get Vicky (my unmarried cousin) married. As I calculated, that letter arrived in New York on a

Friday and the following Monday Vicky called to accept the invitation and asked if he could bring a girl.

With the exception of Vicky none of my mother's cousins was able to come nor did any of her close friends whom I called—all, however, kept the secret, and all sent good wishes. To each person I had sent a list of the names of everyone invited. There were twenty-six people at the party, and the surprise was total. Only one of her siblings did not come, the next oldest brother. He, incidentally, married secretly when young, fifty-five years previously, and came back to live with the family for six months before he announced he was married. He was the only sibling who had two children, the one from this group, as I mentioned before, who was more a part of his spouse's system. I point this out because it has become my experience generally to note with families that brothers and sisters will carry out inter-relational inputs at age seventy as though they were still viewing one another as age seven.

There is one other grouping I should like to mention before talking about the party itself. One of my mother's intimates was not a blood relative but her sister-in-law on my father's side; that is my father's brother's wife. My aunt and uncle had lived in Canada with their only child, a son, for forty years, had been extremely successful in the retail business and were perhaps my nuclear family's closest relatives second to my mother's sister's family. In recent years this aunt had been sickly, alcoholic, depressed, and had growths on her feet that necessitated repeated operations. At any given time, however, she was liable to recover completely from everything and take a trip half way around the world. When my father died, this aunt and uncle had begged my mother to move to Canada to be near them.

This group also would not come to the party because my aunt had become phobic after she finally stopped drinking. And like the group on Northern Manhattan none dared fly away for a day "to the heat of Washington." I learned as much about those who did not come to the party as those who did. For example, the absurd excuses given by this group and the one on Northern Manhattan made their own stuck-togetherness stand out in relief and pointed out directions for follow-up in the future.

The party itself was a complete success, especially considering the logistics. People came from four cities and had to meet at one place at precisely the right hour while my mother was bluffed into going out for an hour. The caterer was precision itself, arriving and setting everything up during that same time. Actually, I felt the success at keeping the secret, that is, the ease with which I was able to get my family to gang up in a conspiracy against my mother did not speak well for my family. Her total surprise, however, confirmed my feeling that I had done something truly unthinkable.

At the party one event in particular was significant. My next older cousin, my mother's sister's son, had been like a complementary sibling to me. Although Walter Toman in his work on sibling constellations recognizes the complementary aspects of sibling relationships, he says only children are "wild cards." It has been my experience generally that if there is enough feedback between their parents, two only children from the same family will produce some kind of complementary system. My cousin is an accountant, very proper in all ways, no maverick opinions, and super-responsible for our two mothers. He became totally, helplessly drunk within one hour after the party started and was walked around outside by his wife for the next three hours. During this time, his son, whom I knew only to be obese and failing in school, told me he had been on hard drugs for the last two years. In the middle of the party when I investigated a strange tinkle of breaking glass downstairs, I found my aunt, seventy-one, who in her concern for her son, had given our glass sliding door something that must have been a karate chop with her knee as she went to look for him. She was uninjured but the entire door had been shattered. Rushing in to keep the party going, I told everyone upstairs that they would never guess what my Aunt Rose had done to upstage my mother, her younger sister. Strangely, maybe because of the way I put it, nobody believed me, and everyone went right on eating and drinking while my unmarried cousin, the dentist, applied iodine.

In the months that followed the party, the following events occurred in rather rapid succession: one month later my conservative cousin had grown a beard; for my aunt, who will clean an ash tray before you have finished your cigarette, this was truly earth-shaking. I wrote him a letter telling him I thought it was a terrible thing to do to his mother and whom would I look up to now? I also wrote my young cousin a letter asking him seriously what his trips were like and received a long exposition about the effects of LSD on coitus—to use his word. He also announced that he had given up drugs because he wanted whole children. Two months later my mother's younger brother, the youngest in this line of cousins, the only one who was not seventy, dropped dead of a heart attack. His wife thereupon came to Washington six months later to live with her married daughter and, as previously noted, the younger cousin enrolled at George Washington University the following year. Precisely between those events my dentist cousin married a Gentile divorcee with two children—the granddaughter of a prominent New York Protestant clergyman. They were to come to Washington for a private marriage ceremony by me, but his father had a heart attack, and they haven't made it yet.

During the following year my Canadian aunt made unsuccessful suicide attempts with drugs. I wrote this aunt a letter, having been told by my uncle and cousin that she couldn't come to the phone. In the letter, I told her that I had always thought of her as my most competent aunt, considering her success in business over the years, and I couldn't understand how she would do such a sloppy job of committing suicide. I followed those lines describing my own life in the most depressing terms I could think of. As I say, I was encouraged to do this by what I had seen with the other group. The reaction of my aunt was most interesting.

As it turned out, my mother arrived in Ottawa two days after the letter. My aunt never revealed the contents, and to this day everyone is saying what a wonderful thing my mother did for my phobic aunt, who had not left the house in two years and was now, "as a result of my mother's visit," back to her old self. Indeed she has since struck up relationships with other relatives in the States and relates to me entirely differently than to anyone else. (It never ceases to amaze me that those who think of "system" as a "cold" approach usually resort to electrical means when it comes to shock.) My aunt has re-established contacts with her own family of origin from which she had become increasingly cut off over the years. I paid a visit to her during the summer two months later, during which time she gave me "hell" for writing such a nasty letter; she came down to Washington in September to hear me preach (for the first time) during the High Holy Days; she went to some weddings on her side of the family the following month. And in December she told my uncle that she could no longer take their forty years of a battling marriage, their separate vacations, etc., and that this time she really was going through with their ten-year-old suspended but constantly threatened separation agreement. My uncle went off to the West Indies for a month and came back with cancer of the liver. He died two months later.

I have, since the party, kept up my own interest in the extended network, paying a trip to Chicago, for example, to visit my mother's and aunt's two girl cousins and wound up in the ridiculous position of having my mother and aunt question me about the family for a change; they had never met the younger one, age seventy-two.

The Hangover

In this last section I should like to describe some of my thoughts and conclusions about doing work in one's own family. I shall sub-divide this section into two parts: technical and personal.

From the point of view of technique I would say I consciously tried five different varieties. Listing them in order of least effectiveness, I would say they were: 1) being straightforwardly analytic about people or relationships, that is, being the expert; 2) telling them a story about one of my clients; 3) performing verbal reversals; 4) performing behavior reversals; and 5) being stupid—this one has to follow, if being expert is at the other end of the scale.

Regarding the straightforward analytical approach, I found that the reaction was almost always one of denial. I was told I didn't understand, or a comment would be made about my playing therapist. On the other hand, when I went to Canada after my aunt's suicide attempt and spent one week with the family, never once making an interpretation, I found by the end of the week they got so scared by this that they began to talk to me in a way that showed they knew more, and maybe thought more, in analytic terminology than I did.

Telling them about a client had some limited effectiveness. On several occasions since the party when members of my family were deeply distressed about something, I found that telling them about a similar situation from my practice helped de-personalize the situation for them. It reminded me of what had worked and not worked with the client and thus helped me know how to behave at that moment. But most of all, I think, it enabled the conversation to continue with me in the position of experienced relative who was not trying to change them but who, from their point of view, despite his experience, didn't seem too anxious about it either.

For example, for about a year my mother's older sister had been obsessed with anxiety about gastrointestinal problems. In her concern over the doctor's failure to find something specific, she had not been eating and was thus losing weight. The loss of weight contributed further to her worry that something sinister was at work. Everyone including the family doctor had been at a loss to reassure her. I had treated a similar case with a "paradoxical intention" barrage: did she know where the cancer was, what progress did she think it had been making and, finally, people didn't just get cancer, she must have done something wrong, perhaps God was punishing her.

Thus I dealt with my aunt by: 1) not attempting any reassurance; 2) figuring, but not mentioning, that it had something to do with her son's involvement elsewhere (which indeed turned out to be the case); and 3) telling her as coldly as possible that I still needed her help in getting my mother straightened out, and I would appreciate it if she could just hang on a bit longer.

The third technique is verbal reversals. The two kinds I have employed most have been to out-kook and to go contrary to my instincts. An example of an out-kooking dialogue might go like this (with my dramatic aunt from Canada and in front of my mother who always feels so sorry for her):

aunt: Eddie, what do you think of me?
me: I never analyze my relatives.
aunt: I have opinions about you.
me: Well, maybe you can get more distance.

aunt: You must have some opinions.

me: Okay, I think you're crazy, but it sure keeps you from being boring.

The other form of the verbal reversal is to follow one's instincts and then do the opposite. Thus when my aunts, who are in their seventies, complain about their sundry ailments, and I find myself thinking "they're old, afraid of dying, lonely, etc.," I immediately tell them they're getting older, or nobody lives forever. Sometimes before they get a chance to complain, say on the phone, I tell them they sound terrible. And then we usually have a delightful conversation. As my mother got close to retiring (at seventy-two), I would take her for a drive and point out the new old folks home and describe how secure she would be there. She is now looking for another job and applying for unemployment insurance!

The effect of the verbal reversal on these relationships is, I believe, that I convey I won't play their games. Consequently they relate in a much more adult manner to me than to those who take the so-called compassionate approach. I believe I sometimes set an example for other members of the family and make unthinkable actions do-able.

The fourth technique, the action reversal, is more effective, I believe, though I must admit that this dichotomy between verbal and action reversals is somewhat artificial. There are two kinds here, also. One is to behave in a situation the way no one in the family ever does, the other is to behave the way you yourself never do. The party was so successful, I believe, because both things happened. I have been doing a lot of research on how widows should invest their money, and sending advice to my mother. My CPA cousin has always done my mother's income tax—for free—and she naturally takes my very professionally-appearing plans to him, who admits to my mother he hasn't done much thinking about this area. My final recommendations are always overly-conservative, and he winds up having to suggest something more speculative in comparison.

Switching means of communication is another good behavior reversal (say phone and letter), but reversing whom one talks to about whom is better. Throughout my life I have had gossipy talks with my mother about my aunts; recently I have been doing this with my aunts about my mother. For example, my mother always took a highly sympathetic and supportive position toward my Canadian aunt despite years of my telling my mother that I thought she was selfish. I got a juicy tidbit from my aunt about how she thought my father secretly liked her and passed it on. My conversations with my mother now are filled with my mother's diatribes about my aunt as I try to explain that you have "to understand her." I find that the more I do this the freer my mother seems to be with me. (My grandfather died six months after I was born, and I believe I replaced him in some original triangle with his two daughters.)

The best reversal I have found, however, is to refuse to be serious about what the family is most uptight about. I would add, however, that being exaggeratedly over-serious sometimes seems to amount to the same thing. (I am also coming to believe there would have been much less possibility that my hypertensive father would have died at 56 if he could have taken my mother's "goodness" less seriously.)

This brings me to the fifth and I believe most powerful way of inducing change in one's family, and primarily I believe because it focuses one most on his own inputs, and that is what I call being stupid. At the beginning of this essay I raised the question if patients were to be considered symptoms of their family system, why not therapists? Maybe the same processes that produce dysfunction create other kinds of functioning. Or, since we are talking about process, if when a member of a family becomes the patient, the other members respond in a way that keeps that person in the patient role even though it is ultimately to their own detriment. Maybe a similar process goes on regarding professionals and their families: that once someone becomes a member of the helping professions the effect on the family is to have them adapt to that person in ways which are not necessarily helpful to that person or themselves. If this is true then the way to get the most change in the homeostasis of such a system is clearly never to play therapist in the system, that is, therapist as they would think of therapist, indeed to play anti-therapist. (Stirring up trouble, not being helpful or responsible, giving pain or at least not rushing in to relieve it)

All forms of reversal help in this matter, of course; I asked my formerly alcoholic aunt to take back a bottle of unusual Scotch as a gift to my cousin. She "forgot" it at my mother's in New York. Until my dentist cousin got married I never missed an opportunity to remind him of his responsibility to his aunts and parents as their only offspring. I have found, however, that asking stupid questions or making obvious common sense interpretations of equally obvious pathological behavior turns relatives into very insightful people. And that gets me asking, "Well, if they knew the answers all along why the hell are they asking me about the problem?"

For myself as rabbi another way I have found to be unprofessional is to fail to go to, no less to perform, weddings and funerals for members of the family. This is producing a very strong reaction: on the other hand you can almost watch the shifts in responsibility among my cousins when I force my family members to find their own rabbis. For example, when I just couldn't make it to an uncle's funeral, another cousin (the oldest in the line) who went, took charge. This has changed his relationship with that uncle's family and I believe had corresponding salutary effects on his own nuclear family.

I find this quite a paradox: that is, by not helping precisely where because of my professional expertise I could have been most helpful, I may have been more useful.

Now I should like to conclude with a few personal observations. This whole paper has been framed in terms of obtaining change in one's extended family. Yet I am quite sure that the person benefiting most from any attempt to induce such change, at least in the ways I have been describing, is the person doing it. In fact, it would be my guess that if one sets about trying to induce change for the sake of inducing the change, or for the sake of helping the relatives primarily, it won't work, or at least it won't work as well. The paradox here is resolved, I think, by remembering that as long as you are doing it for others you would be behaving as a therapist, a role that is hard to get out of and that secretly maintains homeostasis.

The approach I have been taking, therefore, is to do these things to see what it teaches me about my family. This in turn, however, has raised some interesting and serious theoretical questions. First of all, I have been wondering recently if these five techniques do not wind up with exactly the same effectiveness rating when one is working professionally with families. This is an exciting idea for I have never been comfortable with a style of therapy that could not also be a style of life. Thus, I have begun to ask myself if what I have most in common with those who see me professionally is that we have both been the results of similar processes and that, therefore, the more I understand about my family and my position in it the more I will understand family process in general. These are insights I can share.

From the personal point of view I should also like to make a passing comment on what I have most obviously avoided, namely the effect on one's nuclear family if one tries to obtain change in one's extended family. To talk publicly about relationships in this area is to get too personal; on the other hand, I would not want to imply, by ignoring that area, that there are no repercussions.

It may also be worth noting that my wife received several notes of thanks. This was quite surprising since I did not involve her in one single detail, having had the entire affair catered down to the silverware, chairs and tables, and since all correspondence and phone calls to set up the party came only from me; no one had even spoken to my wife during the preparations.

Finally, I should like to enter a disclaimer. When this paper was delivered, some heard it as playing God and suggested that I should have warned my family about what I was trying to do. Let me state clearly, therefore, that I knew I could not be fully aware of the results. This is not to say I had no fears, trepidations, or fantasies. (None of my fantasies about deaths and suicides materialized—perhaps because fantasies come out of the system as it exists. If individuals are to be seen as symptoms of the family, so must their fantasies.) Things had been the way they had been for an awfully long time; members of the family were suffering now because of the irresponsibility (dependency) of others. I decided, therefore, I would take responsibility only for my own feelings and behavior and each other member of the family would have to take responsibility for his.

In no way, therefore, do I take credit for any of the changes I have described in my family, for in no way can I prove that my new inputs produced the new outputs. But I do believe that few of the things I did would have had the same effect on the family if anyone else would have done them, and if that is true, it is not because of any special attribute, talent, or personality factor that resides within me, but because of where I am on the genogram.

Social Network Intervention

ROSS V. SPECK, M.D.
CAROLYN L. ATTNEAVE, Ph.D.

Like the preceding paper, the one that follows by Speck and Attneave, addresses issues of societal significance, though it does so somewhat more explicitly. There is the same concern for the plight of the nuclear family, for the problems engendered by spatial and physical isolation, for the intense loneliness resulting from the ultrarespect accorded privacy in this culture, for the sense of guilt and impotence and shame that stems from the mistaken assumptions on the part of families that the crises they suffer are somehow unique to them.

While its concerns are not substantively different from those of the Bowen group, the goals of Family Network Intervention are that it seeks to (1) provide "an antidote to the aura of depersonalized loneliness characteristic of postindustrial society"; (2) engage naturally existing, but previously untapped, support systems and groups for obtaining this antidote; (3) try to "stimulate, to reflect, and to focus the potential with the (community) network to solve one another's problems"; and (4) enable people to cope, "to share their strengths in coping," to reap "enjoyments and pleasures that restore their potentials and set them up to handle the inevitable next crisis of living."

The methods of intervention are tailored accordingly. There is the use of theatrical staging, the use of "intervention teams," the reliance on "volunteerism," the elicitation of "peak" experiences in a group context, the employment of "encounter" methods. A number of these features are unique to Family Network Intervention, and some deserve closer attention.

The analogy of family intervention with "theater" is not new with Speck and Attneave. We have encountered it before in this volume in the consideration of Minuchin's work (Minuchin, 1967, 1974). Then, too, Kantor and Hoffman (1966) have employed Brechtian principles as a model for conjoint therapy. What distinguishes the contribution of Speck and Attneave is their conception of audience, space, actors, and directors, as well as the intimate relation they posit between these components of theater. Quite literally, their therapy is conceived as "action theater in the round"; the audience is sizable—sometimes upward of seventy—and seated in concentric rings; the theater itself is a family home; the actors are members of the treatment team, the family of focus, and the entire natural community in attendance; the emphasis is participatory—people exchange chairs, places, roles; the therapeutic team consists of persons "representative" of population segments in the audience—there are old for the old, young for the young, middle-aged for the middle-aged, males for males, women for women; mutual identification, and thus participation, is facilitated.

All these distinguishing characteristics of Family Network Intervention would seem, for the typical clinician, to pose some severe limitations on the practicalities of application. The therapist, for example, would seem to need the skills of a theatrical director; the intervention team members are so delineated that graduates of our current clinical training programs are not likely to qualify; space and timing problems may prove inordinate. Yet, much may be said for the approach, particularly insofar as it emphasizes certain underlying principles that may be separated from technique—that is, certain principles which can be extracted and employed in somewhat different contexts. Included here may be the principle of representative-

ness. The Eastern Pennsylvania School of Family Therapy has long advocated that family therapists work in pairs. The Multiple Impact Family Therapy group has compared its working teams of psychiatrists, psychologists, and social workers to families. The team's ability to problem-solve, despite differences of opinion, is sold to serve as a useful model for the families being treated. The presence of adolescents and children as members on a therapeutic team is less reported in the literature, but it is an arrangement that some family therapists have begun to approach (see Leichter and Schulman, 1974, in this volume).

The Family Network Intervention method relies heavily on "volunteerism," and debunks actively the conventional assumption of professional responsibility and patient dependence. In the attempts to demystify professionalism it aligns itself with many of the tenets of the Community Mental Health movement, and concomitantly raises some serious issues for more conservatively oriented therapists to contemplate. Among these are the functions of "privacy" and "deviancy" in American society, to which Speck and Attneave allude without dealing cogently or conclusively with either. Once again, the asociological slant of family clinicians seems to preclude speculation. For example, the authors seem to share with other family therapists the clinical conviction that the maintenance of family secrets is dysfunctional and that they ought, in the interest of healing, to be revealed at some point, although at what point is not precisely delineated. The authors convey this conviction without addressing the cultural or societal underpinnings of "confidentiality" or "secrecy" in a competitive economy and the consequences of revelation are not contemplated. Instead, their intervention method seeks to undo the usual social restrictions on sharing information and more—it attempts to make public revelation a resource, a reservoir of strength and not a liability or invitation to ridicule and abuse. Given the worship of cloisteredness that dominates our society one is tempted to endorse their objectives. Professionals may be overly concerned with matters of privacy, although the obsession may be ours far more than it is that of our clients and patients; if the authors had given active consideration to the societal functions of the privacy code, readers might be more comfortable in endorsing their objectives.

The failure of the authors to deal meaningfully with the social uses of "deviance" in the cultural system is a neglect that this article shares with virtually the entire field. As mentioned earlier, this neglect may be tantamount to a family secret of family therapists. Speck and Attneave reraise the matter of deviance in explicit terms as something required by groups for purposes of boundary maintenance. They then slip away from the issue.

> *. . . this system needs a certain number of persons to scapegoat—to define as sick—in order to define itself. Thus, if one person gets over his needs for being scapegoated he has to be replaced by someone else . . . therapists are apt to find themselves in the middle of a cybernated pegboard game in which, if you press down one peg, sometimes two or three more pop up. Most of the time only one pops up . . .*

The problem of "symptom substitution" could not be stated more clearly in system terms. Similarly, the implication is clear that groups require deviance in order to keep their "shape." Left unclear is just what implications the authors see these insights as having for family therapy.

In social network intervention we assemble together all members of the kinship system, all friends and neighbors of the family, and, in fact, everyone who is of significance to the nuclear family that offers the presenting problem. In our experience, the typical middle-class urban family has the potential to assemble about forty persons for network meetings. These meetings are held in the home. Gathering the network group together in one place at one time provides great therapeutic potential. The assembly of the tribe in a crisis situation probably originated with prehistoric man. Tribal meetings for healing purposes

Reprinted from *Changing Families,* Grune & Stratton, New York, 1971, pp. 312-332. Reprinted by permission of Grune and Stratton, Inc. and the author.

are well known in many widely varying cultures. Social network intervention organizes this group force in a systematic way.

The Intervention Team

When a social network is assembled, they meet with a team of network intervenors. It is doubtful if this type of therapy should routinely be undertaken by one person working entirely alone. The first strategy, then, is the selection of a team. Preferably the team should be made up of two or three people who know one another well enough to have considerable trust in one another and who are familiar with each other's styles of relating and of general behavior. Division of roles and skills is important, but not a prerequisite. A particularly happy combination occurs when one of the team is skilled in large group situations, easily able to command the flow of attention and energy of a network, and knows when and how to turn it loose on itself.

The role of the leader is somewhat like that of a good discussion leader or a good theatrical director (particularly if he or she knows the Stanislavsky techniques). A sense of timing, empathy with emotional highpoints, a sense of group moods and undercurrents, and some charismatic presence are all part of the equipment that is desirable. Along with the ability to dominate, the leader must have the confidence that comes with considerable experience in handling situations and knowing human beings under stress. Equally important is his ability to efface himself, to delegate and diffuse responsibility, emphatically and pointedly, rather than to collect it for himself. This last characteristic is essential and often overlooked. One neophyte team commented that in their networks they did all the talking. By comparison, networks organized by experienced teams deceptively appear to run themselves. In fact, in several instances the team has been known to leave at about 11 o'clock, only to be told the next day, "We didn't even notice you'd gone until after 12 o'clock—and we kept right on talking until about 1:30."

The other team members should also have some of the leaders' characteristics, but many contribute special skills. If the network includes several generations, it is often helpful to have one youth and one grandparent type on the team so that mingling between team and network and participation by many of the network will be facilitated. Also, suppression of manic, overanxious, or inopportune comments is easier if the network member concerned is matched in style and status by a team member. Team members who blend easily with the total network can effectively help focus the smaller groups into which the network divides, such as committees, buzz sessions, or free-floating conversations.

It should be pointed out that if the team has three or more members, one member will often be selected as a scapegoat and be telephoned or vilified whenever the network or any part of it is angry at the leader or frustrated by its own impotence. The scapegoat role may as well be anticipated, even though one cannot always predict before the first meeting whom the network will choose for this sacrificial position.

An important skill that should be represented in the team is familiarity with nonverbal encounter techniques and their impact on groups and individuals. Emphasis on the scientific, cybernated aspect of the world has caused the importance of feelings and emotions to be overlooked to such an extent that most rituals are omitted or even ridiculed while the youth of the land cry out for meaning and for some way of learning how to "feel." Not only are the nonverbal reactions of the group extremely sensitive cues and clues for the intervention team, but when the team plays upon them to build a nonverbal network experience a ritual takes place. The tension released by jumping, shouting, or screaming, the calming effect of group swaying, the solidarity that comes from huddling and handclasping, all of these knot the network together in a way that merely meeting and talking cannot do. One often notes that, if a pattern of nonverbal openers has been utilized in the first meeting, the network members feel uneasy if it is omitted at the next meeting. That newcomers or latecomers are most easily melded into a social setting via informal nonverbal ritual is almost self-evident if one observes the number of rituals that form part of common courtesy, such as offering chairs, moving over, touching, exchanging meaningful looks, etc.

The experienced intervention team scattered in the crowd can respond to the leader's directions spontaneously and dramatically, catalyzing contagion and drawing everyone into participation. If a dignified "doctor" is willing to take off shoes and sit on the floor, or look at the ceiling and let out a rebel yell or war whoop, or close his eyes and sway while the whole group is looking, then it becomes safe for the housewives and husbands, the kids and the parents, the relatives and the neighbors to do so, too.

Also, quick verbal and nonverbal exchanges of information are easier for a team that is used to working together. The leader may need to have a piece of information, understand a relationship, see a development of insight or resistance in some subsection of the network. When space and organization permit, small conferences make information flow easy and help the leader utilize the team to verify impressions, check strategy, switch roles, or just let off steam. However, when conditions are too crowded or the session activities do not permit sub voice team conference, postural and body communications are important and the ability to break in or to toss the ball quickly and deftly about the team becomes more important. Network sessions last three or four hours, and leadership is strenuous. For the team to keep optimally fresh, some spelling off, as well as change of pace, is desirable.

The teamwork exhibited by the professional intervenors is sometimes fundamental as a model for the network. The effect of the teamwork model is most quickly seen in the network's activists, but the more passive members also learn that it is safe to fumble, to stick one's neck out, and to trust one another.

In one first network session involving a teen-age drug user and his friends and family, the network youth group was most reluctant to discuss openly their use of and experience with various drugs, as well as their ideas about drug use, until the matched youth team member spoke up frankly about his own curiosity and experience. While challenging this peer, the network youth found that the network's older generation was both interested in and attentive to their views. Once stereotyped defenses were down, the older members of the network were amazed to find themselves feeling defensive about diet pills and tranquilizers. Discussion was facilitated when the older team members insisted that discussion was relevant and necessary. The leader then capitalized on the commonality demonstrated, instead of the confusion in role reversals, and shifted the pressure away from stereotypes about drug addictions and onto the more pertinent relationships involved. Team member support allowed the leader to capitalize on the mirror-imaging between the generations—a task which otherwise would have been much more difficult.

Goals of the Intervention Team

Naturally the personality, physique, and aura of each individual denote some of the limits of his or her role on the team. The common goal of the team is something else, and whatever the ingredients, the team must be committed to it, regardless of the division of labor.

The goals of all network intervention are to stimulate, to reflect, and to focus the potential within the network to solve one another's problems. By strengthening bonds, loosening binds, opening new channels, facilitating new perceptions, activating latent strengths, and helping to damp out, ventilate, or excise pathology the social network is enabled to become the life-sustaining community within the social matrix of each individual. This does not happen if the intervenors act like therapists toward patients, since implicit in the therapeutic contract is delegation to the therapist of responsibility for healing, even though eventually most therapies provide a terminal phase where responsibility for self is returned to the patient or family.

However, the intervention team must be on guard at every turn to deflect therapist attempts and keep the responsibility within the network itself. This means being able to live with one's own curiosity when the network activists gain enough confidence to take over. It means real, not pseudo, confidence in network members, who know the problems, the landmarks and terrain of the distressed person's life space. They must be free to do the thinking and acting that will evolve more practical and efficient solutions than the professional could. It means the willingness of team members to be available to consult without being drawn in, and it means considerable clinical experience and intuition to be able to make quick and decisive judgments. Above all, it implies a shared working philosophy of faith in human beings and satisfaction in seeing them rise to occasions rather than a faith in a professional mystique and a need to be central and depended upon. If this goal and faith is part of the fiber of the team, it is communicated to the network in a positive and safe manner. Even suicidal and homicidal gestures can usually be controlled and handled by the network. The professional judgment that quickly evaluates both the gesture and the network strengths is important. It takes a good deal of acumen to know when it is safe to say "Leave him out in the rain— when he gets wet he will come in, and he ought to find you drinking coffee in the kitchen, not hanging out the window whining."

We have found that in every network there are members whom we call activists. These network activists perceive the need for someone to take over temporarily, and they require support from the team when filling the breach. It takes guts on the part of a network committee of activists to sit with parents around the clock while they let their boy learn what it is like to earn his own living. It takes compassion to invite a defensive embattled couple to dinner, a card party, or a style show and make them comfortable amongst guests and strangers. It takes reserves of patience to find job after job for an inept and unwilling depressed person, and to help him succeed almost in spite of himself so that he finds out that he can "be somebody." Moreover, it takes considerable courage for most professionals to turn these responsibilities over to someone else who has nothing but his or her humanity, concern, and horse sense to guide him through the traps professionals know so well.

The experienced team has often observed that, if they wanted to, they could shift any network over to individual and family therapy and be busy for the rest of their professional careers. For it is not just the index patient's distress that is dealt with, but that of many other families and individuals in the network. As they bring their distress to the surface, the network deals with it. The network team working through the activists enables the network to begin the important human task of solving one another's problems. The ambivalence of one set of parents is resolved when they find someone dealing with parallel problems down the block. One man's need for manual labor is matched by someone else's inside track to a hideaway that is available. This is the way that society has always functioned best—whether in extended families, small communities, clans, communes, or fraternal organizations. It is this potential within any group of forty or more people related by common concern for one another that can be unchained by the network effect. There is no other single goal—not cure, not treatment, but enabling people to cope and to share their strengths in coping and also in reaping enjoyments and pleasures that restore their potentials and set them up to handle the inevitable next crisis of living.

When these goals are clear, the skills needed by the team are relatively simple to define. The ability to relate to people, to sense group and subgroup moods and strengths, and to facilitate, focus, and reflect back confidence. The particular disciplines and techniques are raw materials, not prerequisites. The intervention team will blend them with experience and use any and all when appropriate.

Sequences and Patterns

With experience, too, comes the sense of an order to the events that transpire, and a pattern falls into shape. This makes it easier to work with the numbers of people involved and their subgroupings. It makes sense of the highs and lows, the ploys and counterploys, and the permutations behind the seemingly infinite changes each network rings on the organizational possibilities of human social relationships.

Not all these patterns have been identified and explored yet. It is part of the fascination of network study and intervention that there are unmapped vistas and old mountains to be climbed before new ones are glimpsed. The sequences and patterning sketched here may after some years seem like the early maps of the new world that showed California as an island and connected the Great Lakes to the western seas. Had the earlier explorers waited for the surveyors, and later perhaps the aerial photographers, before opening trade routes and establishing outposts, the wilderness would remain and the cities of Europe and the coastal plain of the United States would be even more crowded and explosive than they are now.

The assembly of prenetwork phase has already been well described. The opening session is usually one of a series, although on two occasions a single network meeting has been held and subsequent follow up indicated that the network effect had productive effects persisting for well over a year. Theoretically the one session intervention might be the ideal, but it is doubtful that it will be very often approximated when a network has to be assembled and created around the distress of an individual and his family. The experience of many religious groups who rely on the network effect of a conversion experience, as in revival meetings, suggests that even though this is a potent force it has to be renewed periodically or the group falls back into fragmentation. Other groups provide for renewal at a lesser peak through family reunions, seasonal festivals, life cycle celebrations of birth and marriage, and passage from one stage of the life cycle to the next, including death. Network intervenors need to be cognizant of this and, if possible, direct the energy of the network toward some such self-recharging cycle of its own, within whatever context seems appropriate to the group.

The principal reasons for continuing meetings beyond the tossing of the first rock into the pool are the need for practice, learning and development of insight, since one trial learning is usually not very permanent or predictable. The reinforcement that comes with shared coping experiences tends to make the network a stabilized social unit that can continue to function without professional coaching. A series of six meetings seems to be satisfying to all concerned, and practical, although sometimes three or four are adequate. The first session is usually one that ends on a high pitch of excitement and discovery of one another within the group. The reality of the fact that the professionals are not going to take over at some point or another is not always clear to the network at this time, and in fact the illusion of professional protection and sanction may be very important at this point to free the members of the network to explore one another more spontaneously. Hope and communication are both characteristic of this phase.

The strategy for the first session is plotted by the team on the basis of acquaintance with the problem gathered in the prenetwork discussions with the family about its distress. The leader will count on quick feedback from team members of subgroupings and moods as the network gathers. Individual team members arriving early and watching the host family and others can quickly sort out the alignments and the feelings as well as the relationships from the kinesics, the voices, and the clusterings.

New team members often ask "What do I do?" The answer is simple: Set the example of friendly interest, open communication, and unobtrusive returns of the ball whenever anyone moves to put the professional in charge. If asked, identify yourself by name and, if pressed, by occupation or professional role. If not asked, let people assume you are another member of the network, because for the next few weeks that is what you will become. Use whatever social skills seem appropriate, establishing human contact with as many people as possible, but also do a lot of listening and observing. Locate the refreshments, the bathrooms, the cloakrooms, the kitchen, the back door, the fans, the extra chairs, the ashtrays, the telephone and its extensions. Help move furniture if necessary. Get to know the people and the environment thoroughly as quickly as possible. If there are pets, identify them and their names and dispositions. Likewise, the children. Above all, don't get caught with the team standing grouped together staring at the people like zoological specimens. Never seem to be talking at length about any interest that cannot be shared with part of the network. It is not only rude; it is also destructive of morale.

Be prepared for many anxieties and much fear at the first session. Very few people will have any idea why they are there, and there will be many who are apprehensive about the distress of the family who invited them, about the risks they may be taking themselves, and about much that they have read and heard and misinterpreted about the whole profession of psychotherapy. In fact, those who have had experience with such marathons as group or individual therapy may be even more wary than the completely naive. This anxiety has its function, since, as the session relieves it, the relaxation and confidence is a potent reinforcement for continuing with the network intervention model. However, the clinical skill and ability to relieve false fears and to focus feelings realistically can be important at this stage.

Once the group has gathered, the leader takes charge. He needs to introduce himself with an outline of the problem and the network intervention methodology. This is a brief sales pitch and, like many similar openings, has impact beyond the cognitive level. Information may not be retained so much as a sense of purpose and direction.

Almost immediately after this introduction the leader introduced encounter-sensitivity techniques. This rapidly inducts the network into what we have called a group high where enthusiasm, activism, and polarization can break down ordinary social barriers and defenses which isolate each network member prior to the assembly. A fight for control is often noted here as the distressed person, his family, or a network member attempts to not participate. The team scattered through the group stimulates, initiates, and infectiously pulls the fringers into the group. During this prelude the leader often establishes control not merely of the network but through it, of the dissidents and distressed persons in a highly significant fashion. These nonverbal periods need not be long: three, five, or ten minutes at most. But they do seem to be the first big breakthrough that begins the realignment of network bonds and binds.

These nonverbal rituals should end with the group feeling solidified, in contact with one another, and quiet. At this point, the leader quickly forms a structure for dialogue and discussion.

In conducting a new session, the leader's sense of timing is crucial, including his ability to shift the tempo and adapt the rate of change, introduce themes, and provide the staccato and legato marks that build to crescendos of maximum impact.

In introducing dialogue, the leader shifts the members' positions to form an appropriate grouping. The physical arrangements depend on the setting, which are usually the living room and dining room of homes. Frequently, people are seated on the floor as well as chairs, sofas, and stairways. One format that is adaptable to many such settings is the use of concentric circles.

An inner circle of six to ten people is rapidly designated and asked to sit on the floor in the center. These are the more outgoing, often younger members whose talk will stir up ripples and begin to polarize the group. Sometimes an outer group is designated because the older, less immediately involved group have naturally seated themselves on the comfortable peripheral furniture. At times there is a middle group interposed by the apparent vagaries of seating and furniture arrangement. This middle group may serve as a buffer or mediator between the inner and outer groups, which will soon be polarized by the task assignments of the conductor.

The leader not only selects the most communicative group first, but also arranges to polarize issues by dividing along generational lines, or in some other way dramatizing the tensions and differences that exist. He sets a topic for discussion and controls the outside group to prevent interruptions. This keeps the discussion focused, with everyone promised, and later given, their turn for similarly interruption-free expression.

Often a fairly neutral, but subtly loaded question is good for a kick off, like "What do you think of John?" or "How many of you have used drugs?" or "What do you think the basic problem in this family is?" No one is allowed to escape from commentary, but no one is embarrassed. Skill at giving the sanction for open expression is of paramount importance, and both leader and team need to be alert to protect individuals even while encouraging openness.

The purpose of the multiple circles is to produce more intense interaction in smaller subgroups of six to ten persons. The forty-plus group of the assembled network is too large a group for free group discussion. Also, the advantage of multiple polarization (within each subgroup) allows the development and synthesis of various dialectics. It is important to elicit competitive polarities with diverse opinions and resolve some of these. The wide range of topics discussed helps the network begin to select and focus on the major issues to be dealt with in order to resolve the predicament in a nuclear family. Each subgroup is given its turn to interact, with the other subgroups instructed to not interrupt and to listen. Later each will have a chance to criticize what has been said by the other subgroups. An empty chair in the inner circle is an excellent device to use when there is pressure to be heard by peripheral members. If the group is large and active, two empty seats may be placed in the inner circle. Anyone not in the focal group may take the empty chair to signal a desire to speak. Having spoken, he is then obliged to return to the outer group and give way to someone else. Other devices of this nature are within the repertoire of every group leader or skilled teacher who uses discussion techniques. The important thing is to get the group talking to one another rather than holding a socratic dialogue with the professionals or rehashing old arguments among themselves.

As the discussion gets several ideas going and some confrontations emerge, the focal group is shifted off the center stage and another group is brought forward before premature resolutions are frozen into the system. At first it appears that very little is being settled. This phase is a kind of brainstorming. The leader and team are setting the ground rules for widespread participation and much airing of opinions, suggestions, ideas. The objective is to get out in the open misinformation that the group can correct, as well as information that the group can validate.

An important rule is no polite secrets. Indeed, the professional network intervenor not only does not promise confidentiality but establishes the precedent that there will be none. The team helps see to it that this is carried out. At first, the reverse of the usual professional ethics seems to shock everyone. Soon the network members demonstrate their relief at being able to speak openly about things they have already observed but could not deal with. "We knew you and John disagreed, but you would never let us help you understand before. . . . "I was embarrassed after that night you drank too much at my house because you never gave me a chance to say I felt the same way. . . ." "I was angry because you didn't let me know about Aunt Minnie's funeral for three months, so I didn't think you cared. . . ."

It is quite usual for people to think that their secret fears, foibles, and worries are hidden when they are patently obvious. It is also true that often people only know half-truths about one another, when the whole picture makes far better sense. But most heartening of all is not only the way people can take it when truths and secrets are shared, but also how within a social network the resources for supportive acceptance appear, along with a common sense, hardheaded approach to the things that need to be changed.

The sequence of polarizing, shifting, and refocusing, with everybody listening is timed to end again with a restatement of a specific problem. At the end of the session, buzz groups or a free-floating refreshment and visiting period is in order. Before breaking up, the leader designates the next time to meet and sets the assignment of a specific, task-oriented topic with this in mind. This is usually enough to get everyone talking, and as soon as that is assured the team exists with minimal attention to goodbyes, beyond the bare amenities, until the next meeting.

Initiating the Network Process

Consider a case in its initial phases, where decisions as to the strategy to be employed have not yet been made. A nuclear family consisting of a mother and father in their late 40's, a 25-year-old daughter, and an 18-year-old son (Jim) came to the clinic for help following Jim's acute psychotic episode, during which he thought his mind was being tape recorded and his thoughts played over the local radio stations. He also thought that the telephone system in the house was monitored by outside wires and enlisted the aid of his parents in tracing the wiring throughout the house in a frantic effort to cut off this source of outside interference. It was fascinating to learn that the sister worked at a local radio station taping spot announcements and advertisements, and that she resisted the initial efforts to involve her in any family conferences.

At the first session with the whole family, an attempt was made by the intervention team to find out just what kind of help the family was looking for. Among the possibilities were hospitalization for the son, psychotherapy for the whole family conjointly, and the assembly of their loosely knit social network with an attempt at network intervention by our team. A potential goal in the minds of the team was the mobilization of a peer-supporting network that might enable Jim to move out of the house and find employment and social relationships more appropriate for his age and status. The family was opposed to hospitalization, and at first resisted family therapy by using the sister's work as an excuse for all being unable to attend. They were intrigued by, but even more frightened of, the thought of network intervention, insisting that it would be impossible to assemble the forty persons which we gave as a minimum number necessary. Jim began to assert himself at this point and expressed reluctance to include his friends and peers in the same network as his parents' peers and kin.

What we are trying to communicate by this anecdote is that the resistance to any form of therapy or intervention rests on the lack of familiarity with it. People are unable to conceptualize the process and change modalities about to be unleashed. Human beings universally resist change, and those in distress are usually most defensive in the face of a choice about whether to introduce a new element or not. If they have never heard of network intervention, the vast majority of people will want to proceed cautiously.

In fact, both the interventions and the nuclear patient nexus prefer as simple an intervention as feasible. However, where the simple measures such as counseling, individual psychotherapy, group therapy, and family therapy have also been rejected, and where they seem inadequate to solve the family's predicaments, the potential network intervenor has to expand his own horizons and begin formulating strategies around a new theoretical base. This is essential to get himself into a network set. Once he is able to do this, it is not extraordinarily difficult to guide the family into thinking about themselves and their problems in network terms. We believe that this line of thinking does not involve any unusual problem, but we underline the seemingly obvious fact that, unless one thinks in a new frame of reference, the likelihood of the intervenor's being overwhelmed by the difficulties he perceives often prevents him from doing the obvious.

To round off the illustration, the family in question, even before actually completing their own network assembly, discussed the idea with many others. A new family called the clinic and startled the intake worker by saying, "We have a son with a problem just like Jim's, and the Jenkinses have told us about how you assemble networks to help solve it. Do you think you could do one for us?"

The Assembly Process: Advantages of Rapid Assembly

Once again it might be well to examine the predicament, the distress, and the forces suggesting the appropriateness of network intervention. In this case a 42-year-old mother had four children under school age. The oldest, a girl, was not presented as having any problems. The next, a 3-year-old boy, was dramatically frightening everyone, mother, siblings, baby-sitters, neighbors, and kin by grabbing knives and threatening to kill them. He appeared to be trying to avenge his father's murder, which all the children and the mother had witnessed. The killing was the aftermath of a neighborhood quarrel, when an older son of a neighbor, under the influence of drugs, invaded their home and stabbed the father in the presence of his family, who were watching a TV program.

The third sibling was severely damaged from birth defects affecting his central nervous system and was quite hyperactive. The last sibling, born after the father's death, was mongoloid and was in need of corrective plastic surgery.

Although the mother was not overtly depressed, she was drained of energy from coping with the four small children. She had moved from her previous home because of the overwhelming associations of loss and terror. She had lost contact with many of her old friends and had no extended kin since she had grown up in foster homes. However, there were some foster sisters as potential network participants.

The usual rationale for intervention in a case of this sort involves the treatment of the mourning and loss problems of mother and child(ren) and the search for social agencies to relieve the mother of some of the more pressing and energy-draining responsibilities in caring for defective children. One might suggest relieving the mother of her burdens by simply assuring them or handing them on to other professionals, if one were to follow the sick-and-needy-person model. However, a rapid assembly of interested and able friends, neighbors, relatives, and, if indicated, agency personnel, the foster families of the past, and perhaps the church-related persons of the present could provide a large enough group to stimulate considerable change. Presented with the predicaments and given the responsibility to jointly participate in their solution, both mother and network members, under the stimulus of the network effect, may generate some innovative and creative solutions, support the control needed for the abreacting boy, help the mother not only mourn but find and form nexus and clustering relationships. All this could be accomplished in a much more efficient and self-perpetuating fashion than the conventional assumption of professional responsibility and patient dependence.

Slower Assembly: Advantages and Disadvantages

Most reports of the assembly and creation of networks for therapeutic intervention deal with cases in crisis where there is virtually no option but rapid decisive action. We recently had experience with the assembly and creation of a loosely knit social network around a nuclear family with a son who had had an acute psychotic episode and was on the verge of hospitalization because of delusional ideas, erratic behavior, and family turmoil. Unique features in the network preassembly phase included reluctance of the family to do anything about their predicament but call and talk to the social worker for hours. They refused to relinquish control over their own situation; yet they kept asking for help. After accepting (hesitantly) the idea of network assembly, they reasserted this control by disregarding the instructions merely to call and invite all the people that they and their son knew for a meeting at a given time and place. Instead they made a series of visits. They spent a couple of hours with each of about ten such friends, telling them about he network idea and discussing their own problems. Only after several weeks of this did they get into gear and begin phoning and settling specifics of time and place.

This slow-paced use of five or six weeks to mobilize the network is unique in our experience in the assembly and creation of networks and raises the following hypothetical formulations and theoretical questions:

1. Slow assembly, controlled by the rate of dissemination of information which feels most comfortable to the nuclear nexus, sets the network-effect phenomenon into operation before the large assembly. Much of the network interventive action has already occurred before the larger meeting. Assembly in this case could confirm and validate actions and perceptions already shared, and could focus energy displaced by the directions already set in motion. The first actual meeting of the network might somewhat resemble a second- or third-stage meeting of a more rapidly assembled network.

2. Some danger of stasis might occur because the family has already selected its own system out of the available social matrix. In our experience the rapid assembly and creation of the network in a chaotic crisis situation seems to have the advantage of multiple foci which

could be relatively easily rocked or shaken loose by various strategies in order to introduce new structures and form new vincula. The rapid assembly of social networks, within ten days or two weeks of our being consulted about a crisis situation, makes up the largest number of our interventions. It is our clinical impression that more significant changes in occupation, in role performance, and in network relationships (vincula) occurred when crisis situations forced the rapid assembly of the network. However, we have not yet seen enough slow assembly cases to be sure of these speculations.

3. One related type of impasse is the polarization which may result if the nuclear nexus controls the slower process of assembly. If there is sufficient binding, knotting, and stacking of vincula, the assembly presents the intervenors with a dialectic so energized that the task of disalignment and realignment is staggering. One wonders what elements of good fortune would have to be added to technique to implode the plexus and produce the network effect. The potential violence unleashed if the implosion is successful may spill over to involve police action or other disagreeable effects.

This risk is particularly probable if the polarization occurs around two or more clusters within the network. The intervenors are then set up for a large-scale reenactment of the classical situation where a well-meaning mediator attempts to reconcile a battling couple and gets clobbered by each of them.

4. On the positive side, however, the slow assembly process, if contact is maintained with the distressed nexus, allows the intervenors access to more information than is usually available when rapid assembly is utilized. In one particular case, the son with the schizophrenic label revealed that he and his friends had been using a variety of drugs, including marijuana, hashish, barbiturates, amphetamines, and possibly mescaline and LSD. Because of the experience of one of the authors with similar cases on the psychedelic drug scene, he had a strong clinical hunch that the psychotic process would not be as ingrained as in cases where drugs were used in the absence of peer relationships, or in cases where drug use had not been part of the clinical picture.

When the intervention team has advance information, it is possible to set goals for the network assembly that involve other less loaded areas of concern, which may enable the polarized factions to find common elements around which to reform. These might include appropriate employment for the son, who had graduated from high school six months before and was not yet motivated either for work or further education, and possibly moving the youth out of his home into a semi-structured or somewhat loosely peer-supervised living arrangement—a pad in the center of the city, for instance.

At this point in time, there is simply not enough experience to provide the criteria for selecting appropriate cases for slow assembly versus rapid assembly of the network. Nor is there evidence to decisively rule either process in or out as a method of choice.

Invocation of Preexisting Networks

The invocation and utilization of a preexisting group which possesses the membership variety characteristic of a social network is not as common as creating a new social network via the assembly method. It seems applicable where minority group members depend upon tribal-style assemblies, or where the nuclear nexus in distress centers much of its life around some organization such as a church or temple, a cousin's club, a block organization, or the like. If this group provides the heterogeneity of most rapidly assembled networks, much the same process can occur. If, however, it has factions, some of the dangers of the slow assembly process, such as selectivity of polarized clusters and stasis, may apply. In any case, such a group can add impetus to the network effect if it can be properly amalgamated in the network and involved in the task of solving the predicament of the distressed nexus.

Technical differences often center on how to arrange to invoke the network. It is usually not enough for the intervenors and the nuclear family or distressed individual to agree on the network idea. Preferably, one or more members of the intervention team should already be known, by reputation if not personally, to a plexus or authority figure in the group around which the network can be invoked. If it is a rather formal group, at some point the priest, medicine man, club president, or other role-assigned figure will have to be consulted. Usually a clustering person who has vincula with the authorized role representative can effect the team's introduction to the power structure.

Once introduced, the intervention team should demonstrate that they have no desire to take over the group or to reform it, as well as show mild positive empathy for its avowed goals and activities. If the team conveys the idea that the nexus in distress is somehow caught in a bind which prevents full utilization of the supports offered by the group, some expression of need for revitalizing the whole group is called forth from its leaders. From this point on the intervenors are on familiar ground, using their discretion in communicating confidence in the network effect's multiple impact without promising miracles.

Some differences in intervention technique will probably be required because some of the rituals familiar to the group have potential affect-laden charges that can be utilized in place of innovative nonverbal techniques to loosen binds, form bonds, and to stimulate growth of new vincula. Nonuse of a ritual response when it is expected is also effective in developing new perceptions and awareness.

Peer Networks: Special Cases

Peer networks are powerful social agencies in contemporary culture. They seem to be age-graded stratification phenomena with varying limits; probably a maximum span of about fifteen years is typical for older people and a narrower span for youth.

One needs first of all to recognize that peer networks exist and are as potent a force as the multigenerational networks if they can be properly invoked to assemble. They have varying degrees of tightness from a loose network to highly structured groups. When the generally loose-knit associations are assembled, the process is much like that of the creation of a network for a family, but the actual creation of a network of peers from scratch has not seemed feasible. Rather it seems more effective to take advantage of natural groupings, which abound.

Two natural sources of peer networks are adolescents' and work associations. An example of a hippie peer social network and its interventions was seen in the course of a long-term observation in a pad. A group of college students who had formerly been part of a fraternity formed the plexus of the network. A formal fraternity group had been broken up because of the group use of drugs, and this nucleus rented a large old Victorian home and set up a commune living arrangement. Although several members dropped out of college, most of them eventually graduated.

The intervenor gained access to the peer group through the development of a therapeutic relationship with one of its members when he panicked after prolonged use of LSD and other psychedelic drugs plus amphetamines. When he described his living arrangements, he was asked if we could meet with all the persons who customarily assembled in his pad, and the result was our seeing from six to twenty of his peers on typical weekly visits.

Over the course of a year we got acquainted with about a hundred youths at this pad, many of whom comprised peripheral members of the peer system of the original nexus. Some of these peripheral members were connecting links with drug-dealing networks. Others were pad crashers who were freaked out or were runaways looking for a place to hide. At different times the peer network provided for one or more young persons in acute "schizophrenic crisis," who were allowed the isolation and security they needed, a chance to talk about their panic, and generally secure subcultural approval for the "trip" they were on in their personal distress. Network intervention in this instance was a matter of operating largely as part of a validating cluster with those involved at any particular time, and of utilizing the natural setting as innovatively as the youth who had adopted the life style in the first place.

In the case of one young schizophrenic girl who was symbiotically bound to her mother, activation of several network members broke through the usually reticent relationships enough for them to find her an apartment, physically move her into it, and support her through the initial phases of disorientation as the symbiotic bonds gave way to more personal ego boundaries. The ripple effects were observed as the ringleader of this network group, who had been unemployed for several months, spending his time writing poetry, began to look for a job. In a matter of weeks the associated efforts had transformed him from a sloppy-looking, bitter, depressed, and angry young man into a clean-cut business executive type with medium long hair (no value judgment intended). Another member who had participated in breaking the index girl's symbiotic binds temporarily separated from her husband, saying that she had finally found the strength to stand up to him and renegotiate the relationship. The example could be spun out to illustrate the reactions that affected employment, marital, personal, and interactional patterns in the lives of at least a dozen members of the social network over the next six or eight weeks.

It would seem that the network effect begins once members realize that they are now part of a special human cluster. Therapeutic intervention labels this as a network and works within the newly formed associative groupings—tightening vincula, stimulating nexi, and coalescing clusters. The use of this vocabulary illustrates that the professional is not immune to the strong drive observed in most groups to try to develop rules that regularize and give the new associative bonds some permanence in the network-effect experience.

While these definitions will prove of some use later in this discussion, at present the phenomena can be described as first an experience of a new feeling of freedom. There are fewer rules, at least fewer formalized rules, in the new context. The network intervenors try to keep this openness, this sense of new options, alive so that the network members learn for themselves how to be innovative and creative. Learning is rapid as they discard regulations which do not work or which are limiting and begin to cherish a certain looseness of regulations which potentiates freedom. This sense of freedom, validated through shared intimate experience, is a high, a euphoric experience which energizes the group with confidence so that they can begin to tackle their everyday problems. Their success is partially due to the fact that their problems have been redefined by the new group culture, which strips off old labels, collapses old roles, and punctures old bags that are difficult to get out of. This last allusion is particularly apt, since the contemporary rediscovery and reapplication of this network effect in a therapeutic context belongs as much to the hippies and young radicals of today as to the professionals. A never-ending parade of examples of reinvented social values and cultural forms, as well as new realities, confronts anyone who looks for it in the contemporary scene.

When we began to conceptualize in this way we began to get rid of the "sick" model for many patients, and this felt good. We also began to get rid of the "healer" model for the therapist, and this left us uneasy—particularly in figuring out how to collect fees for an as yet undefined service, to a new population in intuitively defined ways. Tradition tells society what is acceptable to the majority of the group by defining what is sick. When called upon, therapists take the sick person and tell him he must become like the majority, for which the system will reward him. What hasn't always been realized in using this model is that this system needs a certain number of persons to scapegoat—to define as sick—in order to define itself. Thus if one person gets over his needs for being scapegoated he has to be replaced by someone else. An alternative left for a patient is to find that being sick is more fun and to remain chronically ill. In either case, therapists are apt to find themselves in the middle of a cybernated pegboard game in which, if you press down one peg, sometimes two or three more pop up. Most of the time, only one pops up—but only occasionally and apparently by chance do no pop-ups occur.

The network effect can scramble the cybernated pegboard, open new feedback connections, make everybody both an experimenter and a validator of new options. Suddenly the only acceptable and needed epithets are WOW! FANTASTIC! RIGHT ON! and no one is sick.

In Conclusion: Some Thoughts About
Human Social Systems

In our world today, some workers in the social sciences have to become organized in their thinking about behavior and the modification of behavior in large human groups. In the McLuhan world of instant tribalization each of us is influenced by mass behaviors—from protests to festivals. We are involved positively or negatively in the characteristics of what Abbie Hoffman has called the Woodstock nation or what Roszak has called the counterculture. This has some implications of a polarization of mankind into youth and adults which may be due to fragmentation of social networks which in the past held generations with a sense of unity in time and space.

Youths fear the destructive potentials of the cybernated technocratic world, which they feel have led to the imminent destruction of both man and nature. Adults, on the other hand, feel that we have an affluent and manageable system which can be exploited further to bring health, happiness, and security to the "motivated." Like it or not, this is the predicament facing mankind today. Therapists need to be willing to begin to experiment and study these human group phenomena at levels which have during the past couple of centuries been thought of as political. Unless we do this, it is questionable how relevant therapy, or indeed the social sciences in general, is going to be. The culture is changing so rapidly that the old methods of intervention with individuals, families, and groups are not meeting the requirements of the situation.

Rapid social change creates identity confusion in both the adult generation and in youth. Prescribed models for behavior no longer function effectively, and results of actions cannot be anticipated with confidence. This is readily seen in the way youth have established radical changes in dress and codes and opened up to public view many relationships that were cloaked in Victorian mystery. They have also shaken up the adults as they have demonstrated their social and political skills in large assemblies, and as they have openly challenged many institutions disliked by the over-thirty generation who felt change could only occur slowly. Granting that there are many variables contributing to effectiveness, and that youth are not always successful in avoiding violence or achieving change, there is still ample evidence that they have established some new forms and uses of social relationships.

Such social mutations create new tensions and precipitate distress which should not be interpreted as a new guise for old pathologies. Clinically, adolescents seen today are not the same as the youth of the past two or three generations. They appear depressed and hopeless, but they admit it rather than blame themselves. They see the world situation as hopeless, and they are hungry—but for dialogue, not therapy. They are suffering from real distress of the soul, and so are their parents, teachers, and peers. Intuitively they sense something more than they can express about this change.

If the psychotherapist is to maintain relationships with human beings in this predicament, if he is to be of any value in relieving distress, he has to innovate.

It seems to us that social network intervention has much promise as a constructive innovation. It provides a chance for the healing of torn bonds and the gentle freeing of binds. Network intervention may be able to evoke the potential capacity of people to creatively and cooperatively solve their own problems as an antidote to the aura of depersonalized loneliness characteristic of postindustrial society.

Multi-Family Group Therapy:
A Multidimensional Approach

ELSA LEICHTER, M.S.S.A.
GERDA L. SCHULMAN, M.S.

The preeminent structure of the middle-class American family is that of the isolated, nuclear household. It is a structural form tailored to the needs of our industrial and postindustrial bureaucratic society. It places a premium on the tenuous construction, ready dissolution, and facile mobility of families. Isolation means privacy as well as independence from families or origin, social networks, and neighborhood. It implies rootlessness, disconnectedness, and alienation, suggesting that most families come to suffer their crises alone in the hothouse atmosphere of their privacy and without the direct emotional support of others.

These sociological characterizations have gained popular currency. Vance Packard has described us a Nation of Strangers *(1972) and Philip Slater has lamented our* Pursuit of Loneliness *(1970). While it would not be fair to say that family therapists have been unmindful of this state of affairs, it is true that as a group, they have not been explicitly sociologically minded. Until the early 1970s (Scheflen and Ferber, 1972; Berman, 1973) they had not addressed themselves with much deliberate focus to the sociological plight of the middle-class family, or, to family therapy as sociologically reactive to that plight. A few family*

*therapists have evolved techniques and therapeutic principles
which challenge the closed, corporate structure of the isolated,
nuclear family without explicitly addressing the sociological
predicament of the modern American middle-class family
(Bowen, 1971; Speck and Attneave, 1973; Speck and Rueveni,
1969; Guerin and Fogarty, 1972; Laqueur, 1969, 1971, 1972,
1973).*

*It would seem they share an implicit recognition that our small,
claustrophobic, isolated nuclear family is explosively and exqui-
sitely oedipal; that it is an emotionally overloaded system, shot
through with ambivalences that make it lock upon itself; that it
leaves little margin for "shock absorption" (Parsons, 1955); that it
provides the fertile soil for weekend neuroses, while the creed of
family privacy ensures that each family resides with consuming
guilt in the unshaken conviction that theirs is a special and lonely
private purgatory.*

*Robert Ardry (1966) remarked, "There is nothing more
moving—not acts of love or hate—than the discovery that one is
not alone." The article that follows by Leichter and Schulman
conveys the same sentiment, for it was a kindred insight that led
H. R. Laqueur (1969, 1972, 1973) to the development of multi-
family group therapy, whose origins he traces to 1951 when irate
diabetics and their families insisted physicians talk to them
together. The result was that families found they had much to
share with each other, and the conveyance of medical information and instructions faded to secondary significance. The
method of multifamily therapy has evolved over the years to the
form presented here by Leichter and Schulman.*

*With the papers by Friedman and Speck and Attneave in this
volume, the paper that follows shares the premise that one gains
much by reaching beyond the boundaries of the nuclear family
for purposes of doing family therapy. In addition, it shares with
Speck and Attneave the belief that exchange, mutual support and
creative problem-solving can come from intense group experiences with "nonprofessional others." Another similarity is the tendency to deprofessionalize therapy and view emotional distur-*

bance in families, not as psychopathology, but as problems in living. The assumption is that there will always be problems of one kind or another, such that the shift of therapeutic effort is accordingly away from fantasies of "cure" and toward the possibilities of increased "coping" capacities.

Like the others reprinted here, the paper that follows seems uninformed sociologically in its adherence to the internal dynamics of families conceptualized as closed corporate structures and bypasses the opportunity to develop in its family groups a sense of communal exchange around culturally induced crises. To the extent this is so, the method described here probably has yet to realize its full potential. Nevertheless, the paper is a solid description—replete with clinical example—of how to do multifamily group therapy.

Multi-family group therapy began to emerge as a new and important treatment modality approximately ten years ago. A number of factors played a part in its development, but the initial impetus came from the first experiments with multi-family group therapy that were carried on within a mental hospital (Creedmore) under the leadership of Dr. Peter Laqueur. The mental health community and more specifically mental hospitals had been aware for a long time that their patients, in spite of some improvement during hospitalization, frequently regressed upon their return home; some did not benefit sufficiently while they were hospitalized. This led to increasing recognition that the families of the identified patients were implicated in the etiology of the schizophrenic illness and that therapeutic work with the families could help the patients improve more reliably during and after hospitalization. The emergence of multi-family group therapy was a natural development, since many families paid regular visits to their hospitalized sons and daughters and often formed spontaneous groups, which gradually were turned into therapeutic groups. Subsequently, many hospitals and out-patient clinics all over the country followed the original model and began to conduct multi-family therapy groups. Due to practical

Reprinted with permission from *Family Process,* Vol. 13 No. 1 (March 1974), pp. 95-110. Copyright © 1974 by *Family Process.*

considerations, these groups were mostly open-ended; the individual family attended the group for a relatively short period, yet the group itself tended to go on for a long, often undefined, time. Although these groups were considered to be multi-family groups, in actuality, only triads, namely the parents and the identified patients, attended, and treatment was to a large extent focused on the patient.

Simultaneous with the above development, a few family agencies began to experiment with multi-family group therapy in which family and group therapy were combined and integrated. Preceding this, married couples group therapy had been practiced for a long time and in fact had been the first "break" with the classical model in which participants in a therapy group were total strangers to each other. In a way, one might say that the first multi-family therapy group, which included parents and the identified patient, carried the idea of couples groups (parents groups) still another step further in that the identified patient was added as a group member to the dyadic subsystem of the parents.

The authors, as a co-therapeutic team, were the first practitioners at the Jewish Family Service of New York to develop multi-family group therapy. In line with the agency's concept of family therapy, multi-family group therapy was viewed from the beginning as needing to include the entire nuclear family. Underlying this concept was the belief that all parts of the family are interdependent, affect each other in a most powerful way, and participate in the perpetuation of their system.

As the authors have become both familiar and more experienced with multi-family group therapy, they have at times expanded the nuclear family by including the extended kinship; e.g., grandparents or divorced spouses may be part of the multi-family therapy group where and whenever they play a significant role in the family transactions. As a rule, three or four families compose the multi-family therapy group.

Selection of Families for Group

As in all therapy groups, the families are selected for multi-family group therapy by a screening process. The family and the therapists come to a mutual decision as to whether the family is interested and able to become part of the multi-family therapy group. Usually the families are seen several times as a unit. This process reflects the authors' orientation that the understanding and the engagement of the whole has to take priority over involvement with parts of the family. To put it differently, the first goal is to obtain a beginning grasp of the family system rather than attempt to come to an understanding of the whole through its parts. The authors prefer to tell the family almost immediately that the purpose of the first meeting is to determine jointly whether a multi-family therapy would be the best method of treatment for them. While this remains as an underlying, open question, the process then concentrates on what the family is all about.

Can they be engaged as a family group? If this question is answered affirmatively, those families are selected for multi-family group therapy for whom this seems to be the treatment of choice. Naturally, there are many families who can benefit from either individual family therapy or multi-family group therapy and the happenstance that a multi-family therapy group is being formed may very well be the determining factor.

There are some families for whom multi-family group therapy is clearly preferable: among these are the isolated family or the family whose system is circulatory and rigidified, especially the symbiotic family. For the latter, particularly, exposure to different systems may be the only way to shake up their own.

Another type of family for whom multi-family group therapy can be very helpful is the family with a missing parent—usually the father— since the group provides parental substitutes.

There are families, however, for whom individual family therapy is clearly preferable to multi-family group therapy, beyond of course, those families who staunchly refuse to enter a group. Multi-family group therapy seems to be counterindicated with certain chaotic families in which the children, out of their deep anxiety, tend to drown out any meaningful discussion and transaction. The authors do not usually consider families with very young children (under the age of six) because of their inability to grasp and tolerate the group process. However, families that additionally have older children are, of course, considered. The young child may be invited to an occasional session so that the group can see the total family in action. Also unsuitable for multi-family group therapy are families in which an important, pertinent fact is kept as a secret from other family members and the keepers of the secret insist on maintaining their controls. The following example will make this point more explicit.

The authors screened the T. family, which consisted of parents and their only son, ten years old. The family wanted help regarding the child's difficulties in school (lack of concentration, restlessness) and with peers (lack of friends). In the course of the initial interview, the T.'s alluded to a secret which they could not discuss in front of their son. Thus, in the second interview, the parents were seen alone and revealed that the child was adopted, but did not know about it. It was obvious to the therapists that a good part of the child's difficulties (pervasive anxiety and isolation) was related to the secrecy around his origin. The parents first fought this connection but after a couple of interviews seemed more ready to accept it. Yet they pleaded strongly that they were unable to overcome their deep fear of sharing the secret with their child.

The therapists felt that the T. family, therefore, would not be suitable for the projected short-term group, as the couple's need to maintain so powerful a secret would not really allow the group to deal helpfully with the family system. This does not mean that a flexible, individual family treatment approach might not eventually enable them to overcome their resistance, and, indeed, they were referred for family therapy. Of course, as in all treatment modalities, secrets emerge in the course of the treatment process as a result of increasing trust, but this does not represent a bind.

The complexity and the size of multi-family therapy groups has led most practitioners to conduct them as co-therapeutic teams. The authors also do their screening jointly, thus giving the families a sense of the therapists as a unit, just as they expect the whole family to get involved with them from the first contact.

As in any other group, the composition of the multi-family group therapy group is important. In most of these groups, the families come originally because of a problem concerning a child. While this in itself represents a certain commonality, the authors see value in heterogeneity along other dimensions. Their groups encompass a wide age range (even, occasionally, a three-generational span), complete as well as incomplete families, and a variety of family types. As the group becomes more cohesive, identifications take place on the basis of universality of human emotions and needs, rather than on the basis of external similarities.

Long-Term and Short-Term Groups

Like other groups, multi-family therapy groups can be set up for long-term or short-term treatment; the groups can be closed or open-ended.

Short-term groups seem to be particularly helpful in the beginning and ending phases of the overall treatment process. With families that have just started treatment, clarification of the family system and its major pathogenic features can be particularly well accomplished within such a framework. After termination of the group, there may be a mutual agreement that some shift of the pathogenic system has taken place so that the family can operate more effectively on its own. Other families may decide to continue therapy in a more differentiated way with a variety of treatment modalities. Some multi-family groups provide the ending phase of the overall treatment. The family may have had individual family therapy, or there may have been prior treatment of some of the subsystems (couples, mother/child, etc.). Multi-family group therapy lends itself exceptionally well to an integrative process in which the group serves as a bridge to the world at large.

For some families, longer term multi-family group therapy is the treatment of choice—usually, families whose systems are particularly difficult to modify, yet who are motivated to work further on their problem.

The authors, who have experimented with both short- and long-term groups, have found that in spite of the more limited goal, short-time groups demand of the therapists more sharply focused and directive interventions. In a group of longer duration, the group itself can carry more of the treatment process, and the therapists' interventions are less pronounced.

Dynamics and Process Phenomena

Reality Testing

Nevertheless, in all types of multi-family therapy groups, the initial goal is to enable the group to achieve some cohesiveness, so that it can become an optimal working instrument for therapeutic purposes. While this is true of all therapy groups, there is a dynamic difference between a therapy group composed of strangers and a group in which some members belong to the same family. In the multi-family therapy group, each family represents a subsystem with a shared history and a shared, current life situation. This makes for an enriching and complex process, as each subsystem interacts with other subsystems at the same time that each individual responds to other individuals, whether members of his family or strangers. The multi-family therapy group serves both as an arena for cross transferences—based on each person's introject—and as a reality tester. Of course, reality testing is considerably more pronounced in multi-family therapy groups than in other therapy groups, because distortions within a family are frequently readily apparent to the other group members.

A family perceived and treated a child as "dumb," an image that was largely internalized by the child. The group was not bound by the family's label, nor by the child's self-image. It had the opportunity to observe the transactions within the family that had led to the child's assumption of the role of the "dumb one" and was, therefore, free to view and treat the child differently. The parents, on the other hand, were witness to the group relating to the "dumb" child as a person who at times had something valuable to offer and who also, in response to the group's different treatment, gradually became more of a person. This whole process was to a large extent played out rather than articulated, and, therefore, evoked less defensiveness.

Transferential reactions occur, of course, not only within one family, but across family lines. These transferential reactions are dealt with in multi-family therapy groups as they are in other therapy groups. However, in multi-family therapy groups, the reality function of the group comes into special focus, since the member of the family with whom the transferred reaction really belongs very often is present, be it a marital partner, a parent, or a child. Based on its experience with this member, the group can often see where the overreaction originated and deal with it.

A man who throughout his long marriage had been a nonparticipatory husband reacted strongly in a most censuring, straight-laced manner to the use of gut language by an adolescent girl of another family. This led to a lot of angry interplay between the man and the girl, including threats to leave the group. The group, however, had frequently experienced the vulgar, almost violent cursing of the man's wife, who was taken on by others but not by the husband. Thus, the group could confront the man with his overreaction to the girl, enabling him eventually to reveal his distaste for his wife's violence.

The authors have been greatly interested in the developing adult-child relationships across family boundaries within the multi-family therapy group. Being troubled about the increasing alienation between adults and young people, one of their goals in starting such groups was to achieve a better mutual understanding and empathy between the generations. This has, indeed, occurred in most of the groups with which the authors have had direct or supervisory contact. While it is very difficult for children and parents to change the image they have of each other, in the multi-family therapy group, adults and young people have a chance to experience the universality of human needs and emotions across family boundaries. The investment of the children in having a "perfect" and "always available" parent is as great as the parents' investment in the "perfect" child, who is an extension of unfulfilled parental hopes and ambitions.

When adults or children who are outside of one's own family reveal vulnerable feelings, the group responds and demonstrates, in general, a greater tolerance than does the individual family. In the freer atmosphere of the group, identifications between adults and children can take place with the accompanying recognition of their mutual humanity. This can have a profound effect on the way in which adults and children perceive each other within their own families.

In multi-family group therapy, adults can use themselves as parent substitutes to children other than their own, even though the adult may be quite defective in his own role as a parent.

Lena, the mother of Florence, an eleven-year-old girl, and the maternal grandparents had imposed a taboo with regard to even mentioning the child's father from whom Lena had been divorced. After some time, in the course of group treatment, the child was freed to bring out her anguish both about the secrecy surrounding the parental separation, and her profound sense of deprivation. Florence, who attended a religious school, sobbingly described the torture she experienced when during the daily morning prayers, she had to "honor thy father" when there was no one to honor! Her anguish about his painful moment was so great that sometimes she could not get herself to school. This child had been brought for help because of an incipient school phobia, among other symptoms.

As Florence cried out her pain, Lena sat stiffly in her seat. The group appealed to her to respond to her daughter. Actually, it was already considerable progress that Florence had been able to express feelings that at first she had totally denied and that her mother, just a little earlier in the process, would have censored angrily. Lena helplessly and unhappily cried out that she did not know what to say, nor what to do. At that point, another woman in the group volunteered to show her. She moved toward Florence and took her in her arms, letting her cry on her shoulder. While the child momentarily seemed comforted, after a while she whispered, "I want my Mommy," and the woman transmitted this message to Lena. The latter now "knew" what to do; mother and child held each other firmly, and both cried. Following this episode, there was increasing closeness between Florence and her mother, who seemed to have gained a better acceptance of, and feeling for, her maternal role.

The "other mother" who ordinarily was not too perceptive about her own daughter's needs (this child was about Florence's age) seemed to sense her child's momentary aloneness. She moved toward her and held her hand for the rest of the session.

A reversal of roles can also be quite productive, meaning that a child can role-play the parent and a grownup can act as the child.

Donald, an adolescent boy, played hooky from the group session. He had not come home from school, and the family did not know where he was. Donald's father, Sam, threatened angrily that he would punish the boy at home.

Ken, an adolescent from another family, who was himself involved in an angry battle with his mother, felt strongly that punishment was not useful. He took on the role of Donald's father, and the latter played Donald. Ken used himself as a model father who tried to make emotional contact with Donald.

Sam played his defiant son using body gestures almost exclusively and could not be reached. Ken then spoke of his rising anger and perhaps for the first time had a glimmer of what can happen to a parent when a child remains impenetrable in his defiance.

Substitute roles can also be performed by a man and a woman, since members of the group frequently can be more nurturing to another person's husband or wife. This happens in married couples groups as well, but it is particularly useful for children to see, as it helps them begin to appreciate their parents' deprivation instead of just witnessing the mutual blame.

Peer Confrontation

The multi-family therapy group offers to both adults and children the advantage of at least a partial peer group. Children can be especially supportive to each other, yet can hold each other responsible and at times even challenge each other quite strongly and more effectively than can be done by adults. The fact that the parents witness this confrontation not only relieves them of an unpleasant task, but enables them to trust the young people's judgment. It decreases the parents' fantasy that children always condone, and even stimulate, each other's wrongdoings. Following is an example of peer confrontation:

> An adolescent girl challenged a younger girl for angrily cursing the girl's grandmother. This grandmother, who often acted like a witch, was not liked by the group and, therefore, did not get any group support. The only one responding to the old woman as a human being who had feelings was the adolescent girl, who had a tender relationship with her own grandmother.

Thus, children relate to each other both as peers and as substitute parents. In the latter role, they often take the "scolding parent" part with each other. If a multi-family therapy group has children of different ages, the younger children tend to relate to the older children as "ego-ideals" whom they would like to emulate.

The "Well" Sibling

Thus far, no differentiation has been made between the "problem child" and the so-called "well" sibling. This polarization occurs more often in families in which one child is treated as a scapegoat. The families that have an investment in making one child the carrier of the family pathology have an equal investment in having another child "well" and "problem free." These children are usually expected to be not only perfect, but "towers of strength" as well. Many of them are perfectionistic, moralistic, and constricted, often displaying obsessional ideations. Frequently, they are achievers, liked by adults, but often shunned by their peers as goody-goodies, teachers' pets, and sissies. Others have a somewhat flattened affect, which makes them appear superficial and shallow. The girls often seem prematurely lady-like, and the boys tend to have considerable difficulty with their masculine identity. These characteristics are not only accepted but needed and approved in their families.

In considerable contrast to single family therapy, the multi-family therapy group, which has no particular investment in the maintenance of a given family system, notices rather quickly "the unrealness" of the good children and the price they pay for their position in the family. The children, in turn, respond rather well to questions and comments, especially when they are put out lightly and humorously. For example, "Gee, you sound even stricter than your parents," or "Do you ever have any fun?" "Now you sound again like the little old lady." In the accepting atmosphere of the group, which values highly the expression of genuine feelings, the "well" children gradually change from a pattern of denial and blandness (superficiality) to an increasing ability to express emotions. These may be feelings of pain and anger, as well as yearnings for personal acceptance and dependency.

Some children, those who come from families in which self-assertion and the expression of normal impulse drives are perceived as bad and dangerous, learn to repress these feelings and drives. They put their energies into pleasing their parents by doing well in school and by being well-behaved, yet they feel intensely jealous of their "problem" siblings who get a lot of attention, albeit negatively, from their parents. In the course of group treatment, some of these "good" children begin to act out more, much to the dismay of their parents, who become frightened and fight this development. It goes without saying that the goal of multi-family group therapy is not to make "a bad child," out of a "good child"; it is rather to establish a healthier balance in which "good" and "bad" are not polarized and the group and the family can learn eventually to differentiate between acting-out and playfulness.

The way in which the group relates to the "well" children cannot help but affect the "problem" children in the sense that it represents a challenge of the total family system. The indirect approach to the "problem" child is diametrically opposed to his usual treatment in his family and, often, also in the community, as well as in other treatment situations.

Differentiation of Families in the Group

In the early phase, it is very hard for almost every family to see and to understand itself in terms of its own system, especially to understand those features that are pathogenic and growth-stunting, since they are "family ego-syntonic," which means that each member in the family has an investment in maintaining the system.

In the group, it is relatively easy for one family to perceive another family's malfunctioning. If the therapists keep the focus on the most prominent features in each family system, the group gradually learns to think in family terms. As time goes on, individuals apply their new thinking to their own family, even though they rarely become as clear about themselves as a family as they are about others.

Initially, the group tends to use cliches, and generalizations; families, as well as individuals, tend to merge with each other. Gradually, however, the group begins to differentiate between each family's needs and realizes that what is good for one may not be good for another family.

In Florence's family, discussed above, the nonmentionable father needed to become "present," whereas in another family, where a separated husband continued to be in and out of the house and thus created confusion for his children, a more final separation was desirable. It was first hard for Florence to perceive this difference since her need to have her father present was overriding. As the pathology of the other family unfolded, however, Florence was able to distinguish between her own situation and the other family's symbiotic stickiness.

Resistance

Any threat to the equilibrium of the family tends to bring out resistance. The threats may be to the structure ((good-bad child axis, marital and other dyadic relationships), as well as to existing family pacts and family myths. The major form of resistance, as in all therapy, is staying away from sessions. This can be acted out by an individual, a pair, or by the whole family. Absence of the whole family cannot help but be intensely experienced by the therapists and the group as a threat to its survival. While the absence of a whole family signifies the existence of a pact, fortunately, some individuals in the family may feel more positively about the group and be able to help the rest of the family return. Since all families in multi-family group therapy go through resistance phases one way or another, they are in a particularly good position to recognize and deal with resistance in an empathetic way.

On occasion, a family leaves the multi-family therapy group for good, in which case a distinction needs to be made between a family that consciously and responsibly faces the fact that the modality of multi-family group therapy is too much for them and between the family who takes the flight.

Withdrawal of Some Family Members from the Group

An interesting phenomenon in multi-family group therapy occurs when some members of a family want to stay in the group and others do not. Some therapists insist on the participation of the whole family as a basic condition for group treatment. The authors use this approach only if the partial withdrawal from the group takes place very early in the process, since this usually means the family fights the concept of wholeness. However, when the family has reached a more differentiated level of operation, the therapists tend to be more permissive and to allow those members of the family who are more motivated to stay in the group. In further treatment, the knowledge of the family system enables the group to deal more productively with the remaining members.

The following examples demonstrate circumstances under which some members of a family may leave the group, while others stay on.

The father, as well as his adolescent son who had been brought for treatment because of his delinquency (stealing), withdrew from the group at a point at which the boy's stealing was seen as linked to the father's clearly emerging, delinquent tendencies. By then, a shift in the family system had occurred. The mother, who had been seductively involved with her son against the father, had begun to extricate herself from the collusive relationship. This allowed the son to turn to his father for greater closeness, but their alliance was at least partially unhealthy. The father, a very brittle man, left the group in some anger because he could not maintain the denial that his delinquent activities, in which he involved his son, had anything to do directly with the boy's stealing. The son followed suit in order to stay in his father's good graces.

The mother, who had a history of many abortive treatment attempts, was highly motivated to see group treatment through for herself, and she continued productively until the group ended. Subsequent contacts showed that the boy was able to achieve actual, as well as emotional, separation from both parents and was functioning well at an out-of-town college.

In another family, a very disturbed but rigidly defended adolescent boy gained sufficient strength in the group to begin to expose his underlying depression and occasional psychotic ideations. As his pathology emerged, he no longer could tolerate the group but was able to move into and utilize individual treatment.

Max, a fifteen-year-old boy who had taken hashish and had been involved in drinking for about a year, was accepted in a multi-family therapy group together with his parents and younger sister. He had staunchly refused individual treatment but agreed to try the group and was a rather willing participant. Initially, the major focus was on the family's severe dysfunctioning and not at all on his problems. As Max's parents began to take increasing responsibility for their own difficulties, Max, who had been very guarded about himself, became more anxious and began to reveal depressed and suicidal feelings. Even though the group was most accepting of the boy, as his defenses decreased, he could no longer tolerate the many stimuli impinging upon him in the sessions. By this time, however, he was no longer denying his problems and was much more in touch with his real anguish. Therefore, he was ready to move into individual treatment, which was essential for him in terms of his need and level of operation. The rest of the family remained in the group, since they no longer needed to hide around Max's problem and continued to work profitably on their difficulties.

Spontaneous Insights

Naturally, not all growth is accompanied by resistance. As a matter of fact, multi-family group therapy provides a particularly fertile ground for the emergence of spontaneous and unexpected attitudes and insights, which occur almost as a byproduct to the consciously pursued goal. This, of course, is a known phenomenon in all therapy groups, but the very structure of the multi-family therapy group and the process flowing from it can have a very strong impact on its members. These spontaneous changes always have an especially exciting quality.

This actually happened within the B. family, which had a mentally sick son and a young daughter. The latter began to show rebellious behavior toward both parents after her brother's placement. It was quite obvious that there was a serious marital disturbance. However, a variety of earlier treatment efforts had not brought about change, and in their own evaluation, the therapists felt pessimistic about the possibility of change in the marriage. Their plan was to attempt to break into the unholy alliance between mother and daughter against the father, so that the daughter would not need to carry her mother's anger.

The presence in another family of a pair of grandparents whose pathological effect on the next two generations was amply played out in the group led Mr. B. to exclaim suddenly and quite spontaneously that he had just "dethroned" his parents for the first time in his forty-odd years. He spoke about their exploitation of him and of his determination to change his pattern of always needing to give in to their demands. His wife, who had been complaining all along about her husband's overinvolvement with his parents, which she felt affected adversely the marital relationship, seemed astounded at her husband's different view.

Subsequently, there was a marked rapprochement in the marital relationship, which was reinforced in the group. In the last group session, Mrs. B. described joyfully the emergence of her husband's "new me."

The above example demonstrated how the structure of the group—namely the presence of grandparents in another family—contributed to an emotional separation between an adult group member and his heretofore idealized parents. On the other hand, the structure of the multi-family therapy group, with its emphasis on the nurturing of children, often brings out secret longings for mothering on the part of the adults.

This occurred quite dramatically with the family in which the three generations were present. The therapists did not particularly aim at improving the relationship between the adult, Lena, and her mother, who seemed quite inaccessible to change. For a long time, Lena acted as if she had accepted the reality of her mother's stark inability to give, but she continued to be quite depressed. Efforts to reach her depression were unsuccessful.

As the end of the group came nearer, Lena's despair seemed to increase. Finally, she revealed with a lot of emotion that in view of the fact that the group was about to end, she realized that she had harbored a secret hope that her relationship with her mother would improve, and now this would never come true. From this point on, Lena became more reachable; she began to deal with her unfulfilled dependency needs and to give up her secret fantasy. As this occurred, her depression lifted.

Ending Phase of the Group

It is significant that Lena's recognition of her secret longings for her mother's love occurred only under the impact of the approaching end of the group. This is not unusual, since the ending phase brings about a critical sense of urgency for the whole group. Each family and each member of the group, including the therapists, have to come to terms with what is and what might have been, but has not come to pass. This, in fact, is the major theme of the ending phase in which families are quite helpful to each other in drawing a sharp differentiation between fantasy and reality. This process, of necessity, evokes deep feelings of pain, disappointment, and some anger, which is often directed against the therapists for not producing the miracles.

The authors are firmly committed to living out in the group all feelings connected with the ending. As this process develops, a new balance gradually occurs. As one family or individual deals with their ending by regression and denial of change, another family is able to acknowledge growth in themselves and questions the degree of denial in the others, often pointing out significant changes. Gradually, most families are able to view themselves more realistically and are, therefore, better prepared to plan their future direction.

As part of the ending phase, the authors have been using one-day Marathon sessions to give the group an opportunity to deepen the ongoing process. During the period of preparation for the Marathon, the group shows anxiety, as well as a good deal of curiosity and even enthusiasm. It may well be that the idea of the Marathon arouses hope that at least for one day, family life will be more satisfying in that there will be meaningful and intimate communication in which nobody looks for the usual escapes. This hope is, indeed, realistic, since in the actual Marathon session—which is usually very well attended—father does not withdraw to the TV, mother does not hang on the telephone, and the children are not a nuisance. In fact, the children are especially enthusiastic and committed to serious participation. Their staying power is amazing, and not infrequently they take the leadership in the session. The Marathon experience usually has a profound impact on the continuing process; it serves especially to sharpen the focus and to enhance integration in the ending phase.

Conclusion

While there are many aspects of multi-family group therapy that are similar to both individual family therapy and to group therapy, there are some features that are distinctly unique to it. It is quite unusual in the ordinary life situation, as well as in the therapeutic world, that families expose themselves to one another and try to have a significant effect on each other's way of life.

It is equally unusual that adults expose themselves to children as people, rather than in their customary roles; that children let their guard down in front of adults; that they engage with each other in meaningful encounters that are quite different from the customary intrusiveness and stereotyped perception commonly existing between the generations. The experience that multi-family group therapy offers help to decrease alienation and isolation between the generations, as they come to see each other in more human and humane terms.

Brief Therapy: Focused Problem Resolution

JOHN H. WEAKLAND
RICHARD FISCH, M.D.
PAUL WATZLAWICK, Ph.D.
ARTHUR M. BODIN, Ph.D.

Some marriages are "made in heaven," others are "fated from birth." The impending marriage between family therapy and behavior modification is viewed by many as anything but "holy matrimony," nonetheless, it is fated. The reasons for its inevitability are simple: Both are at heart environmentalistic and interpersonal, aiming for altered behavioral outcomes and rearranged social contingencies, employing minimal conjecture about the internal workings of individuals, preferring the analogy of social learning theory's "black box" (see Friedman, 1971, in this volume). In addition, they tend to share an opposition to psychodynamic personality theory and disease conceptions of psychopathology, the dominant ethos of the American mental health field. Although marriage seems imminent, there are serious impediments. As is evident in Stuart's behaviorally oriented paper (in this volume) and the family oriented paper that follows by Weakland, Fisch, Watzlawick, and Bodin the destined parties are the last to acknowledge their destiny. Like Stuart, Weakland and his coauthors, who are veteran family therapists from the Mental Research Institute in California, end their paper with a list of references dominated by recent publications with a parochial flavor in its deemphasis of "behavior modification" publications. Also like Stuart's paper, the one that follows hardly betrays that a confluence of forces is at work. Reading it suggests that formal introductions are still to be made; yet it is stunning that the paper, with only a few substantive exceptions, could have been written by a "behavior modifier." Readers who wish to compare statements from the family therapy article that follows with statements from behavior modification articles could consult Patterson and Reid (1971) and Lazarus and Davison (1971).

Perhaps some of the explanation for this state of affairs might be found in the stark differences in the lineage of family therapy and behavior modification. As has been noted, family therapy is a hybrid, maverick, upstart that is shifting and sifting in an effort to locate its footings and premises, while simultaneously uprooting itself from a traditional psychodynamic clinical orientation. In consequence, it constitutes a melange of professedly self-invented ideas and methods which paradoxically impresses some as rediscovering the wheel in the course of amalgamating a unique "systems" perspective on human behavior, that constitutes the core of family therapy's recently consolidated identity.

Behavior modification, on the other hand, is derived from a long-standing respected heritage; steeped in rigorous, exacting, hypotheticodeductive theorizing with a tradition of purism and empiricism. Its identity has long been securely entrenched in academic experimental psychology with attendant neo-Darwinian assumptions about the primacy of the individual as the basic unit of study.

Without being explicit, the article that follows is really far more interventionist than much therapeutic literature. In addition to the behavior modification mode, there is much in the paper stemming from "crisis intervention" practices, e.g., the stress on the fact that most of the problems encountered in families are the result of demand for change, which many families handle poorly. Such a crisis-oriented perspective on family dysfunction shifts the burden from a search for long-standing patterns of disturbed interpersonal functioning, in which a symptom in a single family member is "needed" by the entire family, to a view of family organizations as symptom free until *a crisis (such as illness, death, unemployment, mobility, separation, etc.) induces disequilibrium and taxes the family's flexibility. Hence, one no longer searches out a typology of families based on phenotypic similarities (e.g., schizophrenogenic families, depressive families, reading-problem families, etc.) but one looks to the nature of the crisis or problems the family faces and treatment interventions are arranged accordingly. Significantly, there is the explicit recognition that instead of requiring the symptom and maintaining it because it is in some sense ego-syntonic for the family, the newly arrived symptom is viewed as ego alien by the family, who wish to rid themselves of it and return to a former state of symptom-free stability. As the authors point out, transitions requiring shifts in role expectations are frequently troublesome and this is enhanced by a cultural taboo against recognizing pain in developmental transitions.*

The authors' conviction that behavioral dysfunction is not necessarily *an integral aspect of a social system's organization results in their notion that one does not have to change the entire family system in order to obtain change in a given behavior. This was the claim of many family therapists (e.g., Miller and Westman, 1964, 1966), who asserted that the system required changing before any of its parts could be modified. The approach in the following paper rests on two alternative propositions. Either the dysfunctional behavior is relatively autonomous of the family system's usual organization, or change in the larger system can be achieved from minor modifications which produce a progressive series of rippling effects throughout the family (a concept not unlike Bowen's "domino effect" which retains "systems" thinking while reversing the process of family intervention).*

As a corollary of the foregoing, Weakland et al. present an optimistic perspective regarding change, drawing on Rosenthal's (1966, 1968) concept of the "self-fulfilling prophecy" in social science, but also in its own way not far removed from the positive thinking of Norman Vincent Peale. The authors are unequivocal that failure in treatment is not to be blamed on the victim in the form of focusing on a family's resistant efforts to maintain the status quo (Miller and Westman, 1964, 1966). Instead, reasons for failure are to be sought in the therapist's engrained doubt and professionally inculcated pessimism (Freud, 1937). Hence, the emphasis on a nonconfrontational approach, "thinking small," the "soft sell," minimizing the risk of engendered resistance, and the avoidance of "insight."

While the forgoing issues place Weakland et al. close to the behavioral and/or crisis interventionist frames, other matters separate them from these orientations. One is their deemphasis of methodological rigor, which would be readily feasible in light of their concrete pragmatic behavior premises oriented to modest behavioral change.

Another is their manipulativeness, which, despite the subtleties of their "soft sell," is nonetheless inescapably manipulative. Clearly, the authors recognize that readers might reject their method on this account, which they anticipate by stating that therapists are designed by the public as influencers of people's behaviors, feelings, ideas. Ergo, the authors are not loath to use attributed or obtained authority to rationalize, coax, suggest, persuade et al. (Beruheim, 1888) to "influence toward desirable ends."

Perhaps the crux of many of the distinctions cited above can be encompassed in the differences between a systems perspective as opposed to a focus on the behavior of a single target person, which can make different and sometimes contradictory claims on a therapist. The choice of orientation and clinical strategy should be less a matter of personal taste or persuasion than it is a matter of evidence-based judgment. Hopefully, future volumes in this series will contain articles that will facilitate making such judgments. The promise of doing so should be greatly enhanced by the joining of behavioral methods with family therapy premises. To further this, family therapists may have to become more rigorous in the ways in which they contract for change with families and the means whereby change in the social system of the family is documented. On the other side, clinician-researchers employing behavioral methods of intervention will have to look beyond the target behavior and the focal dyad for ramifications that their intervention might have in other parts of the family system. This entails a reconsideration of the issue of symptom substitution but in a systemic family context. In other words, to what extent might removal of a child's symptom produce effects on altered contingencies elsewhere in the family, e.g., between mother and father? To really assess this would require collection of observational data on all family members. It might also bring the impending marriage between behavior modification and family therapy closer to consummation.

In the last few years, brief treatment has been proliferating—both growing and dividing. As Barten's (1971) recent collection of papers illustrates, "brief therapy" means many different things to many different therapists. The brief therapy we wish to present here is an outgrowth of our earlier work in that it is based on two ideas central to family therapy: (a) focusing on observable behavioral interaction in the present and (b) deliberate intervention to alter the going system. In pursuing these systems further, however, we have arrived at a particular conceptualization of the nature of human problems and their effective resolution, and of related procedures, that is different from much current family therapy.

We have been developing and testing this approach at the Brief Therapy Center for the past six years. During this period the Center, operating one day a week, has treated 97 cases, in which 236 individuals were seen. (We have also had extensive experience using the same approach with private patients, but these cases have not been systematically followed up and evaluated.) These 97 cases reached us through a considerable variety of referral sources, and no deliberate selection was exercised. As a result, although probably a majority of our cases involve rather common marital and family problems, the same covers a wide range overall. We have dealt with white, black, and

Reprinted with permission from *Family Process*, Vol. 13, No. 2 (June 1974), pp. 141-168. Copyright © 1974 by *Family Process*.

oriental patients from 5 to over 60 years old, from welfare recipients to the very wealthy, and with a variety of both acute and chronic problems. These included school and work difficulties; identity crises; marital, family, and sexual problems; delinquency, alcohol, and eating problems; anxiety, depression, and schizophrenia. Regardless of the nature or severity of the problem, each case has been limited to a maximum of ten one-hour sessions, usually at weekly intervals. Under these circumstances, our treatment has been successful—in terms of achieving limited but significant goals related to the patients' main complaints—in about three-fourths of these cases. We have also demonstrated and taught our approach to a number of other therapists in our area.

We present our approach here for wider consideration. Any form of treatment, however, is difficult to convey adequately by a purely verbal account, without demonstration and direct observation. We will, therefore, begin by discussing the significance and nature of our basic premises in comparison with other forms of treatment. Hopefully, this will provide an orienting context for the subsequent description—supplemented with illustrative case material—of our interrelated concepts, plan of treatment, specific techniques and results.

Psychotherapy—Premises and Practices

In characterizing treatment approaches, although some over-simplification may result, outlining basic premises may make their nature—and especially, their implications—more plain. Often, attention is concentrated on what is explicit and detailed, while what is common and general is neglected. Yet, the more general an idea, the more determinative of behavior it is—especially if its existence is not explicitly recognized. This holds for interpersonal influence as well as individual thinking and behavior; Robert Rosenthal's (1966) experiments demonstrate how the beliefs, assumptions, expectations, and biases of an experimenter or interviewer have a profound effect on his subjects. Similarly, the beliefs and theories held by a therapist may strongly influence not only his technique but also the length and outcome of his treatments—by affecting his patient's behavior, his evaluation of that behavior, or both.

For instance, if schizophrenia is conceptualized as a gradual irreversible mental deterioration involving loss of contact with reality, then attempts at psychotherapeutic contact make little sense, and the only reasonable course of action is long-term hospitalization. The hospitalized patient is then likely to react in a way that clearly justifies this initial "preventive" action. Alternatively, if schizophrenia is seen as a manifestation of a dysfunction structure of family relationships, the outlook is different and more hopeful, although basic restructuring of the family system is now likely to be seen as necessary. Again, in terms of the postulates of classical psychoanalytic theory, symptom removal must perforce lead to symptom displacement and exacerbation of the patient's condition, since it deals only with manifestations of deeper problems. The premises of the theory permit no other conclusion, except the alternative of claiming that the problem must no have been a "real" one (Saizman, 1968). On the other hand, in therapies based on learning or deconditioning theories, symptom manipulation is consistent with the theoretical premises. This enables the therapist to try very different interventions—and, to some extent, constrains him to do so.

That is, all theories of psychotherapy (including our own) have limitations, of practice as well as conception, that are logically inherent in their own nature. Equally important, these limitations are often attributed to human nature, rather than to the nature of the theory. It is all too easy to overlook this and become enmeshed in unrecognized, circular explanations. Stating the basic premises of any psychotherapeutic theory as clearly and explicitly as possible at least helps toward perceiving also its implications, limitations, and possible alternatives.

Our Brief Therapy—Bases and Comparisons

Much of the shorter-term treatment that has recently developed in response to the pressure of patient needs and situational limitations consists essentially of briefer versions of conventional forms of individual or family therapy. The same basic assumptions are involved, and, correspondingly, the methods used are similar, except for limited adaptations to the realities of fewer sessions (Barten and Barten, 1972; Bellak and Small, 1965; Rosenthal, 1970). This is expectable, as the usual frameworks naturally offer more restraints to innovation than encouragement and guidance. Within their terms, new methods are apt to appear strange and unreliable (Krohn, 1971). Consequently, "brief therapy" ordinarily connotes an expedient that may be necessary when a preferred treatment is not available or is considered not feasible— since the "best" therapies often require patients equipped with rather exceptional resources of time, money, intelligence, persistence, and verbal sophistication. The goals of such brief therapy correspondingly are conceived as limited "first aid"—such as relief of some pressing but not fundamental aspect of the patient's problem, or a supportive holding action until really thorough treatment becomes possible.

We recognize and value the practical and economic advantages for patients and society of shortening treatment. We do not, however, see our own kind of brief treatment as an expedient, nor is brevity in itself a goal to us, except that we believe setting time limits on treatment has some positive influence on both therapists and patients. Rather the nature of our therapy, including its brevity, is primarily a consequence of our premises about the nature and handling of psychiatric problems.

Our fundamental premise is that regardless of their basic origins and etiology—if, indeed, these can ever be reliable—the kinds of problems people bring to psychotherapists persist only if they are maintained by ongoing current behavior of the patient and others with whom he interacts. Correspondingly, if such problem-maintaining behavior is appropriately changed or eliminated, the problem will be resolved or vanish, regardless of its nature, origin, or duration (Watzlawick, Beavin and Jackson, 1967; Wender, 1968). Our general principles and specific practices of treatment all relate closely to these two assumptions.

This view, like any other, must be judged by its fruits rather than by its seeds. Yet, a brief consideration of two areas of shared prior experience and interest that appear to have had major implications for our present joint position may clarify it and give some due acknowledgement.

Our present brief therapy is visible first as pursuing further two main aspects of family therapy, in which we have all been extensively involved. A decade-and-a-half ago family therapy began to focus attention on observable behavioral interaction and its influence, both among family members and between them and the therapist, rather than on long-past events or inferred mental processes of individuals (Jackson and Weakland, 1961). In line with this, we now see disturbed, deviant, or difficult behavior in an individual (like behavior generally) as essentially a social phenomenon, occurring as one aspect of a system, reflecting some dysfunction in that system, and best treated by some appropriate modification of that system. We differ, however, with those family therapists who consider the dysfunction involved to be necessarily a fundamental aspect of the system's organization and requiring correspondingly fundamental changes in the system. Instead, we now believe that apparently minor changes in overt behavior or its verbal labeling often are sufficient to initiate progressive developments. Further, while we recognize that along with its obvious disadvantages symptomatic behavior usually has some recognizable advantages or "pay-offs"—such as providing leverage in controlling relationships—we no longer consider these especially significant as causes of problems or obstacles to change.

Family therapy also has prompted greater activity by therapists. Once family interaction was seen as significant for problems, it followed that the therapist should aim to change the going system. Extending this, we now see the therapist's primary task as one of taking deliberate action to alter poorly functioning patterns of interactions as powerfully, effectively, and efficiently as possible.

On the matter of how the therapist can actively influence behavior effectively—the strategy and techniques of change—we are especially indebted to the hypnotic work of Milton Erickson and his closely related psychotherapy.[1] Two points have been particularly influential. First, although Erickson is much concerned with how overt behavior affects feelings or states of mind, his moves to change existing behavior usually depends upon implicit or indirect means of influence. Even

---

[1] The work of Jay Haley (1963, 1973, 1969) has been valuable in making Erikson's principles and practices more explicit, as well as in providing additional ideas from Haley's own work in family therapy and brief treatment.

when behavior is explicitly discussed, his aim often is not to clarify the "reality" of a situation but to alter and ameliorate it by some redefinition. Second, both as hypnotist and therapist, Erikson has emphasized the importance of "accepting what the client offers," and turning this to positive use—in ways we will illustrate later—even if what is "offered" might ordinarily appear as resistance or pathology.

While our present approach thus derives directly from basic family therapy, in part, and from Erikson's work, in part, it also differs from both. For example, many family therapists attempt to bring about change largely by explicit clarification of the nature of family behavior and interaction. Such an attempt now seems to us like a family version of promoting "insight," in which one tries to make clear to families the covert rules that have guided them; we ordinarily avoid this. Meanwhile, our conceptualization of problems and treatment appears at least more general and explicit than Erikson's and probably different in various specific respects.

On the other hand, similarities as well as differences are observable between our treatment approach and other approaches with which we have had little interaction. For example, within the general field of family therapy, we share with the crisis-intervention therapy of Pittman, Langsley, and their co-workers (Pittman, Langsley, Flomenhaft, De Young, Machotka and Kaplan, 1971) beliefs in the importance of situational change for the onset of problems and of both directive measures and negotiation of conflicts in promoting better functioning in family systems. Minuchin and Montalvo (1967), together with a number of their colleagues at the Philadelphia Child Guidance Clinic, have increasingly emphasized active intervention aimed at particular reorderings of family relationship structure to achieve rapid problem resolution; we often pursue similar aims. Other family therapists than ourselves, notably Bowen, assign patients homework as part of treatment. Work with families similar to our own is also being developed abroad, for instance, at the Athenian Institute of Anthropos under Dr. George Vassiliou and at the Istituto per lo Studio della Famiglia in Milan, under Prof. Dr. Mara Selvini Palazzoli. In addition, the behavior modification school of therapy involves a number of ideas and interventions rather parallel to ours, although that field still appears to give little attention to systems of interaction. Furthermore, as noted later, a number of the techniques of intervention we utilize have also been used and described, though usually in a different conceptual context, by other therapists.

In sum, many particular conceptual and technical elements of our approach are not uniquely ours. We do, however, see as distinctive the overall system of explicitly stated and integrated ideas and practices that constitute our approach.

Main Principles of Our Work

1. We are frankly symptom-oriented, in a broad sense. Patients or their family members come with certain complaints and accepting them for treatment involves a responsibility for relieving these complaints. Also, since deviant symptomatic behavior and its accompanying vicious circles of reaction and counterreaction can themselves be so disruptive of system functioning, we believe that one should not hasten to seek other and deeper roots of pathology. The presenting problem offers, in one package, what the patient is ready to work on, a concentrated manifestation of whatever is wrong, and a concrete index of any progress made.

2. We view the problems that people bring to psychotherapists (except, of course, clearly organic psychiatric syndromes) as situational difficulties between people—problems of interaction. Most often this involves the identified patient and his family; however, other systems such as a patient's involvement with others in a work situation may be important at times.

3. We regard such problems as primarily an outcome of everyday difficulties, usually involving adaptation to some life change, that have been mishandled by the parties involved. When ordinary life difficulties are handled badly, unresolved problems tend increasingly to involve other life activities and relationships in impasses or crises, and symptom formation results.

4. While fortuitous life difficulties, such as illness, accidents, or loss of a job sometimes appear to initiate the development of a problem, we see normal transitional steps in family living as the most common and

important "everyday difficulties" that may lead to problems. These transitions include: the change from the voluntary relationship of courtship to the commitment of marriage, and from this to the less reversible commitment when the first child is born; the sharing of influence with other authorities required when a child enters school, and with the child himself and his peers in the adolescent period; the shift from a child-oriented marital relationship back to a two-party system when the children leave the home, and its intensification at retirement; and return to single life at the death of one spouse. Although most people manage to handle these transitions at least passably well, they all require major changes in personal relationships that may readily be mishandled. This view is similar to that of Erikson and Haley (1973).

5. We see two main ways by which "problems" are likely to develop; if people treat an ordinary difficulty as a "problem" or if they treat an ordinary (or worse) difficulty as no problem at all—that is, by either overemphasis or underemphasis of difficulties in living.

The first appears related to utopian expectations of life. There are countless difficulties which are part and parcel of the everyday business of living for which no known ideal or ultimate solutions exist. Even when relatively severe, these are manageable in themselves, but can readily become "problems" as a result of a belief that there should or must be an ideal, ultimate solution for them. For instance, there apparently has been a "generation gap" for the past 5000 years that we know of, but its difficulties only became greatly exacerbated into a "problem" when many people became convinced that it should be closed.

Inversely, but equally, "problems" can arise out of the denial of manifest difficulties—which could be seen as utopian assertions. For instance, the husband and wife who insist their marriage was made in heaven, or the parents who deny the existence of any conflicts with their children—and who may content that anyone seeing any difficulty must be either bad or mad—are likely to be laying the foundation for some outbreak of symptomatic behavior.

Two other aspects of this matter need mention. First, over- or under-emphasis of life difficulties is not entirely a matter of personal or family characteristics; this depends also on more general cultural attitudes and conceptions. While these often may be helpful in defining and dealing with the common vicissitudes of social life, they can also be unrealistic and provoke problems. For example, except for the death of a spouse, our own culture characterizes most of the transitions listed earlier as wonderful steps forward along life's path. Since all of these steps ordinarily involve significant and inescapable difficulties, such over-optimistic characterization increases the likelihood of problems developing—especially for people who take what they are told seriously. Second, inappropriate evaluation and handling of difficult situations is often multiplied by interaction between various parties involved. If two persons have similar inappropriate views, they may reciprocally reinforce their common error, while if one over-emphasizes a difficulty and another under-emphasizes it, interaction may lead to increasing polarization and an even more inappropriate stance by each.

    6. We assume that once a difficulty begins to be seen as a "problem," the continuation and often the exacerbation of this problem results from the creation of a positive feedback loop, most often centering around those very behaviors of the individuals in the system that are intended to resolve the difficulty: The original difficulty is met with an attempted "solution" that intensifies the original difficulty, and so on and on (Wender, 1968).

    Consider, for instance, a common pattern between a depressed patient and his family. The more they try to cheer him up and make him see the positive sides of life, the more depressed the patient is likely to get: "They don't even understand me." The action meant to alleviate the behavior of the other party aggravates it; the "cure" becomes worse than the original "disease." Unfortunately, this usually remains unnoted by those involved and even is disbelieved if anyone else tries to point it out.

    7. We view long-standing problems or symptoms not as "chronicity" in the usual implication of some basic defect in the individual or family, nor even that a problem has become "set" over time, but as the persistence of a repetitively poorly handled difficulty. People with chronic problems have just been struggling inappropriately for longer

periods of time. We, therefore, assume that chronic problems offer as great an opportunity for change as acute problems and that the principal difference lies in the usually pessimistic expectations of therapists facing a chronic situation.

8. We see the resolution of problems as primarily requiring a substitution of behavior patterns so as to interrupt the vicious, positive feedback circles. Other less destructive and less distressing behaviors are potentially open to the patient and involved family members at all times. It is usually impossible, however, for them to change from their rigidly patterned, traditional, unsuccessful problem-solving behavior to more appropriate behavior on their own initiative. This is especially likely when such usual behavior is culturally supported, as is often the case: Everyone knows that people should do their best to encourage and cheer up a loved one who is sad and depressed. Such behavior is both "right" and "logical"—but often it just doesn't work.

9. In contrast, we seek means of promoting beneficial change that works, even if our remedies appear illogical. For instance, we would be likely to comment on how sad a depressed patient looks and to suggest that there must be some real and important reason for this. Once given some information on the situation, we might say it is rather strange that he is not even more depressed. The usual result, paradoxical as it may seem, is that the patient begins to look and sound better.

10. In addition to accepting what the patient offers, and reversing the usual "treatment" that has served to make matters worse, this simple example also illustrates our concept of "thinking small" by focusing on the symptom presented and working in a limited way towards its relief.

We contend generally that change can be affected most easily if the goal of change is reasonably small and clearly stated. Once the patient has experienced a small but definite change in the seemingly monolithic nature of the problem most real to him, the experience leads to further, self-induced changes in this, and often also, in other areas of his life. That is, beneficent circles are initiated.

This view may seem insensitive to the "real," "big," or "basic" problems that many therapists and patients expect to be changed by therapy. Such goals are often vague or unrealistic, however, so that therapy which is very optimistic in concept easily becomes lengthy and disappointing in actual practice. Views of human problems that are either pessimistic about change or grandiose about the degree of change needed undermine the therapist's potentially powerful influence for limited but significant change.

11. Our approach is fundamentally pragmatic. We try to base our conceptions and our interventions on direct observation in the treatment situation of what is going on in systems of human interaction, how they continue to function in such ways, and how they may be altered most effectively.

Correspondingly, we avoid the question "Why?" From our standpoint, this question is not relevant, and involvement with it commonly leads toward concerns about "deeper" underlying causes—historical, mental, familial—of problem behavior and about "insight" into these.

That is, the question "Why?" tends to promote an individualistic, voluntaristic, and rationalistic conception of human behavior, rather than one focused on systems of interaction and influence. Moreover, since underlying causes inherently are inferential rather than observable, concern about them distracts a therapist from close observation of the present problem and what behavior may be perpetuating it.

On the basis of this general conception of problems and their resolution, which is discussed more fully in Watzlawick, Weakland, and Fisch (1974), we can now describe the overall practical approach and specific techniques that we utilize.

Operation of the Brief Therapy Center

The Brief Therapy Center was established as one of the projects at the Mental Research Institute in January, 1967. Since the termination of our founding grants, we have continued our work on a somewhat reduced scale on volunteered time. Some direct operating expenses have been met by donations from patients, although we provide free treatment where appropriate.

Our working quarters consist of a treatment room and observation room, separated by a one-way viewing screen, with provision for simultaneously listening to and tape-recording sessions. There is also an intercom phone between the two rooms. At the outset of our work, a therapist and an official observer were assigned, in rotation, to each case. More recently, we have been working as an overall team, with several observers of equal status usually present.

Our handling of all cases follows a six-stage schema, although in practice there may be some overlap among these:

1. Introduction to our treatment set-up.
2. Inquiry and definition of the problem.
3. Estimation of behavior maintaining the problem.
4. Setting goals of treatment.
5. Selecting and making behavioral interventions.
6. Termination.

Each of these will now be considered in order.

Introduction to Our Treatment Set-Up

Patients intentionally are accepted with no screening. A first appointment is set by the project secretary whenever an applicant calls and there is a vacancy in our schedule. No waiting lists are kept; when we have no vacancy, people are referred elsewhere.

At the first meeting, our secretary has the patient or family fill out a form covering basic demographic data and brings him or them to the treatment room. The therapist begins by explaining the physical and organizational arrangements, mentioning the potential advantages for treatment of the recording and observation, and requests written consent to this. Only two patients have ever declined to proceed on this basis. The therapist also tells the patient at once that we work on a maximum of ten sessions per case; this helps to set a positive expectation of rapid change.

Definition of the Problem

Since our treatment focus is symptomatic, we want first to get a clear and explicit statement of the presenting complaint. Therefore, as soon as the therapist has taken a brief record of the referral source and any previous treatment, he asks what problem has brought the patient to see us. If a patient states a number of complaints, we will ask which is the most important. In marital or family cases, since viewpoints may differ, although they often are plainly interrelated, we ask each of the parties involved to state his own main complaint. From the beginning then, we are following a form of the general principle, "Start where the patient is at."

Fairly often, the patient will give an adequate answer—by which we mean a clear statement referring to concrete behavior. In many cases, however, the response will leave the presenting problem still in doubt. Further inquiry is then needed to define more clearly this point of departure for the entire treatment. For example, patients with previous treatment experience or psychological sophistication are likely, after only the briefest mention of any present behavioral difficulty, to launch into discussion of presumed underlying matters, especially intrapsychic factors and family history, presenting these as the "real problem." We then press the question of what particular difficulties in living have brought them to see us now. To make things more specific, we often ask such questions as "What do you now do because of your problem that you want to stop doing, or do differently?" and "What would you like to do that your problem interferes with doing now?" Such inquiries also begin to raise the related question of treatment goals.

Other patients, especially younger ones, may state their complaints in vague terms that lack reference to any concrete behavior or life situation: "I don't know who I really am"; "We just can't communicate." Such patients can be particularly difficult initially. We find it important not to accept such statements as appropriate and informative but to continue inquiry until at least the therapist, if not the patient, can formulate a concrete, behavioral picture of the problem— of which such attachment to vague and often grandiose thinking and talking may itself be a major aspect.

Estimation of Behavior Maintaining the Problem

Our view, as mentioned earlier, is that problem behavior persists only when it is repeatedly reinforced in the course of social interaction between the patient and other significant people. Usually, moreover, it is just what the patient and these others are doing in their efforts to deal with the problem—often those attempts at help that appear most "logical" or unquestionably right—that is most important in maintaining or exacerbating it.

Once behavior is observed and considered in this light, the way this occurs is often rather obvious: The wife who nags her husband and hides his bottle in her efforts to save him from his alcohol problem and succeeds only in continually keeping drinking uppermost in his mind; the forgiving husband who never criticizes his wife until she feels he doesn't care anything about her, whatever she does, and becomes depressed—and he is forgiving of that too; the parents of a child dissatisfied with school who "encourage" him by talking all the more about how important and great education is—instead of it being a necessary drag. In other instances, of course, the reinforcements may be more difficult to perceive, either because they are subtle or complex—nonverbal behaviors, contradictions between statements and actions, different behaviors by several persons—or because even therapists are conditioned to accept cultural standards of logic and rightness without examining whether things really work that way.

In practice, the therapist first simply asks the patient and any family members present how they have been trying to deal with the problem. This alone may lead rapidly to a view of what keeps things going badly. If not, the inquiry, aiming always at concrete behavior, can be pursued at more length and in more detail, but sympathetically—the therapist's aim is to get enough information to understand what is happening, for which he needs cooperation, not to confront people with their mistakes. In addition to what the patient or others state explicitly, it is important to note how they discuss the problem and its handling, including their interaction. Such inquiry is likely to disclose a number of things that play some part in maintaining the problem, but working briefly demands choosing priorities. On the basis of observation and experience, one must judge which behavior seems most crucial.

Setting Goals of Treatment

Setting a goal both acts as a positive suggestion that change is feasible in the time allotted and provides a criterion of therapeutic accomplishment for therapist and patient. We, therefore, want goals stated clearly in terms of observable, concrete behavior to minimize any possibility of uncertainty or denial later. If parents bring us a child because he is failing in school, we ask for an explicit criterion of satisfactory progress—because we want to avoid subsequent equivocations such as "He is getting B's now instead of F's, but he isn't really learning enough." Also, we steer toward "thinking small" for reasons already discussed. Therefore, our usual inquiry is something like "At a minimum, what (change in) behavior would indicate to you that a definite step forward has been made on your problem?"

Concerning goals especially, however, patients often talk in vague or sweeping terms, despite our efforts to frame the question in terms of specific behavior. We then try to get more concrete answers by further discussion, clarification, and presentation of examples of possible goals for consideration. With vague, grandiose, or utopian patients, we have found it helpful to reverse our field, bringing them down to earth by suggesting goals that are too far out even for them. This again involves accepting what the patient offers, and even enlarging on this, in order to change it. For example, a student who was already in his mid-20's and was still being supported by a working mother told us he was studying "philosophical anthropology" in order to bring the light of India and China to bear on the West. He also, however, mentioned some interest in attending a well-known school of Indian music. It was then pointed out to him that this represented a rather limited aim compared to his concern to unite the spirituality of India with the practical communism of China and use both to reconstruct Western society. He then said that, since he was not doing well in his studies and was short of money, if he could secure a scholarship and really learn Indian music, this would be quite enough accomplishment for the present.

We usually are able, directly or indirectly, to obtain a stated goal that appears sufficiently explicit and appropriate to the problem. In some cases, however, we have not been able to do so. Either the patient persisted in stating only vague, untestable goals, or, rarely, the patient stated and stuck to an explicit goal which we judged inappropriate to his problem. Then we do not dispute what the patient insists on but privately set our own goal for the case by joint staff discussion of what sort of behavior would best exemplify positive change for the particular patient and problem. In fact, some such discussion occurs for all cases; at the least, the staff must always judge whether the patient's statement of his goal is adequate. Also, there is always staff discussion of intermediate behavioral goals; how does the patient—or his family members—need to behave so that the specific goal of treatment will follow?[2]

Our aim is to have a definite goal established by the second session, but gathering and digesting the information needed for this sometimes takes longer. Occasionally, we may revise the original goal in the course of treatment or add a secondary goal.

Selecting and Making Interventions

Once we have formed a picture of current behavior central to the problem and estimated what different behavior would lead to the specific goal selected, the task is one of intervening to promote such change. This stage must be discussed at some length, since it ordinarily constitutes the largest, most varied, and probably most unusual part of our treatment.

Change and "insight." We have already stated that our aim is to produce behavior change and that we do not see working toward insight, at either an individual or a family level, as of much use in this. In fact, working toward insight can even be counter-productive. Simple, practical-minded patients are often put off by this, since they want action and results, while more intellectually minded patients are likely to welcome such an approach but use it to delay or defeat any change in actual behavior. However, in addition to suggesting or prescribing changes in overt behavior, we do utilize interpretations. Our aim, though, is simply the useful relabeling of behavior. Patients often interpret their own behavior, or that of others, in ways that make for continuing difficulties. If we can only redefine the meaning or

---

[2] Our schedule is arranged to allow for one half-hour after each session for staff discussion and planning of goals, specific interventions to use, and so on. In addition, new cases and general issues are considered at more length in separate, weekly staff meetings.

implications attributed to the behavior, this itself may have a powerful effect on attitudes, responses and relationships. Such interpretation might look like an attempt to impart insight, but it is not. Using interpretation to promote insight implies that truth can helpfully be disclosed and recognized. This is not our aim or our belief. Rather, our view is that redefining behavior labeled "hostile" as "concerned interest," for example, may be therapeutically useful whether or not either label is "true," and that such truth can never be firmly established. All that is observable is that some labels provoke difficulties, while others, achievable by redefinition, promote adjustment and harmony—but this is enough.

Such relabeling may be especially important with rigid patients. It does not require overt behavior change, and it may even be accomplished without the need for any active cooperation by the patient or any family member. If the therapist's redefinition of an action or situation is not openly challenged—which can usually be arranged— then the meaning and effects of that behavior have already been altered.

Use of idiosyncratic characteristics and motivation. We attempt early in treatment to determine what approach would appeal most to the particular patient—to observe "where he lives" and meet this need, whether it is to believe in the magical, to defeat the expert, to be a caretaker of someone, to face a challenge, or whatever. Since the consequences of any such characteristic depend greatly on the situation in which it operates and how this is defined, we see these characteristics of different individuals not as obstacles or deficiencies, but as potential levers for useful interventions by the therapist.

For example, certain patients appear inclined toward defeating therapists, despite their request for help. This may be indicated by a history of unsuccessful treatment, repeated failure to understand explanations or carry out instructions, and so on. In such cases, the easiest and most effective course may be for the therapist to insist that the patient cannot possibly resolve his problem and that treatment can at most help him to endure it better. The patient is then likely to defeat this stance by improving.

A middle-aged widow first came to us with a complaint about the behavior of her 18-year-old son: delinquency, school failures, anger, and threatened violence toward her. She stated this was her only problem, although she also mentioned that she was an epileptic and was unable to use her right arm as a result of a work injury. Both mother and son had had about two years of previous therapy. We first suggested directly that her son was acting like a difficult, provoking, overgrown kid and, accordingly, she might gain by handling him more firmly in a few simple ways. She quickly thwarted such suggestions by increasing claims of helplessness: Now the epilepsy was emphasized; there was trouble with the other arm, too; a hysterectomy and appendectomy were also reported, along with childhood rheumatic fever, bleeding gums, troubles with her former husband and with her mother-in-law, constant worsening financial crises, and much more. In short, she was already a woman carrying on bravely amidst a sea of troubles that would have totally swamped anyone else; how could we ask her to do more yet? We then changed our approach to utilize this characteristic opposition. We began to insist to her that she was being unduly optimistic, was minimizing her troubles in an unrealistic way, and was not recognizing that the future very probably held even greater disasters for her, both individually and in terms of her son's behavior. It took some doing to surpass her own pessimistic line, but once we were able to do so, she began to improve. She started to oppose our pessimism—which she could only do by claiming and providing that she was not that sick and helpless—and to take a much more assertive attitude with her son, to which he responded well.

Directed behavior change. One of our main stated claims is to change overt behavior—to get people to stop doing things that maintain the problem and to do others that will lead toward the goal of treatment. While we are willing to issue authoritative directions, we find compliant patients rather rare. After all, most patients have already been exposed to lots of advice. If it was good, they must have some difficulty about profiting from advice; if it was bad, some preparation is needed for them to respond to quite different advice. Moreover, again, it is often just that behavior that seems most logical to people that is perpetuating their problems. They then need special help to do what will seem illogical and mistaken. When sitting on a nervous horse, it is not easy to follow the instructor's orders to let go of the reins. One knows the horse will run away, even though it is really the pull on the reins that is making him jump.

Behavioral instructions therefore are more effective when carefully framed and made indirect, implicit, or apparently insignificant. When requesting changes, it is helpful to minimize either the matter or the manner of the request. We will suggest a change rather than order it. If the patient still appears reluctant, we will back off further. We may then suggest it is too early to do that thing; the patient might think about it but be sure not to take any action yet. When we do request particular actions, we may ask that they be done once or twice at most before we meet again. We may request only actions that will appear minor to the patient, although in our view they represent the first in a series of steps, or involve a microcosm of the central difficulty. For example, a patient who avoids making any demands of others in his personal relationships may be assigned the task of asking for one gallon of gasoline at a service station, specifically requesting each of the usual free services, and offering a twenty-dollar bill in payment (*sic*).

This example also illustrates our use of "homework" assignments to be carried out between sessions. Homework of various kinds is regularly employed, both to utilize time more fully and to promote positive change where it counts most, in real life outside the treatment room.

Paradoxical instructions. Most generally, paradoxical instruction involves prescribing behavior that appears in opposition to the goals being sought, in order actually to move toward them. This may be seen as an inverse to pursuing "logical" courses that lead only to more trouble. Such instructions probably constitute the most important single class of interventions in our treatment. This technique is not new; aspects and examples of it have been described by Frankl (1957; 1960), Haley, (1963), Newton (1968) and Watzlawick et al. (Watzlawick, Beavin and Jackson, 1967). We have simply related this technique to our overall approach and elaborated on its use.

Paradoxical instruction is used most frequently in the form of case-specific "symptom prescription," the apparent encouragement of symptomatic or other undesirable behavior in order to lessen such behavior or bring it under control. For example, a patient who complains of a circumscribed, physical symptom—headache, insomnia, nervous mannerisms, or whatever—may be told that during the coming week, usually for specified periods, he should make every effort to increase the symptom. A motivating explanation usually is given, e.g., that if he can succeed in making it worse, he will at least suffer less from a feeling of helpless lack of control. Acting on such a prescription usually results in a decrease of the symptom—which is desirable. But even if the patient makes the symptom increase, this too is good. He has followed the therapist's instruction, and the result has shown that the apparently unchangeable problem can change. Patients often present therapists with impossible-looking problems, to which every possible response seems a poor one. It is comforting, in turn, to be able to offer the patient a "therapeutic double bind" (Bateson, Jackson, Haley and Weakland, 1956), which promotes progress no matter which alternative response he makes.

The same approach applies equally to problems of interaction. When a schizophrenic son used bizarre, verbal behavior to paralyze appropriate action by his parents, we suggested that when he needed to defend himself against the parents' demands, he could intimidate them by acting crazy. Since this instruction was given in the parents' presence, there were two paradoxical positive effects: the son decreased his bizarreness and the parents become less anxious and paralyzed by any such behavior.

Not infrequently, colleagues find it hard to believe that patients will really accept such outlandish prescriptions, but they usually do so readily. In the first place, the therapist occupies a position of advice-giving expert. Second, he takes care to frame his prescriptions in a way most likely to be accepted, from giving a rationale appropriate to the particular patient to refusing any rationale on the grounds that the patient needs to discover something quite unanticipated. Third, we often are really just asking the patients to do things they already are doing, only on a different basis.

We may also encourage patients to use similar paradoxes themselves, particularly with spouses or children. Thus, a parent concerned about her child's poor school homework (but who probably was covertly discouraging him) was asked to teach the child more self-reliance by offering incorrect answers to the problems he was asking help in solving.

Paradoxical instructions at a more general level are often used also. For example, in direct contrast to our name and ten-session limit, we almost routinely stress "going slow" to our patients at the outset of treatment and, later, by greeting a patient's report of improvement with a worried look and the statement, "I think things are moving a bit too fast." We also do the same thing more implicitly, by our emphasis on minimal goals, or by pointing out possible disadvantages of improvement to patients, "You would like to do much better at work, but are you prepared to handle the problem of envy by your colleagues?" Such warnings paradoxically promote rapid improvement, apparently by reducing any anxiety about change and increasing the patient's desire to get on with things to counteract the therapist's apparent overcautiousness.

On the same principle, when a patient shows unusually rapid or dramatic improvement, after acknowledging this change we may prescribe a relapse, on the rationale that it further increases control: "Now you have managed to turn the symptom off. If you can manage to turn it back on during this next week, you will have achieved even more control over it." This intervention, similar to Rosen's "re-enacting the psychosis" (Pittman, Langsley, Flomenhaft, De Young, Machotka and Kaplan, 1971) and related techniques of Erikson, anticipates that in some patients improvement may increase apprehension about change and meets this danger by paradoxically redefining any relapse that might occur as a step forward rather than backward.

Since we as therapists are by definition experts, giving authoritative instructions on both thinking and acting, another pervasive element of paradox is created by the fact that ordinarily we do so only tentatively, by suggestions or questions rather than direct orders, and often adopt a "one-down" position of apparent ignorance or confusion. We find that patients, like other people, accept and follow advice more readily when we avoid "coming on strong."

Utilization of interpersonal influence. Although many of our treatment sessions include directly only one therapist and one patient, we consider and utilize more extended interpersonal relationships constantly in our work. First, even when we see only the "identified patient," we conceive the problem in terms of some system or relationships and problem-maintaining behavior involving his family, his friends, or his work situation. Therefore, we believe that any interventions made with the patient must also take their probable consequences for others into account. Equally, however, useful interventions may be made at any point in the system, and frequently it appears more effective to focus our efforts on someone other than the identified patient. Where a child is the locus of the presenting problem, we very commonly see the whole family only once or twice. After this we see the parents only and work with them on modifying their handling of the child or their own interaction. With couples also, we may see the spouses separately for the most part, often spending more time with the one seen by them as "normal." Our point is that effective intervention anywhere in a system produces changes throughout, but according to what the situation offers, one person or another may be more accessible to us, more open to influence, or a better lever for change in the system.

Second, the therapist and the observers also constitute a system of relationships that is frequently used to facilitate treatment. With patients who find it difficult to accept advice directly from a real live person, an observer may make comments to the therapist over the intercom phone to be relayed to the patient from this unseen and presumably objective authority. When a patient tends to disagree constantly, an observer may enter and criticize the therapist for his "poor understanding" of the case, forming an apparent alliance with the patient. The observer can then often successfully convey re-phrased versions of what the therapist was offering originally. With patients who alternate between two different stances, two members of the treatment team may agree, separately, with the two positions. Then, whatever course the patient takes next he is going along with a therapist's interpretation, and further suggestions can be given and accepted more successfully. Such therapist-observer interaction strategies can bring about change rapidly even with supposedly "difficult" patients.[3]

As may be evident, all of these techniques of intervention are means toward maximizing the range and power of the therapist's influence. Some will certainly see, and perhaps reject, such interventions as manipulative. Rather than arguing over this, we will simply state our basic view. First, influence is an inherent element in all human contact. Second, the functioning necessarily includes this fact of life, but goes much further; professionally he is a specialist at influence. People come to a therapist because they are not satisfied with some aspect of their living, have been unable to change it, and are seeking help in this. In taking any case, therefore, the therapist accepts the assignment of influencing people's behavior, feelings, or ideas toward desirable ends. Accordingly, third, the primary responsibility of the therapist is to seek out and apply appropriate and effective means of influence. Of course, this includes taking full account of the patient's stated and observed situation and aims. Given these, though, the therapist still must make choices of what to say and do, and equally what not to say and do. This inherent responsibility cannot be escaped by following some standard method of treatment regardless of its results, by simply following the patient's lead, or even by following a moral ideal of always being straightforward and open with the patient. Such courses, even if possible, themselves represent strategic choices. To us, the most fundamental point is whether the therapist attempts to deny the necessity of such choices to himself, not what he tells the patient about them. We believe the better course is to recognize this necessity, to try whatever means of influence are judged most promising in the circumstances, and to accept responsibility for the consequences.

Termination. Whether cases run the limit of ten sessions or goals are achieved sooner, we usually briefly review the course of treatment with the patient, pointing out any apparent gains—giving the patient

---

[3] Team work facilitates such interventions but actually is seldom essential. A single therapist who is flexible and not unduly concerned about being correct and consistent can also utilize similar techniques—for example, by stating two different positions himself.

maximum credit for this achievement—and noting any matters unresolved. We also remark on the probable future beyond termination, ordinarily in connection with reminding patients that we will be contacting them for a follow-up interview in about three months. This discussion usually embodies positive suggestions about further improvement. We may remind patients that our treatment was not intended to achieve final solutions, but an initial breakthrough on which they themselves can build further. In a minority of cases, however—particularly with negativistic patients, ones who have difficulty acknowledging help from anyone, or those fond of challenges—we may take an opposite tack, minimizing any positive results of treatment and expressing skepticism about any progress in the future. In both instances, our aim is the same, to extend our therapeutic influence beyond the period of actual contact.

In some cases, we encounter patients who make progress but seem unsure of this and concerned about termination. We often meet this problem by means of terminating without termination. That is, we say we think enough has been accomplished to terminate, but this is not certain; it can really be judged only by how actual life experience goes over a period of time. Therefore, we propose to halt treatment, but to keep any remainder of the ten sessions "in the bank," available to draw on if the patient should encounter some special difficulty later. Usually, the patient then departs more at ease and does not call upon us further.

Evaluation and Results

If psychotherapy is to be taken seriously as treatment, not just an interesting exploratory or expressive experience, its effectiveness must be reliably evaluated. But this is far from easy, and rather commonly therapists offer only general clinical impressions of their results, with no follow-up of cases after termination, while researchers present ideal study designs that seldom get implemented.

We certainly cannot claim to have resolved this problem fully, even though we have been concerned with systematic evaluation of results from the outset of our work. Our method of evaluation still involves some clinical judgments and occasional ambiguities, despite efforts to minimize these. Until very recently, we have not had the resources needed to repeat our short-term follow-ups systematically after longer periods. And our evaluation plan is apt to seem overly simple in comparison with such comprehension schemes as that of Fiske et al. (Fiske, Hunt, Luborsky, Orne, Parloff, Reiser and Tuma, 1970). At most, we can claim only that our method of evaluation is simple, avoiding dependence upon either elaborate manipulation and interpretation of masses of detailed data or elaborate theoretical inference; that it is reasonably systematic and practicable; and most important, that it is consonant with our overall approach to problems and treatment.

We see the essential task of evaluation as systematic comparison of what treatment proposes to do and its observable results. Our treatment aim is to change patients' behavior in specific respects, in order to resolve the main presenting problem. Given the brevity of our work, the past refractoriness of most of the problems presented, and our frequent observation of behavior change immediately following particular interventions, we feel fairly safe in crediting observed changes to out treatment. Our evaluation then depends on answers to the two questions: Has behavior changed as planned? Has the complaint been relieved?

In our follow-up, the interviewer, who has not participated in the treatment, first inquires whether the specified treatment goal has been met. For instance, "Are you still living with your mother, or are you living in your own quarters now?" Next, the patient is asked the current status of the main complaint. This is supplemented by inquiring whether any further therapy has been sought since terminating with us. The patient is also asked whether any improvements have occurred in areas not specifically dealt with in treatment. Finally, to check on the supposed danger of symptom substitution, the patient is routinely asked if any new problems have appeared.

Ideally, such evaluation would divide our cases into two neat piles: successes in which our goal of behavior change was met and the patient's problem completely resolved, and failures in both respects. In reality, our treatment is not perfect; while results in these terms are clear for a majority of cases, several sources of less clear-cut outcomes remain: (a) Fairly often we have had cases in which our goal was reached or approached and considerable improvement was evident, but complete resolution of the presenting problem or problems was not attained. (b) Occasionally we have failed to formulate a goal explicit and concrete enough to check on its achievement with certainty. (c) In a very few cases, achievement of the planned goal and reported relief of the problem have been inversely related—hitting our target of change did not lead to relief, or we somehow got results in spite of missing our specific target.

In terms of our basic principles, all such mixed cases must be considered as failures of either conception or execution that demand further study. In the patients' terms, on the other hand, some of these cases have been completely successful, and many others represent quite significant progress. For the more limited and immediate purpose of evaluating the general utility of our approach, therefore, we have classified our cases into three groups according to practical results, recognizing that these correlate generally but not completely with achievement of our specific goals of behavior change. These groups represent: (a) complete relief of the presenting complaint; (b) clear and considerable, but not complete, relief of the complaint; and (c) little or no such change. For simplicity, the one case in which things were worse after treatment is included in the third group. We have not broken down our sample into subgroups based on common diagnosis, since the conventional system of diagnostic categories and our conception of problems and their treatment are based on different assumptions and the nature of the presenting problem has appeared to make little difference for our rate of success or failure. It should also be noted that this evaluation refers directly only to the major presenting complaint. However, in none of our cases in which this complaint was resolved was there any report of new problems arising, and in many of these, improvements in additional areas were reported. On this basis, then, our overall results for 97 cases, involving an average of 7.0 sessions, are:

Success	39 cases	40 per cent
Significant improvement	31 cases	32 per cent
Failure	27 cases	28 per cent

These results appear generally comparable to those reported for various forms of longer-term treatment.

Conclusion: Implications

In this paper we have set forth a particular conception of the nature of psychiatric problems, described a corresponding brief treatment approach and techniques, and presented some results of their application. Clearly, further clinical research should be done, as important problems obviously remain; goals remain; goals are still difficult to set in certain types of cases, the choice of interventions has not been systematized, evaluation is not perfected. Concurrently, though, there should also be more thinking about the broader significance of these ideas and methods. Our results already give considerable evidence for the usefulness of our general conception of human problems and their practical handling. Since this is both quite different from more common views and potentially widely relevant, we will conclude with a tentative consideration of some broad implications of our work.

The most immediate and evident potential of our work is for more effective use of existing psychiatric facilities and personnel. This could include reduction in the usual length of treatment and a corresponding increase in the number of patients treated, with no sacrifice of effectiveness. In fact, our approach gives promise of more than ordinary effectiveness with a variety of common but refractory problems, such as character disorders, marital difficulties, psychoses, and chronic problems generally. Further, it is not restricted to highly educated and articulate middle-class patients but is applicable to patients of whatever class and educational background.

In addition, our approach is relatively clear and simple. It might therefore be feasible to teach its effective use to considerable numbers of lay therapists. Even if some continuing supervision from professionals should be necessary, the combination of brief treatment and many therapists thus made possible could help greatly in meeting present needs for psychological help. Although this kind of development would have little to offer private practice, it could be significant for the work of overburdened social agencies.

Taking a wider view, it is also important that our model sees behavioral difficulties "all under one roof" in two respects. First, our model interrelates individual behavior and its social context instead of dividing them—not only within the family, but potentially at all levels of social organization. Second, this framework helps to identify continuities, similarities, and interrelations between normal everyday problems, psychiatric problems of deviant individual behavior, and many sorts of socially problematic behavior, such as crime, social isolation and anomie, and certain aspects of failure and poverty. At present, social agencies attempting to deal with such problems at the individual or family level are characterized by marked conceptual and organizational divisions—between psychological vs. sociological, supportive vs. disciplinary orientations, and more specifically, in the division of problems into many categories that are presumed to be distinct and discrete—reminiscent of the "syndromes" of conventional psychiatry. At best, this results in discontinuity; ineffective, partial approaches; or reduplication of efforts. At worst, it appears increasingly likely that such divisions themselves may function to reinforce inappropriate attempts at solution of many kinds of problems, as suggested by Auerswald (1968) and Hoffman and Long (1969). Our work thus suggests a need and a potential basis for a more unified and effective organization of social services.

Finally, our work has still broader implications that deserve explicit recognition, even though any implementation necessarily would be a very long-range and difficult problem. Our theoretical viewpoint is focused on the ways in which problems of behavior and their resolution are related to social interaction. Such problems occur not only with individuals and families, but also at every wider level of social organization and functioning. We can already discern two kinds of parallels between problems met in our clinical work and larger social problems. Problems may be reduplicated widely, as when concern about differences between parents and children becomes, in the large, "the generation gap problem." And conflicts between groups—whether these groups are economic, racial, or political—may parallel those seen between individuals. Our work, like much recent social history, suggests very strongly that ordinary, "common-sense" ways of dealing with such problems often fail, and, indeed, often exacerbate the difficulty. Correspondingly, some of our uncommon ideas and techniques for problem-resolution might eventually be adapted for application to such wider spheres of human behavior.

Stages in the Family Therapy of Adolescents

SIGRID R. McPHERSON, Ph.D.
WALTER E. BRACKELMANNS, M.D.
LAWRENCE E. NEWMAN, M.D.

It is frequently assumed—especially by analytically oriented therapists—that adolescents represent a problem of contraindication for family therapy. The reasoning behind this assumption is that adolescents are in the throes of individuation and separation, a process which mandates their being seen in treatment apart from their parents. To include the adolescent in family work is near tantamount to reimmersing him in a family system from which he is striving to gain distance. This article emphatically registers otherwise. In doing so it is heir to the lineage of early work (e.g., that of Ackerman) which originated in the problems presented to families by departing teenagers.

However, it differs significantly from most of the articles presented in this section on family therapy. It is decidedly less manipulative and more traditional than the approaches described by other authors. Second, it takes care to delineate "stages" in the "education" of the family—how one brings members to a perception of problems as family disturbances and not individual psychopathology. Also, it is virtually the only paper in the series to concern itself seriously with coordination of therapist-family expectations and belief systems. While it contains the family therapist's supposition that problems are not what they seem on the surface, and the belief that ultimately the family will get more than it might have bargained for initially, it also involves a gradual, subtle renegotiation of therapeutic contracts that stops short of conscientious manipulation. Fourth, it delineates in step-by-step process the unfolding of family treatment. Few authors have undertaken an analysis of this sequential movement and change through time.

Some assumptions in the paper may appear naive, e.g., the suggestion that once the adolescent is individuated and freed, the parents will have a second courtship, while neglecting to entertain the possibility that husband and wife may no longer have and maybe never had a basis for enduring bonds. People are not static in their requirements or needs—these shift over time—and it is paradoxical that a paper so sensitive to other developmental issues should deemphasize this vital aspect, especially since an adolescent's crisis may stem from his family's unwillingness to have him individuate because the parents want to avoid facing each other in all their emptiness or incompatible anguish.

Family therapy is a method of treatment used to intervene in certain cases of psychopathology (Ackerman, 1961; Ferber, Mendelsohn and Napier, 1972; Sager and Kaplan, 1972)—a therapeutic tool with limited, yet powerful attributes. It can be characterized as a process having comparatively definitive stages, as well as clear beginning and end points. The stages are transition points in which upheavals occur and the danger of abortion of treatment is highest. The stages can, therefore, be considered crisis points, with specific therapy-related hazards—i.e., treatment events that have the potential to disturb the equilibrium of the family unit.

Each crisis demands the generation of new styles of coping on the part of the family members. It is, thus, a time of upset and stress that brings with it the danger of regression to less effective patterns of adjustment (Caplan, 1961). However, the crisis presents the family with an opportunity to grow and adopt healthier styles of coping.

Reprinted with permission from *Family Process*, Vol. 13, No. 1 (March 1974), pp. 77-94.

Family therapy is especially applicable in the treatment of the emotionally disturbed adolescent who still lives with his family; examples will be drawn here from such cases. Similar concepts apply in helping a latency child achieve greater maturity or in freeing the unemancipated adult who still lives at home.

The concept of distinctive stages or crisis points in the course of family therapy is based on the notion that the family member who is defined as the index patient often is the vehicle for expression and resolution of unconscious family conflicts (Vogel and Bell, 1960). Thus, the family is viewed as a system of interrelating forces that have certain stress points (Bateson, 1971; Lewin, 1965). Different members enact particular roles assigned them by the family system; often such roles are accepted and enacted unconsciously (Sager and Kaplan, 1972). The "disturbed child," as "expressor" (Parsons, 1951) of the family's stress, is also the family member whose unconsciously assigned task is to keep the system in homeostatic equilibrium. Family therapy is the process designed to help make family members aware of, and restructure, such maladaptive roles and to free blocked channels of emotive expression. The task of family therapy may also be to emotionally separate a "fused" (Boszormenyi-Nagy, 1965) family unit. The goal is, thus, to restore the family to a healthy functioning system in which stresses are internally corrected and the ongoing homeostatic balance is one of health and well-being for all family members. Eight stages in the process are outlined below.

Presentation of the Family System

Among the questions a family therapist will ask himself when the family initially presents itself are: What has disturbed this family system? What is the family's view of the present difficulty? Why is outside help sought now? What are the expectations of the family members?

The systems approach (Bateson, 1971) to the request for treatment assumes that stress has desequilibrated the previously stable family system and that treatment is sought in an effort to reestablish homeostatic equilibrium. This attempt at reequilibration frequently takes place through scapegoating (Vogel and Bell, 1960) of a family member, usually, although not always, a child or adolescent.

A fifteen-year-old girl ran away from home and was picked up by the police. When her parents arrived to fetch her, the probation officer suggested that she seemed to be having emotional problems and ought to be seen by a counselor. Thus, Susie was brought to a clinic. Her parents' expectations were that the clinic would accept her as an individual patient, i.e., that the agency would try "to straighten her out"; the parents expected to be involved minimally. During the the intake interview in which the clinic requested that all family members be present, the mother went to great lengths to explain how difficult things have been with Susie, how rebellious she tends to be, how frequently she has run away from home, and how dismaying this is to her two younger brothers. The mother was especially upset about the apparent unpredictability of Susie's behavior, "Susie'll be a wonderful kid, cheerful and kind. She'll promise that she won't ever run away again one minute, yet be gone the next." Inquiries about the particulars of some of the running-away episodes revealed that they were not entirely unpredictable. Susie would usually be especially well-behaved for a few days just before she'd run away again. In the mother's words, "I can begin to relax and tend to other matters, like discussing things with my husband," adding, with a nervous laugh, "maybe even get to know each other again, but no, she's off again. It affects us all."

The therapist noted a possible relation between Susie's good behavior and the emergence of marital difficulty. Perhaps Susie's runaway behavior was her attempt to draw attention away from the threatening marital conflict. Thus, Susie's behavior might be an expression of unconscious parental conflict. When the therapist asked the parents about their relationship, they claimed it was harmonious, yet the communication between them indicated that there were underlying problems. Family therapy, therefore, seemed to be the treatment of choice. The parents knew, however, that it was all Susie's problem.

The therapist planned his intervention strategy in several steps. He would begin with the family "where it was" existentially, and start by seeing Susie alone; he would establish an alliance with her first. Soon, parents and other latency siblings would be invited for occasional sessions that would center in discussions around Susie. Subsequently, the parents must be helped to define themselves as part of the problem so that the whole family could enter the treatment process. This possibility exists once a parent begins to discuss problems not related to the index patient and, thus, makes tentative moves toward identifying other family members as persons in need of treatment. As other family members join in, family therapy gets underway.

The crisis: the family was beginning to recognize that Susie's problem was a family problem.

Preparation for Family Therapy

In preparation for family therapy, the therapist recognizes and accepts the family members "where they are" emotionally, in an existential manner of speaking. This means that when the parents request treatment for the child and clearly imply that they do not wish to be involved, as in the foregoing example, the therapist takes this as a starting point in the intervention. Involvement of other family members can be brought about only cautiously and gradually.

A mother called a therapist in private practice and said, "Cindy needs therapy. She is having problems. She can't communicate with us anymore. Cindy says the problem is with the family, but I know it's her problem." The therapist made the appointment for Cindy, as requested by mother, but extended an invitation to the entire family to come so that he might get to know Cindy's family. He took care to clearly show the mother that he respected her view of the problem, but he also put out tentative feelers to learn if perhaps a little bit more could be gained at the start. The entire family agreed to come. When they arrived at the therapist's office, the therapist made a few mental notes: mother was very well dressed, wore a rigid smile, and appeared to be very strained; the 18-year-old son and the 16-year-old daughter (the index patient) followed behind their mother, both nice-looking, somber youngsters; behind mother and children, and at a much slower pace, came the father, on crutches. All four family members quickly explained that the crutches were regarded matter-of-factly; father had been using them since he had polio when Cindy was just 15 months old. Almost the first words Cindy said to the therapist were, "Dad and I learned to walk together."

The therapist first talked things over individually with each family member. The family's story emerged gradually. Cindy wanted to join a drug-abuse group at school; she complained, ". . . but Mom won't let me. She doesn't want her baby in with those drug fiends, or with the nice counselor." The 18-year-old boy was planning to leave for an out-of-state college in six months. He expressed much concern for his mother and considerable awareness of her emotional distress. He was also very anxious to get away from it all and to live his own life. "I am leaving," he stated firmly. "Even if she's all upset, I need to go away." Both children let the therapist know that their father worked up to twenty hours a day at his own little company. "His job is his life," the mother said, echoing her children. She added, "But that's OK, I have accepted that." The therapist perceived a covert request on the part of the mother to influence her husband and children to help support her crumbling defenses. Underneath the veneer of forced cheerfulness, the therapist sensed much anger and even more sadness and depression. The mother seemed to feel that both children were deserting her just as her husband had already deserted her. Her fixed smile soon gave way to bitter sobs. The husband, on the other hand, expressed his feelings quite matter-of-factly. He was quite aware that he buried himself in his job so as to avoid a more intense involvement with his wife; yes, he missed being close to his children, but the price to pay of being emotionally involved with his wife was one that he found too overwhelming.

The present crisis thus involved not only the daughter, for whom mother sought treatment, but also mother's partially conscious apprehension of how deserted she would feel when her son left for college and when Cindy would become involved in the peer group and look elsewhere for advice and support. The therapist viewed the situation as difficult for both parents, since not only the very depressed mother, but the father perhaps as well, would react strongly to coming events. Ideally, husband and wife would obtain support by being reunited emotionally. But not one of the family members acknowledged a need for help at this time. Only Cindy might conceivably view the therapist as a helping agent, since not only her mother, but the drug-abuse counselor too, had raised questions regarding the appropriateness of her joining the drug-abuse group. Cindy might see the therapist as the one possible agent to get her into that group.

The therapist began by setting up a number of individual sessions with Cindy in order to further explore the drug-abuse group issue. He asked both parents to plan to come in for several discussions relating to the therapy interviews he was planning to have with Cindy.

There were a number of difficulties here in the way of starting family therapy at once. First of all, the therapist felt that the mother was presently so depressed that individual therapy seemed indicated for her; he planned to suggest that to her as soon as possible. He could move actively into family therapy only after the emotional state of the mother was such that she could tolerate the intense feelings that often emerge in family therapy. However, the therapist felt pressed for time; he believed that the entire family needed a number of family therapy sessions prior to the date the son was to leave for college. Only in this way could they be helped to deal with the feelings of anger and guilt about the separation. He openly discussed this issue with Cindy in her individual therapy with the result that Cindy was helping in getting her mother started in therapy of her own. Family therapy proper began when the family decided that all needed help in coping with the son's departure. In this, a crucial part was played by the index patient in actively involving the family in the treatment process.

The crisis: the children's efforts at separating from the family system.

Family Therapy Begins

This step is a major stress point because if the process begins too fast and the family is not ready to identify itself as a patient, at least in part, they may leave the therapy situation altogether. The therapist must be especially aware of danger signals at the time family therapy proper is begun. He may introduce the concept "family therapy" with such remarks as, "In the course of doing therapy with all of you together, I shall be changing hats many times. At one time I may be the staunch supporter of Jimmy, but then you might find that suddenly I'm busy supporting mother's point of view, even though it may be somewhat in opposition to what Jimmy has just said. On a third occasion I might put on the hat that fits the role of being father's ally. I will be doing this as the talk between you flows back and forth, because I want to help you understand what kinds of things you communicate to each other, how you go about doing this, and how you make each other feel. Often that's best accomplished by my playing musical hats." This may be followed by a comment to the effect that often in the course of family therapy the family will feel it's all hard work and no rewards; therefore, at times temptation to leave therapy before the task is done will be strong, but "forewarned is forearmed." Introductions such as these may make it possible for family members to comment later on the process they are experimenting and, thus, perhaps reduce anxiety and confusion and gain insight. It should be noted, however, that neither family members nor the family therapist will experience the gratifying stable transference relationship that often facilitates individual psychotherapy. Absence of this intimate relationship makes everyone's task more strenuous.

As family therapy proper gets under way, the therapist has probably already formulated a number of hypotheses regarding the subsystems that have been formed in a given family. In an "ideal," emotionally healthy family, there is no need for stabilized subsystems, i.e., for splits and alliances (Wynne and Singer) within the family. In the disturbed family system, one parent is often clearly on the outside of an "inner circle" and unable to communicate openly and directly with the other marital partner, while the other parent is in a close emotional alliance (of a positive, negative, or ambivalent nature) with one or several children—most frequently the index patient. Other siblings may be in one or several subsystems. Affective communication in such a family is blocked along one or several lines, depending upon the subsystems formed. As family therapy proceeds, the family therapist must keep clearly in mind what is happening to each subsystem within the family.

A domineering, stubborn husband; his meek, childlike wife; and their 16-year-old daughter Joyce were approaching the point in Joyce's therapy where they were becoming aware that the 16-year-old's repeated behavior of running away and sexually acting-out often occurred after father and daughter had had a particularly intense encounter with one another. In their encounters each usually tried to convince the other of the "rightness" of his or her point of view by means of shouting arguments. When all three came to the therapist's office after a crisis phone call, they began by relating that two days ago Joyce had met a former boyfriend, had spent the night with him at the beach without letting her parents know where she was, and had been "raped" by him. The next morning, i.e., yesterday, Joyce had come home sobbing to tell her parents of the outrage that had befallen her. The father was incensed. He didn't believe Joyce's cry of rape; he accused her of being a slut. Predictably, this triggered Joyce, and father and daughter were into a shouting match. The meek wife spoke up, addressing her husband, "Why object now—it's happened many times before, I don't like it either; but I like it even less that she is getting between you and me again. I had begun to think recently that maybe I was more to you than just the 'child-mother' of your daughter. I don't want her to ruin that."

The crisis: the system's maladaptive equilibrium was being loosened, as the mother began to challenge the father-daughter subsystem.

The Therapist Is Accepted into at Least One Subsystem of the Family

Families will allow the therapist to enter the family system in different ways. Entry may be into one, two, or all subsystems. During the process of gaining acceptance, the therapist may find himself inside one subsystem at one point, outside of it again soon afterward. The family may also encapsulate him within the system by assigning him the role of another subsystem.

The experience of being accepted into the family system is one that is intuitively felt by the therapist; it consists primarily of a feeling of ease within the family unit that enables him to take more "risks." He can communicate less cautiously and express himself more freely. "Gutsy" words and strong-worded interpretations that would have been inappropriate a few weeks ago now seem especially fitting. There is a feeling in the sessions that is analogous to that of the "working alliance" experiences in one-to-one psychotherapy. However, there is a difference: The security of the family therapist's position within the family tends to be much more tenuous than the position of the therapist in one-to-one psychotherapy. The degree of this tenuousness depends to a considerable extent upon the structure of the family and the emotional tone within the family, but also upon the therapist's own nature. Thus, the family therapist may at times find himself suddenly thrust out of a family system, with strong defenses blocking his way to go in, until some particular issue is worked through either in the family system or within the therapist himself. For example, he may find himself unable to escape an assigned constricting role of "family member" within the family because the role happened to fit his own unconscious needs. Until it is resolved, the assumption of such a role may block much of his effectiveness as a therapist.

Acceptance of a therapist into the family system may occur in several steps punctuated by temporary ejections. Acceptance may be by one family member only, such as the index patient, with subsequent, tenuous acceptance by other family members. If there are two therapists, the family may decide to accept one therapist but not the other. Also, a therapist who overidentifies with the patient and overdoes the "rescue work" may suddenly find himself on the outside of the family unit again, sometimes even on the outside of the subsystem, "index patient." From a dynamic point of view, the family system and its defenses are stronger than one or even two therapists. Changes are most possible when the therapist is moving within the system while at the same time functioning as consultant to the system, i.e., by avoiding a rigid system-assigned role. In this fashion, the therapist can best initiate the forces for change, which will occur gradually by the realignment of the forces that operate within the family system.

Pat, a 16-year-old girl had recently run away, taking the family car and two boys who were friends of Pat's former boyfriend. The boyfriend had met death from a drug overdose six months earlier. Just prior to that experience, Pat had overdosed herself accidently. The runaway episode had precipitated the family's request for family therapy, since "that's what the school counselor had recommended." Pat was disinterested in individual psychotherapy; therefore the major emphasis was upon family therapy from the beginning, even though the family was "in therapy" with words only. Weekly meetings had been held for three months. In addition to Pat, there was the angry and depressed older brother, the chronically depressed mother and the jovial-acting, yet hostile, father. The therapist had been very tenuously accepted by the mother only. The family tone during the sessions was laced with sarcasm and contemptuousness toward each other as well as toward the therapist. These themes were best expressed by Pat who refused to become involved in discussions at all with the exception of making biting comments toward the parents and the therapist. Since the runaway episode, Pat had behaved in this sarcastic, noncommunicative fashion at home as well. Both parents presented a united front of outrage, yet the sarcasm was especially trying for Pat's mother. In one particular session, the mother viciously attacked Pat in her turn. She accused Pat of being insensitive, callous, and unable to have or express feelings. Pat remained silent. Into the silence the therapist calmly dropped the comment that perhaps sometimes feelings were so painful that it seemed best to lock them away altogether and to cover them with sarcasm. Soon afterward, she noted that Pat was quietly crying. She invited Pat to put her tears into words. Pat shook her head. Immediately, both parents began to apply pressure by demanding that Pat express her feelings. The therapist intervened firmly, "I asked Pat to put her tears into words if she wanted to, not that she had to." A long silence ensued. Pat pointed her finger toward the therapist, saying slowly, "I think you know what I'm crying about, don't you?" The therapist replied, "I have an idea or two, Pat. However, when you want to, I'd like to talk about it with you." Eventually Pat could talk to the therapist alone about her boyfriend's death. In family therapy this led eventually to an expression of Pat's angry feelings toward her parents and brother for "condemning" the boyfriend because of the drug involvement that had led to his death. "I loved him," Pat insisted.

Soon the family discovered that mother and father did not at all agree on their feelings about the issues involving Pat, the boyfriend, etc., as had been assumed heretofore. The crisis: upheaval of the checks and balances of the family system by the entry of the therapist into the system.

Subsystem Boundaries Are Dissolved

Often, subsystem boundaries are dissolved by a dramatic return to the fold of a family member who emotionally had been outside the "inner circle" of the family system. The isolated family member is often one of the parents. With his or her emotional return, affective communication between the two marital partners begins to be opened up once more. Even though this return can be described in a few words, a great deal of therapeutic work goes into its facilitation. When the return occurs, it often is almost explosive in its intensity.

The road to the emotional return was opened by the revelation of a family myth. An oldest son, the index patient, had been kept at home and away from all sports and activities for over two years during his preadolescent years upon the advice of the family physician. The boy had not been told very clearly why he was suddenly not allowed to be active, ride his bicycle, or play with his friends after school; thus, he tended to view the whole thing as a giant punishment. The needs of the family, especially of the mother, were to keep "upsetting information" from the boy. As a result, the son perceived mother as an agent who suddenly restrained him severely without reason. Randy's father worked long hours; he was perceived as weak and ineffectual by Randy—powerless to oppose such a strong woman as his big (over 200 pounds) mother. Years later, a course of family therapy was initiated because the boy had begun to be in serious acting-out difficulties. In the sessions, Randy accused his mother of being an arbitrary disciplinarian and responsible for spoiling years of his childhood; he blamed her for his lack of athletic skills, which contributed to his present feelings of inadequacy. He felt incompetent and resentful toward his two younger brothers who had not had this kind of punishing experience. At the same time, the boy tended to be very protective of his father. After all, father couldn't help "being stuck" with such a powerful wife who set up such arbitrary rules.

During one therapy hour, mother and Randy were going through a by now familiar ritual of arguing on the theme, "Why is mother chief disciplinarian?' The dyad of mother-index patient formed a subsystem in which the affective communication was powerful, if mostly negative; father was clearly on the outside and considered incompetent and ineffectual by wife and son. Direct communication of feelings between husband and wife was blocked. Presently, the therapist asked father again what, in his opinion, the argument might really be about. In reply, the father turned to the boy and said quietly, "Well, you know, the decision, then, to listen to the doctor and not to let you go out and run and play, that was my decision, too, because that's what the doctor had said. I really felt badly about it, but at that time we just could not afford another costly physical examination like the one you had just had and that had resulted in the doctor saying that you could not be active. After all those illnesses you'd had, it made sense what the doctor said. As a matter of fact, I had a long talk with the doctor; he showed me the X-rays and the cardiogram on the basis of which he had made his decision, and although I'm a lay person and don't understand about medicine, that made sense to me, but I felt awful about it."

The quiet statement of the father exploded the family myth that mother had unnecessarily restrained Randy. Both parents were ready, at this point, to begin talking about their intense feelings of guilt regarding the son's former physical condition. Thus, they had reached the phase in family therapy during which the subsystems were being dissolved and father was allowed to reenter the entire family system.

The crisis: emotional return of the isolated marital partner threatened to bring the marital unit into long-avoided emotional closeness.

The Family Members Sort Out Their Roles

The sorting-out process of who does what to whom, why and how, will take up the family's time during the dissolution of stable subsystems. It is not dissimilar to the process of "working through" in individual therapy. In family therapy, it involves a careful examination of the behavior and communication within the family. Although the isolated family member has now rejoined the family system, some of the behaviors that maintained him or her on the outside will still occur. Now they can be examined openly.

Returning again to the last example, the therapist found during subsequent hours that whenever mother and father had a difference of opinion, Randy would actively attempt to reestablish the old alliance with his mother by provoking an argument with her. But now when it occurred, the therapist was able to point it out, "Mom and dad have a difference of opinion, but Mom and Randy do the arguing." The father at last picked up the therapist's cue. "Yes. That is right. And I'm sick and tired of it. I may not know how, but I'd sure like to discuss some of these things directly with my wife, without you butting in."

The father then requested a series of sessions without the children so that he could talk more freely to his wife. During those sessions, he explained to her that he had always found it extremely difficult to speak up in front of his children because he was very much afraid that he might really lose his temper; he believed that a good father did not show open anger in front of his children. He often felt criticized by her but did not know how to respond to this other than to explode with rage. He was a self-made man with less formal education than his wife. Prior to therapy, the family had had a number of serious financial setbacks that had intensified his feelings of inadequacy. With the support of the therapist, he was able to confront her with these feelings; she could, in turn, communicate her despair about receiving no response, no matter what she said to him. To her this had meant that he had "lost his feelings." The marital partners subsequently continued a sorting-out process with the help of the children. The crisis: discovery of "hidden roles" assigned to family members.

It should be noted that during this phase of therapy, when the family members are sorting out and redefining their roles, the therapist's interventions will often be of a transactional nature. The transactional approach is especially useful in families in which there is a tendency to "parenticize" the child (Zuk and Rubinstein, 1965) or when communication between spouses is not taking place on an adult level. While transactional interpretations always form an integral part of family therapy, they are especially valid during this stage, just as during other stages a focus on affectional needs was of importance. During each stage of family therapy, the therapist must be sensitive to the aspect of the system that presents itself foremost.

The Children Separate Themselves Emotionally from the Marital Relationship

Finally, it is time for the children to separate emotionally from the marital relationship. This is especially true for the index patient who tends to be most involved. In comparatively healthy families, the separation often follows spontaneously from the analysis of the family roles. A discussion of such notions as that it is not the child's job to protect the parents and that in therapy an emotional and open dialogue can safely take place between mother and father may initiate the steps toward separation. However, often the prospect of reestablishing a closer marital relationship is a very frightening prospect for the parents, since it implies vulnerability to the very same disappointments, hurts, and feelings of guilt that in the past necessitated the emotional disengagement and focus on the family's "problem child."

Old fears may still be waiting in the wings. There may be a need to bring up the idea that conflict discussed and examined will not lead to a blowup and divorce but may in fact be helpful in strengthening the relationship. The therapist must communicate repeatedly about the good things he sees in the relationship between mother and father.

A professional man and his wife brought their 15-year-old son, their oldest child, to therapy with the complaint that the son was underachieving in school, would not communicate with them, and was mean toward his younger sisters and brother. Sam had had problems since birth. He had suffered anoxia prior to birth and had been delivered by emergency Caesarian section. During early childhood he had had numerous allergies, intestinal upsets, and infectious illnessess. His early school years had been marred by perceptual problems of one nature or another, necessitating treatment in that area. Thus, Sam had had numerous involvements of a quasi-psychotherapeutic nature; he had also been seen in play therapy by a well-known child therapist. For years he had been considered a very disturbed child.

Sam was angry with his parents for bringing him to the therapist, since to him this meant that they thought there was still something wrong with him, even though he was strong and healthy now and believed that he was performing satisfactorily in school.

While the parents requested therapy for Sam, they expressed a strong desire to involve the entire family. They had heard about family therapy from a close friend who was a therapist and felt it would be useful for them in acquiring "tools to deal with Sam."

In the course of a number of exploratory individual sessions with Sam, the therapist learned that Sam was not very angry, but also genuinely puzzled about finding himself in treatment again. He clearly indicated that he did not wish to deal with his own feelings of rage. Since the therapist had observed that the parental communication style with Sam as one of extreme intrusiveness, the therapist kept the conversation between Sam and himself primarily on topics Sam enjoyed, avoiding any probing and interpreting. Sam seemed to like talking about his interests but at the same time expressed the wish that he'd rather not be in therapy at all. The parents also resisted by refusing to have more than one therapy session per week for anyone. Thus, the therapist decided that weekly family sessions made the most sense, since at least some of the parental pressure upon Sam could be dealt with in that way. He would have preferred, however, to see Sam in additional individual sessions as well. The therapist made every effort to include Sam in the decision-making process regarding family therapy.

Family sessions alternated between parents and Sam, and the parents and all four children. When the entire family was present, sessions were chaotic, with constant disruptions of any meaningful theme. The parents were extreme deniers. Not only did they insist that the primary problem was with Sam and that the other children's behavior was a result of their feelings about Sam, but they also continued to emphasize the goodness of their marriage and their ability to communicate freely with one another. They repeated this theme even while the smallest child, seven-year-old Michael, made frequent comments in sessions such as "How come you're never home, Dad?" and "Why does Mom do all the worrying Dad?"

The underlying marital conflict emerged gradually. First, there was a session for which the parents spontaneously came alone. The issue they wanted to discuss was that during a party the wife had "inexplicably" exploded in rage at her husband. The husband was nonplussed. Yes, she'd exploded like that a few times during the first few years of their marriage, but as she had become "better adjusted," this had ceased. The wife attempted to explain that she often felt "squelched" by her husband. He was domineering and rarely took her seriously—he didn't listen to her and failed to include her when major decisions were being made. The husband was shocked, then angered: "Well, if this is what family therapy leads to—who needs it!" The wife reacted with apprehension to the prospect of losing family therapy and became apologetic. During subsequent family sessions, however, she continued to drop gentle hints about problems relating to the marital dyad. Then, during one family session in which only Sam was present, both parents exploded into a violent argument. Sam confided to the therapist, "They've been fighting all the way here." The father retorted, "We have not, Sam. We were just having a spirited discussion."

In the ensuing discussion, the wife expressed her anger at her husband for again having made a major decision concerning the entire family without consulting her at all. "You're taking advantage of my powerlessness," she said. He responded, "Don't you dare make me feel guilty about things I want to do." Halfway through the session the father suddenly turned angrily to the therapist, "How come you allow this to go on? We are wasting time with this! What about Sam? We're here to talk about Sam!" The therapist replied calmly, "I think Sam's doing just fine, not being the center of attention for once." Sam smiled, mumbling that he was "just listening."

Gradually, Sam was allowed to move to the periphery of the triad; the focus shifted to the couple and their efforts to deal in earnest with their long buried, marital problems. The crisis: the "liberated" child serves no longer as buffer between husband and wife.

Starting the separation of the child is not always readily accomplished, since the index patient often has his identity strongly invested in his assumed role, although unconsciously so, and will resist change. Sometimes the change can be initiated by helping the recently "returned" family member to be in tune with the index patient's needs and wants so that healthier gratifications can take the place of the present neurotic rewards. Often, the index patient needs to be assured that being involved in his own activities will not mean that now Mom and Dad will forget all about him. He may require additional therapy.

Individuation of Family Members

Another difficulty in the separation process is presented by a "fused" family. In such families, even after the marital partners are again communicating, the parents will suddenly be afraid of being abandoned all over again as soon as the child begins to live a life of his own. Before separation can be accomplished, each family member must grow to be an individual who is a member of the family system but who is also striving to be an autonomous person. The notion of "autonomy" and the idea that family members may freely leave and enter a family system is a difficult and frightening concept for certain families. The family therapist may succeed to a degree by engaging in brief portions of individual therapy with each family member in the presence of the other family members. This stage is essentially a process of individuation. Family members can help each other achieve it once they understand what is involved.

In fact, one real reward of family therapy is this chance for greater individuation. However, since the therapist must focus on some painful maladaptive behaviors within the family, a high level of motivation on the part of the family is especially desirable during this stage. Some typical confrontations are over the assumption that family members know each other's private motivations, how family members use each other as "watchdogs," or how they may invalidate each other's emotional experience. For example, when 15-year-old Julie said, "I'm very unhappy about what you and Dad just talked about—I'm afraid you might divorce," Julie's mother replied, "No, you're not unhappy, you're just mad at us." The therapist must clarify and clearly expose such kinds of behavior so that the family may learn how and why it occurs. Moreover, families need to learn about the limits of each person's perception of the other's inner experience, about assuming responsibility appropriately, and about defining the kinds of problems that are shared family problems as opposed to those that are individual ones.

The Family System Realigns Itself, Redefines Its Roles, and Moves Toward Stabilization

Later, affective lines of communication between husband and wife are reestablished in earnest. If all has gone well, almost a second courtship between husband and wife can be observed. The transition from having the feelings expressed by the child to a direct expression of the affectional modes between husband and wife can be an exciting time for the family and the therapist. Husband and wife are relearning to tell each other directly how they feel. The patient-child is outside the dyad and is beginning to be absent from sessions. The negative aspects of the marital relationship—which often are much more easily dealt with than are the positive ones—are partially worked through. Husband and wife have begun the difficult task of talking to each other about tender and caring feelings.

A family consisting of father, mother, index patient—18-year-old daughter Fran—and 15-year-old son Joe had been in family therapy for almost two years. There had been a gradual transition to conjoint marital therapy. Recently, husband and wife had begun to show in a number of ways, such as going out for dinner and dancing, that they had entered a second courtship. Daughter Fran had begun an exciting job and was making plans to move out of the home; son Joe had taken up surfing and had become part of an outgoing group of boys. During one conjoint session, the couple mentioned casually that the wife's younger brother, 27-year-old Tom, had decided to move to California. The wife was excited to have "baby brother" move closer. To be helpful, the couple had invited Tom to live with them for a few months. Both expressed their pleasure about making this offer.

Not long after Tom's arrival, however, there began to be vague complaints about him in sessions, even though they were always followed with reassurances that all would be well soon. Then one day the therapist received an urgent phone call from the husband. Tom really did have a serious problem; he had lined up a number of jobs in the last few weeks but hadn't followed through on any of them. Today he had received a speeding ticket. Tom needed therapy. Would the therapist see him?

The therapist discussed the issue of seeing Tom with the couple first, indicating that while he would not see Tom in ongoing individual psychotherapy, he would try to be of help in assessing the situation.

The therapist's suspicion, namely that Tom had become part of the family system, proved to be accurate. Tom told the therapist about his recent experiences trying to get a job. Whenever he found one that he liked, either his sister or his brother-in-law found all sorts of faults with it. Tom said to the therapist, "I get the feeling that they don't want me to go; it's almost as if I had taken Fran's place since she moved out."

Tom showed considerable insight regarding his own passivity and his intense need to please his sister and her husband. He had come to see the therapist in good part to please them. He knew he had problems, but he did not feel that he wanted to be in therapy at this time; he resented his brother-in-law's pressure in this regard.

The issue at hand was one of effecting a separation. While Tom needed to work on his separation from the couple, the couple needed to deal with their attempt to reestablish the equilibrium of the past. The crisis: a resurrection of the feelings of excessive vulnerability and dependency.

Philosophy of Therapist

In conclusion, the outcome of family therapy may in good part hinge upon the philosophy of the family therapist. A family therapist must truly believe that the people he is treating did not marry only for neurotic maladaptive resons, but also for the good they saw in each other. If he does not firmly believe that the potential exists within the family to give each other needed emotional rewards and supports, he is not doing the family a service by engaging them in family therapy. Unless he himself believes this marriage is one that can be saved and can be a good one, he cannot honestly communicate with the family in the context of doing family therapy.

In Defense of
Child Therapy

BRAULIO MONTALVO

JAY HALEY

*The following article is a remarkable example of the maverick
tradition of family therapy writing. Provocatively challenging,
irreverently disputatious to the extent of being combative and
perhaps even assaultive, it has been seen by some as condescend-
ingly calculated to mock traditional child therapy. It does not
speak of trust, warmth, or concern, and represents to some an icy
disparagement of therapeutic relationships. Regardless of what
one may think, it is a significant article, from the standpoint of
both history and content.*

*The entire paper is "paradoxical," beginning with the title.
Instead of joining those family therapists who have written off
individual treatment as false, useless, without merit, and, worse
yet, destructive and therefore to be rejected out of hand, the
article that follows appears to be saying the traditional may have
had some value, but for reasons other than those advanced by its
practitioners and/or theorists. The authors subsume the merits of
the old under the banner of the new—family theory and therapy.
This amounts to saying child therapists may have all along been
unwitting practitioners of effective family treatment. In order to
absorb and embrace the traditional within the new, Montalvo
and Haley paradoxically relabel the "old" as "avant garde" as well*

as being naively and inadvertently manipulative. Focusing on the child, who is seen as having an internalized conflict and agreeing with the parents that the child needs individual help, becomes for the authors a measure tantamount to family therapists "prescribing the symptom." Similarly, arranging for therapy on a one-to-one basis largely between therapist and child with relative exclusion of the parents is reconstrued as a powerful intervention into the family system. The child's alliance with an adult outside the family dilutes the child's role in cross-generational alliances and integrational splits within the family (e.g., if the child's part in parental struggles is reduced, the parents will be forced together). There are many more intriguing paradoxes in the paper and if readers are stimulated or provoked to the proper frame of mind, they will conjure up additional ones. Inducing the incentive to do just that is one of the remarkable features of the article.

Historically, this paper will well be a signpost, although it can stand on other substantive merits. For instance, it has much to say about the powerful, but hitherto seldom remarked upon, "demand characteristics" of child psychotherapy. And while some readers may deem the analysis of these qualities more clever than compelling and more opportunistic than heart-rendering, the fact that the authors provide additional or alternative rationales for consensually and conventionally accepted explanations of common phenomena indicates that their arguments deserve serious attention, even if they infuriate. Things are seldom all they seem (sometimes by calculation, as in the manipulation that is the forte of many family therapy authors—but more frequently it stems from the non-consciousness created by imbued professional culturalisms and belief systems), and any effort directed at generating doubt and focused awareness is to be welcomed as broadening and enriching.

Thus, this reassessment of the merits of individual therapy with children may be understood as an extension of Bowen's "domino effect" or, relatedly, as an explicit statement of the family therapist's thesis that any therapeutic intervention—be it drug therapy, psychoanalysis, group treatment, or whatever—is inevitably a family intervention, and, the therapist ought, for the sake of all, be aware of this fact. Concomitantly, traditional child treatment is seen as working because it avoids confrontality, explicitness, insight, or the cognitive reasoning out of problems. This is because parents and child believe the "real work" is going on in child therapy, when in reality the crucial factor is the offhand, low-key seemingly secondary and indirect transactions of messages to the parents about handling the child and treatment. It is in the "double-masked" management aspects of the case that success or failure obtains, since the therapist, whether knowingly or not, is really involved in brief therapy, i.e., a family treatment organized around management issues. The arrangement is seen as beneficial because resistance is minimized by permitting the parents and child to operate according to one set of premises (e.g., the disease model and the virtues of individual treatment), while the therapist plays the game and outmaneuvers the family by treating them as a family system without signaling such to them. The parents believe their "sick" child is in individual psychotherapy aimed at reorganizing the child's psychic equilibrium, while the therapist "softsells" the parents without having to "educate" them to their culpability nor to reeducate them to "systems thinking" and away from the "disease model." It is a coup de grace or one-upmanship, that is the quintessence of so much current family therapy literature. It merits extensive consideration.

In their enthusiasm for a new orientation of therapy, many family therapists disregard therapeutic approaches that have a long and respectable history. As family therapy expands and new approaches proliferate, many beginning family therapists seem to argue that, if the whole family is not in the room, the therapy is old-fashioned. They disregard any therapy in which only individuals are interviewed. In doing so, they may overlook the valuable contributions made by earlier therapeutic modes. A glaring example is the way many family therapists regard child therapy, or child analysis. This was once a legitimate form of therapy with many adherents; family therapists talk about it lightly, if not with levity. They assume that a child could not possibly change unless his family changes, and playing with a child will not change his family. Yet even though outcome studies of child therapy are almost non-existent, it is undeniable that children have changed by experiencing play therapy. How is this possible? An explanation of such an occurrence will be offered here with an emphasis upon what can be learned from child therapy that might correct the errors of many family therapists.

Discussing the individual treatment of a child could be setting up a straw man; when a child is given play therapy, his parents are usually also involved in some form of treatment. However, such a discussion is legitimate, since the theory of child psychopathology assumes that only the child has the problem. His parents and other relatives are a stress factor rather than the unit with the problem.

When focusing on the treatment of the child alone, we must discuss a situation that has never been fully described. No research data are available on what child therapists actually do with children and families. Our description, therefore, is in part what is supposed to be done in child therapy, as we try to clarify the process by which a child might change in such a situation. First we will emphasize the structure of the treatment context and later the way the therapist uses the child to intervene in the family.

The Structure of Child Therapy

Often the treatment of a child takes place in a clinic where many factors in addition to the individual interviews are causal to change. A social worker typically sees the parents, and as the parents are helped to resolve some of the basic ways they use the child in their conflicts with one another, the child can change. For example, if a male child must struggle against behaving in effeminate ways so that mother and father can use him in the issue of father's masculinity, the child is able to recover when the issue between father and mother has been resolved. However, what of those cases in which a therapist appears to be treating the child alone?

Clearly, a child is never the only one involved in the treatment, even when he appears to be. A number of important factors are part of the total encounter that occurs in child therapy. To begin with, there is the situation that precipitates the child into treatment. A child must express a family problem in such a way that a limit of tolerance is passed and the family is driven to take action. Either the parents decide upon treatment because of internal stress in the family or because of their concern about a traumatic experience of the child, or they are pressured into such action by school authorities, the family physician, or friends and neighbors. Often, when the parents decide to follow through on a referral for their child, they confront each other with the seriousness of the problem for the first time. This in itself can be therapeutic, since the parents are mutually agreeing that something must be done and so readying themselves for a change. They must also tell the child that they are going to take him to a doctor. When the child realizes that this time it is not merely one of the previous ineffectual threats, he can begin to initiate new behavior. Usually the parents benevolently reassure the child about the nice qualities of the therapist, but he is aware of his parents' concern and anger with him.

The parents make an appointment with the child therapist who arranges to see the child and also to see the parents to set the fee and agree to the contract for treatment. During the interview with the parents, he listens to their complaints about the child, and when he agrees the child is disturbed, he offers treatment. Sometimes he must deal with the parental conflict over treatment, if one or the other parent has arranged it against the opposition of the other. Although these "management" aspects of the case are not usually considered theoretically to be central to the treatment, they are obviously crucial issues. Under the rubric of "management," there exists a range of effective techniques for making an impact upon the family system.

The Effects of Focusing on the Child

One major effect on the family occurs when the child therapist simply agrees with the parents that the child is the problem; this major intervention into the family joins the parents against their problem child. Since the theory of child psychopathology suggests that the child is reacting to his past and to his introjects, the therapist's approach to the parents can be one that frees them from the blame for the child's current problems. Granted that the child therapist is often accused of condemning parents because he identifies with the child, he is still sufficiently guided by his theory to think of the current parental influence as less relevant than the "real" internalized problem of the child.

Some family therapists would argue that focusing on the child as the problem and, therefore, siding with the parents against the child would be disastrous for a good treatment outcome; they believe it is always unwise to join any family members against the others. In fact, family therapists argue that focusing upon the child in this way freezes the child in the pathological system so that change is not possible. However, experienced family therapists also recognize that family therapy is an orientation to a problem and not a method of treatment so that different approaches sometimes have different advantages.

Spontaneous Change

One advantage of the child therapist's approach to families is the "spontaneous" change that can happen. Although parents offer up a child as the problem and claim that all is well with the family, they know on another level that this is not so. In those cases in which the therapist agrees that the child is the problem, the parents must redress the balance by accepting some blame themselves. As an example, a child will not eat all his food but hides it in various places in the house. The child therapist who operates to the basis of his theory circumvents parental resistance, as he assumes that this problem is related to the child's interiorized oral aggression and anal retention. He will imply to the parents that the problem is entirely within the child. However, the parents know that at the dinner table the father insists that the child eat everything on his plate and the mother insists he does not have to. To deal with this conflict, the child hides his food. Since the parents know they are participating in this situation, they must accept part of the blame themselves because the child therapist offers them none. Sensing from him an exonerating stance, they are indirectly freed to privately work on the confict when they might not have done so if the therapist had taken an interest in it.

The parents can leave a first session with a child therapist reassured that the problem resides more within the child than in their parenting, and they can feel relieved that they have taken action to resolve their difficult problem. In some cases the child will immediately improve; it can be argued that this response occurs because so much has happened within the family just by the action of reaching agreement, seeking treatment, and being reassured that they have not been causing the child's problems. Also, one should not underestimate the ability of the child to affect the other members of the family. The child can be a pivotal force for change when he senses his referral to a doctor as parental rejection. Upon feeling himself expelled, he can recoil into attempts to regain his parents' affection. His efforts may be interpreted by the parents as the therapist's success. They bring therapy to an end, and the child is rewarded by reintegration with his family.

The amount of time and effort the family puts into organizing themselves to get the child to the therapy sessions at regular intervals is in itself of importance. Not only is this a concerted activity requiring more efficient family organization, but often parents and child are thrown together for an extended period during the trip. Some parents report this is the only time during the week when they are engaged in a common activity with the child. The parents also experience themselves as being helpful and doing something for their child after living through long periods of feeling hopeless and powerless to help him.

Confidential Interviews with an Outsider

The family also faces the fact that the child is now going to an outsider, an expert, and revealing things about the family. Because of the confidentiality of the sessions, they cannot know what the child is reporting nor can they rebut what he might be saying. This concern about the child "revealing the family" can lead to more concerted effort by the parents to change the family so that what is reported will be more complimentary. Some families report that their most determined efforts to modify their behavior toward the child (becoming more lenient, or firmer, or more respectful) come from a mutual concern over what the child is saying about them.

Another aspect of the structure of the situation is the healthy competition that emerges between the parents and the expert. Parents can feel compelled to recover their child when they suspect that the child is getting more fond of an outsider than of them. Often the child was never previously permitted a relationship with an outsider, and now he has a base outside the family for changing his position within the family. Part of the merit of this outside base is the opportunity he has to help expert and parents compete for his affection. An interesting process can develop in which the therapist becomes a "friendly contender" who lets the parents emerge the winners. (Supervisory sessions often include the problems of dealing with the jealous parent, and poor outcome can occur if the therapist becomes too jealous of the parents.)

At the same time that they are competing for affection, the parents find that the child's therapy also forces them in the opposite direction. As the child in his therapy sessions is given freedom to say and do anything he pleases, he finds that his therapist will try to put up with just about any kind of behavior. (Not only are many child therapists permissive, but to help the child express his fantasies they allow a wide range of undisciplined behavior.) Naturally, the child begins to behave in the same way at home thinking that his parents must approve or they would not have put him into that situation. Yet, even though a child therapist can be permissive with almost any kind of behavior for an hour in the office, no one living with the child twenty-four hours a day can tolerate such impulsive and undisciplined behavior. Therefore, the parents are driven to discipline the child in order to live with him. In many cases they have never effectively disciplined him before, so the child finds a more secure home life. Often, too, the parents could never agree with each other about discipline, and each attempt led to a quarrel. Now they must agree to survive when the child is behaving in such an extreme way. A fundamental rule becomes apparent in the situation—the more permissive the child therapist in the office, the more he provokes the parents to provide discipline at home. Consequently the child undergoes therapeutic change.

Related to questions of discipline and security is the change in the parental relationship with the child when he has been given over to an expert. Since the child has professional support, the parents feel more free to make mistakes and, therefore, more free to make decisions, because the therapist will make it up to the child and work it through with him. For example, parents may become free to expect the child to go to bed at the proper time, instead of having the usual evening battle, because they feel the treatment must be helping him to be more normal. As they expect proper behavior from him, the child delivers it, with consequent changes throughout the family. In this instance, the parents usually find that if they are not quarreling with the child at bedtime, they are quarreling with each other. Now they must resolve their conflicts, because the child won't rescue them as he has done in the past by making trouble in the evening.

Therapist as Extended Kin

Other structural changes occur in the family merely by the act of placing the child in therapy. If the treatment goes on long enough, the child therapist takes his place in the kinship structure by becoming a paid member of the extended family. He becomes built in as a helpful uncle or grandparental figure who emphasizes marital harmony and can, in time, offer advice to everyone in the family and not merely focus upon the child. Even at the start of treatment, the extended family structure is affected. When the parents take the child to an expert, they free themselves from the need to quarrel with their own parents about the child. The mother can say to her mother, "He's in treatment now, so I would rather not discuss his problems with you." Since the child's symptoms reflect not only the parental conflict but the conflict with extended kin as well, the introduction of the outside expert forces a change throughout the total family system. Once the child is shifted outside the focus of family conflict, he is free to change and respond more normally. The exclusion of the in-laws also fosters the cementing of the marital relationship and helps draw a boundary around the nuclear family.

When a child therapist interviews a child, he is inevitably intervening in the marriage of the parents. As one example, he replaces father as the person mother talks to about the child's problem. The complaints that used to go to the father are now directed toward the therapist; the father is displaced from the position of listening to a constantly complaining and harassing wife. With this structural shift, some of the bitterness of the relationship lessens and the spouses reach out to one another. Ultimately, the spouses can form a tighter coalition that puts pressure on the therapist for more success with their child.

As treatment continues, the influence of the child therapist upon the parents often becomes more direct, even though his contact with them is brief. One must emphasize the skill that is necessary to deal effectively with the parents while having only short contacts with them. When the mother delivers and retrieves her child, she must be influenced quickly, as must the father when he discusses the bill and joins his wife in receiving a report on the child's progress. Using what he has learned about the family from the child, the therapist has a series of brief encounters with the parents that have a cumulative effect over time. Full credit must be given to child therapists for their ability to do brief therapy and exert influence upon both the parent, child, and the marital relationship so that the child can change.

A child therapy orientation may prevent one of the most recent and common errors of family therapy—that of overfocusing on the couple and losing the child in the process. Buttressed by the popular theory that if the marital struggle is resolved, the child's symptomatic functions will disappear, some family therapists work unilaterally with the couple, failing to deal with the child as a necessary, integral part of the problem and its resolution. If they lose the child's contributions as regulator of the speed of therapy, as moderator of the pace of change (through his "when and how" of symptom increase or decrease), the child fails to change.

The Therapist's Influence on Parents

At first the child therapist may be influenced by his theory to treat the parents as only the ghosts of past introjects, but later he begins to deal with them as human beings, particularly as he becomes more fond of the child. If the therapist finds that his individual therapy sessions with the child are not effecting behavioral change, he usually feels an empathy and compassion for the parents' similar plight and thus develops a more positive relationship with them. The parents become more relaxed and flexible, and the child can have an atmosphere in which change is more possible.

As he begins to deal with the parents more directly, the therapist finds also that they ask more of him if the child is not changing. Feeling he must offer them something, he gives increasing amounts of advice about how to deal with the child. Sometimes the parents are willing to follow his advice at this stage, partly because the therapist is more friendly but also because they feel pride in their competence at having forced the advice from him. The advice is also more valuable than it would have been if freely offered.

The child therapist deals more directly with the parents when the child has begun to undergo change. The therapist becomes invested in protecting the changes he sees himself as having created. To do this, he is subtly but surely compelled to move into the larger system. This move can dovetail with the changes the child is producing in the system, sustaining and reinforcing them.

The Function of "Play"

Granting the child therapist's skillful use of brief therapy with the parents, his influence on the family does not confine itself to direct contact with the parents. He not only uses the child to gain information about the family, but he effectively uses the child to bring about change in the family. In this sense, child therapy is similar to the approach taken by some family therapists who select a key member and interview him individually, using him as a lever to bring about family change. However, child therapy has developed a unique method of influencing a family with its use of "play" with the child. It is significant that the vehicle used to enter the complicated organization of family life is the child, the most innocent and directly perceptive member.

The private playroom of the child therapist and the child is like a safety zone for both of them, although the content of the play may appear to be about unmastered experiences and the resolution of internalized conflicts. To the extent that play and fantasy mirror the actions of the family, the child learns to deal with harmful family interventions by coping with them in miniature; the therapist, who may have been appalled by the destructiveness evident in the family, becomes more inured to these patterns in play form. The child and his play become the child therapist's way of entering a family on a familiar path, with the play therapy like a decompression chamber that permits the therapist to approach the family later without too much risk and uncertainty.

Play is one of the most important factors in human life, but in child therapy, "play" is a peculiar and deviant form. By definition, play is something that occurs between voluntary participants and has no purpose except the pleasure of the action. This generally accepted definition of play is clearly not applicable to "play therapy." When play is used as a therapeutic tool, it is given a purpose and so by definition becomes something other than play. There is also a question as to how voluntary the play is in therapy; the child is sometimes brought to it unwillingly, and the child therapist is paid money to participate. Clearly it is not a spontaneous occurrence but an arrangement made with an ulterior motive—to induce change in one (or both) of the participants. Another aspect of it is also unusual; although adults sometimes play with children, it is rare to find two people playing with dolls when one of them is old enough to have a moustache.

Seen in this way, play therapy is less play in form and more of a special communication that has different rules from ordinary life. Like other forms of therapy in which patient and therapist can play with ideas and words that would not be proper in other settings, child and child therapist can play with objects in ways that would not be appropriate outside the room. For example, if the child picks up a toy truck and throws it, an adult will ordinarily protest. The adult child therapist might pick up the truck and throw it himself, or if less active, he might at least make a permissive comment or interpretation. The usual rules of adult-child interchange are suspended or treated as a fiction in this setting.

With this kind of freedom established, there is also a suspension of the usual rules for directing someone to behave differently. The unstated task of the child therapist in the play room is to ease the child into behaving differently with adults and particularly with his parents and siblings. This persuasion is not accomplished by explicit directives to behave differently, any more than it is in most methods of therapy, but by indirection, which is more difficult to resist. As the child goes through searching behavior to define his relationship with the therapist and to find out how he is to behave, the toys in the play room become devices for trial-and-error experimentation. They not only become expressions of real family issues that can be resolved (as theory has it) in symbolic form, but more importantly, they can become a vehicle for the therapist's instructions as to how to deal with these family issues in reality. The way the child therapist responds to the child's handling of the family dolls, for example, can be an indirect instruction as to how he is to deal with adults and with the real family at home. In effect, they are remote, indirect communications to the adults as to how to deal differently with the child.

The most typical children's problems involve a contract between parent and disturbed child that the parents will demand certain behavior from the child, which he will not deliver. The child may not talk, or he may not control his bowels and bladder, or he may not learn in school, and the parents put pressure upon him to do these things. Child therapy, with its format of a nonpressured atmosphere, an emphasis on play, a loosening of rules, and so on, not only offers the child a different adult response, and so a new contract, but also a directive for how to deal differently with the parents. For example, a young child is brought to a therapist because he is restless and "doesn't talk yet." At home the parents are locked in a struggle with the child to persuade him to talk. The therapist agrees with the parents that he will deal with the child's mutism, but actually he deals with it by offering other modalities of expression, such as drawing, plastics, and toys. With no pressure on him to talk, the child begins to speak in the play room. The therapist also draws the parents' attention to these alternative ways of dealing with the child, and so the conflict over talking is reduced. When the withdrawn child is offered the opportunity to express himself with toys, he can be less withdrawn in a new modality and proceed to behave more aggressively, first with toys and later at home. As he knocks over the mother doll and survives it in the playroom, the therapist encourages this aggression against the doll. Implicitly he is encouraging more aggression with mother. When the child is then more outspoken with mother and does not deal with her by withdrawing, mother is forced to deal with him differently, and so a different pattern is set up in the family. Yet the therapist has never asked the child directly to assert himself more with mother, he has "merely" directed his play with a mother doll. He has never asked the mother to deal differently with the child either. With older children the therapist will use other devices, such as saying to the child, "Your bad side wants to fight with your parents all the time, but your healthy side wants to be happier." Dividing up the child this way, or joining the healthy part of the ego, is a way of directing the child to behave differently without making a "request" that can be refused.

In those cases in which the child is obviously responding negatively to parental pressures, the child therapist must help the parents deal with him differently. For example, the therapist might ask the parents to be less intrusive and not pump the child but, instead, to let him have some secrets. This is easy to do within his theoretical conviction about the need for confidentiality between himself and his child patient. However, the therapist does not merely make these requests to the parents, he also uses various arts of persuasion. One of his procedures is to explore briefly with the parents their own childhood, with a compassionate view of how it has influenced their behavior with their child in ways beyond their control. Finding themselves being forgiven for their current behavior, the parents are more willing to change it. If the child "regresses" because the loose and permissive setting of child therapy facilitates moments of controlled "regression," the parents become more dependent upon the therapist. This is reinforced by handling the child's regression as a phasic event, if possible even as proof of progress, reassuring the parents in their moments of increased stress. The disappointment of the parents, which initially made them seek treatment, is deepened and so is their need for the therapist's guidance and support. As they lean upon him more, he becomes more relevant to their family system and is more able to influence it.

One should also not overlook the importance of the play therapy setting for the therapist. In the standard therapeutic setting for adults there can be an illusion that people are rational or irrational (although dream interpretation helps overcome this myth), but the child therapist is under no such constraint and can use nonverbal communication, fantasy, etc. when dealing with his child patient. Unlike the modern family, with its emphasis on cognitive solutions to problems, or reasoning with the child, he is free to use means other than intellectual to contact the child. These nonverbal techniques also make him better able than the parents to monitor the child's pace of interpersonal development.

Because "play" is theoretically unacknowledged as a means of communication from the therapist through the child to the parents, and from the parents through the child to the therapist, child therapy respects and utilizes the family's defensive arrangement by its very definition of method. Pretending that the parents are not (through play) being given instructions and circumstances for behaving differently, child therapy avoids many current trends. It avoids frontality, explicitness, "getting to know where you are at," and any confrontative "reasoning out" of the problems. These trends are stressed as important to change in many therapies. But by using "play" and by claiming no direct influence on the parents, child therapy provides a "double masking screen" through which the proper freedom for indirect communications, so essential to outcome, is preserved.

A "modern" error of many family therapists is treating family members as if they are only behavioral contributions in unfolding interpersonal sequences. The possibility of family members feeling a measure of responsibility for their own behavior can be reduced in this format. In play therapy, the framework by itself allows family members to feel always that they are discrete and separate individuals, despite the fact that their behavior can be at the service of obscure forces, like larger multi-generational sequences or "childhood events." Because the framework of child therapy serves ostensibly to enable the child to come to terms with himself as a separate being, most processes through which the significant work occurs can only become incidental or implicit. Since the incidentals entail most communicational relays between parent, child, and therapist, a convenient situation of unguardedness develops; that is, all participants can keep out of the field of conscious preoccupation any rational checking of each other's intentions, while these are modified. The rethreading of parents and child into a different system proceeds then precisely by deemphasizing that they are a system at all.

One should note in passing that one of the dangers of individual play with the child is the possibility that the therapist will become too attached to the child and so threaten to detach him from his parents. As part of the wisdom of the child guidance movement, this effect was balanced by having a social worker deal with parents. Along with many other functions, the social worker could interpret the therapist's ideas and behavior to the parents and serve as a mediator while also influencing the parents to change.

When family therapy fails to change the child, the child therapist who works alone becomes increasingly involved with the parents and requests certain kinds of changes in the parent-child relationship. If this does not produce results, the therapist raises the question of whether the marital relationship should be investigated and treated. This threat often is sufficient to force the parents to deal with each other differently to avoid going into their marital problems further, and consequently the child changes. The more the therapist is thwarted in his attempts to help the child change, the more he begins to inquire incisively into the nuances of the conflict between the spouses. The parents quickly shield themselves by changing their parenting, thus benefiting the child. The child himself can also initiate a fast bootstrap operation to modify his behavior sufficiently so that the parents have an excuse to withdraw him from treatment; thus the child helps protect his parents, with their marital difficulties, by improving instead of by having symptoms as he did previously. This kind of intervention is sometimes done by family therapists, who see the child's problem as largely a product of family conflict, but usually they help the parents work through the conflicts because they are seeking perduring changes in the child and not temporary ones. Obviously, change in the child can only persist if his family has changed.

The Contribution of the Child

Up to this point there has been an emphasis upon the parents' influence upon the child and the therapist's influence upon the family. The important influence of the child upon both parents and therapist should also be dealt with explicitly. An example can partially summarize the child's contribution. In a family with conflict between the parents over who was superior to the other, their child was caught between them as a vehicle for this conflict. The mother insisted that the child be outstanding in school as part of her attempt to set the child up as a competitor to her husband, whom she considered weak and unsatisfactory. The father responded to the child's achievement by indicating that the child was siding with the mother against him and humiliating him. The child responded to this situation by manifesting an acute fear of homework, thereby being unable to achieve in school for reasons outside of his control. When he entered child therapy and began to relate in a positive way to the therapist, his problem was increased. To please the therapist, he must lose the fear of homework in the context of play with this safe and significant person. As happens in many such cases, the child improves, but the family has not significantly changed. The child then either relapses or offers different symptoms, such as other fears, headaches, etc. Often the therapist sees the "regression" of the child as part of the transference aspect of treatment. However, in terms of his actions, the therapist shifts his strategy with the child and also becomes more involved in "management" interviews with the parents, partly to persuade them to deal effectively with the child—"We mustn't rush him so much"—and partly to gather more information about the home setting in order to understand the child's difficulties. In the process of canvasing the field for more information, the therapist can seldom fail to insinuate a paradoxical situation as well. He can talk about the regression in such a way that its implications for signaling therapeutic gains cannot be ignored. Almost everything the child does and alarms the parents can turn out to imply the possibility of immediate or impending progress in an unfolding process. This keeps child and parents firmly bound to the situation. Either the therapist's "brief management" interventions then steer the parents in a radically different direction, or the regression so intensifies that it pulls the parents into behaving differently with the child, or eventually the child's maturation ushers in a new developmental stage changing the regressive behavior.

From the point of view we are describing here, "regression" can be seen as a progression of the child to a more effective way of communicating with the therapist. He is responding to the therapist's lack of understanding by trying other means to influence the therapist to modify his situation, particularly the parental behavior. Symptomatic behavior, and play, are the child's way of indirectly instructing the therapist to shift his strategy of therapy. If the therapist does not understand, the child will communicate by more severe symptoms, as if using a megaphone, until his influence is successful in activating the therapist and the parents to behave differently. His severe symptoms encourage the parents to seek counsel with the therapist and encourage the therapist to enquire further into what is happening at home. When the sensitive therapist picks up the child's cues and modifies his approach to child and parents, the conflicts in the family become resolved and the child is free to give up this form of communication. At this point, neither symptomatic behavior, which the child has learned to use in his family, nor the "play" therapy, which the child has learned from the therapist as a way of communicating, is necessary.

In terms of the relationship between therapist and child, a mutually regulatory pattern becomes established. When the therapist is flexible enough to heed the child's message, he demonstrates his respect for the child's autonomy. He communicates to the child, "Your communications have power." A level of respectful reciprocity within the interdependent relationship is attained, and autonomy is now feasible for both. The autonomy of the therapist, as well as of the child, is in this sense an eventual product of an underlying collaborative dimension. This dimension is achieved by child and therapist testing each other for impact of communications, without perceiving themselves in a complex relay system of more than two persons. Evidence that communicational cues beyond the two of them are being effectively relayed and received may show only in nonverbal indicators or collaboration. There is room for behavior shifts on the part of both— the therapist to modify his strategies, the child to change his deviant behavior, neither feeling necessarily conscious of dealing with more than one person.

The Family Orientation

It was once thought that enduring change in the child could occur only if, in addition to child therapy, both parents were in individual therapy. Sometimes it was assumed that treatment could be coordinated by collaboration among the several therapists of the different family members. Such collaboration usually failed, and typically the individual treatment did not resolve the marital struggle in which the child was entangled. From the view offered here, it would seem that treatment can be more effective and efficient if the person treating the child also "manages" the parents so that change in the different parts of the family system at different stages are coordinated by a single person.

Many child therapists continue with the procedure of alternate interviews with child and parents, and this way of approaching families has many merits. In some cases parents can react with resentment and resistance if they are directly confronted with family conflicts the child is expressing. Advice offered by someone who is clearly not blaming them because he feels the child has a problem inside of himself can often lead the parents to accept directives and respond in new ways with less resistance. In this sense it is the very fact that the child therapist acts naive about family dynamics that sometimes makes his influence upon the family effective.

Why Child Therapy Fails

What has been emphasized here are those aspects of child therapy that have merit if viewed from a family orientation. Yet, if one grants these merits, one must address the question of why child therapy and child analysis do not usually succeed in bringing about therapeutic change. It can be argued that the naivete about the context of the child helps the child therapist correct errors of family therapists who are overfocused upon the marriage and neglect the child's contribution to the problem and to the therapy. Yet being naive also causes change to come about inadvertently instead of predictably, and, therefore, treatment failure is as likely as treatment success.

There are two main handicaps for the child therapist, both of them related to the theory he is taught. The first handicap is, of course, the idea that the problem is within the child. Although this theory helps the child therapist be less blaming of the parents, it is also likely to cause him to neglect the parents after the fee is set. If his theory persuades him that he is trying to change something within the child, he will not communicate to the parents through the child but will merely pass the time playing with the child, and no change will take place.

The second handicap is based upon the child therapist's lack of understanding of the ways the child is responding to his interpersonal context. If the therapist takes the child's communicative behavior only as a report about his inner nature rather than a report about his social situation, the therapist will not direct his efforts toward deliberately influencing the social situation so that the child can change. While it is true that by not forcing the family to deal with the parental conflict, he may avoid the consequent bad feelings among the family members, he will be like the behavioral modifier who brings parents together around a new conditioning program without ever realizing that previously the parents were in conflict about how to deal with the child. Yet, by not knowing that the child is responding to a conflictual family structure, the child therapist will not be able to indirectly influence that structure in any systematic way. If he does have an influence, it will be a chance occurrence, and so therapeutic change will occur by chance.

When a social worker is dealing with the parents while the child therapist treats the child, there is a chance of an influence on the family through the social worker's endeavors. However, there is also a chance that social worker and child therapist will be in covert conflict with each other about the family, taking sides in family struggles, and will merely replicate the conflictual situation that has produced a disturbed child.

Summary

Despite the many theoretically based factors that can cause treatment to fail, one should not overlook the fact that the child therapist approaches symptoms within the newer theoretical model developing in the field. Previously, it was assumed that a patient's symptoms should not be dealt with directly because they are supposed to have "roots." Child therapy offers an alternative view: focus on the child, or symptom, acknowledge the roots of pathology in the family, but do not deal with the roots directly. In the last few years this approach has been considered innovative in the treatment of symptomatic adult behavior, such as phobias or compulsions. Such symptom-oriented therapies as behavioral conditioning, the paradoxical intention approach (1), Milton H. Erickson's methods (2), or Stampful's procedure (3), all assume that the symptom should be dealt with directly. Some of these approaches emphasize not only focusing upon the symptom, but even encouraging it as a way of bringing about change.

Clearly child therapy has anticipated these innovations and is in the avant garde of the field. When the child therapist accepts and encourages the family's presentation of the child as the problem, he is accepting the scapegoat function of the child without arousing resistance in the family. This approach leaves him free to convey effective suggestions in his brief contacts with the parents. Whether he conveys those suggestions to bring about change in the family and consequent change in the child is partly determined by chance since in the nature of child therapy theory it must be unplanned.

References

Aarons, A. Z. (1970). Normality and abnormality in adolescence. *Psychoanalytic Study of the Child*, Vol. 25. New York: International Universities Press.

Ackerman, N. W. (1962). Direct observation.

Ackerman, N. W. (1965). Films available from The Family Institute, New York, N.Y.

Ackerman, N. W. (1961). Emergence of family psychotherapy on the present scene. *Contemporary Psychotherapies*, ed. H. Stein. New York: Free Press.

Ackerman, N. W. (1965). The "depth" question in family psychotherapy. Presented at the annual meeting of the American Orthopsychiatric Association.

Ackerman, N. W. (1966). *Treating the Troubled Family in New York.* New York: Basic Books.

Ackerman, N. W. (1970a). *Family Process.* New York: Basic Books.

Ackerman, N. W. (1970b). *Family Therapy in Transition.* Boston: Little, Brown.

Ackerman, N. W., and Behrens, M. (1956). A study of family diagnosis. *American Journal of Orthopsychiatry* 26:66-78.

Adolescents Grow in Groups (1972), ed. I. Berkovitz. New York: Brunner/Mazel.

Advanced Techniques of Hypnosis and Therapy: Selected Papers of Milton H. Erickson (1967), ed. J. Haley. New York: Grune & Stratton.

Ajuriaguerra, J. de (1971). *Manuel de psychiatrie de l'enfant*. Paris: Masson & Cie.

Albee, G. (1966). The dark at the top of the agenda. *Clinical Psychology* 30:7-9.

Aleksandrowicz, Dov R. (1962). The meaning of metaphor. *Bulletin of the Menninger Clinic* 26:92-101.

Alexander, F. (1963). The dynamics of therapy in the light of learning theory. *American Journal of Psychiatry* 120:440-448.

Alger, I. (1969). Therapeutic use of videotape playback. *Journal of Nervous and Mental Diseases* 148:430-436.

Alger, I. (1972). Television image confrontation in group therapy. *Prognosis in Group and Family Therapy*, ed. C. Sager and H. Kaplan. New York: Brunner/Mazel.

Alger, I. (1974). Audio-visual techniques in family therapy. *Techniques of Family Psychotherapy*, ed. D. Block. New York: Grune & Stratton.

Alger, I., and Hogan, P. (1967). The use of videotape recording in conjoint marital therapy. *American Journal of Psychiatry* 123: 1425-30.

Alger, I., and Hogan, P. (1968). Enduring effects of videotape playback experience on family and marital relationships. Paper read at the annual meeting of the American Orthopsychiatric Association.

Allen, F. H. (1942). *Psychotherapy with Children*. New York: Norton.

Alpern, E. (1956). Short clinical services for children in a child guidance clinic. *American Journal of Orthopsychiatry* 26:314-325.

Aman, M. G. (1972). The effects of methylphenidate and dextroamphetamine on learning and retention. Unpublished master's thesis, University of Illinois.

Anderson, D. (1971). Public institutions: Their war against black youth. *American Journal of Orthopsychiatry* 41:65.

Anderson, R. (1972). The importance of an actively involved therapist. *Adolescents Grow in Groups*, ed. I. Berkovitz, pp. 31-36. New York: Brunner/Mazel.

Anderson, W. M., and Dawson, J. (1965). The variability of plasma 17-hydroxycorticosteroid-levels in affective illness and schizophrenia. *Psychosomatic Research* 9:237-248.

Angrist, B., Sathananthan, G., and Gershon, S. (1973). Behavioral effects of L-dopa in schizophrenic patients. *Psychopharmacologia* 31:1-12.

Annell, A. L. (1955). Insulin shock treatment in children with psychotic disturbances. *Acta Psychotherapeutica Psychoanalytica Orthopoedica* 3:193-205.

Annell, A. L. (1969a). Manic-depressive illness in children and effect of treatment with lithium carbonate. *Acta Paedopsychiatrica* 36:292-361.

Annell, A. L. (1969b). Lithium in the treatment of children and adolescents. *Acta Psychiatrica Scandinavica* 207 (Supp):19-30.

Anonymous (M. Bowen) (1972). Toward the differentiation of a self in one's own family. *Family Interaction = A Dialogue Between Family Researchers and Family Therapists*, ed. J. Framo. New York: Springer.

Anthony, E. J. (1964). Communicating therapeutically with the child. *Journal of the American Academy of Child Psychiatry* 3:106-125.

Anthony, E. J. (1971). The making of a discipline: Introduction to the American edition. *Modern Perspectives in Child Psychiatry*, ed. G. Howells. New York: Brunner/Mazel.

Anthony, E. J., and Koupernik, C. (eds.) (1970). *The Child in His Family*. New York: Wiley-Interscience.

Anthony, E. J., and Koupernik, C. (eds.) (1973). *The Child in His Family: The Impact of Disease and Death*. New York: Wiley-Interscience.

Anthony, E. J., and Koupernik, C. (eds.) (1974). *The Child in His Family: Child at Psychiatric Risk*. New York: Wiley-Interscience.

Anton-Tay, F., and Wurtman, R. J. (1971). Brain monoamines and endocrine function. *Frontiers in neuroendocrinology*, ed. L. Martini and W. F. Ganong. London: Oxford Univ. Press.

Appelberg, E. (1965). The cottage meeting as a therapeutic tool. *Group Work as Part of Residential Treatment*, ed. H. W. Maier. New York: Association of Social Workers.

Arbit, J., Boshes, B., and Blonsky, R. (1970). Behavior and mentation changes during therapy. *L-dopa and Parkinsonism*, ed. A. Barbeau and F. H. McDowell.

Ardry, R. (1966). *The Territorial Imperative*. New York: Atheneum.

Arlow, J. A. (1961). Silence and the theory of technique. *Journal of the American Psychoanalytic Association* 9:44-55.

Arnold, L. E., Kirilcuk, V., Corson, S. A., and Corson, E. O'l (1973). Levoamphetamine and dextroamphetamine: Differential effect on aggression and hyperkinesis in children and dogs. *American Journal of Psychiatry* 130:165-170.

Arnold, L. E., and Wender, P. H. (1974). Levoamphetamine's changing place in the treatment of children with behavior disorders. *Excerpta Medica.* Supplement 1974: 179-191.

Arnold, L. E., Wender, P. H., McCloskey, K., and Snyder, S. H. (1972). Levoamphetamine and dextroamphetamine: Comparative efficacy in the hyperkinetic syndrome. *Archives of General Psychiatry* 27:816-822.

Arthur, A. Z. (1967). Behavior therapy versus psychotherapy and applied science. *Canadian Psychology* 8a:105-113.

Auerswald, E. (1968). Interdisciplinary vs. ecological approach. *Family Process* 7:202-215.

Axline, V. M. (1947). *Play Therapy*. New York: Ballantine Books 1969.

Ayllon, T., and Azrin, N. (1968). *The Token Economy*. New York: Appleton.

Azrin, N., and Holz, W. (1966). Punishment. *Operant Behavior: Areas of Research and Application*, ed. W. Honig. New York: Appleton.

Bach, G. R. (1966). The marathon group: Intensive practice of intimate interaction. *Psychological Reports* 18:995-1005.

Baer, D. M., and Sherman, J. (1964). Reinforcement control of generalized imitation in young children. *Journal of Experimental Child Psychology* 1:37-49.

Baer, D. M., Wolf, M. M., and Risley, T. R (1968). Some current dimensions of applied behavior analysis. *Journal of Applied Behavior Analysis* 1:91-97.

Bailey, J., Phillips, E., and Wolf, M. (1970). Homebased reinforcement and the modification of predelinquents' classroom behavior. Proceedings of the 78th annual convention of the American Psychological Association 5:751-752 (Summary).

Baker, L., and Barcai, A. (1970). Psychosomatic aspects of diabetes mellitus. *Modern Trends in Psychosomatic Medicine*, ed. C. W. Hill. Vol. 2. New York: Appleton.

Balazs, R., Kovacs, S., Cocks, W. A., Johnson, A. L., and Eayrs, J. T. (1971). Effect of thyroid hormone on the biochemical maturation of rat brain: Postnatal cell formation. *Brain Research* 25:555-570.

Balter, M. B., and Levine, J. (1969). The nature and extent of psychotropic drug usage in the United States. *Psychopharmacological Bulletin* 5: 3-13.

Ban, T. A. (1971). Nicotinic acid in psychiatry. *Canadian Psychiatric Association Journal* 16:413-431.

Ban, T. A., and Lehmann, H. E. (1970). Nicotinic acid in the treatment of schizophrenias. *Progress Report I*. Toronto: Canadian Mental Health Association.

Bandura, A. (1969). *Principles of Behavior Modification*. New York: Holt.

Bandura, A., and Walters, R. H. (1963). *Social Learning and Personality Development*. New York: Holt.

Barnett, H. et al. (1949). Renal clearances of sodium penicillin G, procaine penicillin G and insulin in infants and children. *Pediatrics* 3:418.

Barrett-Lennard, G. T. (1965). Professional psychology and the control of human behaviour. *Australian Journal of Psychology* 17:24-34.

Barten, H. (ed.) (1971). *Brief Therapies*. New York: Behavioral Publications.

Barten, H., and Barten, S. (eds.) (1972). *Children and Their Parents in Brief Therapy*. New York: Behavioral Publications.

Bateson, G. (1970/71). A systems approach. *International Journal of Psychiatry* 9:242-244.

Bateson, G. et al. (1971) *The Natural History of an Interview*, ed. N. McQuown. New York: Grune & Stratton. Published only on microfilm.

Bateson, G., Jackson, D., Haley, J., and Weakland, J. (1956). Towards a theory of schizophrenia. *Behavioral Science* 1:251-264.

Bazell, R. J. (1971). Panel sanctions amphetamines for hyperkinetic children. *Science* 171:1223.

Beels, C., and Ferber, A. (1973). What family therapists do. *The Book of Family Therapy*. ed. A. Ferber, M. Mendelsohn and A. Napier. New York: Aronson.

Beiser, H. R. (1955). Play equipment for diagnosis and therapy. *American Journal of Orthopsychiatry* 25:761-770.

Bell, J. 1970 Personal communication.

Bell, J. (1961). Family Group Therapy. Public Health Monograph No. 64. U.S. Dept. of Health, Education and Welfare.

Bell, J. (1963). Promoting action through new insights: Some theoretical revisions from family group therapy. Paper read at the meeting of the American Psychological Association.

Bellak, L., and Small, L. (1965). *Emergency Psychotherapy and Brief Psychotherapy*. New York: Grune & Stratton.

Bender, L. (1947). One hundred cases of childhood schizophrenia treated with electric shock. *Transactions of the American Neurological Association* 72:165-169.

Bender, L., Cobrinik, L., Faretra, G., and Sankar, D. V. S. (1966). The treatment of childhood schizophrenia with LSD and UML. *Biological Treatment of Mental Illness*, ed. M. Rinkel. New York: Page.

Bender, L., and Cottington, F. (1942). The use of amphetamine sulfate (Benzedrine) in child psychiatry. *American Journal of Psychiatry* 99:116-121.

Bender, L., Faretra, G., and Cobrinik, L. (1963). LSD and UML treatment of hospitalized disturbed children. *Recent Advances in Biological Psychiatry*, ed. J. Wortis. New York: Plenum Press.

Bender, L., Goldschmidt, L., and Sankar, D. V. S. (1962). Treatment of autistic schizophrenic children with LSD-25 and UML-491. *Recent Advances in Biological Psychiatry*, ed. J. Wortis. New York: Plenum Press.

Bender, L., and Keeler, W. R. (1952). The body image of schizophrenic children following electroshock therapy. *American Journal of Orthopsychiatry* 22:335-355.

Bender, L., and Nichtern, S. (1956). Chemotherapy in child psychiatry. *New York State Journal of Medicine* 56:2791-2796.

Bergin, A. E. (1966). Some implications of psychotherapy research for therapeutic practice. *Journal of Abnormal Psychology* 71:235-246.

Bergin, A. E. (1971). The evaluation of therapeutic outcomes. *Handbook of Psychotherapy and Behavior Change*, ed. A. Bergin and S. Garfield, pp. 217-270. New York: Wiley-Interscience.

Berkowitz, B. T., and Graziano, A. M. (1972). Training parents as behavior therapists: A review. *Behaviour Research Therapy* 10:297-317.

Berlin, I. N. (1970). Crisis intervention and short term therapy: An approach in a child psychiatric clinic. *Journal of the American Academy of Child Psychiatry* 9:595-606.

Bermann, E. (1973). *Scapegoat: The Impact of Death-Fear on an American Family*. Ann Arbor: Univ. of Michigan Press.

Beruheim, H. (1888). De la suggestion. Paris: Doin.

Bettelheim, B., and Sylvester, E. (1948). A therapeutic milieu. *American Journal of Orthopsychiatry* 18:191-206.

Bijou, S., and Baer, D. (1961). *Child Development I: A Systematic and Empirical Theory*. New York: Appleton.

Bijou, S. W., and Baer, D. M. (1967). *Child Development: Readings in Experimental Analysis*. New York: Appleton.

Blank, M. (1947). Cognitive functions of language in the preschool years. *Developmental Psychology* 10:229-245.

Bloch, D. (ed.) (1973). *Techniques of Family Psychotherapy: A Primer*. New York: Grune & Stratton.

Blom, G. E. (1967a). The community confronts psychoanalysis. Unpublished paper.

Blom, G. E. (1967b). Psychoeducational treatment of emotionally disturbed children. Unpublished paper.

Blom, G. E., Ekanger, C. A., Parsons, P. C., Prodoehl, M., and Rudnick, M. (1972). A psychoeducational approach to day care treatment. *Journal of the American Academy of Child Psychiatry* 11:492-510.

Blos, P. Jr. (1962). On Adolescence. New York: Free Press.

Blos, P. Jr. (1967). The second individuation process of adolescence. *Psychoanalytic Study of the Child* 22:162-186. New York: International Universities Press.

Blos, P. Jr. (1972). Silence: A clinical exploration. *Psychoanalytic Quarterly* 41:348-362.

Bodin, A. (1972). The use of videotapes, ed. A. Ferber, M. Mendelsohn, and A. Napier, Chapter 9, pp. 318-337. *The Book of Family Therapy*. New York: Aronson.

Bodin, A., and Ferber, A. (1972). How to go beyond the use of language, ed. A. Ferber, M. Mendelsohn, and A. Napier, Chapter 8, pp. 272-317. *The Book of Family Therapy*. New York: Aronson.

Bornstein, B. (1951). On latency. *Psychoanalytic Study of the Child* 6:279-285. New York: International Universities Press.

Boszormenyi-Nagy, I. (1965). A theory of relationships: Experience and transaction. *Intensive Family Therapy*, ed. I. Boszormenyi-Nagy and J. Framo. New York: Harper.

Boszormenyi-Nagy, I. (1965). Intensive family therapy as a process. *Intensive Family Therapy*, ed. I. Boszormenyi-Nagy and J. Framo. New York: Harper.

Boszormenyi-Nagy, I., and Spark, G. (1973). *Invisible Loyalties*. New York: Harper.

Boullin, D. J., Coleman, M., and O'Brien, R. A. (1970). Abnormalities in platelet 5-hydroxytryptamine efflux in patients with infantile autism. *Nature* 226:371-372.

Boullin, D. J., Coleman, M., O'Brien, R. A., and Rimland, B. (1971). Laboratory predictions of infantile autism based on 5-HT efflux from platelets and their correlation with the Rimland E-2 score. *Journal of Autism and Childhood Schizophrenia* 1:63-71.

Bowen, M. (1972). Personal communication.

Bowen, M. (1968). Television tapes. Dept. of Psychiatry, Univ. of Virginia College of Medicine.

Bowen, M. (1966). The use of family therapy in clinical practice. *Comparative Psychiatry* 7:345-374.

Bowen, M. (1971). Toward the differentiation of a self in one's own family. In: *Family Interaction*, ed. J. Framo. New York: Springer.

Bowlby, J. (1960). Separation anxiety: A critical review of the literature. *Journal of Child Psychology and Psychiatry* 1:251-269.

Brackelmanns, W., and Berkovitz, I. (1972). Younger adolescents in group psychotherapy: A reparative superego experience. *Adolescents Grow in Groups*, ed. I. Berkovitz, pp. 37-48. New York: Brunner/Mazel.

Bradfield, R. H. et al. (1970). *Behavior Modification: The Human Effort*. San Rafael: Dimensions Publishing.

Bradley, C. (1937). The behavior of children receiving Benzedrine. *American Journal of Psychiatry* 94:577-585.

Bradley, C., and Bowen, M. (1941). Amphetamine (benzedrine) therapy of children's behavior disorders. *American Journal of Orthopsychiatry*, 11:92-103.

Bradt, J., and Moynihan, E. (eds.) (1971). *Systems Therapy—Selected Papers: Theory, Technique, Research*. Washington, D.C.: Authors.

Brady, J. P. (1968). Drugs in behavior therapy. *Psychopharmacology: A Review of Progress*. Washington, D.C.: Government Printing Office, 1957-1967; ed. D. H. Efron, J. O. Cole, J. Levine, and J. R. Wittenborn. U.S. Public Health Service Publication No. 1836.

Brady, J. P. (1971). Drugs in behavior therapy. *Current Psychiatric Therapies*, ed. H. J. Masserman, Vol. 2. New York: Grune & Stratton.

Brambilla, F., and Penati, G. (1971). Hormones and behavior in schizophrenia. *Influence of Hormones on the Nervous System*, ed. D. H. Ford. Basel: Karger.

Breger, L. (1966). Learning theory and behavior therapy. *Psychological Bulletin* 65:170-173.

Breger, L. et al. (1969). The ideology of behaviorism. *Clinical-Cognitive Psychology: Models and Integrations*. Englewood Cliffs: Prentice-Hall, Chapter 2, pp. 25-55.

Breger, L. and McGaugh, J. L. (1965). Critique and reformulation of "learning-theory" approaches to psychotherapy and neurosis. *Psychological Bulletin* 63:338-358.

Breland, K., and Breland, M. (1961). The misbehavior of organisms. *American Psychologist* 16:681-684.

Brody, S. (1964). Aims and methods in child psychotherapy. *Journal of the American Academy of Child Psychiatry* 3:385-412.

Brookover, W. B., Erickson, E., Hamacheck, D., Joiner, L., Lepere, J., Peterson, A., and Thomas, S. (1968). Self-concept of ability and school achievement. *Readings in the Psychology of Adjustment*, 2nd ed., eds. L. Gorlaw and W. Katkovsky. New York: McGraw-Hill.

Browder, J. L. (1972). Appropriate use of psychic drugs in school children. *American Journal of Diseases of Children* 124:606-607.

Brown, J. L. (1960). Prognosis from presenting symptoms of pre-school children with atypical development. *American Journal of Orthopsychiatry* 30:382-390.

Brown-Pembroke Students for a Democratic Society (1970). Mimeographed handout.

Browne, E., Wilson, V., and Laybourne, P. C. (1963). Diagnosis and treatment of elective mutism in children. *Journal of the American Academy of Child Psychiatry* 2:605-617.

Burgess, R. L., and Akers, R. L. (1969). A differential association-reinforcement theory of criminal behavior. *Delinquency, Crime and Social Process*, ed. D. R. Cressley and D. A Ward. New York: Harper.

Burk, H. W., and Menolascino, F. J. (1968). Haloperidol in emotionally disturbed mentally retarded individuals. *American Journal of Psychiatry* 124:1589-1591.

Butcher, L. L., Engel, J., and Fuxe, K. (1970). L-dopa induced changes in central monoamine neurons after peripheral decarboxylase inhibition. *Journal of Pharmacy and Pharmacology* 22:313-316.

Buxbaum, E. (1954). Technique of child therapy. *Psychoanalytic Study of the Child* 9:297-333. New York: International Universities Press.

Byrne, D., and Rhamey, R. (1965). Magnitude of positive and negative reinforcements as a determinant of attractions. *Journal of Personal and Social Psychology* 2:884-889.

Cain, A. C., and Maupin, B. M. (1961). Interpretation within the metaphor. *Bulletin of the Menninger Clinic* 25:307-312.

Camp, B. W. (1971). Remedial reading in a pediatric clinic. *Clinical Pediatrics* 10:36-42.

Campbell, J. D. (1955). Manic-depressive disease in children. *Journal of the American Medical Association* 198:154-157.

Campbell, M. (1973). Psychotic boy with self-mutilating behavior and the antiaggressive effect of lithium. *Journal of the American Academy of Child Psychiatry*, in press.

Campbell, M., Fish, B., David, R., Shapiro, T., Collins, P., and Koh, C. (1972a). Response to triiodothyronine and dextroamphetamine: A study of preschool schizophrenic children. *Journal of Autism and Childhood Schizophrenia* 2:343-358.

Campbell, M., Fish, B., Korein, J., Shapiro, T., Collins, P., and Koh, C. (1972b). Lithium-chlorpromazine: A controlled crossover study in hyperactive severely disturbed young children. *Journal of Autism and Childhood Schizophrenia* 2:234-263.

Campbell, M., Fish, B., David, R., Shapiro, T., Collins, P., and Koh, C. (1973). Liothyronine treatment in psychotic and nonpsychotic children under six years. *Archives of General Psychiatry* 29:602-8.

Campbell, M., Fish, B., Shapiro, T., and Floyd, A., Jr. (1970). Thiothixene in young disturbed children. A pilot study. *Archives of General Psychiatry* 23:70-72.

Campbell, M., Fish, B., Shapiro, T., and Floyd, A., Jr. (1971a). Study of molindone in disturbed preschool children. *Current Therapeutic Research* 13:28-33.

Campbell, M., Fish, B., Shapiro, T., and Floyd, A., Jr. (1971b). Imipramine in preschool autistic and schizophrenic children. *Journal of Autism and Childhood Schizophrenia* 1:267-282.

Campbell, M., and Hersh, S. P. (1971c). Observations on the vicissitudes of aggression in two siblings. *Journal of Autism and Childhood Schizophrenia* 1:398-410.

Campbell, M., Fish, B., Shapiro, T., and Floyd, A., Jr. (1972). Acute responses of schizophrenic children to a sedative and "stimulating" neuropletic: A pharmacologic yardstick. *Current Therapeutic Research* 14:759-766.

Campbell, M., Friedman, E., DeVito, E., Greenspan, L., and Collins, P. J. (1973). Blood serotonin in disturbed and brain damaged children. *Journal of Autism and Childhood Schizophrenia* 4:33-41.

Cantwell, D. P. (1972). Psychiatric illness in the families of hyperactive children. *Archives of General Psychiatry* 27:414-417.

Caplan, G. (1961). *An Approach to Community Mental Health*. New York: Grune & Stratton.

Carlson, C. S., Arnold, C. R., Becker, W. C. et al. (1968). The elimination of tantrum behavior of a child in an elementary classroom. *Behaviour Research Therapy* 6:117-119.

Carson, R. C. (1969). *Interaction Concepts of Personality*. Chicago: Aldine-Atherton.

Cattell, R. B. (1953). New concepts of measuring leadership in terms of group syntality. *Group Dynamics*, ed. Cartwright, Dorwin, and Zander. New York: Harper.

Cerletti, V. (1950). Old and new information about electroshock. *American Journal of Psychiatry* 107:87-94.

Chess, S. (1960). Diagnosis and treatment of the hyperactive child. *New York State Journal of Medicine* 60:2379-2385.

Christensen, D. E., and Sprague, R. L. (1973). Reduction of hyperactive behavior by conditioning procedures alone and combined with methylphenidate (Ritalin). *Behaviour Research Therapy* 11:331-4.

Church, J. (1956). *Language and the Discovery of Reality*. New York: Random House.

Cleckley, H. M., Sydenstricker, V. P., and Geeslin, L. E. (1939). Nicotinic acid in the treatment of atypical psychotic states. *Journal of the American Medical Association* 112: 2107-2110.

Clement, P. W., Fazzone, R. A., and Goldstein, B. (1970). Tangible reinforcers and child group therapy. *Journal of the American Academy of Child Psychiatry* 9:409-427.

Clements, S. D. (1966). Minimal brain dysfunction in children. U.S. Public Health Service Publication No. 1415.

Clements, S. D., and Peters, J. E. (1962). Minimal brain dysfunction in the school-age child. *Archives of General Psychiatry* 6:185-197.

Cohen, J. (1969). *Statistical Power Analysis for the Behavioral Sciences*. New York: Academic Press.

Cohen, N. J., Douglas, V. I., and Morgenstern, G. (1971). The effect of methylphenidate on attentive behavior and autonomic activity in hyperactive children. *Psychopharmacologia* 22:282.

Cole, J. O. (1968). Peeking through the double blind. *Psychopharmacology: A Review of Progress 1957-1967*. U.S. Public Health Service Publication No. 1836, ed. D. H. Efron, J. O. Cole, J. Levine, and J. R. Wittenborn. Washington, D.C.: Government Printing Office, pp. 979-984.

Coleman, M. (1970). Serotonin levels in infant hypothyroidism. *Lancet* 2:365.

Coleman, M. (1973). Serotonin and central nervous system syndromes in childhood: A review. *Journal of Autism and Childhood Schizophrenia* 3:27-35.

Coleman, M., Campbell, M., Freedman, L. S., Roffman, M., Ebstein, R. P., and Goldstein, M. (1974). Serum dopamine-B-hydroxylase levels in Down's syndrome. *Clinical Genetics* 5:312-5.

Colon, F. (1973). In search of one's past: An identity trip. *Family Process* 12:429-438.

Combrinck-Graham, L. (1973). Structural family therapy in psychosomatic illness: Treatment of anorexia nervosa and asthma. Unpublished manuscript.

Comly, H. H. (1970). The use and misuse of psychotropic drugs. *Journal of the Iowa Medical Society* 60:98.

Comly, H. H. (1971). Cerebral stimulants for children with learning disorders. *Journal of Learning Disability* 4:484-490.

Conference on Pediatric Pharmacology (1967). Washington, D.C.: Government Printing Office.

Conners, C. K. (1969). A teacher rating scale for use in drug studies with children. *American Journal of Psychiatry* 126:884.

Conners, C. K. (1970). Psychopharmacologic treatment of children. *Clinical Handbook of Psychopharmacology*, ed. A. D. Dimascio and R. J. Shader. New York: Aronson.

Conners, C. K. (1970). Symptom patterns in hyperkinetic, neurotic and normal children. *Child Development* 41:667.

Conners, C. K. (1970). The use of stimulant drugs in enhancing performance and learning. *Drugs and Cortical Function*, ed. W. L. Smith. Springfield: Charles C Thomas.

Conners, C. K. (1971). Cortical visual evoked response in children with learning disorders. *Psychophysiology* 7:418-428.

Conners, C. K. (1971a). Drugs in the management of children with learning disabilities. *Learning Disorders in Children: Diagnosis. Medication. Education*, ed. L. Tarnopol. Boston: Little, Brown.

Conners, C. K. (1971b). Recent drug studies with hyperkinetic children. *Journal of Learning Disability* 4:476-483.

Conners, C. K. (1972a). Pharmacotherapy of psychopathology in children. *Psychopathological Disorders of Childhood*, ed. H. C. Quay and J. S. Werry. New York: Wiley-Interscience.

Conners, C. K. (1972b). Stimulant drugs and cortical evoked responses in learning and behavior disorders in children. *Drugs, Development, and Cerebral Function*, ed. W. L. Smith, pp. 179-199. Springfield: Charles C Thomas.

Conners, C. K. (1972c). Symposium: Behavior modification by drugs. II. Psychological effects of stimulant drugs in children with minimal brain dysfunction. *Pediatrics* 49:702.

Conners, C. K. (1973). Psychological assessment of children with minimal brain dysfunction. *Annals of the New York Academy of Science* 205: 283-302.

Conners, C. K., and Eisenberg, L. (1963). The effects of methylphenidate on symptomatology and learning in disturbed children. *American Journal of Psychiatry* 120:458-464.

Conners, C. K., Eisenberg, L., and Barcai, A. (1967). Effect of dextroamphetamine on children: Studies on subjects with learning disabilities and school behavior problems. *Archives of General Psychiatry* 17:478-485.

Conners, C. K., Eisenberg, L., and Sharpe, L. (1964). Effects of methylphenidate (Ritalin) on paired-associate learning and Porteus Maze performance
in emotionally disturbed children. *Journal of Consulting Psychology*
28:14.

Conners, C. K., and Rothschild, G. (1968). Drugs and learning in children.
Learning Disorders, ed. J. Hellmuth, Vol. 3. Seattle: Special Child
Publications.

Conners, C. K., Rothschild, G., Eisenberg, I. et al. (1969). Dextroamphetamine sulfate in children with learning disorders. *Archives of General
Psychiatry* 21:182.

Conners, C. K., Taylor, E., Meo, G. et al. (1972). Magnesium pemoline and
dextroamphetamine: A controlled study in children with minimal brain
dysfunction. *Psychopharmacologia* 26:321-36.

Conrad, W. G., Dworkin, E. S., Shai, A. et al. (1971). Effects of amphetamine
therapy and prescriptive tutoring on the behavior and achievement of
lower class hyperactive children. *Journal of Learning Disability* 4:509-517.

Coolidge, J. C., and Gruenebaum, M. G. (1964). Individual and group
therapy of a latency aged child. *International Journal of Group Psycho
Therapy* 14:84-96.

Corson, S. A., Corson, E. O'L., Kirilcuk, V., Knopp, W., and Arnold, L. E.
(1972). Differential interaction of amphetamines and psychosocial factors
in the modification of violent and hyperkinetic behavior and learning
disability. *Federal Proceedings* 31: 820.

Curry, A. E. (1965). Management of multiple family groups. *International
Journal of Group Psychotherapy* 15:90-96.

Cytrin, L., Gilbert, A., and Eisenberg, L. (1963). The effectiveness of
tranquilizing drugs plus supportive psychotherapy in treating behavior
disorders of children: A double blind study of eighty outpatients.
American Journal of Orthopsychiatry 33:431-446.

Daniels, N. (1967). Participation of relatives in a group-centered program.
International Journal of Group Psychotherapy 17:336-342.

Danziger, L. (1958). Thyroid of schizophrenia. *Diseases of the Nervous
System* 19:373-378.

Danziger, L., and Kindwall, J. A. (1953). Thyroid Therapy in some mental
disorders. *Diseases of The Nervous System* 14:3-13.

Davies, I. J., Ellenson, G., and Young, R. (1966). Therapy with a group of
families in a psychiatric day center. *American Journal of Orthopsychiatry*
36:134-146.

Day, W. (1969). Radical behaviorism in reconciliation with phenomenology. *Journal of the Experimental Analysis of Behavior* 12:315-328.

DeLong, A. R. (1972). What have we learned from psychoreactive drug research on hyperactives? *American Journal of Diseases of Children* 123:177-180.

Dimascio, A., Soltys, J. J., and Shader, R. I. (1970). Psychotropic drug side effects in children. *Psychotropic Drug Side Effects: Clinical and Theoretical Perspectives*, ed. R. I. Shader and A. Dimascio. Baltimore: Williams & Wilkins.

Dollard, J., and Miller, N. (1950). *Personality and Psychotherapy.* New York: McGraw-Hill.

Donner, J., and Gamson, A. (1968). Experience with multi-family, time-limited, outpatient groups at a community psychiatric clinic. *Psychiatry* 31:126-137.

Dostal, T. (1972). Antiaggressive effect of lithium salts in mentally retarded adolescents. *Depressive States in Childhood and Adolescence*, ed. A. L. Annell. Stockholm: Almqist & Wiksell.

Doubros, S. G., and Daniels, G. J. (1966). An experimental approach to the reduction of overactive behavior. *Behaviour Research Therapy* 4:251-258.

Douglas, V. I. (1972). Stop, look and listen: The problem of sustained attention and impulse control in hyperactive and normal children. *Canadian Journal of Behavioral Science* 4:259-282.

Drillien, C. M. (1964). *The Growth and Development of the Prematurely Born Infant.* Baltimore: Williams & Wilkins.

Drillien, C. M. (1972). Aetiology and outcome in low-birthweight infants. *Developmental Medicine and Child Neurology* 14:563-574.

Dupree, D. (1971). Pills for learning. New York: *Wall Street Journal*, January 28.

Durell, J., Libow, L. S., Kellam, S. G., and Shader, R. I. (1963). Interrelationships between regulation of thyroid gland function and psychosis. *Association for Research in Nervous and Mental Diseases* 43:387-399.

Dusay, J., and Steiner, C. (1971). Transactional analysis in groups. *Comprehensive Group Psychotherapy*, ed. H. Kaplan and B. Sadock, pp. 198-240. Baltimore: Williams & Wilkins.

Dykman, R. A., Ackerman, P. T., Clements, S. D. et al. (1971). Specific learning disabilities: an attentional deficit syndrome. *Progress in Learning Disabilities,* ed. H. R. Myklebust, Vol. 3. New York: Grune & Stratton.

Dyson, W. L., and Barcai, A. (1970). Treatment of children of lithium-responding parents. *Current Therapeutic Research* 12:286-290.

Easson, W. M. (1969). *The Severely Disturbed Adolescent*. New York: International Universities Press.

Eayrs, J. T. (1968). Developmental relationships between brain and thyroid. *Endocrinology and Human Behavior*, ed. R. F. Michael. New York: Oxford Univ. Press.

Ebaugh, F. G. (1923). Neuropsychiatric sequelae of acute epidemic encephalitis in children. *American Journal of Diseases of Children* 25:89-97.

Editorial (1972). Coffee, tea, cocoa and cola drinks—their contained caffeine as a stimulant. *Clinical Pediatrics* 11:257.

Effron, A. S., and Freedman, A. M. (1953). The treatment of behavior disorders in children with benadryl. *Journal of Pediatrics* 42:261-266.

Eisenberg, L. (1958). School phobia: A study in the communication of anxiety. *American Journal of Psychiatry* 114:712-718.

Eisenberg, L. (1959). The pediatric management of school phobia. *Journal of Pediatrics* 55:758-766.

Eisenberg, L. (1964). Role of drugs in treating disturbed children. *Children* 11:167.

Eisenberg, L. (1966). The management of the hyperkinetic child. *Developmental Medicine and Child Neurology* 8:593.

Eisenberg, L. (1969). Persistent problems in the biopsychology of development. Presented at American Museum of Natural History, New York.

Eisenberg, L. (1971). Principles of drug therapy in child psychiatry with special reference to stimulant drugs. *American Journal of Orthopsychiatry* 41:371-379.

Eisenberg, L., and Conners, C. K. (1963). The effect of a stimulant drug on impulsivity and learning in disturbed children. *American Journal of Psychiatry* 20:458.

Eisenberg, L., and Conners, C. K. (1971). Psychopharmacology in childhood. *Behavioral Science and Pediatric Medicine*, ed. N. B. Talbot, J. Kagan, and L. Eisenberg. Philadelphia: Saunders.

Eisenberg, L., Gilbert, A., Cytrin, L., and Molling, P. A. (1961). The effectiveness of psychotherapy alone and in conjunction with perphenazine or placebo in the treatment of neurotic and hyperkinetic children. *American Journal of Psychiatry* 117:1008-1093.

Eisenberg, L., Lackman, R., Molling, P. A., Lochner, A., Mizelle, J. D., and Conners, C. K. (1963). A psychopharmacologic experiment in a training school for delinquent boys. *American Journal of Orthopsychiatry* 33:431-446.

Eissler, K. R. (1958). Notes on problems of technique in the psychoanalytic treatment of adolescents. *Psychoanalytic Study of the Child* 13:223-254. New York: International Universities Press.

Ekstein, R. (1965). *Children of Time and Space, of Action and Impulse.* New York: Appleton.

Ekstein, R., and Wallerstein, J. (1956). Observations on the psychotherapy of borderline and psychotic children. *Psychoanalytic Study of the Child* 11:303-311. New York: International Universities Press.

Ellis, M. J., Witt, P. A., Reynolds, R. et al. (1974). Methylphenidate and the activity of hyperactives in the informal setting. *Child Development* 45:217-20.

Elson, A., Pearson, C., Jones, C. D., and Schumacher, E. (1965). Follow-up study of childhood elective mutism. *Archives of General Psychiatry* 13:182-187.

Engelhardt, D. M., Polizos, P., and Margolis, R. A. (1972). The drug treatment of childhood psychosis. *Drugs, Development and Cerebral Function*, ed. W. L. Smith. Springfield: Charles C Thomas.

Engelhardt, D. M., Polizos, P., Waizer, J., and Hoffman, S. P. (1973). A double-blind comparison of fluphenazine and haloperidol in outpatient schizophrenic children. *Journal of Autism and Childhood Schizophrenia* 3:128-137.

Epstein, N., and Altman, S. (1972). Experiences in converting an activity group into verbal group therapy with latency-age boys. *International Journal of Group Psychotherapy* 22:93-100.

Epstein, L. C., Lasagna, L., Conners, C. K. et al. (1968). Correlation of dextroamphetamine excretion and drug response in hyperkinetic children. *Journal of Nervous and Mental Disease* 146:136-146.

Erikson, E. H. (1940). Studies in the interpretation of play: Part I. Clinical observations of play disruption in young children. *Genetic Psychology Monographs* 22:557-671.

Erikson, E. H. (1951). Sex differences in the play configuration of pre-adolescents. *American Journal of Orthopsychiatry* 21:667.

Erikson, E. H. (1959). *Identity and the Life Cycle* (Psychological Issues, Monograph 2). New York: International Universities Press.

Erikson, E. H. (1963). *Childhood and Society.* 2nd ed. New York: Norton.

Everett, G. M., and Borcherding, J. W. (1970). L-dopa: Effect on concentrations of dopamine, norepinephrine and serotonin in brains of mice. *Science* 168:849-850.

Eysenck, H. J. (1959). Learning theory and behavior therapy. *Journal of Mental Science* 105:61-75.

Eysenck, H. J. (1964). *Experiments in Behaviour Therapy.* Oxford: Pergamon Press.

Eysenck, H. J. (1965). The effects of psychotherapy. *International Journal of Psychiatry* 1:99-144.

Fant, R. S. (1971). Use of groups in residential treatment. *Healing Through Living,* ed. M. F. Mayer and A. Blum. Springfield: Charles C. Thomas.

Fayol, H. (1970). *General Principles of Management: Social Work Administration,* ed. H. Schatz. New York: Council on Social Work Education.

Feather, B. W., and Rhoads, J. M. (1972). Psychodynamic behavior therapy. *Archives of General Psychiatry* 26:496-511.

Feldmesser-Reiss, E. E. (1958). The application of triiodothyronine in the treatment of mental disorders. *Journal of Nervous and Mental Disease* 127:540-545.

Ferber, A., and Beels, C. (1970). Changing family behavior patterns. *Family Therapy in Transition,* ed. N. Ackerman. Boston: Little, Brown.

Ferber, A., Mendelsohn, M., and Napier, A. (eds.) (1972). *The Book of Family Therapy.* New York: Aronson.

Ferenczi, S. (1950). A little chanticleer. *Contributions to Psychoanalysis.* New York: Brunner/Mazel.

Ferster, C. B. (1961). Positive reinforcement and behavioral deficits of autistic children. *Child Development* 32:437-456.

Ferster, C. B., and DeMyer, M. K. (1961). The development of performances in autistic children in an automatically controlled environment. *Journal of Chronic Diseases* 13:312-345.

Films available from Hillcrest Family Series (1966). Eastern Pennsylvania Psychiatric Institute, Philadelphia.

Finnerty, R. J., Soltys, J. J., and Cole, J. O. (1971). The use of D-amphetamine with hyperkinetic children. *Psychopharmacologia* 21:302-8.

Fish, B. (1960). Drug therapy in child psychiatry: Pharmacological aspects. *Comprehensive Psychiatry* 1:212-227.

Fish, B. (1963). The influence of maturation and abnormal development on the responses of disturbed children to drugs. Proceedings of the Third World Congress of Psychiatry.

Fish, B. (1968). Drug use in psychiatric disorders of children. *American Journal of Psychiatry* 124: (Supp.): 31-36.

Fish, B. (1970). Psychopharmacologic responses of chronic schizophrenic adults as predictors of responses in your schizophrenic children. *Psychopharmacology Bulletin* 6:12-15.

Fish, B. (1971). The "one child, one drug" myth of stimulants in hyperkinesis. *Archives of General Psychiatry* 25:193-203.

Fish, B., Campbell, M., Shapiro, T., and Weinstein, J. (1969). Preliminary findings on thiothixene compared to other drugs in psychotic children under five years. *The Thioxanthenes: Modern Problems of Pharmacopsychiatry*, ed. H. E. Lehmann and T. A. Ban, Vol. 2. Basel: Karger.

Fish, B., Campbell, M., Shapiro, T., and Floyd, A., Jr. (1969a). Comparison of trifluperidol, trifluoperazine and chlorpromazine in preschool schizophrenic children: The value of less sedative antipsychotic agents. *Current Therapeutic Research* 2:589-595.

Fish, B., Campbell, M., Shapiro, T., and Floyd, A., Jr. (1969b). Schizophrenic children treated with methysergide (Sansert). *Diseases of the Nervous System* 30:534-540.

Fish, B., Shapiro, T., and Campbell, M. (1966). Long-term prognosis and the response of schizophrenic children to drug therapy: A controlled study of trifluoperazine. *American Journal of Psychiatry* 123:32-39.

Fiske, D., Hunt, H., Luborsky, L., Orne, M., Parloff, M., Reiser, M., and Tuma, A. (1970). Planning of research on effectiveness of psychotherapy. *Archives of General Psychiatry* 22:22-32.

Fixsen, D., Phillips, E., and Wolf, M. (1972). Achievement place: The reliability of self-reporting and peer-reporting and their effects on behavior. *Journal of Applied Behavior Analysis* 5:19-30.

Ford, D., and Urban, H. (1963). *Systems of Psychotherapy*. New York: Wiley-Interscience.

Foulkes, S., and Anthony, E. (1965). *Group Psychotherapy: The Psychoanalytic Approach*. 2d ed. Harmondsworth, Eng.: Penguin Books.

Fox, W., Gobble, I. R., Clos, M., and Denison, E. (1964). A clinical comparison of trifluperidol, haloperidol and chlorpromazine. *Current Therapeutic Research* 6:409-415.

Framo, J. (1965). Rationale and techniques. *Intensive Family Therapy*, ed. I. Boszormenyi-Nagy and J. Framo. New York: Harper.

Framo, J. (1972). Book review of "Systems Therapy" by J. Bradt and C. Moynihan. *Family Process* 11:515-518.

Framo, J. (ed.) (1972). *Family Interaction: A Dialogue Between Family Researchers and Family Therapists.* New York: Springer.

Frank, G. (1965). The role of the family in the development of psychopathology. *Psychological Bulletin* 64:191-205.

Frank, J. D. (1973). *Persuasion and Healing.* Revised ed. Baltimore: Johns Hopkins Press.

Frankl, V. (1957). *The Doctor and the Soul.* New York: Knopf.

Frankl, V. (1960). Paradoxical interventions. *American Journal of Psychotherapy* 14:520-535.

Franks, C. (1969). *Behavior Therapy Appraisal and Status.* New York: McGraw-Hill.

Freedman, A. M., Ebin, E. V., and Wilson, E. A. (1962). Autistic schizophrenic children. An experiment in the use of D-lysergic acid diethylamide (LSD-25). *Archives of General Psychiatry* 6:203-213.

Freedman, D. X. (1971a). Report of the conference on the use of stimulant drugs in the treatment of behaviorally disturbed young children. *Psychopharmacology Bulletin* 7:23.

Freedman, D. X. (1971b). Report of the conference on the use of stimulant drugs in the treatment of behaviorally disturbed young school children. Sponsored by the Office of Child Development and the Office of the Assistant Secretary for Health and Scientific Affairs, Dept. of Health, Education and Welfare, Washington, D.C., Jan. 11-12.

Freeman, R. D. (1966). Drug effects on learning in children. A selective review of the past thirty years. *Journal of Special Education* 1:17-44.

Freeman, R. D. (1967). Special education and the electroencephalogram: Marriage of convenience. *Journal of Special Education* 2:61.

Freeman, R. D. (1970a). Psychopharmacology and the retarded child. *Psychiatric Approaches to Mental Retardation*, ed. F. Menolascino. New York: Basic Books.

Freeman, R. D. (1970b). Review of medicine in special education: Another look at drugs and behavior. *Journal of Special Education* 4:337.

Freeman, R. D. (1970c). Use of psychoactive drugs for intellectually handicapped children. *Diminished People: Problems and Care of the Mentally Retarded*, ed. N. R. Bernstein. Boston: Little, Brown.

Freeman, W. (1959). Psychosurgery. *American Handbook of Psychiatry*, ed. S. Arieti, Vol. 2. New York: Basic Books.

Freud, A. (1946). *The Psychoanalytic Treatment of Children.* London: Imago Publishing Co.

Freud, A. (1966). *The Ego and the Mechanisms of Defense*. Rev. ed. New York: International Universities Press.

Freud, S. (1909). Analysis of a phobia in a five year old boy. Standard edition 10:1-149. London: Hogarth Press, 1955.

Freud, S. (1913). The occurrence in dreams of material from fairy-tales. Collected Papers 4:236-243. London: Hogarth Press, 1949.

Freud, S. (1926). *The Problem of Anxiety*. New York: Norton, 1936.

Freud, S. (1937). Analysis terminable and interminable. Standard Edition 23:209-253. London: Hondard edition 10:1-149. London: Hogarth Press, 1964.

Friedlander, K. (1941). Children's books and their function in latency and prepuberty. *American Imago* 3:129-150.

Friedman, A. et al. (1965). *Psychotherapy for the Whole Family*. New York: Springer.

Friedman, E. (1971). The birthday party: An experiment in obtaining change in one's own extended family. *Family Process* 10:345-359.

Frommer, E. A. (1967). Treatment of childhood depression with antidepressant drugs. *British Journal of Medicine* 1:729-732.

Frommer, E. A. (1968). Depressive illness in childhood. *Recent Developments in Affective Disorders. A Symposium. British Journal of Psychiatry*, ed. A. Copper and A. Walk, Special Publication No. 2, pp. 117-136.

Furman, E. (1957). Treatment of under fives by way of parents. *Psychoanalytic Study of the Child* 12:250:262. New York: International Universities Press.

Furman, S., and Feighner, A. (1973). Video feedback in treating hyperkinetic children. *American Journal of Psychiatry* 130:792-6.

Gallagher, C. E. (1970). News release. House Office Building, Washington, D.C., Sept. 21.

Gallagher, C. E. (1970). Federal involvement in the use of behavior modification drugs on grammar school children of the right to private inquiry. Hearing before a Subcommittee of the Committee on Government Operations. House of Representatives. Ninety-first Congress. Second Session. Washington, D.C.: Government Printing Office. No. 52-268.

Gallant, D. M., and Bishop, M. P. (1968). Molindone: A controlled evaluation in chronic schizophrenic patients. *Current Therapeutic Research* 10:441-447.

Gallant, D. M., Bishop, M. P., Nesselhoff, W., Jr., and Sprehe, D. J. (1965). Further observations on trifluperidol: A butyrophenone derivative. *Psychopharmacologia* 7:37-43.

Gallant, D. M., Bishop, M. P., and Shelton, W. (1966). A preliminary evaluation of P-4657B: A thioxanthene derivative. *American Journal of Psychiatry* 123:345-346.

Gallant, D. M., Bishop, M. P., Timmons, E., and Gould, A. R. (1966). Thiothixene (P-4657B): A controlled evaluation in chronic schizophrenic patients. *Current Therapeutic Research* 8:153-158.

Ganter, G., Yaekel, M., and Polansky, N. (1967). *Retrieval from Limbo*. New York: Child Welfare League of America.

Gardner, G. (1966). Residential Treatment for Children with Specific Educational and Emotional Problems. Paper read at Shady Brook School Seminar, October 13, 1966.

Gelfand, D. M., and Hartmann, D. P. (1968). Behavior therapy with children: A review and evaluation of research methodology. *Psychological Bulletin* 69:204-215.

Geller, M. (1972). Reflections on selection. *Adolescents Grow in Groups*, ed. I. Berkovitz, pp. 49-62. New York: Brunner/Mazel.

Gendlin, E. (1963). A theory of personality change. *Personality Change*, ed. P. Worchel and D. Byrne. New York: Wiley-Interscience.

Gergen, K. J. (1969). *The Psychology of Behavior Exchange*. Reading: Addison-Wesley.

Gershon, S., Holmberg, G., Mattson, E., and Marshall, A. (1962). Imipramine hydrochloride. Its effects on clinical autonomic and psychological functions. *Archives of General Psychiatry* 6:96-101.

Gibson, W. (1960). *The Miracle Worker*. New York: Bantam Books.

Ginott, H. (1961). *Group Psychotherapy with Children: The Theory and Practice of Play Therapy*. New York: McGraw-Hill.

Gittelman, M. (1965). Behavioral rehearsal as a technique in child treatment. *Journal of Child Psychology and Psychiatry* 6:251-255.

Gittelman-Klein, R., and Klein, D. F. (1971). Controlled imipramine treatment of school phobia. *Archives of General Psychiatry* 25:204-207.

Gjessing, R. (1932). Beiträge zur Kenntnis der Pathophysiologie des katatonen Stupors. *Archiv für Psychiatrie und Nervenkrankheiten* 96:319-392.

Gjessing, R. (1938). Disturbances of somatic functions in catatonia with a periodic course, and their compensation. *Journal of Mental Science* 84:608-621.

Gjessing, R. (1953). Beiträge zur Somatologie der periodischen Katatonie. *Archiv für Psychiatrie und Zeitschrift Neurologie* 191:191-326.

Glasser, P., and Glasser, L. (eds.) (1970). *Families in Crisis*. New York: Harper.

Glick, I., and Haley, J. (1971). *Family Therapy and Research: An Annotated Bibliography*. New York: Grune & Stratton.

Glover, E. (1959). Critical notice. *British Journal of Medicine and Psychology* 32:68-74.

Gluck, M. R., Tanner, M. M., Sullivan, D. F. and Erickson, P. A. (1964). Follow-up and evaluation of 55 child guidance cases. *Behaviour Research and Therapy* 2:131-134.

Goldings, C. R. (1968). Some new trends in children's literature from the perspective of the child psychiatrist. *Journal of the American Academy of Child Psychiatry* 7: 377-397.

Goldings, H. J. (1974). Focus on feelings: Mental health books for the modern child. *Journal of the American Academy of Child Psychiatry* 13:374-377.

Goodman, L. S., and Gilman, A. (1970). *The Pharmacological Basis of Therapeutics*. 4th ed. New York: Macmillan.

Goodwin, F. K., Murphy, D. L., Brodie, H. K. H., and Bunney, W. E. (1970). L-dopa catecholamines and behavior: A clinical and biochemical study in depressed patients. *Biological Psychiatry* 3:341-366.

Gouldner, A. W. (1960). The norm of reciprocity: A preliminary statement. *American Sociological Review* 25:161-178.

Graham, F., Ernhart, C., Thurston, D. et al. (1962). Development three years after perinatal anoxia and other potentially damaging newborn experiences. *Psychological Monographs* 76(3):1-53.

Gram, L. F., and Rafaelsen, O. J. (1972). Lithium treatment of psychotic children and adolescents. A controlled clinical trial. *Acta Psychiatrica Scandinavica* 48:253-260.

Grant, Q. R. (1962). Psychopharmacology in childhood emotional and mental disorders. *Journal of Pediatry* 61:626-637.

Graziano, A. M. (ed.) (1971). *Behavior Therapy with Children*. Chicago: Aldine-Atherton.

Green, R. (1968). Childhood cross-gender identification. *Journal of Nervous and Mental Disease* 147:500-509.

Green, R. (1969). Psychiatric management of special problems in transsexualism. *Transsexualism and Sex Reassignment*, ed. R. Green and J. Money. Baltimore: Johns Hopkins Press.

Greenacre, P. (1970). Youth, growth and violence. *Psychoanalytic Study of the Child* 25:340-359. New York: International Universities Press.

Greenbaum, G. H. (1970). An evaluation of niacinamide in the treatment of childhood schizophrenia. *American Journal of Psychiatry* 127:129-132.

Greenberg, L. M., and Lipman, R. S. (1971). Pharmacotherapy of hyperactive children: Current practices. *Clinical Proceedings, Children's Hospital (Washington, D.C.)* 27:101.

Greenson, R. (1966). A transvestite boy and a hypothesis. *International Journal of Psychoanalysis* 47:396-403.

Greenwald, A. G. (1966). Nuttin's neglected critique of the law of effect. *Psychoanalytic Bulletin* 65: 199-205.

Grossman, H. A. (1966). Psychopharmacology in learning and behavioral disorders of children. *The Teacher of Brain-Injured Children*, ed. W. N. Cruickshank. Syracuse: Syracuse Univ. Press.

Group for the Advancement of Psychiatry. *Treatment of Families in Conflict*. New York: Aronson.

Guerin, P., and Fogarty, T. (1972). Study your own family. *The Book of Family Therapy*, ed. A. Ferder, M. Mendelsohn, and A. Napier. New York: Aronson.

Guey, J. C., Charles, C., Coquery, J. R., and Soulayral, R. (1967). Study of the psychological effects of ethosuximide (Zarontin) in 25 children suffering from petit mal epilepsy. *Epilepsia* 8:129-41.

Gurewitz, S., and Helme, W. H. (1954). Effects of electroconvulsive therapy on personality and intellectual functioning of the schizophrenic child. *Journal of Nervous and Mental Disease* 120:213-226.

Haley, J. (1959). The family of the schizophrenic: A model system. *Journal of Nervous and Mental Disease* 129:357-374.

Haley, J. (1962). Whither family therapy? *Family Process* 1:69-100.

Haley, J. (1963). *Strategies of Psychotherapy*. New York: Grune & Stratton.

Haley, J. (1966). Review of intensive family therapy, ed. I. Boszormenyi-Nagy and J. Framo. *Family Process* 5:284-289.

Haley, J. (1967a). Comment. *Family Process* 6:121-124.

Haley, J. (1967b). Toward a theory of pathological systems. *Family Therapy and Disturbed Families*, ed. G. Zuk and I. Boszormenyi-Nagy. Palo Alto: Science & Behavior Books.

Haley, J. (ed.) (1969). *Advanced Techniques of Hypnosis and Therapy: Selected Papers of Milton H. Erickson, M.D.* New York: Grune & Stratton.

Haley, J. (ed.) (1971). *Changing Families: A Family Therapy Reader*. New York: Grune & Stratton.

Haley, J. (1972). Beginning and experienced family therapists. *The Book of Family Therapy*, ed. A. Ferber, M. Mendelsohn, and A. Napier. New York: Aronson.

Haley, J. (1973). *Uncommon Therapy: The Psychiatric Techniques of Milton H. Erickson.* New York: Norton.

Haley, J., and Hoffman, L. (1967). *Techniques of Family Therapy.* New York: Basic Books.

Hall, R., Axelrod, S., Tyler, L., Grief, E., Jones, F., and Robertson, R. (1972). Modification of behavior problems in the home with a parent as observer and experimenter. *Journal of Applied Behavior Analysis* 5:53-64.

Hallgren, B. (1950). Specific dyslexia: A clinical and genetic study. *Acta Psychiatrica Neurologica Scandinavica* (Supp.) 65:1-287.

Hallsten, E. A. (1970). State-dependent recognition with methylphenidate and thioridazine in retarded children. Unpublished doctoral dissertation, Univ. of Illinois.

Handlon, J., and Parloff, M. (1962). Comparisons between family treatment and group therapy. Unpublished monograph. See also: Treatment of patient and family as a group. *International Journal of Group Psychotherapy* 12:132-141.

Haring, N. G., and Phillips, E. L. (1962). *Educating Emotionally Disturbed Children.* New York: McGraw-Hill.

Harlow, E. (1970). Intensive intervention: An alternative to institutionalization. *Crime and Delinquency Literature* 2:3-46.

Hartmann, H. (1964). *Essays on Ego Psychology.* New York: International Universities Press.

Havelkova, M. (1968). Follow-up study of 71 children diagnoses as psychotic in preschool age. *American Journal of Orthopsychiatry* 38:846-857.

Haworth, M. R., and Keller, M. D. (1962). The use of food in the diagnosis and therapy of emotionally disturbed children. *Journal of the American Academy of Child Psychiatry* 1:4:548-563.

Henry, J. (1971). *Pathways to Madness.* New York: Random House.

Hentoff, N. (1970). The drugged classroom. *Evergreen Review* 14:31-33.

Hersov, L. A. (1960). Persistent non-attendance at school. *Journal of Child Psychology and Psychiatry* 1:130-136.

Hersov, L. A. (1960). Refusal to go to school. *Journal of Child Psychology and Psychiatry* 1:137-145.

Heuscher, J. E. (1963). *A Psychiatric Study of Fairy Tales.* Springfield: Charles C Thomas.

Heuyer, G., Lang, J. L., and Rivaille, C. J. (1956). Aspects cliniques des schizophrenies traitees par l'insuline. *Revue de Neuropsychiatrie Infantile et d'Hygiene Mentale de l'Enfance* 4:390-396.

Hewett, F. M. (1965). Teaching speech to an autistic child through operant conditioning. *American Journal of Orthopsychiatry* 35:927-936.

Hewett, F. M. (1968). *The Emotionally Disturbed Child in the Classroom.* Boston: Allyn & Bacon.

Himwich, H. E., Kety, S. S., and Smythies, J. R. (1967). *Amines and Schizophrenia.* New York: Pergamon Press.

Hoffer, A. (1970). Childhood schizophrenia: A case treated with nicotinic acid and nicotinamide. *Schizophrenia* 2:43-53.

Hoffer, A. (1973). Mechanisms of action of nicotinic acid and nicotinamide in the treatment of schizophrenia. *Orthomolecular Psychiatry*, ed. D. Hawkins and L. Pauling. San Francisco: Freeman.

Hoffman, L., and Long, L. (1969). A systems dilemma. *Family Process* 8:211-234.

Hollister, L. (1970). Quoted in Associated Press dispatch. *Providence Evening Bulletin*, Nov. 26.

Homme, L. (1966). Contingency theory and contingency management. *Psychology Record* 16:233-241.

Homme, L., Csanyi, A., Gonzales, M., and Rechs, J. (1969). How to use contingency contracting in the classroom. Champaign: Research Press.

Hora, T. (1959). Existential group psychotherapy. *American Journal of Psychotherapy* 13:83-92.

Hoskins, R. G. (1946). The biology of schizophrenia. New York: Norton.

Howells, J. (ed.) (1971). *Theory and Practice of Family Psychiatry.* New York: Brunner/Mazel.

Huessey, H. R., and Wright, A. L. (1970). The use of imipramine in children's behavior disorders. *Acta Paedopsychiatrica* 37:194-199.

Huetteman, M. J., Briggs, J., Tripodi, T., Stuart, R. B., Heck, E. T., and McConnell, J. V. (1970). A descriptive comparison of three juvenile populations of adolescents known to the Washtenaw County Juvenile Court: Those referred for or placed in psychiatric hospitals, those placed in correctional settings, and those released following hearings. Unpublished manuscript, Family and School Consultation Project, Ann Arbor, Mich.

Hug-Hellmuth, H. V. (1921). On the technique of child analysis. *International Journal of Psychoanalysis* 2:287-305.

Hutt, C., and Ounsted, C. (1966). The biological significance of gaze aversion with particular reference to the syndrome of infantile autism. *Behavioral Science* 11:346-356.

Itard, J. (1801). *The Wild Boy of Aveyron*, ed. F. and M. Humphrey. New York: Appleton, 1962.

Jackson, D. (1962). Family therapy in the family of the schizophrenic. *Contemporary Psychotherapies*, ed. M. Stein, pp. 272-287. New York: Free Press.

Jackson, D. (1965). Family rules. *Archives of General Psychiatry* 12: 589-594.

Jackson, D. (1965). The marital quid pro quo. *Archives of General Psychiatry* 12:589-594. See also: The study of the family. *Family Process* 4:1-20.

Jackson, D. (1967). Lecture before Washington Psychological Society.

Jackson, D., and Weakland, J. (1961). Conjoint family therapy: Some considerations on theory, technique and results. *Psychiatry* 24:(Supp.)2:30-45.

Jackson, D., and Yalom, I. (1963/64). An example of family homeostasis and patient change. *Current Psychiatric Therapies*, ed. J. Massermann, Vol. 4. New York: Grune & Stratton.

Johnson, D. L., and Gold, S. R. (1971). An empirical approach to issues of selection and evaluation in group therapy. *International Journal of Group Psychotherapy* 21:321-339.

Joint Commission on Mental Health of Children (1969). *Crisis in Child Mental Health*. New York: Harper.

Jones, D. (1966). Psychopharmacological therapy with the mentally retarded. *Mental Retardation Abstracts* 3:21-27.

Jones, E. (1931). The problem of Paul Morphy: a contribution to the psychoanalysis of chess. *International Journal of Psycho-Analysis* 12:1-23.

Jungreis, J. (1965). The active role of the therapist. *Psychotherapy for the Whole Family*, ed. A. Friedman, pp. 187-196. New York: Springer.

Kadzin, A., and Bootzin, R. (1972). The token economy: An evaluative review. *Journal of Applied Behavior Analysis* 5:343-372.

Kanner, L., and Eisenberg, L. (1955). Notes on the follow-up studies of autistic children. *Psychopathology of Childhood*, ed. P. H. Hoch and J. Zubin, pp. 227-239. New York: Grune & Stratton.

Kantor, R., and Hoffman, L. (1966). Brechtian theater as a model for conjoint therapy. *Family Process* 5:218-229.

Katz, E., and Lazarsfeld, P. F. (1955). *Personal Influence*. New York: Free Press.

Kawi, A. A., and Pasamanick, B. (1959). Prenatal and paranatal factors in the development of childhood reading disorders. *Monographs on Social Research and Child Development* 24:1-80.

Keith, C. R. (1968). The therapeutic alliance in child psychotherapy. *Journal of the American Academy of Child Psychiatry* 7:31-43.

Keller, H. A. (1954). *The Story of My Life.* Garden City: Doubleday.

Kelly, D., Guirguis, W., Frommer, E., Mitchell-Heggs, N., and Sargant, W. (1970). Treatment of phobic states with antidepressants: A retrospective study of 246 patients. *British Journal of Psychiatry* 116:387-398.

Kemeny, J. C., Mirkil, H., Snell, J. L., and Thompson, G. L. (1959). *Finite Mathematical Structures.* Englewood Cliffs: Prentice-Hall.

Kenward, J. Personal communication. 1974.

Kernberg, O. (1966). Structural derivatives of object relationships. *International Journal of Psycho-Analysis* 47:236-253.

Kety, S. S. (1972). Toward hypotheses for a biochemical component in the vulnerability to schizophrenia. *Seminars in Psychiatry* 4:233-238.

Klein, D. F. (1964). Delineation of two drug-responsive anxiety syndromes. *Psychopharmacologia* 5:397-408.

Klein, D. F., and Davis, J. H. (1969). *Diagnosis and Drug Treatment of Psychiatric Disorders.* Baltimore: Williams & Wilkins.

Klein, D. F., and Fink, M. (1962). Psychiatric reaction to imipramine. *American Journal of Psychiatry* 119:432-438.

Klein, M. (1932). *The Psychoanalysis of Children.* London: Hogarth Press.

Klein, M. (1963). On identification. *Our Adult World, and Other Essays.* New York: Basic Books.

Klein, M. (1964). Notes on some schizoid mechanisms. *International Journal of Psycho-Analysis* 27:99-100.

Knights, R. M., and Hinton, G. (1969). The effects of methylphenidate (Ritalin) on the motor skills and behavior of children with learning problems. *Journal of Nervous and Mental Disease* 148:643-653.

Knobel, M. (1962). Psychopharmacology for the hyperkinetic child. *Achives of General Psychiatry* 6:198-202.

Kornetsky, C. (1970). Psychoactive drugs in the immature organism. *Psychopharmacologia* 17:105-136.

Kraft, I. (1968). An overview of group therapy with adolescents. *International Journal of Group Psychotherapy* 18:461-480.

Kraft, I. A., Ardali, C., Duffy, J. H., Hart, J. T., and Pearce, P. (1965). A clinical study of chlordiazepoxide used in psychiatric disorders of children. *International Journal of Neuropsychiatry* 1:433-437.

Krantz, J. C., Jr., Truitt, E., B., Jr., Speers, L., and Ling, A. S. O. (1957). New pharmacoconvulsive agent. *Science* 126:353-354.

Krech, D. (1969). Psychoneurobiochemeducation. *Phi Delta Kappan* 7:370-375.

Krohn, A. (1971). Beyond interpretation. (a review of M. D. Nelson et al., *Roles and Paradigms in Psychotherapy*). *Contemporary Psychology* 16:380-382.

Kugelmass, I. (1956). Psychochemotherapy of mental deficiency in children. *International Record of Medicine and General Practice Clinics* 169:323.

Kupietz, S., Bialer, I., and Winsbert, B. G. (1972). A behavior rating scale for assessing improvement in behaviorally deviant children: A preliminary investigation. *American Journal of Psychiatry* 128:1432.

Kurtis, L. B. (1966). Clinical study of the response to nortriptyline on autistic children. *International Journal of Neuropsychiatry* 2:298-301.

Kwiatkowska, H., Harris, G., and Smith, J. (1967). The use of drawing and painting as a primary medium for communication in the family therapy of schizophrenia. Presented at National Institute of Mental Health, Bethesda, Md.

Lake, A. (1974). Scapegoat: a behavioral critique of methodology and interpretation. Unpublished manuscript, Univ. of Michigan.

Langsley, D., Pittman, F., Machotka, P., and Felder, R. (1968). Family crisis therapy—results and implications. *Family Process* 7:145-158.

Lapin, I. P., and Oxenkrug, G. F. (1969). Intensification of the central serotoninergic processes as a possible determinant of the thymoleptic effect. *Lancet* 1:132-136.

Laqueur, H. (1969). General systems theory and multiple family therapy. *Current Psychiatric Therapies*, ed. J. Masserman, Vol. 8. New York: Grune & Stratton.

Laqueur, H. (1971). Systems therapy. *Current Psychiatric Therapies*, ed. J. Masserman, Vol. 2. New York: Grune & Stratton.

Laqueur, H. (1972). Mechanisms of change in multiple family therapy. *Progress in Group and Family Therapy*, ed. C. Sager and H. Kaplan. New York: Brunner/Mazel.

Laqueur, H. (1973). Multiple family therapy: Questions and answers. *Techniques of Family Therapy Psychotherapy*, ed. D. Bloch. New York: Grune & Stratton.

Lasagna, L. (1969). The pharmaceutical revolution: Its impact on science and society. *Science* 166:1227.

Laufer, M. W. (1971). Long-term management and some follow-up findings on the use of drugs with minimal cerebral syndrome. *Journal of Learning Disability* 4:518-522.

Laufer, M. W., Conners, C. K., and McCarthy, P. (1970). Unpublished manuscript.

Laufer, M. W., Denhoff, E., and Solomons, G. (1957). Hyperkinetic impulse disorder in children's behavior problems. *Psychosomatic Medicine* 19:38-49.

LaVeck, G. D., and Buckley, P. (1961). The use of psychopharmacologic agents in retarded children with behavior disorders. *Journal of Chronic Diseases* 13:174-183.

Lazarus, A., and Davison, G. (1971). Clinical innovation in research and practice. *Handbook of Psychotherapy and Behavior Change: An Empirical Analysis*, ed. A. E. Bergin and S. L. Garfield. New York: Wiley-Interscience.

Leichter, E., and Schulman, G. L. (1968). Emerging phenomena in multi-family group treatment. *International Journal of Group Psychotherapy* 18:59-69.

Leichter, E., and Schulman, G. L. (1972). Interplay of group and family treatment, techniques in multi-family group therapy. *International Journal of Group Psychotherapy* 22:167-176.

Leichter, E., and Schulman, G. L. (1974). Multi-family group therapy: A multi-dimensional approach. *Family Process* 13:95-110.

Lennard, H. L., Epstein, L. J., Bernstein, A. et al. (1970). Hazards implicit in prescribing psychoactive drugs. *Science* 169:438.

Lester, E. P. (1968). Brief psychotherapies in child psychiatry. *Canadian Psychiatric Association Journal* 13:301-309.

LeVann, L. J. (1962). Chlordiazepoxide, a tranquilizer with anticonvulsant properties. *Canadian Medical Association Journal* 86:123-126.

LeVann, L. J. (1969). Haloperidol in the treatment of behavioural disorders in children and adolescents. *Canadian Psychiatric Association Journal* 14:217-220.

Levin, S., and Wermer, H. (1966). The significance of giving gifts to children in therapy. *Journal of the American Academy of Child Psychiatry* 5:630.

Levine, S., and Mullins, R. (1966). Hormonal influences on brain organization in infant rats. *Science* 152:1585.

Levitt, E. E. (1971). Research on psychotherapy with children. *Handbook of Psychotherapy and Behavior Change*, ed. A. E. Bergin and S. L. Garfield, pp. 474-494. New York: Wiley-Interscience.

Levy, D. M. (1939). Release therapy. *American Journal of Orthopsychiatry* 9:713-736.

Lewin, K. (1965). Group decision and social change. *Basic Studies in Social Psychology*, ed. H. Poshansky and R. Seidenberg. New York: Holt.

Lewis, J., and Leberman, H. (1970). The use of videotape to diagnose and treat an unexceptional child. *Social Casework* 51: 417-420.

Liebman, R., Minuchin, S., and Baker, L. (1974a). An integrated treatment program for anorexia nervosa. *American Journal of Psychiatry* 131:4:432-436.

Liebman, R., Minuchin, S., and Baker, L. (1974b). The use of structural family therapy in the treatment of intractable asthma. *American Journal of Psychiatry* 131:535-540.

Liebman, R., Minuchin, S., and Baker, L. (1974c). The role of the family in the treatment of anorexia nervosa. *Journal of Child Psychiatry* 13:2:364-374.

Lindemann, E., and Dawes, L. G. (1952). The use of psychoanalytic constructs in preventive psychiatry. *Psychoanalytic Study of the Child* 7:429-447. New York: International Universities Press.

Lindsley, D. B., and Henry, C. E. (1942). Effect of drugs on behavior and EEG of children with behavior disorders. *Psychosomatic Medicine* 4:140-149.

Lipman, R. S. (1970). The use of psychopharmacological agents in residential facilities for the retarded. *Psychiatric Approaches to Mental Retardation*, ed. F. J. Menolascino. New York: Basic Books.

Lipton, M. A., Ban, T. A., Kane, F. J., Levine, J., Mosher, L. R., and Wittenborn, R. (1973). *Megavitamin and Orthomolecular Therapy in Psychiatry*. Washington, D.C.: American Psychiatric Association.

Loewenstein, R. M. (1956). Some remarks on the role of speech in psychoanalytic technique. *International Journal of Psycho-Analysis* 37:460-468.

London, P. (1964). *The Modes and Morals of Psychotherapy*. New York: Holt.

Looker, A., and Conners, C. K. (1970). Diphenylhydantoin in children with severe temper tantrums. *Archives of General Psychiatry* 23:80-89.

Loomie, L. S. (1961). Some ego considerations in the silent patient. *Journal of the American Psychoanalytic Association* 9:56-78.

Loomis, E. A., Jr. (1957). The use of checkers in handling certain resistances in child therapy and child analysis. *Journal of the American Psychoanalytic Association* 130.

Loranger, A. W., Goodell, H., Lee, J. H., and McDowell, F. (1972). Levodopa treatment of Parkinson's syndrome. Improved intellectual functioning. *Archives of General Psychiatry* 26:163-168.

Lovaas, O. I. (in preparation). Teaching language to psychotic children.

Lovaas, O. I. (1969). Behavior modification: Teaching language to psychotic children. Instructional film, 45-min., 16 mm-sound. New York: Appleton.

Lovaas, O. I., Schaeffer, B., and Simmons, J. A. (1965). Experimental studies in childhood schizophrenia: Building social behaviors by use of electric shock. *Journal of Experimental Studies in Personality* 1:99-109.

Lovaas, O. I., Freitag, G., Gold, V. J., and Kassorla, I. C. (1965). Recording apparatus and procedure for observation of behaviors of children in free play settings. *Journal of Experimental Child Psychology* 2:108-120.

Lovaas, O. I., Berberich, J. P., Perloff, B. F., and Schaeffer, B. (1966). Acquisition of imitative speech in schizophrenic children. *Science* 151:705-707.

Lovaas, O. I., Freitag, G., Kinder, M. I., Rubenstein, B. D., Schaeffer, B., and Simmons, J. Q. (1966). Establishment of social reinforcers in two schizophrenic children on the basis of food. *Journal of Experimental Child Psychology* 4:109-125.

Lovaas, O. I., Freitag, L., Nelson, K., and Whalen, C. (1967). The establishment of imitation and its use for the establishment of complex behavior in schizophrenic children. *Behaviour Research and Therapy* 5:171-181.

Lovaas, O. I., Koegel, R., Simmons, J., and Long, J. (1973). Some generalizations and follow-up measures on autistic children in behavior therapy. *Journal of Applied Behavior Analysis* 6:131-166.

Lovaas, O. I., Litrownik, A., and Mann, R. (1971). Response latencies to auditory stimuli in autistic children engaged in self-stimulatory behavior. *Journal of Abnormal Psychology* 9:39-49.

Lovaas, O. I., Schreibman, L., Koegel, R. L., and Rehm, R. (1971). Selective responding by autistic children to multiple sensory input. *Journal of Abnormal Psychology* 77:211-222.

Lovaas, O. I., and Simmons, J. Q. (1969). Manipulation of self-destruction in three retarded children. *Journal of Applied Behavior Analysis* 2:143-157.

Love, L., Kaswan, J., and Bugental, D. E. (1972). Differential effectiveness of three clinical interventions for different socioeconomic groupings. *Journal of Clinical and Counseling Psychology* 39:347-360.

Lovibond, S. H., and Coote, M. A. (1970). Enuresis. *Symptoms of Psychopathology*, ed. C. G. Costello. New York: Wiley-Interscience.

Lowenfeld, M. (1935). *Play in Childhood*. London: Gollancz.

Lowenfeld, M. (1939). The world pictures of children. *British Journal of Medical Psychology* 18:65-101.

Lundin, R. W. (1963). Personality theory in behavioristic psychology. *Concepts of Personality*, ed. J. M. Wepman and R. W. Heine, pp. 257-290. Chicago: Aldine-Atherton.

Lytton, G. J., and Knobel, M. (1958). Diagnosis and treatment of behavior disorders in children. *Diseases of the Nervous System* 20:1.

MacDonough, T., and Forehand, R. (1973). Response-contingent time-out: Important parameters in behavior modification with children. *Journal of Behavior Therapy and Experimental Psychiatry* 4:231-236.

MacGregor, R. (1967). Communicating values in family therapy. *Family Therapy and Disturbed Families*, ed. G. Zuk and I. Boszormenyi-Nagy. Palo Alto: Science & Behavior Books.

MacGregor, R. et al. (1964). *Multiple Impact Therapy with Families*. New York: Grune & Stratton.

MacKay, J. (1967). The use of brief psychotherapy with children. *Canadian Psychiatric Association Journal* 12:269-279.

Madsen, C. H., Jr., Becker, W. C., and Thomas, D. R. (1968). Rules, praise and ignoring elements of elementary classroom control. *Journal of Applied Behavioral Analysis* 1:139-150.

Madsen, C. H., Jr., Becker, W. C., Thomas, D. R., Kosar, L., and Plager, E. (1968). An analysis of the reinforcing function of "sit down" commands. *Readings in Educational Psychology*, ed. R. K. Parker. Boston: Allyn & Bacon.

Mahler, M. S. (1963). Thoughts about development and individuation. *Psychoanalytic Study of the Child*. New York: International Universities Press 18:307-324.

Maier, H. W. (ed.) (1965). *Group Work as Part of Residential Treatment*. New York: National Association of Social Workers.

Malan, D. (1973). The outcome problem in psychotherapy research. *Archives of General Psychiatry* 29:719-729.

Malone, T. P., Whitaker, C. A., Warkentin, J., and Felder, R. E. (1961). Rational and nonrational psychotherapy: A reply. *American Journal of Psychotherapy* 15:212-220.

Mann, J. (1967). Personal communication.

Mann, J. (1969). The specific limitation of time in psychotherapy. *Seminars in Psychiatry* 1:375-379.

Mann, J. (1971). Monograph in preparation.

Marks, I. M. (1969). *Fears and Phobias*. New York: Academic Press.

Marks, I. M., and Gelder, M. G. (1966). Common ground between behaviour therapy and psychodynamic methods. *British Journal of Medical Psychology* 39:11-23.

Marmor, J. (1971). Dynamic psychotherapy and behavior therapy. *Archives of General Psychiatry* 24:22-28.

Martin, F. (1963). Technical problems in the treatment of adolescents: Beginning psychotherapy. *Journal of Child Psychology and Psychiatry* 4:109-124.

May, J. G., Jr., Sachs, D. A., Hindman, D., and Howard, S. (1966). Control of tantrum behavior in a retarded girl. Presented at Florida Psychological Association, Ft. Lauderdale.

Mayer, M. F. (1972). The group in residential treatment of adolescents. *Child Welfare* 51:482-493.

Maynard, R. (1970). Omaha pupils given "behavior" drugs. *The Washington Post*, June 29.

McAndrew, J. B., Case, Q., and Treffert, D. A. (1972). Effects of prolonged phenothiazine intake on psychotic and other hospitalized children. *Journal of Autism and Childhood Schizophrenia* 2:75-91.

McCann, S. (1971). Mechanism of action of hypothalmic-hypophyseal stimulating and inhibiting hormones. *Frontiers in Neuroendocrinology*, ed. L. Martini and W. F. Ganong. London: Oxford Univ. Press.

McDermott, J. F. (1965). A specific placebo effect encountered in the use of Dexedrine in a hyperactive child. *American Journal of Psychiatry* 121:923-924.

McDermott, J. F., Fraiberg, S., and Harrison, S. I. (1968). Residential treatment of children: The utilization of transference behavior. *Journal of the American Academy of Child Psychiatry* 7:169-192.

McGrath, S. D., O'Brien, P. F., Power, P. J., and Shea, J. R. (1972). Nicotinamide treatment of schizophrenia. Report of a multi-hospital controlled trial. *Schizophrenia Bulletin* 5:74-76.

Meeks, J. E. (1968). Psychiatric aspects of learning disorders. *Texas Medicine* 64:74-79.

Meeks, J. E. (1970). Children who cheat at games. *Journal of the American Academy of Child Psychiatry* 9:157-170.

Meeks, J. E. (1973). Adolescent developmental and group cohesion. *Adolescent Psychiatry* 3: 289-297.

Mehrabian, A., and Ksionsky, S. (1970). Models of affiliative behavior. *Psychological Bulletin* 74:110-126.

Meissner, W. (1964). Thinking about the family—psychiatric aspects. *Family Process* 3:1-40.

Mendelson, W., Johnson, N., and Steward, M. A. (1971). Hyperactive children as teenagers: A follow-up study. *Journal of Nervous and Mental Diseases* 153:273-279.

Metz, J. R. (1965). Conditioning generalized imitation in autistic children. *Journal of Experimental Child Psychology* 2:389-399.

Millar, T. P. (1968). Limit setting and psychological maturation. *Archives of General Psychiatry* 18:214-221.

Miller, D. R., and Westman, J. C. (1964). Reading disability as a condition of family stability. *Family Process* 3:66-76.

Miller, D. R., and Westman, J. C. (1966). Family treatment and psychotherapy. *Family Process* 5:49-59.

Millichap, J. G. Unpublished observations.

Millichap, J. G. (1968a). Drugs in management of hyperkinetic and perceptually handicapped children. *Journal of the American Medical Association* 206:1527-1530.

Millichap, J. G. (1968b). Hyperkinetic behavior and learning disorders. III. Battery of neuropsychological tests in controlled trial of methylphenidate. *American Journal of the Diseases of Children* 116:235-244.

Millichap, J. G. (1969). Management of hyperkinetic behavior in children with epilepsy. *Modern Treatment* 6:1233-1246. New York: Hoeber.

Millichap, J. G., and Boldrey, E. E. (1967). Studies in hyperkinetic behavior, II. Laboratory and clinical evaluations of drug treatments. *Neurology* 17:467.

Millichap, J. G., Egan, R. W., Hart, Z. H., and Sturgis, L. H. (1969). Auditory perceptual deficit correlated with EEG dysrhythmias. Response to diphenylhydantoin sodium. *Neurology* 19:870-872.

Millichap, J. G., and Fowler, G. W. (1967). Treatment of "minimal brain dysfunction" syndromes. Selection of drugs for children with hyperactivity and learning disabilities. *Pediatric Clinics of North America* 14:767-777.

Millichap, J. G., Fowler, G. W., and Egan, R. A. Unpublished observations.

Millichap, J. G., and Johnson, F. H. (in press). Methylphenidate in hyperkinetic behavior: relation of response to degree of activity and brain damage. *Pediatrics* (Supp.)

Millichap, J. G., and Millichap, P. A. (1966). Circadian analysis of phenobarbital-induced hyperkinesia in mice and hamsters. *Proceedings of the Society for Experimental Biology and Medicine* 121:754.

Millichap, J. G., and Schrimpf, J. (n.d.) Unpublished observations.

Minde, K., Webb, G., and Sykes, D. (1968). Studies on the hyperactive child. VI. Prenatal and paranatal factors associated with hyperactivity. *Developmental Medicine and Child Neurology* 10:355-363.

Minde, K. K., and Weiss, G. C. (1970). The assessment of drug effects in children as compared to adults. *Journal of the American Academy of Child Psychiatry* 9:124-133.

Mintz, E. E. (1967). Time-extended marathon groups. *Psychotherapy: Theory, Research and Practice* 4:65-70.

Minuchin, S. (1970). The use of an ecological framework in the treatment of a child. *The Child in His Family*, ed. E. J. Anthony and C. Koupernik. New York: Wiley-Interscience.

Minuchin, S. (1971). Anorexia nervosa: Interactions around the family table. Presented at Institute for Juvenile Research, Chicago.

Minuchin, S. (1974). *Families and Family Therapy*. Cambridge: Harvard Univ. Press.

Minuchin, S., Baker, L., Roseman, B., Liebman, R., Milman, L., and Todd, T. (1973). Psychosomatic illness in children: A new conceptual model. Prepared for the Study Group on Mental Illness and Behavior Disorders, National Institute of Mental Health, Bethesda, Md.

Minuchin, S., and Montalvo, B. (1967). Techniques for working with disorganized low socioeconomic families. *American Journal of Orthopsychiatry* 37:880-887.

Minuchin, S., Montalvo, B., Guerney, B. G., Rosman, B. L., and Schumer, F. (1967). *Families of the Slums—An Exploration of Their Structure and Treatment*. New York: Basic Books.

Mischler, E., and Waxler, N. (1966). Family interaction processes and schizophrenia. *International Journal of Psychiatry* 2:375-430.

Modell, W. (1967). FDA Censorship. *Clinical Pharmacology and Therapeutics* 8:359-361.

Molling, P. A., Lochner, A. W., Sauls, R. J., and Eisenberg, L. (1962). Committed delinquent boys: The impact of perphenazine and of placebo. *Archives of General Psychiatry* 7:70-76.

Moniz, E. (1936). *Tentative Operatoires dans le traitement de certaines psychoses*. Paris: Masson et Cie.

Monkman, M. (1972). *A Milieu Therapy Program For Behaviorally Disturbed Children*, pp. 113-124. Springfield: Charles C Thomas.

Morrison, J. R., and Stewart, M. A. (1971). A family study of the hyperactive child syndrome. *Biological Psychiatry* 3:189-195.

Morrison, J. R., and Stewart, M. A. (1973). Psychiatric status of parents adopting hyperactive children. *Archives of General Psychiatry* 28:888-891.

Mosher, L. R. (1970). Nicotinic acid side effects and toxicity. A review. *American Journal of Psychiatry* 126:1290-1296.

Mowrer, O. H. (1950). *Learning Theory and Personality Dynamics*. New York: Ronald Press.

Muller, C. (1972). The overmedicated society: Forces in the marketplace for medical care. *Science* 176:488.

Murphy, D. L. (1972a). L-dopa, behavioral activation and psychopathology. *Neurotransmitters*, ed. I. J. Kopin. Baltimore: Williams & Wilkins.

Murphy, D. L. (1972b). Amine precursors, amines and false neurotransmitters in depressed patients. *American Journal of Psychiatry* 129:141-148.

Murphy, L. B. (1962). *The Widening World of Childhood: Paths Toward Mastery*. New York: Basic Books.

Murray, E. J. (1963). Learning theory and psychotherapy: Biotropic versus sociotropic approaches. *Journal of Counseling Psychology* 10:250-255.

Neubauer, P. B. (1963). Current advances and problems in child therapy. *Professional School Psychology*, ed. M. B. Gottsegen and G. B. Gottsegen, Vol. 2. New York: Grune & Stratton.

Neubauer, P. B. (1963). Psychoanalytic contributions to the nosology of childhood psychic disorders. *Journal of the American Psychoanalytic Association* 11:595-604.

Newman, L. (1970). Transsexualism in adolescence: Problem in evaluation and treatment. *Archives of General Psychiatry* 23:112-121.

Newton, J. (1968). Considerations for the psychotherapeutic technique of symptom scheduling. *Psychotherapy: Theory, Research, and Practice* 5:95-103.

Nichamin, S. J. (1972). Recognizing minimal cerebral dysfunction in the infant and toddler. *Clinical Pediatrics* 11:255.

Nichamin, S. J., and Comly, H. M. (1969). The hyperkinetic or lethargic child with cerebral dysfunction. *Michigan Medicine* 63:790-791.

Noshpitz, J. D. (1957). Opening phase in the psychotherapy of adolescents with character disorders. *Bulletin of the Menninger Clinic* 21:153-164.

Ny, K. Y., Chase, T. N., Colburn, R. W., and Kopin, I. J. (1970). L-dopa-induced release of cerebral monoamines. *Science* 170:76-77.

O'Brien, C. P., DiGiacomo, J. N., Fahn, S., and Schwarz, G. A. (1971). Mental effects of high-dosage levodopa. *Archives of General Psychiatry* 24:61-64.

Odell, G. (1959). The dissociation of bilirubin from albumin and its clinical implications. *Journal of Pediatry* 55:268.

O'Leary, K., and Drabman, R. (1971). Token reinforcement programs in the classroom: a review. *Psychological Bulletin* 75: 379-398.

O'Leary, K., and O'Leary, S. G. (1972). *Classroom Management: The Successful Use of Behavior Modification.* New York: Pergamon Press.

O'Leary, K., Turkewitz, H., and Taffel, S. (1973). Patient and therapist evaluation of behavior therapy in a child psychological clinic. *Journal of Consulting and Clinical Psychology* 41:279-283.

Olsson, P., and Myers, I. (1972). Nonverbal techniques in an adolescent group. *International Journal of Group Psychotherapy* 22:186-191.

Osmond, H. (1973). The background to the niacin treatment. *Orthomolecular Psychiatry,* ed. D. Hawkins and L. Pauling. San Francisco: Freeman.

Osmond, H., and Hoffer, A. (1962). Massive niacin treatment in schizophrenia. Review of a nine-year study. *Lancet* 1:316-319.

Overton, D. A. (1966). State-dependent learning produced by depressant and atropine-like drugs. *Psychopharmacologia* 10:6-31.

Overton, D. A. (1968). Dissociated learning in drug state (state-oriented learning). *Psychopharmacology: A Review of Progress* 1957-1967, ed. D. H. Efron, J. O. Cole, J. Levine, and J. R. Wittenborn. U.S. Public Health Service Publication No. 1836. Washington, D.C.: Government Printing Office.

Overton, D. A. (1970). Discriminative control of behavior by drug states. *Stimulus Properties of Drugs,* ed. G. T. Heistad, T. Thompson, and R. Pickens, pp. 87-110. New York: Appleton.

Packard, V. (1972). *A Nation of Strangers.* New York: McKay.

Paine, R. S. (1962). Minimal chronic brain syndromes in children. *Developmental Medicine and Child Neurology* 4:21-27.

Palkes, H., Stewart, M., and Kahana, B. (1968). Porteus maze performance of hyperactive boys after training in self-directed verbal commands. *Child Development* 39:817-826.

Palkes, H., and Stewart, M. (1972). Intellectual ability and performance of hyperactive children. *American Journal of Orthopsychiatry* 42:418-426.

Parad, L. G., and Parad, H. J. (1968). Intellectual ability and performance of hyperactive children. *American Journal of Orthopsychiatry* 42:35-39.

Park, C. C. (1967). *The Siege.* New York: Harcourt.

Parker, B. (1972). *A Mingled Yarn: Chronicle of a Troubled Family.* New Haven: Yale Univ. Press.

Parker, E. B., Olsen, T. F., and Throckmorton, M. C. (1960). Social casework with elementary school children who do not talk in school. *Social Work* 5:64-70.

Parsons, T. (1951). *The Social System.* New York: Free Press.

Parsons, T., and Bales, R. (1955). *Family, Socialization and Interaction Process.* New York: Free Press.

Pasamanick, B. (1951). Anticonvulsant drug therapy of behavior problem children with abnormal EEGs. *Archives of Neurology and Psychiatry* 65:752.

Pasamanick, B., and Lilienfeld, A. M. (1955). Association of maternal and fetal factors with the development of mental deficiency. I. Abnormalities of the prenatal and paranatal periods. *Journal of the American Medical Association* 159:155-160.

Patterson, G. R. (1974). Intervention for boys with conduct problems: Multiple settings, treatments and criteria. *Journal of Consulting and Clinical Psychology* 42:471-481.

Patterson, G. R. (1971). *Families.* Champaign: Research Press.

Patterson, G. R.,and Bechtel, G. G. (1970). Formulating the situational environment in relation to states and traits. *Handbook of Modern Personality Study*, ed. R. B. Cattell. Chicago: Aldine-Atherton.

Patterson, G. R., and Gullion, M. E. (1968). Living with children: New methods for parents and teachers. Champaign: Research Press.

Patterson, G. R., Jones, R., Whittier, J. et al. (1965). A behaviour modification technique for the hyperactive child. *Behavior Research Therapy* 2:217-226.

Patterson, G. R., and Reid, J. (1971). Reciprocity and coercion: Two facets of social systems. *Behavior Modification in Clinical Psychology*, ed. C. Neuringer and J. Michael. New York: Appleton.

Paul, N. (1966). Effects of playback on family members of their own previously recorded conjoint therapy material. *Psychiatric Research Reports* 20:175-187.

Paul, N. (1970). Personal communication.

Paul, N. (1967). The role of mourning and empathy in conjoint marital therapy. *Family Therapy and Disturbed Families*, ed. G. Zuk and I. Boszormenyi-Nagy. Palo Alto: Science & Behavior Books.

Paul, N., and Broom, J. D. (1970). Multiple-family therapy: Secrets and scapegoating in family crisis. *International Journal of Group Psychotherapy* 20:37-47.

Paul, N., and Grosser, G. (1965). Operational mourning and its role in conjoint family therapy. *Community Mental Health Journal* 1:339-345.

Pauling, L. (1968). Orthomolecular psychiatry. *Science* 160:265-271.

Peller, L. E. (1954). Libidinal phases, ego development and play. *Psychoana-*

lytic Study of the Child 9:178-198. New York: International Universities Press.

Peller, L. E. (1958). Reading and daydreams in latency: Boy-girl differences. *Journal of the American Psychoanalytic Association* 6:57-70.

Peller, L. E. (1959). Daydreams and children's favorite books. *Psychoanalytic Study of the Child* 14:414-433. New York: International Universities Press.

Persky, H., Zuckerman, M., and Curtis, G. C. (1968). Endocrine function in emotionally disturbed and normal men. *Journal of Nervous and Mental Disease* 146:488-497.

Pflaum, S. W. (1974). *The Development of Language and Reading in the Young Child.* Columbus: Charles E. Merrill.

Pharmacotherapy of Children (Special Issue) (1973). *Psychopharmacology Bulletin,* National Institute of Mental Health, Bethesda, Md.

Phillips, E. L., and Johnston, M. S. H. (1954). Theoretical and clinical aspects of short-term parent-child psychotherapy. *Psychiatry* 17:267-275.

Phillips, E. L., Phillips, E. A., Fixsen, D., and Wolf, M (1971). Achievement place: Modification of the behaviors of pre-delinquent boys within a token economy. *Journal of Applied Behavior Analysis* 4:45-59.

Pickard, P. M. (1961). *I Could a Tale Unfold: Violence, Horror and Sensationalism in Stories for Children.* London: Tavistock Humanities.

Pilkington, T. L. (1961a). Comparative effects of librium and taractan on behavior disorders of mentally retarded children. *Diseases of the Nervous System* 22:573-575.

Pilkington, T. L. (1961b). The effects of librium and taractan on behavior of psychotically disturbed mentally retarded children. *Psychopharmacology Abstracts* 1:572.

Pitcher, E. G., and Prelinger, E. (1963). *Children Tell Stories.* New York: International Universities Press.

Pittman, F. et al. (1966). Family therapy as an alternative to psychiatric hospitalization. *Family Structure, Dynamics, and Therapy,* pp.188-195. Psychiatric Research Reports of the American Psychiatric Association, No. 20.

Pittman, F. S., Langsley, D. G., Flomenhaft, K., De Young, C. D., Machotka, P., and Kaplan, D. M. (1971). Therapy techniques of the family treatment unit. *Changing Families: A Family Therapy Reader,* ed. J. Haley, pp. 259-271. New York: Grune & Stratton.

Plank, E. N., and Plank, R. (1954). Emotional components in arithmetical learning as seen through autobiographies. *Psychoanalytic Study of the Child* 9:274-293.

Polizos, P., Engelhardt, D. M., Hoffman, S. P., and Waizer, J. (1973). Neurological consequences of psychotropic drug withdrawal in schizophrenic children. *Journal of Autism and Childhood Schizophrenia* 3:247-253.

Pollack, M., Klein, D. F., Willner, A., Blumberg, A., and Fink, M. (1965). Imipramine-induced behavioral disorganization in schizophrenic patients: Physiological and psychological correlates. *Recent Advances in Biological Psychiatry*, ed. J. Wortis. New York: Plenum Press.

Polsky, H. S., and Claster, D. S. (1968). *The Dynamics of Residential Treatment: A Social System Analysis*. Chapel Hill: Univ. of North Carolina Press.

Porter, R. (ed.) (1968). *The Role of Learning in Psychotherapy*. London: Churchill.

Prange, A. J., Jr., and Lipton, M. A. (1972). Hormones and behavior: Some principles and findings. *Psychiatric Complications of Medical Drugs*, ed. R. I. Shader. New York: Raven Press.

Prange, A. J., Jr., Wilson, I. C., Rabon, A. M., and Lipton, M. A. (1969). Enhancement of imipramine antidepressant activity by thyroid hormone. *American Journal of Psychiatry* 126:457-469.

Prince, G. S. (1968). School phobia. *Foundations of Child Psychiatry*, ed. E. Miller. London: Pergamon Press.

Proskauer, S. (1969). Some technical issues in a time-limited psychotherapy with children. *Journal of the American Academy of Child Psychiatry* 8:154-169.

Pustrom, E., and Speers, R. W. (1964). Elective mutism in children. *Journal of the American Academy of Child Psychiatry* 3:287-297.

Rabiner, C. J., and Klein, D. F. (1969). Imipramine treatment of school phobia. *Comprehensive Psychiatry* 10:387-390.

Rabkin, R. (1970). Inner and outer space. New York: Norton.

Rachman, A. W. (1969a). Talking it out rather than fighting it out: Prevention of a delinquent gang war by group therapy intervention. *Journal of the American Academy of Child Psychiatry* 19:518-521.

Rachman, A. W. (1969b). The role of "fathering" in group psychotherapy with adolescent delinquent males. Presented at 26th annual convention of the American Group Psychotherapy Association, New York.

Rachman, A. W. (1971). Encounter techniques in analytic group psychotherapy with adolescents. *International Journal of Group Psychotherapy* 21:319-329.

Rachman, S., and Eysenck, H. J. (1966). Reply to a critique and reformulation of behavior therapy. *Psychological Bulletin* 65:165-169.

Ramsey, R. A., Ban, T. A., Lehman, H. E., Saxena, B. M., and Bennett, J. (1970). Nicotinic acid as adjuvant therapy in newly admitted schizophrenic patients. *Canadian Medical Association Journal* 102:939-942.

Rank, B., and Haskins, J. (1946). Case 3: Jerry Haskins. *Psychiatric Interviews with Children*, ed. H. L. Witmer, pp. 136-156. Cambridge: Harvard Univ. Press.

Rapaport, D. (1953). On the psychoanalytic theory of affects. *International Journal of Psychoanalysis* 34:177-198.

Rapaport, D. (1957). The theory of ego autonomy. *The Collected Papers of David Rapaport*, ed. M. M. Gill, pp. 722-744. New York: Basic Books 1967.

Rapoport, J. L. (1965). Childhood behavior and learning problems treated with imipramine. *International Journal of Neuropsychiatry* 1: 635-642.

Rapoport, J. L., Abramson, A., Alexander, D. F. et al. (1971). Playroom observations of hyperactive children on medication. *Journal of the American Academy of Child Psychiatry* 10:524-534.

Rapoport, J. L., Lott, I. T., Alexander, D. F. et al. (1970). Urinary noradrenaline and playroom behaviour in hyperactive boys. *Lancet* 2:1141.

Redl, R., and Wineman, D. (1957). *The Aggressive Child*. New York: Free Press.

Reed, G. F. (1963). Elective mutism in children: A re-appraisal. *Journal of Child Psychology and Psychiatry* 4:99-107.

Rees, L., Butler, P. W. P., Gosling, C. et al. (1970). Adrenergic blockade and the corticosteroid and growth hormone responses to methylamphetamine. *Nature* 228:565-566.

Reese, E. (1966). The analysis of human operant behaviour. *Introduction to Psychology: A Self-selection Text*, ed. J. Vernon. Dubuque: William C. Brown.

Reiss, M. (1954). Correlations between changes in mental states and thyroid activity after different forms of treatment. *Journal of Mental Sciences* 100:687-703.

Reiss, M. (1958). *Psychoendocrinology*. New York: Grune & Stratton.

Reiss, M. (1971). Clinical and basic neuroendocrine investigations in some states of mental retardation. *Influence of Hormones on the Nervous System*, ed. D. H. Ford. Basel: Karger.

Richard, R. (1972). Drugs for children—miracle or nightmare? *Providence Sun Journal*, February 6.

Rimland, B. (1964). *Infantile Autism*. New York: Appleton.

Rimland, B. (1973). High-dosage levels of certain vitamins in the treatment of children with severe mental disorders. *Orthomolecular Psychiatry*, ed. D. Hawkins and L. Pauling. San Francisco: Freeman.

Rinsley, D. B., and Inge, G. P., III (1961). Psychiatric hospital treatment of adolescents: Verbal and nonverbal resistance to treatment. *Bulletin of the Menninger Clinic* 25:249-263.

Risley, T., and Wolf, M. (1967). Establishing functional speech in echolalic children. *Behaviour Research and Therapy* 5:73-88.

Ritvo, E. R., Yuwiler, A., Geller, E., Kales, A., Rashkis, S., Schicor, A., Plotkin, S., Axelrod, R., and Howard, C. (1971). Effects of L-dopa in autism. *Journal of Autism and Childhood Schizophrenia* 1:190-205.

Ritvo, E. R., Yuwiler, A., Geller, E., Ornitz, E. M., Saeger, K., and Plotkin, S. (1970). Increased blood serotonin and platelets in early infantile autisms. *Archives of General Psychiatry* 23:566-572.

Robins, L. (1966). *Deviant Children Grown Up*. Baltimore: Williams and Wilkins.

Rodgers, R. (1973). *Family Interaction and Transaction*. Englewood Cliffs: Prentice-Hall.

Rodman, H., and Grams, P. (1967). Juvenile delinquency and the family: A review and discussion. President's Commission on Law Enforcement and Administration of Justice, Task Force on Juvenile Delinquency. *Task Force Report: Juvenile Delinquency and Youth Crime*. Washington, D.C.: Government Printing Office.

Rogers, J. (1971). Drug abuse—Just what the doctor ordered. *Psychology Today* 5:16-24.

Rolo, A., Krinsky, L., Abramson, H., and Goldfarb, L. (1965). Preliminary method study of LSD with children. *International Journal of Neuropsychiatry* 1:552-555.

Rose, S. D. (1973). *Treating Children in Groups*. San Francisco: Jossey-Bass.

Rosen, J. (1953). *Direct Analysis*. New York: Grune & Stratton.

Rosenthal, A. J. (1970). *Report on brief therapy research to the clinical symposium*, Department of Psychiatry, Stanford Univ. Medical Center, November 25.

Rosenthal, A. J., and Levine, S. V. (1970). Brief psychotherapy with children: a preliminary report. *American Journal of Psychiatry* 127: 646-651.

Rosenthal, A. J., and Levine, S. V. (1971). Brief psychotherapy with children: Process of therapy. *American Journal of Psychiatry* 128:141-146.

Rosenthal, R. (1966). *Experimenter Effects in Behavioral Research.* New York: Appleton.

Rosenthal, R. (1968). Experimenter expectancy and the reassuring nature of the null hypothesis decision procedure. *Psychological Bulletin Monograph Supplement* 70:30-47.

Rutter, M. (1967). Prognosis: psychotic children in adolescence and early life. *Early Childhood Autism: Clinical Educational and Social Aspects,* ed. J. K. Wing. London: Pergamon Press.

Rutter, M. (1967). A children's behavior questionnaire for completion by teachers. *Journal of Child Psychology and Psychiatry* 8:1-11.

Rutter, M. et al. (1969). A tri-axial classification of mental disorders in childhood. *Journal of Child Psychology and Psychiatry* 10:41-61.

Rutter, M., Tizard, J., and Whitmore, K. (1970). *Education, Health and Behaviour.* London: Longmans.

Sachar, E. J. (1963). Psychoendocrine aspects of acute schizophrenic reactions. *Psychosomatic Medicine* 25:510-537.

Sachar, E. J., Harmatz, J., Bergen, H., and Cohler, J. (1966). Corticosteroid responses to milieu therapy of chronic schizophrenics. *Archives of General Psychiatry* 15:310-319.

Sachar, E. J., Hellman, L., Roffwarg, H. P., Halpern, F. S., Fukushima, D. K., and Gallagher, T. F. (1973). Disrupted 24-hour patterns of cortisol secretion in psychotic depression. *Archives of General Psychiatry* 28:19-24.

Sachs, D. (1973). The efficacy of time-out procedures in a variety of behavior problems. *Journal of Behavior Therapy and Experimental Psychiatry* 4:237-242.

Safer, D. J. (1971). Drugs for problem school children. *Journal of School Health* 41:491-495.

Safer, D. J., Allen, R., and Barr, E. (1972). Depression of growth in hyperactive children on stimulant drugs. *New England Journal of Medicine* 287:217-220.

Sager, C. J., and Kaplan, M. (1972). *Prognosis in Group and Family Therapy.* New York: Brunner/Mazel.

Saizman, L. (1968). Reply to the critics. *International Journal of Psychiatry* 6:473-478.

Sakel, M. (1938). *The Pharmacological Shock Treatment of Schizophrenia.* New York: Nervous and Mental Diseases Publishing Co.

Sandler, J., Holder, A., and Dare, C. (1970a). Basic psychoanalytic concepts: II—The treatment alliance. *British Journal of Psychiatry* 116:555-558.

Sandler, J., Holder, A., and Dare, C. (1970b). Basic psychoanalytic concepts: III—Transference. *British Journal of Psychiatry* 116:667-672.

Sandler, J., Holder, A., and Dare, C. (1970c). Basic psychoanalytic concepts: V—Resistance. *British Journal of Psychiatry* 117:215-221.

Sandler, J., Holder, A., and Dare, C. (1971). Basic psychoanalytic concepts: X—Interpretations and other interventions. *British Journal of Psychiatry* 118:53-59.

Sands, R., and Golub, S. (1974). Breaking the bonds of tradition: A reassessment of group treatment of latency-age children. *American Journal of Psychiatry* 131:662-665.

Satir, V. (1964). *Conjoint Family Therapy*. Palo Alto: Science & Behavior Books.

Satir, V. (1967). Workshop in family therapy, Falls Church, Va.

Satir, V. (1972). Peoplemaking. Cupertino: Science & Behavior Books.

Satterfield, J. H., Cantwell, D. P., Lesser, L. I. et al. (1972). Physiological studies of the hyperkinetic child: I. *American Journal of Psychiatry* 128:1418-1424.

Satterfield, J. H., and Dawson, M. E. (1971). Electrodermal correlates of hyperactivity in children. *Psychophysiology* 8:191-197.

Schachter, S. (1964). The interaction of cognitive and physiological determinants of emotional state. *Psychobiological Approaches to Social Behavior*, ed. P. H. Leiderman and D. Shapiro, pp. 138-173. Stanford: Stanford Univ. Press.

Schaefer, J. W., Palkes, H. S., and Stewart, M. A. (1974). Group counseling for parents of hyperactive children. *Child Psychiatry and Human Development* 5:89-94.

Schafer, W. E., and Polk, K. (1967). Delinquency and the schools. President's Commission on Law Enforcement and Administration of Justice, Task Force on Juvenile Delinquency. *Task Force Report: Juvenile Delinquency and Youth Crime*. Washington, D.C.: Government Printing Office.

Schaffer, L., Wynne, L., Day, J., Ryckoff, I., and Halperin, A. (1962). On the nature and sources of the psychiatrist's experience with the family of the schizophrenic. *Psychiatry* 25:23-45.

Schain, R. J., and Freedman, D. X. (1961). Studies of 5-hydroxyindole metabolism in autistic and other mentally retarded children. *Journal of Pediatrics* 58:315-320.

Schapiro, S. (1971). Influence of hormones and environmental stimulation of brain development. *Influence of Hormones on the Nervous System*, ed. D. H. Ford. Basel: Karger.

Scheflen, A. (1964). The significance of posture in communication systems. *Psychiatry* 27:316-331.

Scheflen, A. (1966). *Stream and Structure of Communicational Behavior*. Behavior Science Monograph, I. Philadelphia: Eastern Pennsylvania Psychiatric Association Press.

Scheflen, A. (1968). Human communications: Behavioral programs and their integration in interaction. *Behavior Science* 13:44-55.

Scheflen, A. and Ferber, A. (1972). Critique of a sacred cow. IN: Ferber, A., Mendelsohn, M. and Napier, A. *The Book of Family Therapy*. New York: Aronson.

Scheidlinger, S. (1953). *Freudian Concepts of Group Relations in Group Dynamics*. New York: Harper.

Schildkraut, J. J., and Kety, S. S. (1967). Biogenic amines and emotion. Pharmacological studies suggest a relationship between brain biogenic amines and affective state. *Science* 156:21-30.

Schmideberg, M. (1949). Short-analytic therapy. *Nervous Child* 8:281-290.

Schnachenberg, R. C. (1973). Caffeine as a substitute for Schedule II stimulants in hyperkinetic children. *American Journal of Psychiatry* 130:796-798.

Schou, M. (1972). Lithium in psychiatric therapy and prophylaxis. A review with special regard to its use in children. *Depressive States in Childhood and Adolescence*, ed. A. L. Annell. Stockholm: Almqist & Wiksell.

Schulman, J. L., and Clarinda, M. (1964). The effect of promazine on the activity level of retarded children. *Pediatrics* 33:271-275.

Schwartz, W. (1971). Groups in social work practice. *The Practice of Group Work*, ed. W. Schwartz and Z. R. Zalba. New York: Columbia Univ. Press.

Scott, W. C. M. (1961). Differences between the playroom used in child psychiatric treatment and in child analysis. *Canadian Psychiatric Association Journal* 6:281-285.

Searles, H. F. (1963). The place of neutral therapist-responses in psychotherapy with the schizophrenic patient. *International Journal of Psycho-Analysis* 44:42-56.

Shader, R. I., and Dimascio, A. (1970). *Psychotropic Drug Side Effects*. Baltimore: Williams & Wilkins.

Shapiro, T. (1975). Personal communication.

Shaw, W. H. (1971). Aversive control in the treatment of elective mutism. *Journal of the American Academy of Child Psychiatry* 10:572-581.

Sheard, M. H. (1970a). Effect of lithium on foot shock aggression in rats. *Nature* 228:284-285.

Sheard, M. H. (1970b). Behavioral effects of *p*-chlorophenylalanine in rats. Inhibition by lithium. *Communications in Behavioral Biology* 5:71-73.

Sheard, M. H. (1971a). Effect of lithium on human aggression. *Nature* 230:113-114.

Sheard, M. H. (1971b). The effect of lithium on behavior. *Communications in Contemporary Psychiatry* 1:1-6.

Sherman, M., Ackerman, N., Sherman, S., and Mitchell, C. (1965). Nonverval cues and reenactment of conflict in family therapy. *Family Process* 4:133-162.

Sherwin, A. C., Flach, F. F., and Stokes, P. E. (1958). Treatment of psychoses in early childhood with triiodothyronine. *American Journal of Psychiatry* 115:166-167.

Shetty, T. (1971). Phobic responses in hyperkinesis of childhood. *Science* 174:1356-1357.

Shirkey, H. (1968). Therapeutic orphans. *Journal of Pediatry* 72:119.

Shopper, M. (1969). The use of children's literature and toys in the teaching of child development to medical students in the preclinical years. *Journal of the American Academy of Child Psychiatry* 8:1-15.

Silver, A. A. (1955). Management of children with schizophrenia. *American Journal of Psychotherapy* 9:196-215.

Simeon, J., Saletu, B., Saletu, M., Itil, T. M., and DaSilva, J. (1973). Thiothixene in childhood psychoses. Presented at Third International Symposium on Phenothiazines, Rockville, Md.

Simmons, J. Q., III, Leiken, S. J., Lovaas, O. I., Schaeffer, B., and Perloff, B. (1966). Modification of autistic behavior with LSD-25. *American Journal of Psychiatry* 122:1201-1211.

Simpson, G. M., Cranswick, E. H., and Blair, J. H. (1963). Thyroid indices in chronic schizophrenia. *Journal of Nervous and Mental Disease* 137:582-590.

Simpson, G. M., Cranswick, E. H., and Blair, J. H. (1964). Thyroid indices in chronic schizophrenia: II. *Journal of Nervous and Mental Disease* 138:581-585.

Simpson, G. M., and Igbal, J. (1965). A preliminary study of thiothixene in chronic schizophrenics. *Current Therapeutic Research* 7:310-314.

Simpson, G. M., and Krakov, L. (1968). A preliminary study of molindone (EN-1733A) in chronic schizophrenia. *Current Therapeutic Research* 10:41-46.

Skinner, B. F. (1957). *Verbal Behavior*. New York: Appleton.

Skolnick, A. (1973). *The Intimate Environment: Exploring Marriage and the Family*. Boston: Little, Brown.

Skolnick, A., and Skolnick, J. (1971). *Family in Transition*. Boston: Little, Brown.

Skynner, A. C. R. (1961). Effect of chlordiazepoxide. *Lancet* 1:1110.

Slater, P. (1970). *The Pursuit of Loneliness*. Boston: Beacon Press.

Slavson, S. (1950). *Analytic Group Psychotherapy*. New York: Columbia Univ. Press.

Slavson, S. (1964). *Para-analytic Group Psychotherapy: A Treatment of Choice for Adolescents*. Pathways in Child Guidance, Vol. 6, No. 7.

Sloan, N. H., Johnston, M. K., and Bijou, S. W. (1967). Successive modification of aggressive behavior and aggressive fantasy play by management of contingencies. *Journal of Child Psychology and Psychiatry* 8:217-226.

Sloane, R. B. (1969). The converging paths of behavior therapy and psychotherapy. *International Journal of Psychiatry* 7:493-503.

Small, A., Hibi, S., and Feinberg, I. (1971). Effects of dextroamphetamine sulfate on EEG sleep patterns of hyperactive children. *Archives of General Psychiatry* 25:369-380.

Smith, J. M., and Smith, D. E. P. (1966). *Child Management*. Ann Arbor: Ann Arbor Publishers.

Snow, D. L., and Brooks, R. B. (1970). Issues in school consultation: The role of the consultant and the use of behavior modification techniques. Unpublished paper.

Snyder, S. H., Taylor, K. M., Coyle, J. T., and Meyerhoff, J. L. (1970). The role of brain dopamine in behavioral regulation and the actions of psychotropic drugs. *American Journal of Psychiatry* 127:199-207.

Sokoloff, L., and Roberts, P. (1971). Biochemical mechanism of the action of thyroid hormones in nervous and other tissues. *Influence of Hormones on the Nervous System*, ed. D. H. Ford. Basel: Karger.

Solomons, G. (1972). Drug therapy, initiation and follow-up. Presented at Conference on Minimal Brain Dysfunction, New York.

Sonne, J., Speck, R., and Jungreis, J. (1965). *Psychotherapy for the Whole Family*, ed. A. Friedman. New York: Springer.

Speck, R., and Attneave, C. (1973). *Family Networks*. New York: Pantheon.

Speck, R., and Attneave, C. (1973). Network therapy. *The Book of Family Therapy*, ed. A. Ferber, M. Mendelsohn. New York: Aronson.

Speck, R., and Bowen, M. (1966). Lecture at Georgetown Univ.

Speck, R., and Rueveni, U. (1969). Network therapy: A developing concept. *Family Process* 8:182-191.

Spiegel, H. (1967). Is symptom removal dangerous? *American Journal of Psychiatry* 123:1279-1283.

Sprague, R. L. (1972). Psychopharmacology and learning disabilities. Presented at Child Development and Child Psychiatry Conference, Columbia, Mo., October.

Sprague, R. L. (1973). Minimal brain dysfunction from a behavioral viewpoint. *Annals of the New York Academy of Science* 2:349-361.

Sprague, R. L., Barnes, K. R., and Werry, J. S. (1970). Methylphenidate and thioridazine: Learning, reaction time, activity and classroom behavior in emotionally disturbed children. *American Journal of Orthopsychiatry* 40:615-628.

Sprague, R. L., Christensen, D. E., and Werry, J. S. (in press). Experimental psychology and stimulant drugs. *Excerpta Medica*.

Sprague, R. L., and Toppe, L. K. (1966). Relationship between activity level and delay of reinforcement. *Journal of Experimental Psychology* 3:390-397.

Sprague, R. L., and Werry, J. S. (1971). Methodology of psychopharmacological studies with the retarded. *International Review of Research in Mental Retardation*, ed. N. R. Ellis, Vol. 5. New York: Academic Press.

Sprague, R. L., Werry, J., and Davis, K. (1969). Psychotropic drug effects on learning and activity level of children. Presented at Gatlinburg Conference on Research and Theory in Mental Retardation. Gatlinburg, Tenn., March.

Sroufe, L. A. (1975). Drug treatment of children with behavior problems. *Review of Child Development Research*, ed. F. Horowitz, Vol. 4. Chicago: University of Chicago Press.

Sroufe, L. A., Sonies, B. C., West, W. D. et al. (1973). Anticipatory heart rate deceleration and reaction time in children with and without referral for learning disability. *Child Development* 44:267-273.

Staats, A. W., and Butterfield, W. H. (1965). Treatment of nonreading in a culturally deprived juvenile delinquent: an application of reinforcement principles. *Child Development* 36:925-942.

Stedman, J., Patton, W., and Walton, K. (1973). *Clinical Studies in Behavior Therapy with Children. Adolescents and Their Families*. Springfield: Charles C Thomas.

Stedman, J., Peterson, T., and Cardarelle, J. (1971). Application of a token system in a preadolescent boys' group. *Journal of Behavior Therapy and Experimental Psychiatry* 2:23-29.

Stein, M. (1970). The function of ambiguity in child crises. *Journal of the American Academy of Child Psychiatry* 9:462-476.

Stein, M. I., Kliman, A. S., Rosenfeld, R., and Harbur, A. (1970). Brief treatment of preschoolers. Workshop presentation at meetings of the American Association of Psychiatric Services for Children.

Steinberg, G. G., Troshinsky, C., and Steinberg, H. R. (1971). Dextroamphetamine-responsive behavior disorder in school children. *American Journal of Psychiatry* 128:174-179.

Stevens, D. A., Boydstun, J. A., Ackerman, P. T. et al. (1968). Reaction time, impulsivity and autonomic lability in children with minimal brain dysfunction. *Proceedings of the 76th Annual Convention of the American Psychological Association*, pp. 367-368. Washington, D.C.: American Psychological Association.

Stewart, M. A., Pitts, F. N., Craig, A. G. et al. (1966). The hyperactive child syndrome. *American Journal of Orthopsychiatry* 36:861-867.

Stoller, F. H. (1968). Accelerated interaction: A time-limited approach based on the brief, intensive group. *Journal of the American Academy of Child Psychiatry* 18:220-235.

Stoller, R. J. (1968). *Sex and Gender: The Development of Masculinity and Femininity*. New York: Aronson.

Stoyva, J. M. (1970). Approaches to mind-body problems: the public (scientific) study of private events. *International Psychiatric Clinics* 7: 355-367.

Strauss, A. A., and Kephart, N. C. (1955). *Psychopathology and Education of the Brain-Injured Child*. Vol. 2. *Progress in Theory and Clinic*. New York: Grune & Stratton.

Strauss, A. A., and Lehtinen, L. E. (1947). *Psychopathology and Education of the Brain-Injured Child*. New York: Grune & Stratton.

Strupp, H. H. (1973). *Psychotherapy: Clinical, Research and Therapeutic Issues*. New York: Aronson.

Stuart, R. B. (1969). Operant-interpersonal treatment for marital discord. *Journal of Consulting Clinical Psychology* 33:675-682.

Stuart, R. B. (1970a). Assessment and change of the communicational patterns of juvenile delinquents and their parents. *Advances in Behavior Therapy, 1969*, ed. R. D. Rubin. New York: Academic Press.

Stuart, R. B. (1970b). Behavior modification techniques for the education technologist. *Proceedings of the National Workshop on School Social Work, 1969-70*, ed. R. C. Sarri. New York: National Association of Social Workers.

Stuart, R. B. (1970c). Situational versus self control in the treatment of problematic behaviors. *Advances in Behavior Therapy*, ed. R. D. Rubin. New York: Academic Press.

Stuart, R. B. (1971). Behavioral contracting within the families of delinquents. *Journal of Behavior Therapy and Experimental Psychiatry* 2:1-11.

Sugerman, A. A., and Herrmann, J. (1967). Molindone: An indole derivative with antipsychotic activity. *Clinical Pharmacology and Therapeutics* 8:261-265.

Sugerman, A. A., Stolberg, H., and Herrmann, J. (1965). A pilot study of P-4657B in chronic schizophrenics. *Current Therapeutic Research* 7:310-314.

Sulzer, E. S. (1962). Research frontier: Reinforcement and the therapeutic contract. *Journal of Counseling Psychology* 9:271-276.

Sykes, D. H., Douglas, V. I., and Morgenstern, G. (1972). The effect of methylphenidate (Ritalin) on sustained attention in hyperactive children. *Psychopharmacologia* 25:262-274.

Sykes, D. H., Douglas, V. I., Weiss, G. et al. (1971). Attention in hyperactive children and the effect of methylphenidate (Ritalin). *Journal of Child Psychology and Psychiatry* 12:129-139.

Taft, J. (1933). *The Dynamics of Therapy in a Controlled Relationship*. New York: Macmillan.

Taylor, K. M., and Snyder, S. H. (1970). Amphetamine: Differentiation by D- and L-isomers of behavior involving brain norepinephrine or dopamine. *Science* 168:1487-1489.

Tharp, R. G. (1963). Dimensions of marriage roles. *Marriage and Family Living* 25:389-404.

Tharp, R. G., and Otis, G. (1965). Toward a theory for therapeutic intervention in families. Presented before Western Psychological Association, Honolulu.

Tharp, R. G., and Wetzel, R. J. (1969). *Behavior Modification in the Natural Environment*. New York: Academic Press.

Thibaut, J. W., and Kelley, H. H. (1959). *The Social Psychology of Groups*. New York: Wiley-Interscience.

Thomas, D. R., Becker, W. C., and Armstrong, M. (1968). Production and elimination of disruptive classroom behavior by systematically varying teacher's behavior. *Journal of Applied Behavior Analysis* 1:35-45.

Thomas, E., and Walter, C. (1973). Guidelines for behavioral practice in the open community agency: procedure and evaluation. *Behaviour Research and Therapy* 11:193-205.

Thompson, T. I., and Pickens, R. (1971). *Stimulus Properties of Drugs.* New York: Appleton.

Toussieng, P. W. (1971). Child psychotherapy in a new era. *American Journal of Orthopsychiatry* 41:58-64.

Treating Children in Groups, (1972), ed. S. D. Rose. San Francisco: Jossey Bass.

Tupin, J. P., and Smith, D. B. (1972). The long-term use of lithium in aggressive prisoners. Presented at meeting of Early Clinical Drug Evaluation Unit, Psychopharmacology Research Branch, NIMH, Catonsville, Md., June.

Ullmann, L., and Krasner, L. (1965). *Case Studies in Behavior Modification.* New York: Holt.

United States Department of Health, Education and Welfare (1971). *Report on the Conference on the Use of Stimulant Drugs in the Treatment of Behaviorally Disturbed Young School Children.* Sponsored by the Office of Child Development and the Office of the Assistant Secretary for Health and Scientific Affairs. Washington, D.C.: Office of Child Development, January 11-12.

Van Scoy, H. (1972). Activity group therapy: A bridge between play and work. *Child Welfare* 51:528-534.

Vogel, E. F., and Bell, N. W. (1960). The emotionally disturbed child as the family scapegoat. *The Family*, ed. N. W. Bell and E. F. Vogel. New York: Free Press.

Waelder, R. (1962). Psychoanalysis, scientific method and philosophy. *Journal of the American Psychoanalytic Association* 10:617-638.

Wahler, R. G. (1969). Setting generality: Some specific and general effects of child behavior therapy. *Journal of Applied Behavior Analysis* 2:239-246.

Waizer, J., Polizoes, P., Hoffman, S. P., Engelhardt, D. M., and Margolis, R. A. (1972). A single-blind evaluation of thiothixene with outpatient schizophrenic children. *Journal of Autism and Childhood Schizophrenia* 2:378-386.

Walker, C. F., and Kirkpatrick, B. B. (1947). Dilantin treatment for behavior problem children with abnormal EEGs. *American Journal of Psychiatry* 103:484-492.

Warkentin, J., and Whitaker, C. (1966). Serial impasses in marriage. *Psychiatric Research Reports* 20:73-7.

Watzlawick, P., Beavin, J., and Jackson, D. (1967). *Pragmatics of Human Communication*. New York: Norton

Watzlawick, P., Weakland, J., and Fisch, R. (1974). *Change: Principles of Problem Formation and Problem Resolution*. New York: Norton.

Weed, L. (1969). Medical records, medical evaluation and patient care. Cleveland: Case Western Reserve Univ.

Weischer, M. L. (1969). On the antiaggressive effect of lithium. *Psychopharmacologia* 15:245-254.

Weiss, B., and Laties, V. G. (1962). Enhancement of human performance by caffeine and the amphetamines. *Pharmacological Review* 14:1-36.

Weiss, G., Minde, K., Werry, J. S. et al. (1971). Studies on the hyperactive child. VIII. Five-year follow-up. *Archives of General Psychiatry* 24:409-414.

Weitzman, B. (1967). Behavior therapy and psychotherapy. *Psychological Review* 74:300-317.

Wender, P. H. (1968). The role of deviation-amplifying feedback in the origin and perpetuation of behavior. *Psychiatry* 31:317-324.

Wender, P. H. (1971). *Minimal Brain Dysfunction in Children*. New York: Wiley-Interscience.

Werner, E., Bierman, J. M., French, F. E. et al. (1968). Reproductive and environmental casualties: A report on the 10-year follow-up of the children of the Kauai pregnancy study. *Pediatrics* 42:112-127.

Werry, J. S. (1968) Studies of the hyperactive child, IV. An empirical analysis of the minimal brain dysfunction syndrome. *Archives of General Psychiatry* 19:9-16.

Werry, J. S. (1972). Organic factors in childhood psychopathology. *Psychopathological Disorders of Childhood*, ed. H. C. Quay and J. S. Werry, pp. 83-121. New York: Wiley-Interscience.

Werry, J. S. (1973). Diagnosis for psychopharmacological studies in children. *Pharmacotherapy of Children, Psychopharmacology Bulletin* (Special Issue), National Institute of Mental Health, Bethesda, Md.

Werry, J. S., and Quay, H. C. (1969). Observing the classroom behavior of elementary school children. *Exceptional Child*. 35:461-470.

Werry, J. S., and Sprague, R. L. Methylphenidate in children—Effect of dosage. Unpublished paper.

Werry, J. S., and Sprague, R. L. (1970). Hyperactivity. *Symptoms of Psychopathology*, ed. C. G. Costello. New York: Wiley-Interscience.

Werry, J. S., and Sprague, R. L. (1972). Psychopharmacology. *Mental Retardation IV*, ed. J. Wortis. New York: Grune & Stratton.

Werry, J. S., Weiss, G., and Douglas, V. (1964). Studies on the hyperactive child I. Some preliminary findings. *Canadian Psychiatric Association Journal* 9:120-130.

Werry, J. S., Weiss, G., Douglas, V. et al. (1966). Studies on the hyperactive child III. The effect of chlorpromazine upon behavior and learning ability. *Journal of the Academy of Child Psychiatry* 5:292-312.

Werry, J. S., and Wollersheim, J. P. (1967). Behavior therapy with children: A broad overview. *Journal of the American Academy of Child Psychiatry* 6:346-370.

Wetzel, R. J., Baker, J., Roney, M., and Martin, M. (1966). Outpatient treatment of autistic behavior. *Behavior Research and Therapy* 4:169-177.

Whitaker, C. (1958). Psychotherapy with couples. *American Journal of Psychotherapy* 12:18-23.

Whitaker, C. (1965a). Acting out in family psychotherapy. *Acting Out: Theoretical and Clinical Aspects*. New York: Grune & Stratton.

Whitaker, C. (1965b). Psychotherapy of married couples. Lecture No. 2, Cleveland Institute of Gestalt Therapy.

Whitaker, C., and Warkentin, J. (1965). Countertransference in the family treatment of schizophrenia. *Intensive Family Therapy*, ed. I. Boszormenyi-Nagy and J. Framo. New York: Harper.

White, G., Nielson, G., and Johnson, S. (1972). Time out duration and the surpression of deviant behavior in children. *Journal of Applied Behavior Analysis* 5:111-120.

White, R. W. (1963). *Ego and Reality in Psychoanalytic Theory* (Psychological Issues, Monograph 2) New York: International Universities Press.

White, R. W. (1964). *The Abnormal Personality*, 3d ed. New York: Ronald Press.

Whitehead, P. L., and Clark, L. D. (1970). Effect of lithium carbonate, placebo and thioridazine on hyperactive children. *American Journal of Psychiatry* 127:824-825.

Williams, J. M., and Freeman, W. (1953). Evaluation of lobotomy with special reference to children. Association for Research in Nervous and Mental Disease, *Proceedings* 31:311-318.

Wilson, I. C., Prange, A. J., Jr., and Lara, P. P. (1972). T3 alone in depressed adults. Presented at annual meeting of American College of Neuropsychopharmacology, San Juan, December.

Wilson, M. B., Prange, A. J., Jr., McClane, T. K., Rabon, A. M., and Lipton, M. A. (1970). Thyroid hormone enhancement of imipramine in nonretarded depressions. *New England Journal of Medicine* 282:1063-1067.

Winnicott, D. W. (1971a). *Playing and Reality*. New York: Basic Books.

Winnicott, D. W. (1971b). *Therapeutic Consultations in Child Psychiatry*. New York: Basic Books.

Winsberg, B. G., Bialer, I., Kupietz, S. et al. (1972). Effects of imipramine and dextroamphetamine on behavior of neuropsychiatrically impaired children. *American Journal of Psychiatry* 128:1425-1431.

Witmer, H. L. (1946). *Psychiatric Interviews with Children*. New York: Commonwealth Fund.

Witt, P. A. (1971). Dosage effects of methylphenidate on the activity level of hyperactive children. Unpublished doctoral dissertation, Univ. of Illinois.

Wittenborn, J. R., Weber, E. S. P., and Brown, M. (1973). Niacin in the long-term treatment of schizophrenia. *Archives of General Psychiatry* 28:308-315.

Witter, C. (1971). Drugging and schooling. Trans-Action 8:31.

Wolf, A. (1949). The psychoanalysis of groups. *American Journal of Psychotherapy* 3:525-558.

Wolf, M., Risley, T., Johnston, M., Harris, R., and Allen, E. (1967). Application of operant conditioning procedures to the behavior problems of an autistic child: A follow-up and extension. *Behaviour Research and Therapy* 5:103-112.

Wolf, M., Risley, T., and Mees, H. (1964). Application of operant conditioning procedures to the behavior problems of an autistic child. *Behaviour Research and Therapy* 1:305-312.

Wolff, S. (1967). Behavioral characteristics of primary school children referred to a psychiatric department. *British Journal of Psychiatry* 113:885-893.

Wolpe, J. (1969). *The Practice of Behavior Therapy*. New York: Pergamon Press.

Woltmann, A. G. (1955). Concepts of play therapy techniques. *American Journal of Orthopsychiatry* 25:771-783.

Woody, R., and Woody, J. (1973). *Sexual, Marital and Familial Relations: Therapeutic Intervention for Professional Helping*. Springfield: Charles C Thomas.

Wright, H. L., Jr. (1968). A clinical study of children who refuse to talk in school. *Journal of the Academy of Child Psychiatry* 7:603-617.

Wynne, L. C. (1961). The study of intrafamilial alignments and splits in exploratory family therapy. *Exploring the Base for Family Therapy*, ed. N. Ackerman, F. Beatman, and S. Sherman. New York: Family Service Association.

Wynne, L. C. (1965). Some indications and contraindications for exploratory family therapy. *Intensive Family Therapy*, ed. I. Boszormenyi-Nagy and J. Framo. New York: Harper.

Wynne, L. C., Singer, M. T. et al. (1963). Thought disorder and family relations of schizophrenics: I. A research strategy. *Archives of General Psychiatry* 9:191-206.

Yaffe, S. J. (1970). An evaluation of the pharmacologic approaches to learning impediments. *Pediatrics* 46:142.

Yates, A. J. (1970). *Behavior Therapy*. New York: Wiley-Interscience.

Young, G. C., and Turner, R. K. (1965). CNS stimulant drugs and conditioning treatment of nocturnal enuresis. *Behavior Research Therapy* 3:93-101.

Zelings, M. A. (1961). The psychology of silence: Its role in transference, counter-transference and the psychoanalytic process. *Journal of the American Psychoanalytic Association* 9:7-43.

Zilbach, J., Bergel, E., and Gass, C. (1972). The role of the young child in family therapy. *Progress in Group and Family Therapy*, ed. C. Sager and H. Kaplan. New York: Brunner/Mazel.

Zimmerman, F. T. and Burgemeister, B. B. (1958). Action of methylphenidy-lacetate (Ritalin) and reserpine in behavior disorders in children and adults. *American Journal of Psychiatry* 115:323-328.

Zinner, J., and Shapiro, R. (1972). Projective identification as a model of perception and behavior in families of adolescents. *International Journal of Psychoanalysis* 53:523-530.

Zuk, G. H. (1965). On the pathology of silencing strategies. *Family Process* 4:32-49.

Zuk, G. H. (1966). The go-between process. *Family Process* 5:162-178.

Zuk, G. H. (1967a). Family therapy: Formulations of a technique and its theory. *Archives of General Psychiatry* 16:71-79.

Zuk, G. H. (1967b). The victim and his silencers: Some pathogenic strategies against being silenced. *Family Therapy and Disturbed Families*, ed. G. H. Zuk and I. Boszormenyi-Nagy, pp. 106-115. Palo Alto: Science & Behavior Books.

Zuk, G. H. (1971). *Family Therapy: A Triadic-Based Approach*. New York: Behavioral Books.

Zuk, G. H. (1973). Comments on *What Family Therapists Do* by C. Beels and A. Ferber. *The Book of Family Therapy*, ed. A. Ferber, M. Mendelsohn, and A. Napier. New York: Aronson.

Zuk, G. H., and Rubinstein, D. (1965). A review of concepts in the study and treatment of families of schizophrenics. *Intensive Family Therapy*, ed. I. Boszormenyi-Nagy and J. Framo. New York: Harper.

Zwerling, I., Scheflen, A., Jackson, D., Boszormenyi-Nagy, I. (1967). Communication within the family: a panel discussion. *Expanding Theory and Practice in Family Therapy*, ed. N. Ackerman et al. New York: Family Service Association.

Index